CITATION CLASSICS FROM SOCIAL INDICATORS RESEARCH

Social Indicators Research Series

Volume 26

This new series aims to provide a public forum for single treatises and collections of papers on social indicators research that are too long to be published in our journal *Social Indicators Research*. Like the journal, the book series deals with statistical assessments of the quality of life from a broad perspective. It welcomes the research on a wide variety of substantive areas, including health, crime, housing, education, family life, leisure activities, transportation, mobility, economics, work, religion and environmental issues. These areas of research will focus on the impact of key issues such as health on the overall quality of life and vice versa. An international review board, consisting of Ruut Veenhoven, Joachim Vogel, Ed Diener, Torbjorn Moum, Mirjam A.G. Sprangers and Wolfgang Glatzer, will ensure the high quality of the series as a whole.

The titles published in this series are listed at the end of this volume.

CITATION CLASSICS FROM
SOCIAL INDICATORS RESEARCH

The Most Cited Articles Edited and Introduced
by Alex C. Michalos

Edited by

ALEX C. MICHALOS

University of Northern British Columbia,
Canada

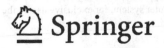

A C.I.P. Catalogue record for this book is available from the Library of Congress.

ISBN 1-4020-3722-8 (PB)
ISBN 978-1-4020-3722-1 (PB)
ISBN 1-4020-3742-2 (ebook)
ISBN 978-1-4020-3742-9 (ebook)

Published by Springer,
P.O. Box 17, 3300 AA Dordrecht, The Netherlands.

www.springeronline.com

Printed on acid-free paper

Table of Contents

vi

PREFACE

The idea of publishing some sort of a volume celebrating the first thirty years of publishing *Social Indicators Research* came to me some time early in the twenty-ninth year. When I shared the idea with the publisher's representative, Welmoed Spahr, she was very enthusiastic about it. We both thought we should try to produce a volume in 2004, preferably in time for the November meeting of the International Society for Quality of Life Studies. That implied that the publisher would need the complete manuscript by May 2004. So, we had a clear time frame for getting the job done.

As I reflected on the variety of volumes we might produce, I thought it would be particularly helpful for contemporary and future social indicators researchers to assemble a set of papers that would represent the best that had come out of our journal. The question was: How should we define 'best'? A few fairly elaborate decision procedures based on different criteria were constructed, and each seemed to require more time and other resources than we could spare. I rapidly settled on the idea of using article citation counts as a measure of article quality. I knew it was problematic, but so was everything else I could think of, and citation counts had four distinct advantages. First, such counts were relatively easy to obtain and objectively observable by other researchers. Second, there were about 40 years' of constructive and critical research on the strengths and weaknesses of the use of citation counts as indicators of the quality of research publications. Third, it was possible to provide an overview of that research which would be sufficient to allow readers to make their own judgments about my decision to use this approach. Finally, it would be wonderful if anyone unhappy with this approach would undertake an alternative analysis that would provide some confirmation or disconfirmation of the results reported here.

All the papers reprinted here appear as they were originally published, except for minor corrections of typos. In 1978, at the ninth World Congress of Sociology in Uppsala, I presented a short paper describing the origins of the journal. Because most of the people interested in the papers in this collection will have some interest in knowing how it all started and that paper has never been published, I have included it immediately following my introductory essay. Since it was written over 25 years ago, both its author and the publisher (D. Reidel) have changed quite a bit. I must say that it gives me considerable pleasure to be able to report that I have enjoyed our long relationship immensely, and I look forward to many more years of collaboration. When I read that John Maynard Keynes took over the *Economic Journal* from F.Y. Edgeworth in 1912 and edited it for the next 33 years, it occurred to me that 30 years is not too long a time to edit a journal.

viii

Besides, for me, next to writing up my own research, editing other people's research is the most enjoyable academic activity I do.

I would like to thank Welmoed Spahr and Kluwer Academic Publishers for helping me produce this volume. Also, I would like to thank Bob Cummins and Ruut Veenhoven for providing me with electronic versions of their papers, which helped reduce our production costs.

1. Citation Classics: The Idea and the Collection

ALEX C. MICHALOS

After about three years in graduate school studying the history of religions, my interests turned to logic and the philosophy of science. My doctoral thesis was on a dispute between Karl Popper and Rudolf Carnap over the construction of quantitative measures of the acceptability of scientific theories (Michalos, 1971). For most of the 40 years that I was a university teacher, I taught courses in the philosophy of science, always including issues related to the evaluation of the activities and products of social and natural scientists. Since there are no generally accepted definitions of such key concepts as science, scientific explanation, scientific laws, scientific theories and scientific acceptability, but there are particular groups of researchers that tend to accept certain concepts while rejecting others (Michalos 1980), I take a fairly pragmatic approach to the construction of my own scientific vocabulary. For present purposes, the only part of that vocabulary that requires explanation concerns the term 'citation classic'.

I first encountered the term some years ago reading something by Eugene Garfield, the founder of the Institute for Scientific Information (ISI), the *Science Citation Index*, *Social Sciences Citation Index* and several other important works. According to Garfield (1985), "By definition, a *Citation Classic* is a paper or book that has been highly cited in its field" (p.404). From 1977 to 1993 the ISI publication *Current Contents* regularly featured an article called Citation Classics Commentary, which was subsequently replaced by In-Cites. Because different fields are characterized by different institutional arrangements (e.g., numbers and kinds of communication media, practitioners, standardized practices and rules of procedure), different numerical thresholds are used to identify classics in each field. In an earlier paper, Garfield (1976) wrote that

> ". . .less than 25% of all papers will be cited ten times in all eternity! . . . any paper cited ten times in one year is *ipso facto* significant. Occasionally there is an anomaly. But a paper cited ten times in each of two successive years is well on its way to citation stardom. Whether the author is on the way to immortality depends on how well he or she does in other papers" (p.419).

An average paper in the *Science Citation Index* is cited about 1.7 times per year (Garfield, 1972). For the years 1955-1987, Garfield (1989) claimed that for the whole *Index* database,

> ". . .more than 56 percent of the source items are uncited – not even self-cited. (Many of these source items are abstracts, letters, and editorials, of limited interest; nevertheless, a huge number of papers go uncited.)" (p.7).

1

Alex C. Michalos (ed.), Citation Classics from Social Indicators Research, 1–56.
© 2005 *Springer. Printed in the Netherlands.*

In 1973 Garfield distinguished three kinds of "uncitedness", namely, "the incitedness of the mediocre, the unintelligible, the irrelevant", then that "of the meritorious but undiscovered or forgotten", and finally that

> "of the *distinction* that comes to those whose work has become so well known (and presumably been previously so heavily cited) that one finds it at first tedious, then unnecessary, and finally actually gauche to cite such men at all" (p.413).

Hamilton (1990) reported that ISI data revealed that about 55% of the "papers published between 1981 and 1985 in journals indexed by the institute received no citations at all in the 5 years after they were published" (p.1331). In response, Pendlebury (1991) wrote that the precise figures were "47.4% uncited for the sciences, 74.7% for the social sciences, and 98.0% for the arts and humanities". However, more importantly, he explained that

> "These statistics represent every type of article that appears in journals indexed by the Institute for Scientific Information (ISI) in its *Science Citation Index*, *Social Sciences Citation Index*, and *Arts & Humanities Citation Index*. The journals' ISI indexes contain not only articles, reviews, and notes, but also meeting abstracts, editorials, obituaries, letters like this one, and other *marginalia*, which one might expect to be largely un-cited. In 1984, the year of the data quoted by Hamilton, about 27% of the items indexed in the *Science Citation Index* were such *marginalia*. The comparable figures for the social sciences and arts and humanities were 48% and 69%, respectively.

> If one analyzes the data more narrowly and examines the extent of uncited articles alone (this information was not yet available when Hamilton wrote his articles), the figures shrink, some more than others: 22.4% of 1984 science articles remained uncited by the end of 1988, as did 48.0% of social sciences articles and 93.1% of articles in arts and humanities journals. . .Only 14.7% of 1984 science articles by U.S. authors were left uncited by the end of 1988. . .articles published in the highest impact journals like Science are almost never left uncited" (pp.1410-1411).

Exhibit 1 illustrates a few thresholds for citation classics from different fields, ranging from papers with 50 or more citations covering the fields of geography and marine biology to 500 or more citations covering all fields listed in the *Science Citation Index*. Plomp (1990) used a threshold of 25 citations to identify "highly cited papers", which is a more modest label than 'citation classic' and perhaps not quite the same idea. His rationale for the figure was interesting.

> "Considering the (average) number of references in a paper as its 'input' and the number of citations achieved by that paper as its 'output', the ratio citations/references may be interpreted as the 'gain factor' of the paper; it sounds reasonable that a gain factor of 1 is a sort of watershed between papers recognized by the scientific community as important and papers not recognized as important. As the average number of references in scientific articles is about 20 (according to the 1986 SCI), I consider

N = 25 a good compromise for a paper to be considered as a highly cited paper (from here on labeled as HCP). This category includes only 3% of all articles cited between 1961 and 1980 (Garfield, 1984). Extensive explorations by the author have confirmed that by using HCP rather than the total number of citations as an indicator of scientific impact, the injustice to the many excellent scientists working in small scientific fields, so abundantly clear in lists of most cited authors (e.g., Garfield, 1981a), is greatly eliminated" (p.187).

As others had before him (e.g., Garfield, 1972), Plomp noticed, for example, that because in 1982 the 40 core biochemistry journals produced 13,500 articles while the 25 core astrosciences journals produced 4,500 articles, there were many more opportunities for citations in the former field than in the latter. In fact, "the most cited biochemistry papers obtained ten times as many citations as the most cited astrosciences papers".

In the *Encyclopedia of Library and Information Science*, the entry for 'citer motivations' says

> "Citations are examples of unobtrusive or nonreactive social science measures. Unobtrusive measures are physical evidences of activity that exist independently of their source: the private act of authorship produces citations that are public objects available for scrutiny and analysis. As with many of these unobtrusive measures, it is difficult to ascertain in any given application what social or psychological construct the citation counts are measuring" (Brooks, 1988, p.48).

For social indicators researchers, this quotation has a remarkably familiar ring. In our terms the author was saying that citations are objective indicators providing unclear indications. They must be supplemented by subjective indicators revealing not only the motivation or aims of authors/citers, but also the meaning or interpretation of citations for those who read them. People like Garfield shared the view of sociologists of science like Merton (1977), who believed that the status of any scientist's research output

> ". . .resides only in the recognition accorded his work by peers in the social system of science through reference to his work. . .Since recognition of the worth of one's work by qualified peers is, in science, the basic form of reward (all other rewards deriving from it) and since it can only be widely accorded within the social system of science when the attributed work is widely known, this provides institutional incentive for the open publication, without direct financial reward, of scientific work" (pp.47-48, as quoted by Lawani and Bayer, 1983).

Lawani and Bayer (1983) go on to say that

> "The pressure for public diffusion of one's work through open publication is accompanied by the obligation within the institutional structure of science for the user of that freely published knowledge to make open reference to the sources to which he is indebted. 'Not to do so is to incur the sanctions visited upon those judged guilty of stealing another's intellectual property (i.e., plagiary)' [Merton 1997, p.48]. This reflects the origin of the practice of citing and is a basic justification for

its application in studies of the sociology and history of science. . .
Despite the ambiguities of citation practices, the difficulties of
ascertaining why a paper is or is not cited, and the potential malpractices
in citing, considerable evidence has been accumulated to suggest that
citations do indeed provide an objective measure of what is variously
termed "productivity," "significance," "quality," "utility," "influence,"
"effectiveness," or "impact" of scientists and their scholarly products"
(pp.60-61).

The evidence takes many forms. For example, Narin (1976) reviewed 24
studies published between 1957 and 1975 that generally confirmed the
hypothesis that citation counts are positively correlated with peer rankings of
the quality of scientific articles, eminence of scientists, graduate schools,
graduate departments, editor evaluations, Nobel prizes and other awards,
authors' incomes, access to resources, initial appointments and mobility. Eight
of 12 studies that provided correlation coefficients had values of at least 0.6,
with 5 of those above 0.7. The lowest value was 0.2. Brooks (1985) reported
that Virgo (1977)

". . .found citation analysis to be a consistent and accurate predictor of
important scientific papers, better on the average than the individual
scientist's judgment which 'is a reasonable conclusion if one considers
that citations actually reflect a consensus of a large group of readers as
compared to the evaluation of a single individual' [Virgo, 1977, p.423]".

Lawani and Bayer (1983) undertook a very thorough study comparing peer
assessments of cancer research papers with the papers' citation rates and
concluded that "Highly rated papers are more highly cited than average papers".
Notwithstanding such supporting evidence for the usefulness of citation
counts in the evaluation of published research, Garfield has often published
cautionary remarks about the use of such counts. For example, he wrote that

"Counts of this sort are strictly quantitative and objective. But even
admitting this limitation, an author's or a paper's frequency of citation
has been found to correlate well with professional standing. It is
certainly not the *only* measure, nor one that can be used, for any purpose,
in isolation. We do not claim for it the absolute reliability that critics of
citation analysis have wrongly imputed to us when they have attacked it.
The fact does remain, however, that it provides a useful objective
criterion previously unavailable" (Garfield, 1981, p.135, reprinted in
Garfield 1983).

Among the problems with using citation counts in the ISI databases to evaluate
publications, Garfield (1983) mentioned the following.

". . .there are undoubtedly highly useful journals that are not cited
frequently [e.g., Scientific American]. Scientists read many such journals
for the same reason people read newspapers and other non-scientific
periodicals – to keep up with what is going on generally. . .Another
consideration is that citation frequency is sometimes – indeed to some
extent must be – a function of variables other than scientific merit. Some
such variables may be an author's reputation, the controversiality of

subject matter, a journal's circulation and its cost, reprint dissemination, its coverage by current-awareness and indexing and abstracting services, society memberships, the availability and extent of libraries' journal collections, national research priorities" (p.137); see also Garfield (1977, 1988).

In a series of papers, MacRoberts and MacRoberts (1986, 1987, 1989, 1989a) challenged the use of citation counts on a variety of grounds. From their papers and others I constructed the following list of criticisms. (1) Many individuals and works that have had an influence on the development of published papers are not cited in those papers (they estimated that "about 15 percent of the influence on a paper is contained in its references"; (2) sometimes important influences are mentioned in the text of published papers but not in their bibliographies; (3) the motivation for self-citations is suspect (Self-citations are generally estimated to be about 10% to 30% of all citations; Bonzi and Snyder (1991) surveyed 51 self-citing authors and found "very few differences in motivation" between self- and other-citations.); (4) when review papers are cited, it is unclear exactly who is being "rewarded"; (5) general references within a text also have unclear referents, e.g., "Mendelian genetics"; (6) ISI indexes contain many errors, e.g., when authors' names are spelled in different ways, or written sometimes with and sometimes without middle initials, separate entries may made for the same document; when page and/or volume numbers are changed, separate entries may be made; when page numbers alone or page numbers and volume numbers are inverted, new entries may be made; (7) ISI indexes cover only about 10% of scientific literature; (8) "English language journals and western science are clearly over-represented, whereas small countries, non-western countries, and journals published in non-Roman scripts are under-represented."; (9) different disciplines are more or less well represented (e.g., 6% of biology journals are included, compared to 14% of clinical medicine journals); (10) politics seems to have influenced inclusions and exclusions (e.g., *Review of Radical Political Economy* is excluded, but *Public Interest* is included); (11) later proponents of views may be cited as the views' inventers; (12) proponents of views may be cited as opponents, and vice-versa; (13) people often cite material that "they have not seen or that they have seen but have not read"; (14) people make ceremonial and perfunctory citations (Moravcsik and Murugesan (1975) estimated about 40% of the references in a sample of high energy physics papers were perfunctory); (15) private communications are often influential but do not provide a published title to cite; (16) authors are notorious for repeating themselves in different papers, each of which may be cited as an additional contribution to research; (17) people sometimes select only one of several similar papers that influenced them; (18) they also redundantly cite several similar papers because they are similar, although they may have read and/or been influenced by one (Moravcsik and Murugesan (1975) estimated about one-third of the references in their sample were redundant); (19) they may cite a well-known or fail to cite a relatively unknown author because these practices are perceived to impress their readers; (20) about 70% of citations appear to be "multi-motivated"; (21) different disciplines have different typical rates of citation, which are typically neglected by citation analysts (e.g., engineering and mathematics papers average 5 to 6 references per publication, psychology and biology average 8 to 10, earth and space science, physics, chemistry and clinical medicine average 12 to 15 and biomedical research papers average 18 to 20); (22) citation rates vary with countries of origin; (23) rates vary with the "size of the pool of available citers"; (24) methods and review papers "receive disproportionately more citations than theoretical or empirical papers"; (25) citation counts cannot allocate credit for papers with several authors; (26) researchers from some countries tend to be aware of and cite papers coming from their countries (e.g., Americans tend to cite papers by Americans); (27) citation counts do not distinguish positive or negative reasons for the citations; (28) authors tend to search the literature for and cite those papers that agree with their views; (29) citation rates vary with the physical accessibility of cited material; (30) changes in editors and editorial boards have produced changes in citation patterns (Sievert and Haughawout, 1989); (31) recent papers are cited more than older ones because there are relatively more of the former (Oppenheim and Renn, 1978); (32) rapidly developing fields like molecular biology and biochemistry are "more dependent on fresh data" and therefore generate relatively more citations (Vinkler, 1987).

Summarizing their criticisms, MacRoberts and MacRoberts, 1989a) wrote

> "Apparently, the pioneers of citation analysis were so intent on finding an 'objective' measure of quality that, in their enthusiasm, they neglected to check their assumptions against events. . .What is the consequence of this discovery for the practical application of citation analysis? It alone should suffice to exclude evaluative citation analysis from the arena of science policy. Add to this our empirical findings, and those of others, and the claims made for citation analysis largely collapse. It would therefore be the better part of wisdom to place a moratorium on the use of citations in science policy until the problems are thoroughly aired, which means attending to critics rather than ignoring or dismissing them as uninformed and misguided 'non-believers'" (p.10).

While I believe that most of the criticisms listed above are accurate and should not be ignored or dismissed, I feel the same way about all the correlational studies indicating some validity in the use of citation counts for evaluative purposes. In fact, I believe that many of the problems and limitations of citation counts are similar to problems and limitations encountered with objective indicators in other fields. While research by sociologists and psychologists of science (scientometricians) has not progressed as rapidly as that of other social indicators researchers into explorations of the subjective side of citation behaviour and motivations, it has certainly progressed. Good investigations and literature reviews of citer motivations may be found in Smith (1981), Prabha (1983), Cronin (1984), Brooks (1985, 1988), Puder and Morgan (1987), Moravcsik (1988) Cozzens (1989), Bonzi and Snyder (1991) and Liu (1993). Today, anyone writing an essay like this one relying heavily on citation counts must be aware of, and make readers aware, of their limitations. I hope that this brief overview of some of the literature has at least accomplished that.

More importantly, I hope that other researchers will regard this review of the citation classics from *Social Indicators Research* as merely a first step toward an evaluation of our research literature. Additional steps involving survey research and detailed, systematic appraisals of publications must be taken, and the sooner the better.

Given the background information just reviewed, and especially that summarized in Exhibit 1, it is obvious that we have some flexibility in specifying a threshold figure for citation classics. I exchanged some ideas with people at Kluwer and at ISI regarding a list of the top 50 most frequently cited papers or, alternatively, papers with 50 or more citations. David Pendlebury provided us first with a list of all papers with 35 or more citations, and then with a complete list of every cited paper from the journal for the whole period from March 1974 to December 2003. I cleaned up the material a bit, entered the whole dataset into an SPSS file and produced the statistics in Exhibit 2. There were a total of 1392 titles published in the first 30 years. Since the journal seldom published book reviews, editorials or letters, most of those titles represented articles. Eight hundred and twenty articles (58.9%) were not cited at all, which is a bit higher than the 55%-57% general average for the whole *Index* database, lower than the 74.7% for all social sciences material and higher than the 48% for social science articles alone. The 572 (41.1%) cited articles generated 4979 citations, with a classic hyperbolic distribution curve in which relatively few articles attract many citations and relatively many articles attract few citations. The mean number of citations per published article was 3.6, with a mode and median value of zero, and a standard deviation of 11.8. There were 34 articles with 35 or more citations each, and those 34 (2.4%) articles attracted 2208/4979 = 44.4% of all citations. The top 68 (4.9%) articles attracted 2997/4979 = 60.2% of all citations. Given their extraordinary contribution to the journal's total citation count, and the fact that articles with 35 or more citations were nearly three standard deviations above the mean, those articles form a fairly distinguished lot. Therefore, I decided to use 35 as the threshold figure for designating citation classics from *Social Indicators Research*. Of course, other researchers may prefer to use other figures.

The Appendix to this introduction contains the complete list of cited articles with their citation figures. The articles are divided into the decades of their publication, 1974-79, 1980-89, 1990-99 and 2000-03, and each is listed alphabetically by first authors' names. After spending some hours cleaning up the list, I became convinced that I would never be able to catch all the errors in the time that was available to me. But it is a pretty good list for others to begin with. At the end of the Appendix there is a short table summarizing publication and citation figures.

Exhibit 3 lists our 34 citation classics with their citation figures. Because it takes some time for articles to be discovered, used and cited, there are no classics from the 2000-03 period. There are 10 articles (29.4%) each from 1974-79 and 1990-99, and 14 (41.1%) from 1980-89. By authors' countries of origin, there are 16 (47.1%) from the USA, 5 (14.7%) each from Canada and Australia, 3 (8.8%) from the Netherlands, 2 (5.9%) from the UK and 1 (2.9%) from Israel.

By first authors' names, there are 5 (14.7%) by Andrews, 4 (11.8%) by Diener, 3 (8.8%) each by Veenhoven and Headey, 2 (5.9%) each by Cummins, McKennell and Michalos, and one each by all other authors. Collectively, 37 authors produced the 34 papers, and there are 16 single-authored papers. Using Plomp's threshold for highly cited papers, only 8 more papers would be added to the 34.

Nineteen (55.9%) of the 34 articles appeared as the lead article in some issue. This seemed quite remarkable to me because I was responsible for sequencing the set of articles for every issue and I always put what I regarded as the best available article first. Since we know that only 2.4% of all articles ended up as classics, either (a) I was a pretty good judge of quality, (b) the lead articles tend to be read more than others (like newspaper articles), or (c) both.

Examining the content of the articles, I was shocked to discover that all but one of them (McCall, 1975) focused on some aspect of subjective indicators. In view of the historical facts that the field was originally dominated by researchers interested in objective indicators and that today practically all researchers agree that objective and subjective indicators are equally important, the near total dominance of subjective indicators research in our classics is both surprising and disturbing. I would guess that the main reason for the dominance of subjective indicators research is that there are relatively more psychologists and people interested in personal reports about a good quality of life than there are others. While "Others" would include a wide variety of people, e.g., sociologists, demographers, gerontologists, geographers, environmentalists, economists, political scientists and population health researchers, each group would have a relatively narrow range of interests compared to those interested in the psychological structure of perceived well-being. Whether or not there is anything to that explanation, it would be a pity if objective indicators research came to be relatively neglected in the future. Hopefully, this publication can serve as a wake up call for researchers to redirect attention to redressing the balance.

Although the articles in this collection are assembled chronologically, they are discussed below in an order that emphasizes their interrelations and reveals the gradual expansion of the frontier of research in subjective well-being. Only 17 articles are included because they seemed to be sufficient to reveal the progress made over the past 30 years, with a minimum of duplication.

The article by McCall (1975) contains a brief but historically instructive account of the state of the discussion in the early 1970s about the definition of the phrase 'quality of life'. There are several nice distinctions drawn and some arguments are given in favour of a definition of 'quality of life' based on objective indicators. First, he claimed that "to define QOL in terms of the general happiness, of 'the greatest happiness of the greatest number,' would be merely to repeat Mill's work". If one's analysis went no further than the definition, that might be true, but no contemporary proponent of Mill's formula ends his or her analysis at that point, e.g., see the paper in this collection by Veenhoven (1994). Second, he claimed that a society that looked good on the basis of objective indicators (e.g., full employment, low crime rates) would have a higher QOL than one that looked bad on the same basis even though people in the latter society were happier (had higher subjective well-being ratings) than those in the former. This is patently question-begging, and he offers nothing stronger in its defence than "intuitively, one would think that the QOL of" the society with the superior objective indicators is superior. It has, in his view, "the *necessary conditions* for happiness", and it is these conditions that he regards as defining QOL. In my view, people's perceived well-being measured by subjective indicators constitutes a complementary and equally necessary defining condition of QOL. That is, the quality of life of an individual or a community should be defined and measured by both objective indicators of their living circumstances (Veenhoven's 'livability indicators') and subjective indicators of their perceived well-being (happiness, satisfaction or subjective well-being) (Michalos 2003, 2004). (It must be remembered, of course, that some evaluation by someone is necessary in order to determined exactly what objective indicators indicate evaluatively.) While McCall allowed that subjective indicators might be *signs* of but not *constitutive* of QOL, my view is that high levels of perceived well-being, measured by subjective indicators, are *partly constitutive* of QOL, the other part being people's living circumstances broadly construed. I regard my view as socially constructed and subject to revision. I think it is generally representative of the views of the majority of social indicators researchers today, but I have not done any systematic research to support that belief.

With some oversimplification, we might use the two necessary conditions to characterize four states of affairs. If one's living conditions and perceived well-being are good, then the overall quality of one's life is good. This we may call Real Paradise. If one's living conditions are bad and one's perceived well-being is good, then the overall quality of one's life is not good. This would be the proverbial Fool's Paradise. If one's living conditions are good and one's perceived well-being is bad, then the overall quality of one's life is still not good. It might be called a Fool's Hell. Finally, if one's living conditions and perceived well-being are bad, then the overall quality of one's life would certainly be bad. That, I suppose, could be called Real Hell. Since living conditions and perceived well-being admit of diverse levels or degrees of goodness or desirability in some sense, these blunt distinctions could easily be made more sophisticated and subtle. Fortunately, there is no need to pursue such complications here.

In another section of McCall's paper he claims that because human needs may be objectively determined and are in principle limited while human wants may only be subjectively determined and are in principle unlimited, a notion of quality of life defined in terms of need fulfillment is preferable to one defined in terms of want fulfillment. He relied heavily on Maslow's (1954) theory of a hierarchy of needs, and the strength of his position is directly proportionate to the persuasiveness of his case for the objectivity of needs versus wants. In Michalos (1978) I devoted a considerable amount of space to providing fairly rigorous definitions of 'needs' and 'wants', and concluded that it would be impossible to make such a case persuasive. I thought that if anyone could have made such a case, Braybrooke (1987) would have done it, but a careful reading of that volume only reinforced my earlier view. A definition of 'quality of life' based on some set of objectively determined needs seems to me to be unachievable and, in the light of my views explained in the preceding two paragraphs, undesirable.

The first and last articles in the collection were published 22 years apart, but they addressed the same basic problem, with some different additional hypotheses and methodologies. The basic problem was to empirically determine the total number of domains required for a full assessment of the perceived quality of life of individuals and communities.

The paper by Andrews and Withey (1974) was followed by several articles and by their fine book, Andrews and Withey (1976). They began by creating a "list of items which, ideally, would include all the significant 'concerns' of people". They found 800 items by examining published lists from national and international bodies, 8 different national samples of Americans, representative data from 12 other countries, structured interviews of a dozen people with diverse backgrounds and lists of published values. Using "some *ad hoc* clustering to combine concerns", they found 123 items that seemed to cover about 100 concerns. Then they applied Guttman (1968) Smallest Space Analysis to a 62-item subset of the 123 items, which was possible because the 62 items were used in the US national survey of May 1972 (N = 1297). The "62 items were reduced to 30 semi-independent domains", and finally to 12, on the basis of three criteria, namely, (1) predictive power, (2) dispersion in multi-dimensional space and (3) policy relevance. The 12 domains were house/apartment, spare time activities, things done with family, your health, amount of fun, time to do things, job index, national government index, efficacy index, family index, consumer index and money index. To test the robustness of the dozen domains, Andrews and Withey undertook separate analyses on 10 subgroups, including, ". . .men, women, blacks, four different age groups, two groups extreme with respect to socio-economic status, and a group of married, white, employed men in their middle years with children living at home". Summarizing their work, they wrote,

> "A series of analyses, some of them replicated in more than one survey, showed that a particular subset of 12 domains could explain 50% to 60% of the variance in sense of overall life quality, that neither other domains nor standard classification variables contributed anything additional to this explanatory power, and that this level of explanation could be achieved in each of 22 different subgroups of the American population (defined in demographic terms) as well as in the population considered as a whole. . .one wonders how close to the actual upper limit is the achieved explanatory power of 50% -- 60%. Given the unreliability of the measures the upper limit is certainly not 100%. Further work will attempt to assess the reliability of the measures employed" (p.23).

The dependent variable used to measure "overall life quality" was called "Life #3", whose values were equal to the mean score resulting from asking "How do you feel about your life as a whole?" at two points of time 8 to 12 minutes apart in each interview. The two responses to the same question (Life #1 and Life #2) usually correlated with each other in the 0.6 to 0.7 range. The response scale used was the now-famous 7-point Delighted-Terrible scale (DT scale). For reasons that will be made clear below (in the discussion of Andrews and McKennell, 1980), the DT scale contains two words specifically designed to elicit an affect-based response, i.e., "pleased" and "unhappy". The "explanatory power" of the 12 domains was measured by Multiple Classification Analysis, which is a kind of ordinary least-squares regression, using the various mean DT scores for each domain as predictors. In a footnote the authors explained that they tried weighting domain DT scores with "importance scores", but "no predictive gain could be achieved". They also "thought there might be substantial interactions in the data, but so far, none of marked effect has been found". The "standard classification variables" included respondents' income, sex, race, family life cycle, age and education.

Cummins (1996) began by scanning 1,500 articles providing data on life satisfaction, looking for "different terms that had been used to describe domains of life satisfaction". For an article's terms to be used, the article had to have at least three domains purporting to "represent a broad indication of life quality", and a detailed description of the scales used and average scores obtained for each domain. Most importantly, in contrast to Andrews and Withey, "Responses to criteria of happiness were excluded". All together, Cummins found 32 studies meeting his criteria, and those studies used 351 different domain names. The 68 samples described in those studies were "of four broad types: general population probability or quota samples, general population samples based on a variety of specific criteria, samples of people with chronic medical conditions, and samples comprising people with a chronic psychiatric impairment". The inclusion of samples of people with chronic physical and mental health problems was a notable step beyond Andrews and Withey.

His first aim was to determine how many domain names could be categorized under one of the seven domain headings of his Comprehensive Quality of Life Scale (ComQol). The latter's domains include material well-being, health, productivity, intimacy, safety, community and emotional well-being. He found that 83% of the 351 domain names could be reasonably classified into one or another of ComQol's seven domains. For example, ComQol's category of "intimacy" includes things like family life, family relations, friendships, marriage, living partner and spouse. He listed the 56 domain names that did not fit into the ComQol categories and indicated that "the question as to the appropriate number of domains must remain open". Nevertheless, he expressed reservations about adding the particular domain of government because "Not only would the inclusion of such a domain exert a strong negative bias on life satisfaction measurement, but also people generally report these aspects of life to be unimportant to them personally".

His second aim was to see if "a hierarchy of domain satisfaction could be established" and, if so, third, to see if it was invariant among groups with high or low levels of life satisfaction. Examining mean values for each domain across four levels of reported life satisfaction, he found that there was indeed a hierarchy with the two domains of intimacy and health "consistently above the study mean [of Z-scores], while the other five domains lay consistently below.

Most remarkable in this respect was intimacy which lay from 1.29 to 1.53 standard deviations above the mean for each of the four levels of overall life satisfaction". While the hierarchy was invariant with respect to membership in the top two and bottom five domains, among the latter there was considerable shuffling about. For example, productivity and community occupied the third and fourth places, respectively, for those in the group with the highest levels of life satisfaction, sixth and third places for those in the group with the second highest levels of life satisfaction, fourth and seventh for those in the next group, and sixth and fifth for those with the lowest levels of life satisfaction. Contrary to Cummins's claim, it does not seem to me that "the data in Table IV indicate a high level of inter-domain consistency" for five of the seven domains.

Considering the results for his samples of people with chronic health problems, Cummins found that those with chronic physical problems had life satisfaction scores much like those in "normal population samples", while those with chronic psychiatric problems "had significantly lower overall life quality scores than either of the other two groups. Moreover, . . .the domain of intimacy no longer retained its pre-eminence. These data are consistent with the loss of intimacy as a buffer against diminished life circumstances".

Since the procedures and criteria for success used by Andrews and Withey and Cummins were different, one would not have expected both approaches to yield identical results. It is perhaps worthwhile to mention that while Cummins treated all the terms used by other researchers in the context of domain identification as domain names, Andrews and Withey distinguished (unfortunately without rigorous definitions) domains or "role situations" from values. As illustrated in the first exhibit of their paper, these authors had the idea that people might, for example, look for beauty (a value in their terms) in several domains (on the job, at home, in one's friends). Then, using many values and many domains, one could generate a matrix of value-by-domain satisfaction levels, which in the aggregate would constitute one's overall satisfaction with life. Inspection of the first table in Cummins's paper reveals that some of his domain names were regarded as value names by Andrews and Withey. For example, 'safety' is a domain name for Cummins but a value name for Andrews and Withey. Since there is no generally accepted rule book for determining what one ought to regard as a value versus a domain, one need not take sides on which approach is most appropriate. The bottom line is that the two approaches yielded fairly similar results.

I suppose anyone reading the philosophic literature since *The Republic* of Plato would have expected to see fairly similar results. A good overview may be found in Tatarkiewicz (1976). Around the world and across time, people regard good health, family and friends, beautiful things, financial and other forms of security as important features of a good life. Andrews and Withey and Cummins showed us that the core of important life domains is not as broad as the great numbers of possible domain names or items might suggest. Cummins's observations that "The larger the proportion of scale items that relate to satisfaction with family and friends, the higher will be the overall life satisfaction score" and that "the inclusion of items relating to 'Government'. . .

will produce a lower life satisfaction score" in aggregated indexes are well worth remembering.

Although the paper by Levy and Guttman (1975) was not included in Cummins's study, the problem addressed in the paper was closely related. Methodologically, the paper is closer to Andrews and Withey. Levy and Guttman began with what I would call a semantic view of theories (Michalos 1980). According to this view, a scientific theory is a system of definitions that one hypothesizes will match some aspect of the real world, and then one makes empirical observations to test one's hypothesis. The elaborate network of definitions contained in Levy and Guttman's comprehensive mapping sentence includes 6 facets identifying (A) a type of assessment (cognitive versus affective), (B) type of state or treatment, (C) group, (D) environmental framework, (E) level of specificity, and (F) life area (domain) according to some level of satisfactoriness. I suppose their life areas of security and communication would be values for Andrews and Withey. In any case, multiplying the elements available for each facet times all the others, Levy and Guttman could generate 5824 items ("structuples"), from which they selected 24 to test in their 1973 spring survey in Israel. Applying Smallest Space Analysis to correlation coefficients for pairs of variables in their data-set, they were able to obtain geometrical representations of relationships among the variables. The representations are difficult for me to interpret and to compare with the representations constructed by Andrews and Withey (1974, 1976) using similar software. While it is clear that the mapping sentence provided a useful heuristic device for generating items that corresponded to features of relationships among attitudes of their respondents, it is unclear what good the geometrical representations are in themselves or for explaining the relationships. One can look at the figures and see that this or that attitude/item is literally in space nearer or farther from some others, but the correlation coefficients themselves gave us information about their conceptual closeness and additional statistical analyses without geometrical representations could give us information about likely causal connections among the variables. I suppose proponents of the geometrical representations would say that the figures make it easier to "see" relationships and craft explanatory hypotheses, but in fact very few hypotheses seem to have been generated from all the figures presented, for example, in Andrews and Withey (1976).

Andrews and Inglehart (1979) applied Smallest Space Analysis to the U.S. survey data from May 1972 and data from national surveys in nine European countries in order to see how comparable the structure of subjective well-being was in the 10 countries. At the time they wrote, "the cross-cultural comparability of the phenomenon of perceived well-being [was] largely unexplored". In their view, there were "important practical uses of such structures". In particular, Andrews and Inglehart thought

> "They provide guides to the adequacy of coverage and statistical
> efficiency of indicators of perceived well-being. To the extent that
> people in different societies organize their thinking about well-being in
> basically similar ways, it is feasible and potentially productive to

undertake cross-cultural research with standardized instruments and to make well-grounded comparative statements based on the results" (p.74).

Fortunately, they discovered that

". . .(a) there seems to be a basic similarity in structures among all nine of these western societies; (b) within this basic similarity the European structures are distinct from the American structure; (c) even within Europe there is modest heterogeneity; and (d) if one averages out the differences among the individual European structures, the result is a structure that is closer to the American structure than are most of the individual European structures" (p.83).

Besides these general conclusions, Andrews and Inglehart reported that the American structure was "most similar to that of The Netherlands. . .and least similar to the structures in Great Britain, France and Denmark".

Schneider (1975) provided data addressing a fundamental problem for all social indicators researchers in the 1960s and 1970s. As he put it,

"It is certainly possible that individuals or social groups may be exposed to objectively better conditions of health care, environment, employment, etc. than other individuals or groups but subjectively feel that the quality of their personal life experiences are no better. Despite the often found assumption that objective social indicators data actually reflect the quality of life experienced by people, we have no reason *a priori* to assume that such a correlation exists. The connections between the 'quality of life' as measured by objective social indicators and the 'quality of life' subjectively experienced by people is really open to question. . .(pp.496-497)."

Comparing data on "objective life conditions" in 13 U.S. cities from a 1972 study with "measures of subjective life quality" in those cities obtained from a 1968 social survey, Schneider boldly concluded that

". . .no relationship exists between the level of well being found in a city as measured by a wide range of commonly used objective social indicators and the quality of life subjectively experienced by individuals in that city. Cities that are most well off as measured by objective indicators are not necessarily the same cities in which people are subjectively most satisfied with their life situations. Conversely, cities that are worst off objectively are not necessarily the same cities where subjective satisfaction is highest. . .Objective social indicators cannot be taken as direct measures of the welfare or the quality of life actually experienced by individuals" (p.505).

It is difficult to confirm this very strong statement on the basis of the data provided in the article. We are told that of some 416 correlations calculated for two racial groups, "11% (9% for whites, 13% for blacks) [were] significant at the 0.10 level". We are not given the full list of subjective indicators or any justification for each of the objective indicators. So it is unclear how 416 correlations were generated. Presumably Schneider counted percent changes in indicator values as negative or positive if the indicators themselves were negative or positive, e.g., if robbery rates are negative indicators, then increases in such rates are negative and decreases are positive indicators. It may be asking too much to expect percent changes in a single year to show a significant correlation with some relevant subjective indicator for that year, e.g., to have a negative percent change in air quality in 1968-69 (annual reduction in air pollution) show a significant correlation with residents' satisfaction with air quality, especially since we do not know exactly when the attitudes were measured and when the pollution levels were measured. It is indeed unclear why satisfaction with housing would be negatively correlated with United Fund contributions for "whites" (-0.48) but positively correlated for "blacks" (0.51), but it is also unclear to me why one would expect any correlation at all between housing satisfaction and such contributions. I suppose it may have been assumed that such contributions would be positively related to incomes which would be positively related to objective housing quality which was finally to be positively related to housing satisfaction. If that is the chain of reasoning, one would have thought a simple income-to-housing satisfaction correlation would have been more direct and therefore preferable. I was unable to figure out which half of the significant correlations were "in the wrong direction".

Although the interpretation of Schneider's evidence is a bit difficult, there is plenty of other evidence supporting the view that the association between people's objectively measured life conditions and their subjective assessments of those conditions is relatively weak. Personal disposable income, as self-reported in surveys or as estimated from a nation's National Income and Product Accounts in the form of Gross Domestic Product (GDP) per capita, is probably the best single, overall objective measure of people's access to good life conditions. Generally speaking, access to both public and private goods and services are increased as a population's GDP per capita increases, although every segment of the population may not enjoy an equal share of the increase. The UNDP's annual *Human Development Report* reveals that around the world, as per capita incomes increase, so do people's opportunities for better housing and house furnishings, better hospitals and schools, health care and education, longer lives free of disability, food and food security, jobs and job security, social safety nets (e.g., old age pensions), roadways and other means of communication, greater social and economic mobility, greater control over government and over their own lives. Thus, using personal disposable income as a good surrogate objective indicator of life conditions, one might regard the association between this indicator and a subjective indicator like reported life satisfaction (or happiness or subjective well-being) as central for confirming or disconfirming Schneider's view.

The relative insignificance to life satisfaction of half a dozen "standard classification variables", including income, in the presence of a dozen domain satisfaction variables was already documented by Andrews and Withey (1974, 1976), and similar results were reported by Inglehart and Rabier (1986) for 8 west European countries. Duncan (1975) put the question bluntly when he asked: Does money by satisfaction? To answer this question, he examined associations between respondents' reported family incomes and satisfaction with their "standard of living. . .the kind of house, clothes, care, and so forth" from the Detroit Area Studies of 1955 and 1971. He found that although respondents' median family "income in constant dollars increased by a factor of 1.42" in the period from 1955 to 1971, their mean levels of satisfaction with their standard of living did not significantly change. Nevertheless, he also noticed·that "individual satisfaction typically increases with increasing incomes *in cross-section data*". Thus, he concluded (roughly as Aristotle concluded 2400 years earlier) that "the relevant source of satisfaction with one's standard of living is having more income than someone else, not just having more income" (p.273). These conclusions confirmed those of Easterlin (1973).

Diener and Biswas-Diener (2002) published an excellent review of a substantial chunk of the literature around this question and provided the following convenient summary.

> "Four replicable findings have emerged regarding the relation between income and subjective well-being (SWB): 1. There are large correlations between the wealth of nations and mean reports of SWB in them, 2. There are mostly small correlations between income and SWB within nations, although these correlations appear to be larger in poor nations, and the risk of unhappiness is much higher for poor people, 3. Economic growth in the last decades in most economically developed societies has been accompanied by little rise in SWB, and increases in individual income lead to variable outcomes, and 4. People who prize material goals more than other values tend to be substantially less happy, unless they are rich. Thus, more money may enhance SWB when it means avoiding poverty and living in a developed nation, but income appears to increase SWB little over the long-term when more of it is gained by well-off individuals whose material desires rise with their incomes. Several major theories are compatible with most existing findings: A. The idea that income enhances SWB only insofar as it helps people meet their basic needs [Maslow 1954], and B. The idea that the relation between income and SWB depends on the amount of material desires that people's income allows them to fulfill. We argue that the first explanation is a special case of the second one. A third explanation is relatively unresearched, the idea that societal norms for production and consumption are essential to understanding the SWB-income interface. In addition, it appears high SWB might increase people's chances for high income" (p.119).

Additional information on the theories "compatible with most existing findings" and the "relatively unresearched" explanation will be considered below in Michalos (1985) and Veenhoven (1994).

Beginning with the assumptions that measures of perceived well-being are measures of attitudes, and that attitudes are composed of cognitive, affective and conative elements, Andrews and McKennell (1980) applied structural equation modeling (LISREL III, Joreskog and Sorbom, 1976) to British and American data-sets to assess the average distribution of these elements in 23 measures of life-as-a-whole. Their effort represented

". . .a conceptual and statistical refinement over a common past practice of considering that all global measures are simply reflections (perhaps to differing degrees) of a single underlying factor, feelings about life-as-a-whole. Measures that ask about happiness, fun, and enjoyableness (in addition to Bradburn's scales of positive and negative affect) fall in the group for which relatively high affect-cognition ratios were observed. On the other hand, items that employ the term 'satisfaction' and/or that involve comparisons with implicit or explicit criteria tend to have lower affect-cognition ratios. . .satisfaction measures tend to tap more negative than positive affect and. . .in the United States (but not in Great Britain) the reverse is true for happiness measures. . .There was a rather consistent tendency for measures employing 3-point response scales to show lower validities than measures with scales having more response categories" (pp.150-151).

A better idea of the significance of their analyses may be grasped by considering their results for two life satisfaction scales mentioned earlier, namely, the DT version including the words 'pleased' and 'unhappy', and the 7-point satisfaction scale running from 'completely satisfied' to 'completely dissatisfied'. Although the DT version (Life #1) and the 7-point satisfaction scale each had affect-to-cognition ratios of 0.8, the DT version had a more even balance of positive and negative affect than the 7-point satisfaction scale. The validity coefficients for each measure were similar (0.77 versus 0.75, for the DT version and the 7-point satisfaction scale, respectively).

In a later paper, Andrews (1984) used the same structural equation modeling techniques to estimate the construct validity, method effects and residual error for a comprehensive set of survey research measures. I think it is the best paper he published, and perhaps the best paper in the field, although it was not published in *Social Indicators Research*. He examined 13 aspects of survey design, including characteristics of the response scales (e.g., number of scale categories, off scale options, explicit midpoint), item characteristics (e.g., length of introduction and question, absolute vs. comparative), questionnaire design (e.g., item positions, single items vs. sets), topic characteristics (e.g., social desirability sensitivity, content specificity), and data collection procedures (e.g., telephone, face-to-face interview). His overall assessment was that

". . .the 'typical' survey measure examined in this research consisted of 66 percent valid variance, 3 percent method variance, and 28 percent residual variance. . .Although no claim is made that the set of survey items examined here is representative of all items used in current surveys, this set of items is broader and more heterogeneous than any other we know of whose quality has been estimated, and hence these estimates for the quality of our 'typical' item probably provide the best available information about these aspects of measurement quality for single-item survey measures tapping rather specific attitudes and behaviors. . .For the validity estimates, which have a standard deviation of .10, one can infer that about two-thirds of all validity estimates fell in the range .71 to .91. Hence, about two-thirds of the survey measures

examined here contained between 50 percent and 83 percent valid
variance; roughly one-sixth contained more than 83 percent valid
variance, and about one-sixth had less than 50 percent valid variance"
(pp.424-425).

The papers by Kammann, Farry and Herbison (1984) and Fordyce (1988)
are similar insofar as they each provide comparative assessments of a wide
array of measures of subjective well-being. Their main difference is that the
former paper is focused on showing that there is a "single general well-being
factor", while the latter is focused on showing the virtues of a single measure of
happiness.

Kammann and his colleagues developed an affect-balance scale that was
similar to Bradburn's (1969) in having separate items for positive and negative
affect, and in using a "balance or net scoring formula to obtain the overall well-
being score". While Bradburn's scale has 10 items, Kammann's has a 96-item
version called Affectometer 1 and a 40-item version called Affectometer 2.
With Bradburn's scale, respondents are asked *whether or not* they have had a
particular feeling "during the past few weeks", while with the affectometers
they are asked *how often* they have had a feeling in that period, with five
options: not at all, occasionally, some of the time, often, all the time. Many
researchers, using many different samples, found that Bradburn's Negative
Affect (NA) and Positive Affect (PA) scales were relatively independent, while
the affectometers' NA and PA scales had an average association of $r = -0.66$.
Thus, in contrast to Andrews and Withey (1974, 1976) and Andrews and
McKennell (1980), Kamman, Farry and Herbison (1984) claimed that

"Psychologically. . .we must expand or enrich the sense of satisfaction
[with life as a whole] into the experience of really enjoying life, as
having a high preponderance of positive feelings and few if any negative
ones. In fact, our data suggest that global life satisfaction and the balance
of affect come very close to an identity of meaning and that both of these
interpret the phrase 'sense of well-being'. . .The most important finding,
however, is that this dimension of well-being overlaps strongly with the
well-known dimension of neuroticism that regularly arises as a primary
factor in the factor analysis of personality items. To this it may be added
that scales of depression and trait anxiety also seem to be measuring the
negative region of an overall well-being spectrum. . .The hypothesis that
positive and negative affect are two independent processes is now shown
to be less than a universal structure for well-being. As an empirical result
this orthogonality may depend very closely on the particular ten items
and test format used in Bradburn's method; on the other hand, the
general incompatibility of PA and NA reported here could be a
peculiarity of the affectometer technique. . .Researchers who wish to
defend the model of independence of positive and negative affect should
now demonstrate that independence can be demonstrated by methods
other than Bradburn's original procedure" (pp.111-113).

Fordyce (1988) reviewed results of several years of testing his 2-item
Happiness Measures which, he claimed, revealed that the simple index showed
"good reliability, exceptional stability, and a record of convergent, construct,

and discriminative validity unparalleled in the field". The index is constructed of an 11-point happy/unhappy scale measuring the *intensity* of affect, and a *frequency* scale measuring the percent of time "on the average" that respondents feel happy, unhappy or neutral. The formula used to obtain a single combination score from the two items is "*combination* = (*scale score* x 10 + *happy %*)/2".

In support of his own results, Fordyce noted that Diener's examination of twenty well-being indexes led the latter to conclude that

". . .the 11-point Fordyce scale showed the strongest correlations with daily affect and with life satisfaction of any measure we assessed. . ." and that the HM's ". . .positive and negative frequency estimates provide convergent, construct and criteria validities that are equal to or superior to those found for the Bradburn scale. . ." (p.364, quoted from Diener (1984)).

Based on those results, Fordyce was able to construct the familiar profile of a happy person as one who has low levels of

". . .fear, hostility, tension, anxiety, guilt, confusion, anger. . .a high degree of energy, vitality and activity; a high level of self-esteem. . .emotionally stable personality; a strong social-orientation. . .healthy, satisfying and warm love and social relationships; a life-style typified as involved, active, social and meaningfully productive. . .optimistic, worry-free, present-oriented, internally-locused, and well-directed. . .But beyond this, this description also closely approximates what the literature in psychology views as the major criteria of optimal mental health" (pp.365-370).

Having illustrated the fact that our field has a vast variety of measures of subjective well-being emphasizing one or more of its many dimensions or elements, it should not be surprising to discover that someone tried to find a 'gold standard' to bring some order to the apparent disorder. That is what Cummins (1995) tried to accomplish, not only for whole populations (of western countries) but also for ten subgroups, namely, females, those over 65 years of age, physically disabled, intellectually disabled, those with chronic medical problems, post-organ transplant recipients, low and high income people, U.S. "whites" and "blacks".

Looking for appropriate samples, he scanned over 1,000 articles and books according to a set of criteria that were generally reasonable. The only criterion that I found questionable was the one excluding all scales measuring happiness. He did not indicate why they were all excluded, but I would have included at least some of them on the grounds of their high correlations with most measures of life satisfaction. He included the life satisfaction DT scale of Andrews and Withey although, as mentioned earlier, that scale explicitly includes the terms 'pleased' and 'unhappy' to elicit affective responses. Results based on the Satisfaction with Life Scale of Diener, Emmons, Larson and Griffin (1985) were excluded because the scale routinely yielded "data which fall at least 10%SM [Scale Maximum] points below those of comparable scales". The 17 data-sets finally used were drawn from Australia, Canada, England, Norway,

Sweden and the U.S.A., and they employed 14 different measures of life satisfaction. The common statistic he constructed is called "the Percentage of Scale Maximum" (%SM) and is generally defined as "(score – 1) x 100/(number of scale points – 1)".

Examining the reported results from the various studies, he found that "The arithmetic mean and standard deviation of the %SM values is 75.02 ± 2.74". So, he ". . .proposed that, as a working hypothesis, the life satisfaction gold standard be considered as 75.0 ± 2.5%SM". Using that standard as the norm, he found, for example, that (1) the mean scores for "females, people who have survived an organ transplantation for a number of years, and people with a mild or moderate level of intellectual disability living in the community" did not differ from the normative range, (2) the mean scores for "people over the age of 65 years, people with a physical disability, or with a low income, are on the lower margins of the normal range", (3) "people with a chronic medical condition. . .have a mean value well below the two standard deviation range" and (4) people with a high income have means scores "above the normal range".

Atkinson (1982) presented results from a longitudinal (panel) study involving "a representative sample of 2162 Canadians interviewed in 1977 and again in 1979". Apart from some results dealing with a subset (N = 285) of the national sample used in Campbell, Converse and Rodgers (1976), this was the first published report "on the stability of QOL measures over time". The particular measures employed included an 11-point life satisfaction item similar to those used in Great Britain and in the European Community, a self-anchoring ladder scale adapted from Cantril (1965), the Gallup 3-point happiness scale and domain satisfaction scales for five domains; job, finances, housing, health and marriage/romance. A General Quality of Life Index was formed by combining responses for the life satisfaction, happiness and Cantril scales, and a Domain Satisfaction Index was formed by combining domain satisfaction scores. In order to assess levels of change in people's lives from the first to the second survey, respondents were asked in the second wave if their current status was the same, better or worse, for life in general and for specific domains. They were also asked which of 16 significant life events they had experienced in that period, e.g., divorce/separation, serious injury, new job or house.

His most important conclusions were admirably summarized as follows.

> "Opinions have been expressed in some quarters that subjective measures such as satisfaction are poor social indicators because they were so conditioned by expectations and restricted awareness as to be insensitive to changing circumstances. It is also argued that expectations and aspirations adjust very quickly to new situations and that satisfaction and other measures revert to their original levels immediately. This position would have led to predictions that (a) very few individuals would indicate any change in their situation, and/or (b) virtually no adjustment in subjective indicators would occur when changes did occur.

> Our findings contradict both hypotheses in that significant numbers of respondents perceive changes in their lives and those changes were reflected, for better or worse, in their satisfaction levels. The fact that

these changes took place over a two year period indicates that, while adaptation probably does occur, it is not instantaneous and will be detected by an indicator series which utilizes fairly frequent measurements" (pp.128-129).

Because the questionnaire included respondents' perceived changes (subjective indicators) and numbers of specific life events experienced (objective indicators), Atkinson was able to compare levels of association between each of these measures and satisfaction measures. He found that

"The hypothesis that the No Change group would have more stable QOL scores than those reporting change is supported when the perceptual indicator of change is used as the independent variable but not when the event measures are involved. . .[As well] Relationships between self-reported change and satisfaction levels are always higher than between events and changes in satisfaction" (pp.122, 126).

This phenomenon is especially interesting to people working with discrepancy theories (e.g., Michalos 1985) because it has been found that perceived discrepancies between what one has and wants, for example, are better predictors of satisfaction than researcher-calculated discrepancies (i.e., difference scores between things actually possessed and wanted), e.g., see Oliver and Bearden (1985), Wright (1985), and Michalos (1991). Rice, McFarlin and Bennett (1989) compared the predictive power of perceived discrepancy scores with calculated discrepancy scores for job satisfaction and concluded

"It appears that the components of a discrepancy are not capable of totally capturing the psychological comparison process represented by have-want discrepancies. Rather, it seems that have-want discrepancies have a power to predict and explain facet satisfaction that goes above and beyond the predictive power of the two components" (p.597).

Appealing to the different ways to measure changes in people's lives (perceived changes versus numbers of significant life events), Atkinson thought that the often observed low correlations between objective and subjective indicators might be the result of the fact that "the objective event is too gross a measure to lead to a prediction of its effects". Furthermore, he noted that the long- and short-term consequences of events may be very different.   For example,

"Divorce and separation appear to have neutral or negative short-term impacts followed by a positive long-term consequence. Most analyses of the impact of changing conditions have not considered the possibility of time dependent effects and have assumed that the impact of change is constant, or at least in the same direction, over time" (pp.129-130).

Most have also assumed that the impact of certain kinds of events is the same for all individuals, which is contrary to what we know about "individual differences in values and judgement standards".

Headey, Veenhoven and Wearing (1991) reported results from four waves of an Australian panel study conducted in the state of Victoria, involving samples ranging from 942 in 1981 to 649 in 1987. In the original linear model employed by Andrews and Withey (1974) and many others, global well-being measured by life satisfaction, happiness or, more broadly, subjective well-being is explained by (regressed on) measures of satisfaction in several domains, e.g., satisfaction with one's family life, job, housing and health. Diener (1984) called this the Bottom-Up (BU) model. However, because all of the key domain satisfaction variables are highly intercorrelated, some people have suspected that the original model might have the causal story completely backwards. They think that global well-being is like a personality trait or stable disposition that influences people's individual assessments of every domain of their lives. Diener called this the Top-Down (TD) model. The paper by Veenhoven (1994) in this collection provides a thorough review of all the evidence for and against the TD model. Besides these two possibilities, there is a Bi-Directional (BD) model that posits the causal arrows running in both directions (Mallard, Lance and Michalos, 1997), and a Spurious Causation (SC) model that posits some other variable(s) as the cause of the observed correlations among domain and global variables (Costa and McCrae, 1980).

Headey, Veenhoven and Wearing provided some evidence for the top-down (TD), two-way (BD) and spurious causation (SC) models. Their global dependent variable was a 9-point version of Life #3 from Andrews and Withey (1994), and their 9-point domain satisfaction variables were for the domains of marriage, work, standard of living, leisure, friendship and health. They had two personality variables, extraversion and neuroticism, from Eysenck and Eysenck (1964), and gross family income, main breadwinner's occupational status, respondent's educational level, age and sex. Like Andrews, Atkinson and others, the software employed was a version of LISREL (Joreskog and Sorbom, 1978).

For the domain of marriage, they found two-way causation.

> "Being happily married increases one's life satisfaction ($BU = 0.18$), but it is also true that happy people are more likely to maintain happy marriages. . .while miserable people tend to have miserable marriages ($TD = 0.12$). . .Costa and McCrae's (1980) hypothesis that stable personal characteristics account for apparent causal relationships between domain satisfactions and life satisfaction appears incorrect in regard to the marriage domain" (pp.90-91).

Regarding the domains of work and standard of living, they found only a TD model was confirmed. Part of the relationship between leisure and life satisfaction was from the latter to the former (TD), and part of it was spurious (SC). The relationship between friendship and life satisfaction was spurious (SC), resulting from the influence of extraversion on both variables, while the relationship between health and life satisfaction was also spurious (SC), driven by both extraversion and neuroticism.

These interesting results are difficult to square with the conclusions of Kammann, Farry and Herbison (1984). If those authors were right in their assessment that scales for neuroticism and extraversion are "only half-asked well-being questionnaires", and that properly measured global life satisfaction and affect balance capture a single general well-being factor, then the allegedly spurious causal relationships found by Headey, Veenhoven and Waring would be little more than the effects of questionnaire design. Strictly speaking, the work done by extraversion and neuroticism on leisure and health satisfaction would really have been done by life satisfaction, and would have been further evidence for a Top-Down model. Without trying to resolve this problem, it is worthwhile to briefly review results of an even broader examination of the issues raised in Headey, Veenhoven and Wearing's paper.

Headey, Veenhoven and Wearing (1991) remarked that it was useful to have panel data to address the issues of the relative strength of the four models "(a) because no instrumental variables are required (and the search for appropriate instruments is often fruitless) and (b) because few restrictive assumptions are required" (p.85). As luck would have it, the rich data-set developed for the *Global Report on Student Well-Being* (Michalos 1991, 1991a, 1993, 1993a) provided a few variables that could satisfy the conditions for instrumental variables (James and Singh, 1978). Mallard, Lance and Michalos (1997) used the have-want discrepancy variable for that purpose, and examined the relative strength of three models (BU, TD and BD) for explaining satisfaction in 11 domains of life using samples drawn from undergraduate populations in 32 countries. The 11 domains were health, finances, family, paid employment, friendships, housing, living partner, recreation, religion, transportation and formal education. The 32 countries were Austria, Bahrain, Bangladesh, Belgium, Brazil, Cameroon, Canada, Chile, Egypt, Finland, Germany, Greece, Israel, Japan, Jordan, Kenya, Korea, Mexico, Netherlands, New Zealand, Norway, Philippines, Puerto Rico, South Africa, Spain, Sweden, Tanzania, Thailand, Turkey, United Kingdom, United States of America and Yugoslavia. The software employed was LISREL VII (Joreskog and Sorbom, 1989).

This is how they summarized their results.

> "The first purpose of this paper was to provide additional competitive tests between the BU, TD, and BD models. Overwhelmingly, results supported the BD model, as this model provided the best fit to the data for all but three of the 32 samples examined. In the remaining three samples [Belgium, Jordan and Sweden] the TD model received the strongest support. Importantly, the BU model received the *least* support in all 32 samples. This finding runs counter to a majority of satisfaction research whose theoretical assumptions have been rooted in the BU perspective (Diener, 1984; Lance *et al.*, 1995; Sloan, 1990). Thus, findings reported here now provide global support *counter* to the idea that some subjectively weighted composite of LFSs [life facet satisfactions] determines OLS [overall life satisfaction], and in support of the idea that OLS-LFS relationships are multidirectional.
>
> The second purpose of this paper was to determine whether culture moderates the OLS-LFS relationship. . .The fact that the BD model

received overwhelming support in 29 of the 32 samples studied points to the answer 'no'. On the other hand, the fact that different patterns of OLS-LFS relationships were found in each sample points to the answer 'yes'. However, since none of the clusters of samples could be clearly defined by some (set of) cultural factor(s) [it] makes the answer even more difficult" (pp.278-279).

There were many different explanatory paths revealed in the 32 countries. For example, in Canada the BD model had the best fit for the OLS-LFS relationships for the domains of health, finances, family, friendships, living partner, recreation and education, while in Cameroon, this model fit best for only the domains of finances, family and friendships, and in the United States, it fit best for the domains of finances, family, friendships, housing, living partner, recreation and transportation. Nevertheless, when Ward's (1963) hierarchical agglomerative clustering method was applied to all the samples, it was found that Cameroon, Canada and the United States clustered together, with 52% of the OLS-LFS relationships fitting the BD model, 36% fitting TD, 9% BU and one not statistically significant. All together, there were 7 distinct clusters.

Support for a Top-Down model may be regarded as evidence that subjective well-being has some kind of a relatively stable, enduring aspect, which some researchers describe in fairly minimalist terms while others prefer stronger language, referring to the enduring aspect as a disposition or, perhaps even stronger, a personality trait. For reasons related to logical problems defining disposition-designating terms generally and personality traits in particular (Michalos 1980, 1991), I am inclined to use minimalist language. Veenhoven (1994) was less circumspect. In a paper that I rank along side Andrews (1984), he asked bluntly "Is happiness a trait?", and answered unequivocally, "happiness is no immutable trait". Veenhoven uses the term 'happiness' in a very broad sense that is close to Diener's 'subjective well-being', although I think that for most English-speaking people 'happiness' has a narrower sense. In any case, Veenhoven's analysis seems straightforward enough.

"Happiness does *not* meet the classic three definitions of trait.

Firstly, *happiness is not temporally stable*. Individuals revise their evaluation of life periodically. Consequently their happiness rises and drops, both absolutely and relatively. Average happiness of nations appears not immutable either. Though stability prevails, there are cases of change.

Secondly, *happiness is not situationally consistent*. People are not equally happy in good and bad situations. Improvement or deterioration of life is typically followed by changes in the appreciation of it. This is also reflected at the collective level. Average happiness is highest in the countries that provide the best living conditions. Major changes in condition of the country affect average happiness of its citizens.

Lastly, *happiness is not entirely an internal matter*. It is true that happiness roots to some extent in stable individual characteristics and collective orientations, but the impact of these inner factors is limited.

They modify the outcome of environmental effects rather than dominating them.

These findings knock the bottom out of the argument that happiness is too static a matter to be influenced by social policy. There is thus still sense in pursuing greater happiness for a greater number.

The findings also refute the related claim that happiness is not a useful social indicator. Though happiness may be a slowly reacting instrument, it does reflect long-term change for better or worse" (pp.145-146).

The two papers by Michalos (1980a, 1985) are closely related to each other, and also to Veenhoven (1994). They are related to the latter paper insofar as both are evidently rooted in some sort of pragmatic moral consequentialism. There is not only "sense in pursuing greater happiness for a greater number", there is also a moral obligation to do so. Since many types of moral consequentialist theories and critiques of such theories have been around for a few hundred years, and I have explained my particular views in other places (e.g., Michalos 1995, 2001), there is no need to review those issues here. Here it only has to be recorded that in the 1980a and 1985 papers, as in many of my other scientific investigations, the primary motive was an interest in finding a reliable and valid general theory of human well-being that could be the foundation for a naturalistic moral theory.

In Michalos (1980a) I cited a couple remarks by Campbell, Converse and Rodgers (1976) indicating their recognition that they did not have a "very elaborated theory" and that it was "quite conceivable" that standards of comparison and aspiration levels might be different for different domains of life and for life as a whole. As a review of the papers in this collection reveals, the plain fact is that social indicators research has never had an abundance of theories or theoreticians. On the contrary, a lot of our work has been in the positivistic tradition that generally underemphasized the importance of theories and overemphasized the importance of good measurement (Michalos 1971). Although I was a teenage positivist and shades of the boy remain in the man, I do think that many of the positivist views about what science is and ought to be are not tenable (Michalos 1980). However, with regard to the structure of scientific theories, I believe the positivist idea of constructing them in the form axiomatic systems is worthwhile. Among other things, such systems have the virtues of making the basic concepts, postulates and immediate implications of theories relatively transparent (Michalos 1980). That is why I tried to give Multiple Discrepancies Theory (MDT) such a form, although it came a few years after the 1980a paper.

In the 1980a paper I assumed that a respondent's *perceived* gap between some current status and some comparison standard should be more closely related than a *researcher-calculated* gap to the respondent's reported satisfaction. The only gaps considered were those regarding respondents' comparisons with their own aspirations, average people of their age and their best previous experiences. The only models considered were one called "the Michigan model" and another called "its most plausible competitor". In the former, the goal-achievement gap served as a mediating variable between satisfaction or happiness and the other two gap variables, while in the latter the dependent variables were directly regressed on the three gap variables. The two models were tested for life satisfaction and happiness, and satisfaction in 12 domains, namely, health, financial security, family life, friendships, housing, job, free time activity, education, self-esteem, area lived in, ability to get around and security from crime. In every case, the Michigan model looked superior to its competitor, from which I concluded

> "The implications of confirmation of most of the postulated relations in the Michigan model are profound. Insofar as this type of model can be substantiated, human satisfaction is not just a brute fact to be accommodated like the wind and rain. . . .Insofar as satisfaction is generated as the Michigan model indicates, education and individual initiative have a fundamental role to play in the development of the good life for individuals and societies. Accurate perceptions of the real world have a vital role to play in the determination of satisfaction with that world. The proverbial Fool's Paradise may be regarded as the result of experiencing uninformed or misinformed satisfaction. Thus, if knowledge is a reasonable thing (i.e., something to which principles of sound reasoning are applicable), then so is satisfaction, taste, etc. Here the dreams of all naturalistic value theorists loom large" (pp.406-411).

A nice attitude to be sure. Unfortunately, things soon got more complicated. In the 1985 paper I reviewed the evidence revealing the influence of 7 comparison standards (yielding 7 potential discrepancies or gaps) on people's reported satisfaction and happiness. Briefly, these were the gaps between what people have and want, relevant others have, the best one has had in the past, expected to have 3 years ago, expects to have after 5 years, deserves and needs. I assumed that by rolling these 7 standards into one theory, the latter would enjoy the explanatory power of the lot. Since there was also evidence that satisfaction and happiness were determined to some extent by people's age, sex, education, ethnicity, income, self-esteem and social support, I called the latter variables 'conditioners' and rolled them into my theory as well. The most important feature of the theory was the assumption that 6 of the gap variables and all 7 of the conditioners would have *both direct and indirect effects* on satisfaction and happiness. The primitive models that I regarded as competitors in the 1980a paper were really parts of a bigger integrated model, which I finally described in 6 basic hypotheses or postulates and called Multiple Discrepancies Theory (MDT).

MDT was supposed to provide a new foundation for all kinds of utility theories. While utility theories generally and philosophical utilitarianism in particular typically begin with revealed preferences or some sort of a *given* affect-laden attitude or interest, MDT was "designed to break through and explain" those preferences, attitudes or interests. Insofar as MDT explained satisfaction and happiness as the *effects* of other things (perceived discrepancies and conditioners), satisfaction and happiness were not just *incorrigible givens* but could be altered by altering those other things. What's more, as indicated in the paper, MDT's explanatory power was considerable. For the convenience sample of 682 undergraduates described in the paper, MDT explained 49% of the variation in scores for reported happiness, 53% for life satisfaction and on average 57% for satisfaction in the 12 domains. The theory explained as much as 79% of the variance in reported satisfaction with family relations and as little as 35% of the variance in satisfaction with education.

The most extensive testing of MDT was based on a sample of over 18,000 undergraduates in 39 countries (Michalos 1991, 1991a, 1993, 1993a). In broad strokes, the theory explained on average 52% of the variance in scores for the 14 dependent variables used in the 1985 paper, including 51% for males and 53% for females. The theory worked best on samples of undergraduates from Austria and Finland (64% variance explained on average), and worst on the sample from Mexico (36% variance explained). Samples from Bangladesh, Sweden and Switzerland also had average explanatory figures in the 60s, while the average figures for Egypt and Thailand were in the 30s. For the group as a whole, on average the goal-achievement gap was exactly as influential as the social-comparison gap, while for males the social-comparison gap and for females the goal-achievement gap, respectively, were most influential. Of the 6 gaps influencing the goal-achievement gap, the social-comparison gap was by far the most influential.

Diener (1994) provided a fine summary of the field of subjective well-being studies as late as the summer of 1993, although the material it reviewed and the agenda for research that it recommended is much more contemporary than its date of origin would suggest. The aim of the paper was to alert social indicators researchers to relevant recent research from the field of psychology, especially research related to the affective aspects of subjective well-being, including the pleasantness and unpleasantness experienced in feelings, emotions and moods. He was particularly interested in reminding us of the variety of emotions that people experience (e.g., sadness, fear, anger, guilt, affection, joy) and showing us the variety of methods available to measure them. "It is now widely agreed", he said, "that emotion is composed of behavioral, nonverbal, motivational, physiological, experimental, and cognitive components." Emotions may be revealed through facial expressions (e.g., smiling), action readiness, coping activities and self-reports. Self-reports are the standard instruments used by survey researchers, but such reports lack precision because (1) different people identify and name different experiences in different ways, (2) some people deny or ignore some kinds of emotions, (3) some are reluctant to report what they feel, and (4) people experience and remember diverse emotions with different levels of intensity, different frequencies and durations. In short,

> "Contributions in other areas of psychology lead us to conceive of subjective well-being in a more differentiated, less monolithic way. The goal will then be, not to discover *the* cause of SWB, but rather to understand the antecedents of various types of SWB parameters. Subjective well-being cannot be considered to be a brute, incontrovertible fact, but will, like all scientific phenomena, depend on the types of measures used to assess it" (p.140).

Among other things, researchers' methods might include a variety of assessments of nonverbal behaviors (e.g., sleeping and eating habits, alcohol consumption), reports from significant others, electromyographic facial recording, diverse priming protocols, experience sampling of moods, video and audio records, self-reports of goals, self-worth and helplessness, and in-depth interviews. In the future, subjective well-being research will be characterized by multiple measures of the multiple components of the construct.

Reflecting on the array of more or less subtle techniques that are currently available for measuring perceived well-being, one must be concerned about the political and moral implications of our expanding opportunities. Among the "uses and abuses of social indicators and reports" reviewed in Michalos (1980b), I mentioned the possibility that our efforts might lead to a technocratic and elitist society which would be subversive for democracy. As our understanding of the complex roots of human judgments and evaluations of their lives become more sophisticated, there is a danger of paralysis. In the presence of great uncertainty about exactly what personal reports about people's own lives are worth, people may become reluctant to engage in social and political activities, even those that appear progressive. While that is certainly possible, we should remember and find comfort in things like Andrews's reliability and validity studies, Veenhoven's research on the good consequences of happiness and Fordyce's profile of happy people. It is reasonable to believe that a better world is possible, and that our best weapons against imperfect democracies driven by imperfect understanding and appreciation are improved understanding and appreciation, leading to improved personal and public decision making and action, in short, to more perfect democracies.

Exhibit 1. Citation classics, diverse definitions and fields

Required Cites, ≥	N of Classics	Maximum Cites	Fields/Journals	Source
500	3	1255	All Sci.Cit.Index	Johnston 2003
100	36	1255	All Sci.Cit.Index	Johnston 2003
50	150	Na	Geography Js	Bodman 2003
158[a]	100	705	J Am. Med. A	Garfield 1987
100[b]	50		Anaesthesia & Pain Js	Terajima & Åneman 2003
75	28	405	Chesap. Bio. Lab	Waring 2000
50	21	868	Marine Bio. Js	Fuseler-McDowell 1988
25[c]	na	Na	Medicine	Plomp 1990

a Top 100 most cited articles selected, minimum citation frequency was 158
b Top 50 most cited articles selected, minimum citation frequency was 100
c Highly cited articles

Exhibit 2. Frequency and percentage distributions of citation values.*

Number of Citations	Frequency	Percent	Cumulative Percent
162	1	.1	.1
139	1	.1	.1
137	1	.1	.2
121	1	.1	.3
109	1	.1	.4
99	1	.1	.4
81	1	.1	.5
80	1	.1	.6
71	1	.1	.6
68	1	.1	.7
59	1	.1	.8
58	1	.1	.9
57	1	.1	.9
56	1	.1	1.0
55	1	.1	1.1
53	1	.1	1.1
52	1	.1	1.2
50	3	.2	1.4
49	1	.1	1.5
48	1	.1	1.6
46	2	.1	1.7
45	1	.1	1.8
44	3	.2	2.0
43	1	.1	2.1
42	1	.1	2.2
40	1	.1	2.2
39	1	.1	2.3
36	1	.1	2.4
35	1	.1	2.4
32	1	.1	2.6
30	1	.1	2.7
29	2	.1	2.8
27	1	.1	2.9
25	3	.2	3.1
24	3	.2	3.3
23	5	.4	3.7
22	1	.1	3.7
21	3	.2	4.0
20	1	.1	4.0
19	1	.1	4.1
18	3	.2	4.3

Exhibit 2. Contintued

Number of Citations	Frequency	Percent	Cumulative Percent
17	2	.1	4.5
16	3	.2	4.7
15	8	.6	5.2
14	9	.6	5.9
13	8	.6	6.5
12	12	.9	7.3
11	13	.9	8.3
10	9	.6	8.9
9	17	1.2	10.1
8	13	.9	11.1
7	18	1.3	12.4
6	29	2.1	14.4
5	28	2.0	16.5
4	40	2.9	19.3
3	54	3.9	23.2
2	75	5.4	28.6
1	174	12.5	41.1
0	820	58.9	100.0
Total	1392	100.0	

* Total number of citations = 4979; mean number of citations per article = 3.6, mode = 0, median = 0, Std. Deviation = 11.8.

Exhibit 3. **Citation Classics, 1974-2003***

<u>Cites</u>

162   Andrews, F.M. and S.B. Withey
Measures of perceived life quality: results from several
national surveys
1974   v.1   n.1   1-26

139   Diener, E.
Assessing subjective well-being: progress and opportunities
1994   v.31   n.2   103-157

137   Michalos, A.C.
Multiple discrepancies theory (MDT)
1985   v.16   n.4   347-413

121   Michalos, A.C.
Satisfaction and happiness
1980   v.8   n.4   385-422

109   Andrews, F.M. and A.C. McKennell
Measures of self-reported well-being: their affective,
cognitive and other components
1980   v.8   n.2   127-155

99   Abbey, A. and F.M. Andrews
Modeling the psychological determinants of life quality
1985   v.16   n.1   1-34

81   Larsen, R.J., E. Diener and R.A. Emmons
An evaluation of subjective well-being measures
1985   v.17   n.1   1-17

80   Veenhoven, R.
Is happiness relative?
1991   v.24   n.1   1-34`

71   Levy, S. and L. Guttman
On the multivariate structure of wellbeing
1975   v.2   n.3   361-388

68   Shin, D.C. and D.M. Johnson
Avowed happiness as an overall assessment of the quality of
life
1978   v.5   n.4   475-492

59   Schneider, M.
            The quality of life in large American cities: objective and
            subjective social indicators
            1974   v.1   n.4   495-509

58   Diener, E., E. Sandvik, L. Seidlitz and M. Diener
            The relationship between income and subjective well-being:
            relative or absolute
            1993   v.28   n.3   195-223

57   Fordyce, M.W.
            A review of research on the Happiness Measures: A sixty
            second index of happiness and mental health
            1988   v.20   n.4   355-381

56   Andrews, F.M.
            Social indicators of perceived life quality
            1974   v.1   n.3   279-299

55   Diener, E., E. Suh
            Measuring quality of life: economic, social and subjective
            indicators
            1997   v.40   ns.1-3   189-216

53   Duncan, O.D.
            Does money buy satisfaction?
            1975   v.2   n.3   267-274

52   Andrews, F.M. and R. Crandall
            The validity of measures of self-reported well-being
            1976   v.3   n.1   1-19

50   McKennell, A.C.
            Cognition and affect in perceptions of well-being
            1978   v.5   n.4   389-426

50   Headey, B., R. Veenhoven and A. Wearing
            Top-down versus bottom-up theories of subjective well-being
            1991   v.24   n.1   81-100

50   Veenhoven, R.
            Developments in satisfaction research
            1996   v.37   n.1   1-46

49   Chamberlain, K.
            On the structure of subjective well-being
            1988   v.20   n.6   581-604

48   Atkinson, T.
            The stability and validity of quality of life research
            1982   v.10   n.2   113-132

46   McCall, S.
            Quality of life
            1975   v.2   n.2   229-248

46   Andrews, F.M. and R.F. Inglehart
            The structure of subjective well-being in nine western
            societies
            1979   v.6   n.1   73-90

45   McNeil, J.K., M.J. Stones and A. Kozma
            Subjective well-being in later life: issues concerning
            measurement and prediction
            1986   v.18   n.1   35-70

44   McKennell, A.C. and F.M. Andrews
            Models of cognition and affect in perception of well-being
            1980   v.8   n.3   257-298

44   Headey, B., E. Holmstrom and A. Wearing
            Models of well-being and ill-being
            1985   v.17   n.3   211-234

44   Cummins, R.A.
            The domains of life satisfaction: an attempt to order chaos
            1996   v.38   n.3   303-328

43   Emmons, R.A. and E. Diener
            Factors predicting satisfaction judgments: a comparative
            examination
            1985   v.16   n.2   157-167

42   Headey, B., E. Holmstrom and A. Wearing
            Well-being and ill-being: different dimensions?
            1984   v.14   n.2   115-139

40   Veenhoven, R.
            Is happiness a trait? Tests of the theory that a better society
            does not make people any happier
            1994   v.32   n.2   101-160

39   Cummins, R.A.
            On the trail of the gold standard for subjective well-being
            1995   v.35   n.2   179-200

36   Kammann, R., M. Farry and P. Herbison
            The analysis and measurement of happiness as a sense of
            well-being
            1984   v.15   n.2   91-115

35   Diener, E., E. Sandvik, W. Pavot and D. Gallagher
            Response artifacts in the measurement of subjective well-
            being
            1991   v.24   n.1   35-56

* Articles cited 35 times or more, in the top 2.4% of cited articles.

REFERENCES

Andrews, F.M.: 1984, "Construct validity and error components of survey measures: a structural modeling approach", *Public Opinion Quarterly*, 48, pp.409-442.

Andrews, F.M. and S.B. Withey: 1976, *Social Indicators of Well-Being* (Plenum Press, New York).

Bodman, A.R.: 2003, "Citation classics in geography journals" (Abstract), Association of merican Geographers (http://convention.allacademic. com/aag2003/view_paper_info.html?pub_id=2274). Accessed 12/19/2003)

Bonzi, S. and H.W. Snyder: 1991, "Motivations for citation: a comparison of self-citation and citation to others", *Scientometrics*, 21(2), pp.245-254.

Bradburn, N.M.: 1969, *The Structure of Psychological Well-Being* (Aldine, Chicago).

Braybrooke, D.: 1987, *Meeting Needs: Studies in Moral, Political and Legal Philosophy* (Princeton University Press, Princeton).

Brooks, T.A.: 1985, "Private acts and public objects: an investigation of citer motivations", *Journal of the American Society for Information Science*, 36(4), pp.223-229.

Brooks, T.A.: 1988, "Citer motivations", in A. Kent (ed.), *Encyclopedia of Library and Information Science* (Marcel Dekker, New York), pp.48-59.

Campbell, A., P.E. Converse and W.L. Rodgers: 1976, *The Quality of American Life: Perceptions, Evaluations, Satisfactions* (Russell Sage Foundation, New York).

Cantril, H.: 1965, *The Pattern of Human Concerns* (Rutgers University Press, New Brunswick).

Costa, P.T. and R.R. McCrae: 1980, "Influence of extraversion and neuroticism on subjective well-being", *Journal of Personality and Social Psychology*, 38, pp.668-678.

Cozzens, S.E.: 1989, 'What do citations count? The rhetoric-first model", *Scientometrics*, 15(5-6), pp.437-447).

Cronin, B: 1984, *The Citation Process: The Role and Significance of Citations in Scientific Communication* (Taylor Graham, London).

Diener, E.: 1984, "Subjective well-being", *Psychological Bulletin*, 95(3), pp.542-575.

Diener, E. and R. Biswas-Diener: 2002, "Will money increase subjective well-being?", *Social Indicators Research*, 57(2), pp.119-169.

Easterlin, R.A.: 1973, "Does money buy happiness?", *The Public Interest*, 30, pp.3-10.

Eysenck, H.J. and S.B.G. Eysenck: 1964, *Manual of the Eysenck Personality Inventory* (Hodder and Stoughton, London).

Fuseler-McDowell, E.: 1988, "Documenting the literature of marine biology", in Winn, Burkhart and Burkhart (eds.) *Marine Science Information Throughout the World* (International Association of Aquatic and Marine Science Libraries and Information Centers, Charleston).

Garfield, E.: 1972, "Citation analysis as a tool in journal evaluation", *Science*, 178, pp.471-479.

Garfield, E.: 1973, "Uncitedness III – the importance of *not* being cited", *Current Contents*, 24, February 21, pp.413-414.

Garfield, E.: 1976, "Is the ratio between number of citations and publications cited a true constant?", *Current Contents*, 6, February 9, pp.419-421.

Garfield, E.: 1977, "Restating the fundamental assumptions of citation analysis", *Current Contents*, 39, September 26, pp.232-239

Garfield, E.: 1981, "Why the *Journal Citation Reports*?", in E. Garfield (ed.), *Science Citation Index: Journal Citation Reports* (Institute for Scientific Information, Philadelphia).

Garfield, E.: 1981a, "The 1,000 contemporary scientists most-cited 1965-1978. Part 1. The basic list and introduction", *Current Contents*, 24, October 12, pp.3-12.

Garfield, E.: 1983, "How to use *Journal Citation Reports*, including a special salute to the *Johns Hopkins Medical Journal*", *Current Contents*, 17, April 25, pp.131-138.

Garfield, E.: 1984, "The 100 most-cited papers ever and how we select citation classics", *Current Contents*, 27, June 4, pp.3-9.

Garfield, E.: 1985, "Uses and misuses of citation frequency", *Current Contents*, 43, October 28, pp.403-409.

Garfield, E.: 1987, "100 citation classics from the Journal of the American Medical Association", *Journal of the American Medical Association*, 257 (1), pp.52-59.

Garfield, E.: 1988, "The impact of citation counts – a UK perspective", *Current Contents*, 37, September 12, pp.296-298.

Garfield, E.: 1989, "Citation behavior – an aid or a hindrance to information retrieval?", *Current Contents*, 18, May 1, pp.3-8.

Hamilton, D.P.: 1990, "Publishing by – and for? – the numbers", *Science*, 250, pp.1331-1332.

Inglehart, R. and J.-R. Rabier: 1986, "Aspirations adapt to situations – but why are the Belgians so much happier than the French? A cross-cultural analysis of the subjective quality of life", in F.M. Andrews (ed.), *Research on the Quality of Life* (Institute for Social Research, University of Michigan), pp.1-56.

James, L.R. and B.K. Singh: 1978, "An introduction to the logic, assumptions, and basic analytical procedure of two-stage least squares", *Psychological Bulletin*, 85, pp.1104-1122.

Johnston, G.A.R.: 2003, "Citations in Science Citation Index", (http://www.usyd.edu.au/pharmacology/aalab/Citations.html). Accessed 12/19/2003.

Joreskog, K.G. and D. Sorbom: 1976, *LISREL III: Estimation of Structural Equation Systems by Maximum Likelihood Methods* (National Educational Resources, Inc., Chicago).

Joreskog, K.G. and D. Sorbom: 1978, *LISREL IV* (International Educational Services, Chicago).

Joreskog, K.G. and D. Sorbom: 1989, *LISREL 7: A Guide to the Program and Applications* (SPSS Inc., Chicago).

38   ALEX C. MICHALOS

Lance, C.E., A.G.C. Mallard and A.C. Michalos: 1995, "Tests of the causal
    directions of global-life facet satisfaction relationships", *Social Indicators
    Research*, 34, pp.69-92.
Lawani, S.M. and A.E. Bayer: 1983, "Validity of citation criteria for assessing
    the influence of scientific publications: new evidence with peer
    assessment", *Journal of the American Society for Information Science*,
    34(1), pp.59-66.
Liu, M.: 1993, "Progress in documentation, the complexities of citation
    practice: a review of citation studies", *Journal of Documentation*, 49(4),
    pp.370-408.
MacRoberts, M.H. and B.R. MacRoberts: 1986, "Quantitative measures of
    communication in science: a study of the formal level", *Social Studies of
    Science*, (16), pp.151-172.
MacRoberts, M.H. and B.R. MacRoberts: 1987, "Testing the Ortega hypothesis:
    facts and artifacts", *Scientometrics*, 12(5-6), pp.293-295.
MacRoberts, M.H. and B.R. MacRoberts: 1989, "Problems of citation analysis:
    a critical review", *Journal of the American Society for Information Science*,
    40(5), pp.342-349.
MacRoberts, M.H. and B.R. MacRoberts: 1989a, "Citation analysis and the
    science policy arena", *Trends in Biochemical Sciences*, 14(1), pp.8-10.
Mallard, A.G.C., C.E. Lance and A.C. Michalos: 1997, "Culture as a moderator
    of overall life satisfaction – life facet satisfaction relationships", *Social
    Indicators Research*, 40(3), pp.259-284
Maslow, A.H.: 1954, *Motivation and Personality* (Harper, New York).
Merton, R.K.: 1977, "The sociology of science: an episodic memoir", in R.K.
    Merton and J. Gaston, (eds.), *The Sociology of Science in Europe* (Southern
    Illinois University Press, Carbondale), pp.3-141.
Michalos, A.C.: 1971, *The Popper-Carnap Controversy* (Martinus Nijhoff, The
    Hague).
Michalos, A.C.: 1980, "Philosophy of science: historical, social and value
    aspects", in P.T. Durbin (ed.), *The Culture of Science, Technology and
    Medicine* (The Free Press, New York), pp.197-281.
Michalos, A.C.: 1980a, "Satisfaction and happiness
Michalos, A.C.: 1980b, *North American Social Report: Volume 1, Foundations,
    Population and Health* (D. Reidel, Dordrecht).
Michalos, A.C.: 1991, *Global Report on Student Well-Being: Volume 1, Life
    Satisfaction and Happiness* (Springer-Verlag, New York).
Michalos, A.C.: 1991a, *Global Report on Student Well-Being: Volume 2,
    Family, Friends, Living Partner and Self-Esteem* (Springer-Verlag, New
    York).
Michalos, A.C.: 1993, *Global Report on Student Well-Being: Volume 3,
    Employment, Finances, Housing and Transportation* (Springer-Verlag,
    New York).
Michalos, A.C.: 1993a, *Global Report on Student Well-Being: Volume 4,
    Religion, Education, Recreation and Health* (Springer-Verlag, New York).
Michalos, A.C.: 1995, *A Pragmatic Approach to Business Ethics* (Sage
    Publishers, Thousand Oaks).

Michalos, A.C.: 2001, "Ethics counselors as a new priesthood", *Journal of Business Ethics*, 29, pp.3-17.

Michalos, A.C.: 2003, *Essays on the Quality of Life* (Kluwer Academic Publishers, Dordrecht).

Michalos, A.C.: 2004, "Social indicators research and health-related quality of life research", *Social Indicators Research*, 65(1), pp.27-72.

Moravcsik, M.J.: 1988, "Citation context classification of a citation classic concerning citation context classification", *Social Studies of Science*, 18, pp.515-521.

Moravcsik, M.J. and P. Murugesan: 1975, "Some results on the function and quality of citations", *Social Studies of Science*, 5, pp.86-92.

Narin, F.: 1976, Evaluative Bibliometrics: *The Use of Publication and Citation Analysis in the Evaluation of Scientific Activity* (Computer Horizons, Washington).

Oliver, R.L. and W.O. Bearden: 1985, "Disconfirmation processes and consumer evaluations in product usage", *Journal of Business Research*, 13, pp.235-246.

Oppenheim, C. and S.P. Renn: 1978, "Highly cited old papers and the reasons why they continue to be cited", *Journal of the American Society for Information Science*, 29(3), pp.225-231.

Pendlebury, D.A.: 1991, "Science, citation and funding", *Science*, 251, pp.1410-1411.

Plomp, R.: 1990, "The significance of the number of highly cited papers as an indicator of scientific prolificacy", *Scientometrics*, 19(3-4), pp.185-197.

Prabha, C.G.: 1983, "Some aspects of citation behavior: a pilot study in business administration", *Journal of the American Society for Information Science*, 34(3), pp.202-206.

Puder, K.S. and J.P. Morgan: 1987, "Persuading by citation: an analysis of the references of fifty-three published reports of phenylpropanolamine's clinical toxicity", *Clinical Pharmacology and Therapeutics*, 42(1), pp.1-9.

Rice, R.W., D.B. McFarlin and D.E. Bennett: 1989, "Standards of comparison and job satisfaction", *Journal of Applied Psychology*, 74, pp.591-598.

Sievert, M.E. and M. Haughawout: 1989, "An editor's influence on citation patterns: a case study of *Elementary School Journal*", *Journal of the American Society for Information Science*, 40(5), pp.334-341.

Sloan, C.E.: 1990, *Relations Between Global Life and Domain Satisfaction: The Role of Domain Scope and Criticality* (Unpublished doctoral dissertation, University of Georgia, Athens).

Smith, L.: 1981, "Citation analysis", *Library Trends*, 30(1), pp.83-106)

Tatarkiewicz, W.: 1976, *Analysis of Happiness* (M. Nijhoff, Hague).

Terajima, K. and A. Åneman: 2003, "Citation classics in anaesthesia and pain journals: a literature review in the era of the internet", *Acta Anaesthesiologica Scandinavica*, 47 (6), pp.655-.

Vinkler, P.: 1987, "A quasi-quantitative citation model", *Scientometrics*, 12(1-2), pp.47-72.

Virgo, J.A.: 1977, "A statistical procedure of evaluating the importance of scientific papers", *Library Quarterly*, 47(4), pp.415-430.

Waring, E.: 2000, "Citation classics Chesapeake Biological Laboratory, 1925-2000", UM Center for Environmental Science Libraries, Summer. (http://www.cbl.umces.edu/Library/history.php3). Accessed 12/19/2003.

Wright, S.J.: 1985, "Health satisfaction: a detailed test of the multiple discrepancies theory model", *Social Indicators Research*, 17, pp.299-314.

APPENDIX

1970s (1974-79)

Cites	Cited Author	Volume	Page	Year
162	Andrews FM	1	1	1974
52	Andrews FM	3	1	1976
1	Andrews FM	33	1	1976
56	Andrews FM	1	279	1974
46	Andrews FM	6	73	1979
1	Bibby RW	5	169	1977
1	Bunge M	2	65	1975
5	Chen M	3	257	1976
2	Chen MK	5	245	1978
7	Citrin J	4	381	1977
19	Cohen LE	6	251	1979
2	Dever GEA	2	453	1976
53	Duncan OD	2	267	1975
2	Evans W	5	181	1978
2	Fagnani F	3	37	1976
2	Fienberg SE	2	153	1975
3	Fitzsimmons SJ	2	389	1975
1	Gerhmann F	5	78	1978
9	Harwood PD	3	471	1976
2	Horowitz IL	6	1	1979
1	Kennedy L	5	457	1978
71	Levy S	2	361	1975
5	Lippman L	3	181	1976
15	Liu BC	1	187	1974
1	Madduri S	3	429	1976
46	McCall S	2	229	1975
3	McGinnis R	6	163	1979
50	McKennell AC	5	389	1978
1	Milbrath LW	1	397	1974
1	Pineault R	2	465	1976
1	Pollard WE	5	279	1978
59	Schneider M	1	495	1974
68	Shin DC	5	475	1978
1	Ziller RC	34	301	1974

1980s (1980-89)

Cites	Cited Author	Volume	Page	Year
99	Abbey A	16	1	1985
15	Ackerman N	12	25	1983
1	Anderson BJ	14	165	1984
1	Andorka R	26	243	1982
109	Andrews FM	8	127	1980
1	Andrews FM	16	1	1985
48	Atkinson T	10	113	1982
18	Badura B	14	295	1984
1	Bell PA	16	181	1985
2	Berman Y	16	213	1985
2	Berman Y	13	419	1983
3	Bertrand WE	7	237	1980
7	Bibby RW	13	1	1983
1	Borg I	9	256	1981
5	Brinkerhoff MB	18	153	1986
7	Brinkerhoff MB	14	177	1984
8	Broadway MJ	21	531	1989
1	Chamberlain	17	345	1985
50	Chamberlain K	20	581	1988
1	Ciechocinska M	20	59	1988
4	Ciechocinska M	14	333	1984
7	Clogg CC	21	559	1989
23	Clogg CC	18	375	1986
32	Clogg CC	12	117	1983
4	Cnaan RA	21	297	1989
12	Connerly CE	17	29	1985
10	Connidis I	15	117	1984
2	Currie RF	21	481	1989
2	Currie RF	18	95	1986
4	Curtis SE	19	255	1987
14	Davis JA	15	319	1984
11	Dehaes JCJM	19	367	1987
22	Diener E	16	263	1985
1	Dorsey SD	20	69	1988
1	Drewnowski J	18	339	1986
1	Dsa ER	18	285	1986
1	Eaglstein AS	20	103	1988

2	Eaglstein AS	15	281	1984
1	Eaglstein AS	13	59	1983
1	Elgie RA	8	175	1980
43	Emmons RA	16	157	1985
21	Faden RR	7	313	1980
9	Fletcher CN	16	333	1985
57	Fordyce MW	20	355	1988
11	Fordyce MW	18	1	1986
1	French C	20	79	1988
9	Gauthier B	19	229	1987
4	Gee EM	21	611	1989
13	Gee EM	18	263	1986
9	Glatzer W	19	15	1987
5	Glatzer W	19	25	1987
2	Glatzer W	19	39	1987
1	Grabosky	7	63	1980
3	Gratton LC	7	463	1980
6	Gruber KJ	19	303	1987
44	Headey B	17	211	1985
21	Headey B	17	267	1985
25	Headey B	15	203	1984
42	Headey B	14	115	1984
1	Headey B	21	445	1989
16	Homel R	21	133	1989
20	Horley J	17	189	1985
13	Irwin PH	10	187	1982
4	Kamler H	14	69	1984
36	Kammann R	15	91	1984
1	Kirschenbaum A	17	73	1985
11	Kozma A	17	49	1985
3	Krebs D	21	113	1989
1	Kurup KB	15	165	1984
1	Land K	7	1	1980
1	Largen R	17	1	1985
81	Larsen RJ	17	1	1985
8	Latten JJ	21	599	1989
1	Lee T	6	47	1980
1	Levy AB	8	441	1980
4	Levy S	21	455	1989

2	MacKellar FL	21	517	1989
2	Martin E	9	197	1981
14	Mastekaasa A	14	141	1984
18	Mastekaasa A	14	385	1984
7	Maxim P	13	39	1983
44	McKennell AC	8	257	1980
1	McCrae D	8	15	1980
45	McNeil JK	18	35	1986
2	Meredith WH	14	83	1984
5	Mesalago C	16	275	1985
121	Michalos AC	8	385	1980
2	Michalos AC	21	293	1989
15	Michalos AC	18	349	1986
137	Michalos AC	16	347	1985
23	Michalos AC	13	225	1983
1	Milbrath L	19	173	1987
6	Moller V	21	279	1989
9	Moller V	12	225	1983
3	Moon CJ	18	129	1986
1	Moum T	20	177	1988
1	Mukherjee R	20	555	1988
1	Murray A	21	229	1989
1	Nagel SS	21	193	1989
10	Near JP	19	383	1987
13	Near JP	15	351	1984
1	Okafor FC	16	69	1985
1	Okafor FC	17	115	1985
1	Omuta GED	20	417	1988
9	Oppong JR	20	605	1988
5	Ostroot NM	17	243	1985
6	Pablo RY	18	205	1986
3	Perry CS	11	193	1982
1	Porter AL	11	207	1982
5	Potvin L	18	409	1986
2	Ray AK	21	35	1989
3	Relyea H	7	137	1980
6	Roos JP	20	141	1988
6	Rosseel E	17	171	1985
1	Salau AT	18	193	1986

13	Seligson MA	12	1	1983
1	Sheret M	15	289	1984
2	Shin DC	12	393	1983
3	Shin DC	15	1	1984
5	Shye S	21	343	1989
2	Smith AW	13	395	1983
2	South SJ	15	389	1984
4	Staats SR	17	235	1985
4	Stevens JB	14	53	1984
13	Stipak B	12	311	1983
11	Stjohn C	15	43	1984
2	Stones MJ	19	275	1987
29	Stones MJ	17	19	1985
5	Straus MA	20	229	1988
4	Tan G	14	29	1984
2	Tepperman L	16	51	1985
29	Thorslund M	16	77	1985
12	Tipps HC	16	35	1985
1	Trent RB	15	417	1984
1	Ujimoto KV	17	253	1985
2	Vaughan DA	16	315	1985
24	Veenhoven R	20	333	1988
17	Veenhoven R	12	49	1983
1	Veenhoven R	19	329	1986
4	Vermunt R	21	1	1989
3	Verwayen H	14	1	1984
8	Walterbusch E	12	337	1983
1	Waltz M	20	303	1988
8	Waltz M	18	71	1986
2	Wasserman IM	13	281	1983
1	Wasserman IM	11	167	1982
1	Whiteside MM	16	113	1985
1	Whorton JW	15	297	1984
10	Williamson JB	19	205	1987
11	Wood LA	21	379	1989
3	Wright S	16	169	1985
9	Wright SJ	17	299	1985
12	Young FW	12	65	1983
3	Young RC	14	421	1984

1	Young RC	8	299	1980
4	Zagorski K	16	131	1985
1	Zapf W	19	5	1987

1990s (1990-99)

Cites	Cited Author	Volume	Page	Year
1	Adams VH	42	205	1997
5	Adebayo A	22	213	1990
7	Alfonso VC	38	275	1996
4	Altergott K	23	367	1990
4	Andorka R	23	1	1990
25	Andrews FM	25	1	1991
7	Arias E	38	53	1996
2	Ascoli U	40	299	1997
1	Asensookyere WK	39	167	1996
30	Balatsky G	28	225	1993
5	Beckie TM	42	21	1997
4	Benjamin M	31	205	1994
2	Berger AR	44	255	1998
4	Bihagen E	47	119	1999
9	Boehmer U	37	333	1996
4	Boelhouwer J	48	51	1999
1	Brinkerhoff MB	42	245	1997
1	Burr JA	34	339	1995
3	Burton RPD	28	137	1993
3	Carlucci F	36	145	1995
3	Casas F	42	283	1997
1	Chakravarty SR	46	125	1999
24	Chamberlain K	26	101	1992
1	Cicerchia A	46	273	1999
1	Cicerchia A	39	321	1996
6	Clark SM	23	337	1990
2	Clifton RA	38	29	1996
1	Corder CK	41	183	1997
1	Corrie BP	34	395	1995
3	Crooker KJ	44	195	1998
25	Cummins RA	43	307	1998
44	Cummins RA	38	303	1996
39	Cummins RA	35	179	1995

2	Dannehl CR	27	59	1992
8	Davis EE	25	103	1991
1	Denbutter FAG	35	27	1995
1	Dershem LD	39	89	1996
55	Diener E	40	189	1997
35	Diener E	24	35	1991
15	Diener E	36	107	1995
13	Diener E	36	275	1995
27	Diener E	34	7	1995
139	Diener E	31	103	1994
58	Diener E	28	195	1993
11	Dietz T	26	353	1992
10	Dillbeck MC	22	399	1990
14	Douthitt RA	26	407	1992
10	Efraty D	22	31	1990
1	Eglite P	30	109	1993
2	Elliott DH	23	395	1990
8	Emmons RA	45	391	1998
4	Estes RJ	42	1	1997
5	Estes RJ	37	119	1996
18	Evans DR	33	47	1994
5	Eyles J	22	139	1990
2	Fosu GB	28	45	1993
15	Fox CR	27	221	1992
7	French SL	35	1	1995
2	Frey RS	47	73	1999
1	Frey RS	42	77	1997
2	Fyrand L	40	285	1997
1	Genov N	43	197	1998
2	Geurts J	30	245	1993
1	Gitmez AS	31	77	1994
1	Glatzer W	27	375	1992
3	Glorieux I	30	149	1993
5	Groenland E	22	367	1990
2	Hagedorn JW	38	139	1996
3	Hagelin JS	47	153	1999
1	Hagerty MR	47	343	1999
2	Hagerty MR	46	249	1999
3	Halpern AS	33	193	1994

3	Hambleton RK	45	153	1998
3	Harris M	41	279	1997
8	Harvey AS	30	197	1993
8	Harvey AS	23	309	1990
5	Harvey EB	22	299	1990
2	Harwood MK	27	1	1992
1	Hashimoto A	40	359	1997
8	Headey B	47	233	1999
3	Headey B	36	247	1995
3	Headey B	31	1	1994
23	Headey B	29	63	1993
7	Headey B	28	97	1993
50	Headey B	24	81	1991
8	Headey B	22	327	1990
3	Helmes E	45	371	1998
5	Heyink JW	29	291	1993
4	Higgins NC	45	319	1998
3	Higgins NC	42	299	1997
1	Hirschowitz R	41	169	1997
6	Hodge T	40	5	1997
3	Hoppe RA	24	123	1991
9	Horley J	34	275	1995
3	Horley J	26	205	1992
9	Horley J	24	113	1991
1	Horley J	20	383	1988
14	Huebner ES	46	1	1999
15	Huebner ES	38	129	1996
4	Huebner ES	34	315	1995
23	Huebner ES	30	71	1993
3	Illner M	43	141	1998
1	Indrayan A	46	91	1999
1	Ivanova I	46	157	1999
1	Jacob JC	46	341	1999
2	Jacob JC	42	171	1997
7	Jacob SG	32	161	1994
2	Jameton A	40	125	1997
6	Jeffres LW	34	181	1995
1	Jerusalem M	38	229	1996
6	Johnston RJ	27	235	1992

1	Jordan TE	48	299	1999
2	Jordan TE	37	47	1996
11	Jordan TE	30	17	1993
1	Jordan TE	29	183	1993
5	Jordan TE	27	257	1992
2	Kalfs N	44	267	1998
6	Kaplan RM	33	121	1994
11	Kempen GIJM	35	303	1995
4	Khaleque A	27	187	1992
3	Khan H	24	153	1991
12	Klasen S	41	51	1997
3	Kousha M	40	329	1997
1	Kozma A	27	293	1992
13	Kozma A	22	119	1990
14	Lance CE	34	69	1995
5	Lance CE	30	1	1993
7	Land KC	24	209	1991
7	Landua D	26	221	1992
1	Larsen RJ	17	1	1995
5	Larson JS	38	181	1996
6	Larson JS	28	285	1993
3	Lee YJ	31	63	1994
3	Leelakulthanit O	30	49	1993
6	Leelakulthanit O	27	41	1992
1	Leonardi F	48	187	1999
3	Lepper HS	44	367	1998
1	Lerner S	40	217	1997
1	Levine E	22	287	1990
6	Lind NC	28	267	1993
12	Lind NC	27	89	1992
1	Lipshitz G	29	161	1993
2	Louw A	41	137	1997
1	Lukovits I	36	91	1995
11	Lundberg O	37	165	1996
12	Lyubomirsky S	46	137	1999
2	Macphail F	45	119	1998
2	Magen Z	37	235	1996
2	Majumder A	34	325	1995
7	Makkai T	27	169	1992

9	Mallard AGC	40	259	1997
10	Man P	24	347	1991
1	Marginean I	42	353	1997
6	Marks GN	46	301	1999
2	Markus KA	45	7	1998
2	Masse R	45	475	1998
12	Mastekaasa A	29	249	1993
1	Matutinovic I	43	97	1998
1	May J	41	95	1997
4	Mazumdar K	47	1	1999
4	Mazumdar K	38	245	1996
4	Mazumdar K	34	261	1995
2	McAllister I	27	169	1992
6	McCoy M	37	149	1996
11	Meadow HL	26	23	1992
14	Mercier C	33	165	1994
2	Messick S	45	35	1998
6	Michalos AC	48	125	1999
9	Michalos AC	40	221	1997
2	Michalos AC	39	121	1996
2	Michelson W	30	121	1993
5	Michelson W	23	353	1990
3	Millar JS	40	147	1997
8	Miller D	27	363	1992
1	Miller DD	27	415	1992
4	Moller V	47	245	1999
6	Moller V	43	27	1998
1	Moller V	41	1	1997
1	Moller V	37	303	1996
10	Moller V	26	309	1992
4	Morrison MA	48	39	1999
1	Moss PA	45	55	1998
4	Moum T	45	279	1998
8	Moum T	32	1	1994
15	Mullis RJ	26	119	1992
3	Muoghalu LN	25	63	1991
1	Napolitano CL	46	191	1999
12	Near JP	29	109	1993
15	Neto F	35	93	1995

3	Neumayer E	48	77	1999
12	NG YK	38	1	1996
16	Niemi I	30	229	1993
1	Njoh AJ	32	263	1994
1	Obrien M	24	301	1991
4	Okun MA	22	419	1990
5	Olson GI	28	173	1993
6	Ormel J	46	61	1999
11	Ory MG	33	89	1994
2	Ostlin P	23	231	1990
6	Ouellettekuntz H	23	283	1990
1	Pagliccia N	34	367	1995
12	Parmenter TR	33	9	1994
32	Pavot W	28	1	1993
1	Peacock JR	48	321	1999
3	Pilcher JJ	43	291	1998
25	Paloma MM	22	255	1990
5	Pychyl TA	45	423	1998
1	Rahman T	39	59	1996
3	Ram B	29	83	1993
4	Rampichini C	44	41	1998
12	Raphael D	39	65	1996
1	Ravaneral ZR	47	99	1999
1	Reckase MD	45	45	1998
2	Requena F	35	271	1995
3	Rettig KD	47	307	1999
6	Rettig KD	24	269	1991
9	Ringdal GI	38	193	1996
2	Roberge R	48	217	1999
5	Roberts LW	27	113	1992
2	Romney DM	33	1	1994
4	Romney DM	33	237	1994
1	Roth EA	22	385	1990
1	Rothenbacher F	44	291	1998
2	Rothenbacher F	29	1	1993
1	Salisbury PS	48	1	1999
2	Salisbury PS	43	261	1998
1	Sanik MM	30	175	1993
4	Saris WE	45	173	1998

3	Sastre MTM	47	203	1999
6	Scherpenzeel A	38	161	1996
1	Schlemmer L	41	15	1997
1	Schrecker T	40	1	1997
1	Schrecker T	40	99	1997
4	Schulz W	34	153	1995
9	Schyns P	43	3	1998
6	Semyonov M	46	225	1999
2	Shen SM	44	225	1998
14	Sherkat DE	26	259	1992
23	Shmotkin D	23	201	1990
11	Singer E	28	117	1993
3	Sireci SG	45	83	1998
15	Sirgy MJ	43	227	1998
7	Sirgy MJ	34	237	1995
4	Smith CL	24	367	1991
2	Staats S	34	93	1995
4	Staats S	29	229	1993
5	Stevans LK	27	327	1992
1	Stones MJ	37	75	1996
7	Stones MJ	36	129	1995
1	Stones MJ	32	251	1994
1	Stones MJ	31	47	1994
4	Stones MJ	31	159	1994
3	Stones MJ	27	103	1992
5	Stones MJ	25	31	1991
2	Stones MJ	24	317	1991
6	Sullivan O	38	81	1996
2	Suzuki H	42	151	1997
7	Sweetmen ME	29	153	1993
4	Tahlin M	22	155	1990
2	Tang KL	43	69	1998
3	Taylor AA	35	313	1995
16	Terry T	35	39	1995
6	Thomas DR	45	253	1998
1	Thomsen K	35	53	1995
3	Toivonen T	26	277	1992
2	Travis R	28	71	1993
3	Ujimoto KV	23	381	1990

9	Vanschuur Wh	36	49	1995
10	Veenhoven R	48	157	1999
1	Veenhoven R	43	211	1998
21	Veenhoven R	39	1	1996
49	Vecnhoven R	37	1	1996
6	Veenhoven R	36	1	1995
5	Veenhoven R	34	299	1995
40	Veenhoven R	32	101	1994
80	Veenhoven R	24	1	1991
1	Verkuyten M	47	281	1999
13	Verkuyten M	32	21	1994
1	Vingilis E	40	159	1997
1	Vingilis E	6	1	1997
1	Vogel J	48	245	1999
4	Vogel J	42	103	1997
2	Waddell S	34	213	1995
1	Watten RG	36	287	1995
6	Watten RG	35	289	1995
3	Weerasinghe J	32	199	1994
1	Weiss D	26	367	1992
1	Werkuyten M	47	281	1999
7	Wheeler RJ	24	71	1991
9	Wikman A	22	199	1990
6	Wood CH	23	247	1990
1	Wood LA	27	345	1992
5	Xu XH	37	189	1996
10	Yardley JK	24	101	1991
9	Yetim U	29	277	1993
12	Ying YW	26	1	1992
1	Ying YW	26	243	1992
4	Young FW	31	27	1994
3	Young FW	22	351	1990
3	Zagorski K	36	227	1995
1	Zamfir E	42	41	1997
2	Zekeri A	39	203	1997
1	Zekeri AA	36	177	1995
1	Zimmerman DW	45	69	1998
1	Zumbo BD	45	1	1998

2000s (2000-03)

Cites	Cited Author	Volume	Page	Year
3	Benarieh A	52	235	2000
1	Bergerschmitt R	58	403	2002
2	Berman Y	50	329	2000
5	Biswasdiener R	55	329	2001
1	Bittman M	52	291	2000
2	Booysen F	59	115	2002
1	Bostic TJ	52	313	2000
1	Chan A	57	263	2002
1	Chen CN	54	57	2001
1	Cohen EH	53	63	2001
1	Cohen EH	50	83	2000
1	Cummins RA	64	159	2003
17	Cummins RA	52	55	2000
2	Delhey J	56	205	2001
2	Diener E	57	119	2002
2	Dijkstra Ag	57	301	2002
1	Doyle KO	52	195	2000
1	Eckermann L	52	29	2000
4	Eckersley R	52	3	2000
1	Ferriss AL	49	1	2000
1	Fiadzo ED	53	137	2001
1	Gee EM	51	309	2000
14	Gilman R	52	135	2000
4	Greenspoon PJ	54	81	2001
1	Gregg PM	54	1	2001
2	Groot W	50	315	2000
6	Hagerty MR	55	1	2001
1	Hagerty MR	49	347	2000
1	Hazelrigg LE	49	147	2000
1	Headey B	50	115	2000
1	Huebner ES	60	115	2002
3	Huebner ES	55	167	2001
1	Jordan TE	57	73	2002
1	Jordan TE	55	199	2001
1	Keng KA	49	317	2000
4	Lai D	51	331	2000
1	Lever JP	50	187	2000

1	Makinen	53	1	2001
1	Mazumdar K	49	335	2000
1	Mcintosh CN	54	37	2001
2	Michalos AC	54	239	2001
1	Michalos AC	53	189	2001
9	Michalos AC	51	245	2000
6	Michalos AC	50	245	2000
3	Mishra GD	56	73	2001
1	Moller V	55	97	2001
1	Njoh AJ	52	161	2000
1	Noll HH	58	47	2002
2	Parkins JR	56	43	2001
1	Plaza D	51	75	2000
7	Price J	3	11	2000
1	Quadrado L	56	21	2001
1	Richardson CG	51	171	2000
1	Richmond L	50	159	2000
2	Ryan L	55	185	2001
2	Sam DL	53	315	2001
1	Saris WE	53	117	2001
1	Sarliolahteenkorva S	54	329	2001
3	Sastre MTM	49	69	2000
11	Schmuck P	50	225	2000
2	Seligson JL	61	121	2003
1	Sirgy MJ	56	125	2001
1	Sirgy MJ	55	241	2001
3	Sirgy MJ	49	279	2000
1	Turksever ANE	53	163	2001
1	Veenhoven R	58	33	2002
1	Vitterso J	57	89	2002
1	Vogel J	59	275	2002
1	Walterbusch E	50	1	2000
1	Wittebrood K	59	153	2002
1	Young FW	55	223	2001
3	Zapf W	51	1	2000

Summary publication and citation statistics

	1974-1979	1980-1989	1990-1999	2000-2003
Total cited	35	157	308	72
Classics cited	10	14	10	0
Vols. published	1-6 (6)	7-21 (14)	22-48 (26)	49-64 (45*)
Issues per vol.	4	7-19=4, 20-21=6	22-27=4,28-48=3	3
Pages per vol.	500	500, 750	500, 330	330

*Total projected for the decade 2000-2009.

2. Social Indicators Research: A Case Study of the Development of a Journal*

By
ALEX C. MICHALOS
DIRECTOR, SOCIAL INDICATORS RESEARCH
UNIVERSITY OF GUELPH
GUELPH, ONTARIO, CANADA

*An earlier version of this paper was presented at the 9th World Congress of Sociology in Uppsala, Sweden August 14 – 19, 1978.

ABSTRACT. This is a review of the birth and development of one social science journal. I explain how it began, why I became the editor, why Reidel became the publisher, and why it has the format and style that it has. Operating policies and procedures are reviewed. Profiles of our output according to areas of concern and countries of origin are presented. Acceptance and rejection rates are considered. Problems with book reviews, marketing and complaints are described, and some future prospects are outlined.

Introduction

Inviting me to talk about *Social Indicators Research* (SIR) is like inviting me to talk about my family. I don't carry a wallet full of photographs, but otherwise the sentiment is practically the same. I'm sure I can't recall all of the details of the birth and development of SIR, but I will reconstruct as much of the history as accurately as I can. I imagine that the report's failures as objective history will be compensated by its success as personal therapy.

Throughout the report I use the abbreviated company name 'Reidel' to refer to any employee of the company, e.g., I mention letters from Reidel, instead of from particular persons who wrote the letters. Occasionally I have a little bit of fun at Reidel's expense, which I hope will be regarded lightly. In all fairness I must say that the total financial risk for SIR has been assumed by Reidel, and I'm grateful for it. But that doesn't make me grateful for everything they do, nor should it.

The Little Red Hen

As I remember it, there's a children's story about a Little Red Hen who repeatedly tried to get others to help with the chores and repeatedly found herself saying "Very well, I'll do it myself." That's about how I began SIR.

57

Alex C. Michalos (ed.), Citation Classics from Social Indicators Research, 57–73.
© 2005 *Springer. Printed in the Netherlands.*

I spent the 1969-70 academic year teaching at the University of Pittsburgh and came to know Nicholas Rescher very well. He was finishing his book *Welfare* while I was there and I had the opportunity to go over the manuscript with him. Rescher had been and still is an inspirational force in my life. His discussions of poverty and social indicators really whetted my appetite for things to come. There was an enormous and fantastic story to be told in that area of research, but neither of us had the time to tell it. Still, the seeds were sown there and sprouted as soon as I finished my *Foundations of Decision-Making.*

The first draft of the *Foundations* manuscript was completed at the end of 1971. While working on the final chapters of that manuscript, I read a lot of the current literature on cost-benefit analysis, planning-programming and budgeting and public choice generally. That included things like *Toward a Social Report* (USGPO, 1969) and the U.S. Senate *Hearings on the Full Opportunity and Social Accounting Act* (USGPO, 1968). The idea of a social report or, rather, what I would today call a social accounting system captured my imagination. I agreed with Ray Bauer and others who saw the first payoffs at least 30 years down the road, but to a man of 36 that was not a long time.

So, before the ink was dry on my *Foundations* manuscript, I began planning a comparative social report for Canada and the United States. The problem I had, however, was that there was no recognized authoritative source for current research in social indicators. Important papers might turn up anywhere. More often than not unpublished dittoed manuscripts were being circulated in non-intersecting circles of researchers.

Working within an establish discipline, one has a good sense of where the frontiers are or at least how to find them. But social indicators research was not and is not a discipline. Nevertheless, people working in the area had a feeling that they were up to something that was roughly recognizable to others up to the same things. What was required was some coordination or organization of efforts.

The response of workers around the world was almost the same. They formed committees. Those that could find funding held conferences. The interesting thing about conferences on social indicators was the wide variety of expertise one found at them. People came from quite different backgrounds and each meeting began like Vince Lombardi's training camps. The late coach of the Green Bay Packers professional football team used to begin with "Gentlemen, this is a football." Speakers at social indicators conferences began with, "By a social indicator I mean …". With all the flurry of activity, committees and conferences in the early 1970's, I thought someone was bound to start a journal. I was content to let nature take its course. I had my research, was a co-editor of *Theory and Decision* and taught a full load of courses every term. When the U.S. Social Science Research Council set up its Washington Center, I thought a journal was bound to be just around the corner. They had the expertise, the money, influence, everything apparently but the inclination. They put out their *Newsletter* and were content.

In 1971 or 1972 I suggested to someone in Canada's Department of Regional Economic Expansion that we needed something like a clearinghouse for current research in social indicators. Nothing happened. Several months went by. I met Mancur Olson at the University of Maryland. I had admired his work in public choice and was delighted to get to know him personally. We agreed that a journal would be a useful research tool and both hoped someone would start one. I remember talking to him on a couch in the hall of some conference center hosting a meeting of the Public Choice Society. At one point I said something like "Would you be interested in editing a journal on social indicators?" and he replied, "No, but I think you would be perfect for the job." I was flattered, but not interested.

I don't remember when I got interested, but some time in 1972 I became the Little Red Hen and decided to do it myself. I haven't been able to find my first letter of inquiry to a publisher, D. Reidel Co. However, I do have Reidel's first response to my letter and it refers to my letter of November 14, 1972. (Reidel's letter is dated November 30, 1972.) Among other things, Reidel said:

> "As the idea looks attractive I would appreciate it to receive from you a detailed outline of the journal as well as a proposal with respect to the editors you intend to invite and a list of prospective members for the Editorial Board."

I replied on December 6, 1972 with a prospectus. I also informed Reidel that I had Olson's help and that I would try to have representatives from all O.E.C.D. countries on the Editorial Board.

From Initial Inquiry to Contract

My working association with Reidel began in 1970 when I became a co-editor of *Theory and Decision*. Since that journal already had three co-editors, I had a small role to play. I approached Reidel first with my proposal because I knew the people there and they knew me. I saw no conflict between the journal I was proposing and *Theory and Decision*. While we would have an area of interest in common in public choice broadly conceived, the new journal would accommodate all kinds of empirical research and would focus on research relevant to measuring aspects of the quality of life. From a marketing perspective, my proposal represented an opportunity to reach an audience that none of their other journals even attempted to reach.

In April or May 1973 I was invited to a meeting of the steering committee of the U.S. Center in Washington. I explained my proposal to them and told them that if they had objections to my editing the journal or if they knew of someone else who would be better suited, I would be glad to step aside. I think I was quite serious. There is a point of no-return in the development of new projects, but when I made that trip to Washington I don't think I had reached that point. I wanted to see the journal come into being in much the same way that others around the table did. But like them, I had my own research. Given my connection with Reidel and my own expertise, I was confident that I could get the thing off the ground as easy as anyone, but I was still the Little Red Hen.

When I offered to step aside, O. Dudley Duncan, who was chairing the meeting, rocked back on his chair, half chuckled and blushed, and said roughly that that wasn't the role of the committee. I took that as an indication that he, at least, was happy to let me get on with it. In fact, everyone seemed satisfied. So on May 15, 1973 I wrote the following to Reidel.

> "At a meeting of the U.S. Social Science Research Council committee on social indicators saturday in Washington, I informed the group of our intention to move forward with *Social Indicators Research*. In response they offered to put a notice of the journal in their bimonthly *Social Indicators Newsletter*. This will also include a call for papers. This group is 100 percent behind our effort and anxious to insure that we get off to a good start. I do not know what the circulation of their *Newsletter* is, but I imagine it is less than 200. Still, I may be flooded shortly with enquiries and subscription orders. Thus, I hope you will prepare the necessary publicity material as soon as possible. At present we have 27 people agreed to join our editorial board, and we are pursuing further lines in India, China, Japan, South America and Australia."

On May 18, 1973 Reidel replied with "As a confirmation of our interest I enclose the agreement, based on what we discussed previously."

That seemed straightforward enough, but by August of that year nothing happened. So I wrote to Reidel, saying among other things, that "If there is any question about Reidel's commitment to the project now, I would very much like to know it." (August 23, 1973) A couple weeks later I received a long letter informing me of "some mutations" in Reidel's staff, "a huge backlog" and continued commitment to the project. (August 31, 1973)

Format and Style

For new journals, questions concerning format and style can be technologically formidable. One can't use any old kind of paper, in any old size and shape, with any old type. This month's product ought to look a lot like last month's product, and all the products ought to be esthetically attractive.

I solved virtually all these problems by signing with Reidel, and Reidel in turn solved virtually all of them in the same way. They had several similar looking journals, e.g. *Synthese* and *Theory and Decision*. They are all 6 by 8 inches in size, 500 pages long, in 4 quarterly 125 page issues. SIR is exactly like the others except for its red cover. In fact, when people ask me to characterize the style and format of SIR, I often say it's a red *Synthese* or a red *Theory and Decision*.

In August 1973 I received a letter from Reidel asking me if I could stop in Dordrecht while I was in Europe. The letter mentioned the names of various department directors in the company and said they would have "a lot of questions and remarks" of a technical sort. I had the suspicion that no matter what I suggested, they would produce yet another journal in the style of all the others. Moreover, I was going to be in Stockholm, not exactly around the corner from Dordrecht. So I replied that "unless something marvelous happens, I will not be visiting you in November. But I certainly hope something marvelous does happen." (September 5, 1973).

Something marvelous did happen. Wolfgang Zapf invited me to a conference in Bod Hamburg, Germany. So I stopped off in Dordrecht, cautiously and optimistically thinking Reidel might have plans for a whole new line of publicatins. I met the people, had a nice discussion and went my merry way. Later on when my wife asked me how it went, I said: "It's going to be like *Synthese* but with a red cover."

Operating policies

In some respects the operation of SIR is more like that of a guerrilla band than a regular army. I had several operating principles that are all subject to temporary suspension in the light of a general Principle of Bcnevolence. This Principle is roughly that one always ought to try to act so as to produce more good than evil for everyone. I don't think I can order my working principles in any non-arbitrary way, but I can certainly list them.

First, the aim of the journal is to provide a public forum for discussion of issues related to measuring aspects of the quality of life. I interpret the phrase "quality of life" very broadly to include virtually all forms of systemic well-being, where the systems may be psychological, biological, social, economic, or whatever. Just as I do not put constraints on the sorts of things whose well-being may be discussed in SIR, I do not put constraints on the notion of well-being used.

Second, any apparently reasonable methodology is acceptable. In particular, I welcome papers proceeding from positions that are theoretic, atheoretic or anti-theoretic; formal or informal; experimental or clinical; speculative or empirical.

Twenty years of work in the philosophy of science has persuaded me that it is pointless to try to distinguish disciplines. Broadly speaking, I think of SIR as a journal whose main constituency is formed by social scientists. That is our primary constituency now and I think it ought to be so permanently. Given my views about the fuzzy nature of disciplines, nothing spectacular follows from these assumptions.

Third, the Editorial Board should be made up of scholars from all parts of the world. From the beginning I have seen the journal as an international project. More personally, I regard the journal as a personal effort to unite nations, i.e., to help people from different countries exchange views on the quality of their lives. Martin Luther King was fond of the Negro spiritual which went "We are all in the same boat brother, so you can't rock one end without rockin' the other." To a large extent, that summarizes my own view about human existence, and to a small extent my insistence on an international board institutionalizes this view. Formally, at least, *Social Indicators Research* is an internationally collective project.

Of course, it's one thing to want an international board and something else to get it. Moreover, once one gets it, it's something else again to get it to work. Fuzzy as the boundaries of disciplines are, they still provide researchers with rough paradigms of good practice and a pecking order of reputable practitioners. It's no trick, for example, to identify leading economists,

sociologists and so on even at an international level. But for a movement-in-
the-making like the social indicators movement, it is difficult to know where to
begin. I needed all the help I could get.

Fortunately, I had the help of Mancur Olson, the group at the U.S. Center
and Sten Johansson. I also had some literature from the O.E.C.D. and the U.N.
Inspection of our original list of Board Members reveals a broad range of
research and policy interests. Some people, like Sylvia Ostry, had done
important related research and had moved on to administrative posts.

Most of the original Members were trained as economists, though their
interests and responsibilities often pressed beyond academic economics. Most
of them were very busy people, so busy that their names were little more than
window dressing on our jacket. I think some window dressing is almost
inevitable in a new venture. After all, in the beginning practically all a journal
has going for it are the reputations of its Editorial Board. After a few years of
operation, the project will stand or fall on the quality of its contents in
comparison to alternatives. But in the beginning, for better or worse, people
tend to consider the source. So I tried to get an illustrious group of people on
the Board. [See Appendix for a complete list of Members of the first Board.]

Although it was supposed to be standard practice at Reidel to have Board
Members replaced about every three years, I figured to make routine
replacements at five year intervals. Our first five year period ended shortly
after the 1978 World Congress of Sociology in Uppsala. Several excellent
papers on social indicators were presented at the Congress, and I had the
opportunity to meet many of the authors. In fact, I invited many of them to join
our Editorial Board, especially those from outside North America. A measure
of the success I had in extending our international connections is the fact that
36% came from this source in the second Board, I continue to look for good
researchers abroad.

Fourth, authors should be able to have a decision made on their
manuscripts within three months. This is obviously an arbitrarily selected turn-
around time, but I think it is manageable, good for research and kind to authors.
The trouble is, when you have an Editorial Board full of stars, it's difficult to
get them to deliver within the preferred time frame. What's more, it's
occasionally difficult to get them to commit themselves to such action.

Fifth, although this is not really an operating policy, I should say that my
model of a first rate journal is the AAAS *Science*. The Rapid Review system
that I have encouraged but not insisted upon has been adopted from the other
AAAS publication, *Science Books*.

Finally, I try to expand the areas of research and discussion at every
opportunity. The frontiers of social indicators research are probably not clear to
anyone. So I try to accommodate everyone's views about what is relevant.
Occasionally this leads to the acceptance of papers of dubious quality.
Nevertheless, if an author can only see dimly what no one else has seen at all
then I will try to give him or her space in SIR. Unfortunately, there is no clear
line of demarcation between the accommodation of novelty which is so vital to
healthy development and the acceptance of nuttiness which is a sure road to
oblivion.

Reviewing procedures

My reviewing process typically begins within 48 hours of receiving a manuscript. I used to read every manuscript that came to me on the day it arrived or the next day. As the number of technical niceties of manuscripts increased, I found I had to skim some and rely more on my reviewers. If I feel reasonably confident about my ability to judge a paper, then I judge it myself. I write immediately to the author indicating acceptance, acceptance with revisions or rejection. Usually I try to estimate the time of publication. Since we can't tell exactly how long a manuscript will be when it's type-set and peculiar things occasionally happen to manuscripts and page proofs in the mail, these first estimates are often pretty rough.

If I don't feel reasonably confident about my ability to judge a manuscript, then I write to a Member of the Board. I have a form letter that asks people if they can read it and give me a decision within one month. It ends with a check list of three options, namely, "send it to me," "send it if I can have ____ weeks to deliver" and "don't send it." If I send it and don't hear within a couple of weeks of the promised delivery date then I write again. Sometimes I telephone, but in one way or another I try to maintain some presence in the reviewer's life until I get delivery. I try to become a psychological nuisance without being at all nasty.

I don't have a clearly articulated set of acceptance criteria. Generally, I look for originality, external and internal coherence, sound methodology and so on. Length means nothing. What happens between the first and last sentences of the paper means everything. I can always divide long manuscripts or run two numbers of a volume together.

Some manuscripts are obviously central to the field, written by well-known scholars and of excellent quality. Those are an absolute delight to receive. (I remember writing Frank Andrews that the paper he had just sent was so exciting that I wished I could duplicate it immediately and deliver it to everyone.) Problems arise in the first place when one or another of the above-mentioned virtues is not present or its opposite is present. For example, I sometimes receive good or at least respectable manuscripts that don't seem to have anything to do with the quality of anyone's life – except perhaps the author's. In such cases I usually explain my position to the authors and reject them.

I have occasionally accepted manuscripts that seem to be only marginally related to the interests of SIR readers, but are excellent. My operating principle in such cases is that excellence in any form tends to breed excellence in some form. Excellent articles tend to be cited more often than mediocre articles and that means more visibility for the journal that carries the articles. Moreover, excellent authors often want to have their work published in the most prestigious journals, and one way to develop a prestigious journal is to attract excellent authors. The system feeds upon itself once it gets going. The trick is to get it going.

Output profile

The results of implementing the policies and procedures described in the preceding two sections are summarized in Tables 1, 3 and 4. Table 1 contains a summary of the numbers of papers received, accepted, rejected and published in our seven full years of operation. The average rejection rate is 34%, which must be lower than average for social science journals. If you look at the summary Table 2 from Zuckerman and Merton (1971, p. 76), you will see that our rate is roughly similar to that of their chemistry and geography journals. It is a long way from the average in sociology, psychology, economics and political science, which are the original disciplines of most of our authors.

The trend of our rejection rates is interesting. In the first five years, the highest rate (38%) came in the very first year and the lowest rate (17%) came in the very last year. The new Board was in place in 1979 and the rejection rate jumped 177% over the 1978 figure. In 1980 it rose to 56%, an increase of 229% over its lowest point.

I'm not sure how one should interpret rejection rates. It would be silly to suppose that journals with high rejection rates publish papers that are uniformly better than those published in journals with low rejection rates. On that interpretation, papers in history and philosophy would typically be better than papers in physics and biology. Rejection rates are clearly a function of a wide variety of variables including operating policies and procedures, constituency size, composition and quality, journal visibility and prestige. With a relatively low rejection rate one can at least be assured that "what you see is roughly what we got." All readers finally have the opportunity to see the bulk of what I have seen. So they can make a fairly valid estimate of the sort of material I have received.

If I had to bet on the single most important influence on our rejection rate, I would say it is my own expansionist policy. I deliberately try to get everyone into the conversation who seems to have something to offer. Given the essentially elitist nature of the scientific enterprise, my attitude may strike some people as dangerously democratic. Needless to say I will be glad to give the latter group a public forum to make their case.

Table 3 summarizes our output according to area of concern (in a broader sense of the phrase as it's used by O. E.C.D.). A priori I guess one would have expected to see more papers of a theoretical-methodological sort than any other kind. One also would have expected to see the health area very high on the list. Both of these expectations are fulfilled. The areas most frequently discussed were health (12.5%), satisfaction (11.4%), national objective indicators (10.8%) and theory or methods (10.2%). Most of the work on satisfaction measures has come out of the researchers at the University of Michigan. I expected to receive more papers related to education and environmental studies than I have received.

I don't have an area preference and am not conscious of being biased for some over others. I would prefer a better balance and greater scope, but that preference is subordinate to my desire to have good papers in any area.

There are a couple kinds of papers that I began rejecting on principle over a year ago. These are state of the art papers and mere conceptual frameworks. The art is not changing so rapidly that it calls for a new review every year, especially since about 80 percent of every review I have seen is like every other review. Moreover, long lists of area of concern or alternative ways to cut the pie of easily accessible time series do not seem to be useful now. The general principle leading to the rejection of these two types of papers is just that of avoiding redundancy. I'm not sure that most of our readers would share my perception of the redundancy of these kinds of papers at this time. So I would welcome feedback on this score. (I would welcome feedback on *any* score.) I do suspect, however, that most of our readers are fairly beyond square one and want to press on.

Table 4 summarizes our output by the home country of the author, i.e., the home address used by the author. SIR has been dominated by North Americans generally (87%) and Americans in particular (75%). No doubt that's a function of language, size, proximity, visibility, research expertise and other things. I have invited papers from people in other countries, especially developing countries, but there have been very few acceptances. I have also received some papers in which the English was so poor that I could not read it. In the latter case, if the paper seemed to have any promise at all and I had a Board Member in the country of its author, then I contacted that member for advice.

Book Reviews

The book reviewing operation of SIR has not developed into the useful sort of research instrument that I had planned. I have sent for and received plenty of good books to review, and I have sent out plenty of books to be reviewed. But the returns are abominable. Table 5 lists the numbers of books reviewed as of December 1980.

I think that half of all the books that I send out for review never get reviewed. Some of them disappear in the mail. Canada's postal service is notoriously unreliable. I have had four book-length manuscripts (my own) lost in the mail since 1970. Some of these were supposed to be returning from the United States. They just disappeared.

But I'm pretty sure that the main culprits are the alleged reviewers themselves. People promise to write the reviews and don't. If a book seems especially important then I try to get a well-known scholar to review it. You know how that goes. The best people are typically up to their ears in their own projects. Sometimes they will agree to write the review, but usually not. Moreover, when they do agree, it frequently gets put on a perennial back-burner. So I'm frequently faced with the choice of a very untimely (late) review of a very important book by a very important reviewer or a timely review of the book by a relatively unknown reviewer. Sometimes I go one way and sometimes the other. (One of the best reviews I have had written came from a graduate student.)

I think that the low esteem given to book reviews (e.g., on tenure and promotion committees) is partly responsible for the sort of returns I have been receiving. I try to maintain a fairly relaxed attitude toward reviews, but I really don't think most reviewers think about what they are up to when they write a review. In particular, one should remember that there are over 70,000 titles published every year, and that the usefulness of a review as an information-sorting device tends to decrease as its usefulness as an appraising device increases. What most reviewers are inclined to do is start right out appraising without ever summarizing the book.

Marketing

Generally when people have asked me how Reidel markets its products, I have answered "Just barely." However, I am happy to report that the firm has been more active than I realised, though still not as active as I would like. In a letter to me commenting on the first draft of this paper, I was informed that

"... through the years we have mailed over 37000 promotional leaflets for SIR to libraries all over the world, subscription agents and booksellers, and to addresses received from the Social Sciences Research Council, Urban Studies Research Center, Deutsche Gesellschaft fur Soziologie, and the International Sociological Association. Sample copies of the journal were also mailed with a covering letter to target markets such as all participants of the UNESCO International Conference on Indicators of Social and Economic Change. And all of these formal mailings do not include numerous pamphlets and sample copies distributed at conferences, colloquia, congresses and book fairs attended by Reidel over the years." (June 19, 1978)

Reidel also exchange journal announcements with several journals. These arrangements are made in a variety of ways. My own strategy has been to try to identify journals with readers representing potential purchasers, for example *Public Choice, Social Science and Medicine, Social Theory and Practice, Social Issues, Policy Studies Journal, Accounting, Organizations and Society.* These announcement exchanges are inexpensive and have a sharper focus than the general mailings.

Our growth path in terms of subscription sales is summarized in Table 6. In our first year (1974) we sold 405 subscriptions, compared to 620 in the last full year (1980) of sales. That's an increase of 53 percent in seven years.

Complaints

I have received relatively few complains about SIR. That is, the ratio of letters of complaint to all other letters I have received concerning the journal is something in the order of 1/200. I believe I have all the letters of complaint that I have received and there are six, not counting my own complaints to Reidel. All but two of the complaints are about subscriptions. People paid, waited, inquired, complained, waited, complained, etc. I have practically nothing to do with subscriptions, though I am occasionally a middleman in the sales transaction. Reidel looks after the subscriber list, the money and the distribution, and that suits me fine.

There are several interesting things about subscription complaints. Horowitz mentions these sorts of problems more often than any others. "Our failure to quickly solve the problem of subscriber complaints and subscription fulfillment" he wrote, "cost us dearly. We still suffer from the bad publicity of those errors." (Horowitz (1972, p.63) He solved his problem by letting a professional distributing firm handle their subscription service.

Some of SIR's strongest supporters have had the most trouble. For example, Statistics Canada carries three subscriptions and apparently had a hard time getting all of them. Our most frequent contributor, Frank Andrews, waited over a year and sent several irate letters to Reidel before his subscription order was fulfilled. The U.S. Social Science Research Council Center had a terrible time. The Director of the Center, Robert Parke, sent me a detailed letter of complaint and I sent another to Reidel's Order Department. My letter ended with "I urge you to put your house in order. You are our subscriber's main link to SIR and you must give us better performance. Everyone is prepared to pay the high price but then they expect excellent service, and I believe they are entitled to it." (February 9, 1976)

On April 19, 1976 I received the following ditty from Nancy Carmichael, Chief Librarian at the U.S. Center.

> "Reidel has come through at last,
> Their slackness apparently past.
> They've sent us by air,
> With copies to spare,
> Volume I, number 1, through the last."

I don't have a copy of my reply, but I remember I answered in kind and the last line was something like "It's nice to know that the schnooks with the books are not crooks – Burma Shave."

So far as I know all subscription complaints have been and will be settled to the satisfaction of subscribers. Of course there's no way to compensate people for the nuisance involved.

I received one complaint informing me that SIR's price was about four standard deviations higher than ten others in its class, e.g., *Urban Affairs Quarterly, The Annals* and *Policy Studies Journal*. Reidel's prices may be higher than average, but not as high as four standard deviations. If one compares SIR with other journals that are not official organs of some association (providing a captive audience), are not endowed (e.g., with grant money) and are not photocopied typescript, then SIR's price does not look so bad. I don't think it ever looks good, certainly not for institutions, but it's tolerable. I'm enough of a free enterpriser to believe that if the price goes too high, then SIR will disappear. What's more, I have enough confidence in Reidel to believe that they will not let that happen. They have been in business for a very long time.

Future Prospects

Judging from our current number of subscribers and the continued quality of submitted manuscripts, there seems to be no doubt that SIR has a future. The Editorial Board still needs a wider range of expertise and of international representation. I am not at all satisfied with the number of subscribers we have attracted so far, and I know that Reidel is continuing their efforts on this score.

It's probably obvious that my commitment to the project has grown over the past years. What began roughly as a public service by a reluctant Little Red Hen, has become very much a private practice. Socrates said that a philosopher is like a midwife giving birth to new ideas. I guess I have passed through the midwife, the nursemaid, and kindergarten, and I'm around Grade 2. I know the kid (SIR) is a bit frail and homely, but he's very much family, and I intend to stick with him.

References

Horowitz, Irving Louis (1972). "On Entering the Tenth Year of Transaction: The Relationship of Social Science and Critical Journalism," *Society*, 10, 49-79.

Zuckerman, H. and R.K. Merton (1971). "Patterns of Evaluation in Science: Institutionalisation, Structure and Functions of the Referee System," *Minerva*, 9, 66-100.

Table 1
Manuscript Profile: Acceptance and Rejection

Year	Accepted	Rejected	Total Received	Rejection Rate %	Published
1974	15	9	24	38	18[a]
1975	25	7	32	22	24
1976	25	11	36	31	21
1977	27	10	37	27	16
1978	39	8	47	17	21
1979	19	17	36	47	28
1980	19	25	44	56	48
Total	169	87	256	34	176

a 3 accepted in 1973

Table 2
Rates for Rejecting Manuscripts for Publication in Scientific and
Humanistic Journals, 1967

	Mean Rejection rate %	No. of Journals
History	90	3
Language and literature	86	5
Philosophy	85	5
Political Science	84	2
Sociology	78	14
Psychology (excluding experimental and physiological)	70	7
Economics	69	4
Experimental and physiological psychology	51	2
Mathematics and statistics	50	5
Anthropology	48	2
Chemistry	31	5
Geography	30	2
Biological sciences	29	12
Physics	24	12
Geology	22	2
Linguistics	20	1
Total		83

Source: Zuckerman and Merton (1971, p. 76).

Table 3
Manuscripts Published by Area of Concern as of Vol. 8, No.4,
December 1980

General Area	Number of Manuscripts	Percent
Health	22	12.5
Satisfaction	20	11.4
National (objective) indicators	19	10.8
Theory / methods	18	10.2
Public policy / planning	16	9.1
Rural	8	4.6
Environment	7	4.0
Economics	7	4.0
Developing countries	7	4.0
Occupation	6	3.4
Urban	6	3.4
Housing	6	3.4
Criminal justice	5	2.8
Consumption / marketing	5	2.8
Time use	4	2.3
Education	4	2.3
Religion	3	1.7
Geography	3	1.7
Science	3	1.7
Politics	3	1.7
Family studies	2	1.1
Ethnic relations	2	1.1
Total	176	100.0

Table 4
Manuscripts Published by Country of Author, to December 1980

Country	Number of Manuscripts	Percent
U.S.A.	132	75.0
Canada	21	11.8
U.K.	5	2.7
Israel	4	2.3
F.R. of Germany	2	1.1
The Netherlands	2	1.1
Austria, France, Ghana, Sweden, Poland, Belgium, Hungary, Chile, Philippines, India	1*	0.6
Total	176	100.0

* Each country had one paper.

Table 5
Number of Books Reviewed Per Volume to December 1980

Volume	Number
I	6
II	8
III	11
IV	10
V	14
VI	8
VII	8
VIII	11

Table 6

Subscriptions (To December 1980)

Volume	Year	Total Subscribers	Private	Percent Change Over 1974 of Total Subscribers
Vol. 1	1974	405	78	0.0
Vol. 2	1975	422	44	4.2
Vol. 3	1976	523	30	29.1
Vol. 4	1977	538	37	32.8
Vol. 5	1978	555	45	37.0
Vol. 6	1979	623	55	53.8
Vol. 7	1980	620	NA	53.1
Vol. 8	1980	620	NA	53.1

Appendix

SIR Editorial Board, 1974
Patrick N. Troy, Australia
Lore Scheer, Austria
D.A. Chant, Canada
Sylvia Ostry, Canada
Paul Reed, Canada
Fred Schindeler, Canada
Marshall Wolfe, Chile
Erling Jørgensen, Denmark
Erkki Laatto, Finland
Bernard Cazes, France
Gerald Eberlein, Germany
H.P. Widmaier, Germany
Wolfgang Zapf, Germany
M.S. Gore, India
Yehezkel Dror, Israel
Itzhak Galnoor, Israel
Chanan Rapaport, Israel
Yoshihiro Kogane, Japan
Robert A. Obudho, Kenya
Pablo Gonzales Casanova, Mexico
H. Brasz, The Netherlands
Jan Drewnowski, The Netherlands
Jan Tinbergen, The Netherlands
A.D. Robinson, New Zealand
Gudmund Hernes, Norway
Sten Johansson, Sweden
E.J. Mishan. United Kingdom
Alan Williams, United Kingdom
Daniel Bell, USA
James T. Bonnen, USA
James S. Coleman, USA
Otis D. Duncan, USA
Bertram Gross, USA
Irving L. Horowitz, USA
F. Thomas Juster, USA
Mancur Olson, USA
Robert Parke, USA
Nicholas Rescher, USA
J.R. Revenga, Venezuela

SIR Editorial Board, 1979
Carlos A. Mallmann, Argentina
Patrick N. Troy, Australia
Lore Scheer, Austria
Rudolf Rezohazy, Belgium
Tom Atkinson, Canada
Ronald J. Burke, Canada
Erling Jørgensen, Denmark
Erik Allardt, Finland
Bernard Cazes, France
Erwin Solomon, France
Henri Verwayen, France
Friedhelm Gehrmann, Germany
Wolfgang Zapf, Germany
Rudolf Andorka, Hungary
Ramkrishna Mukherjee, India
Itzhak Galnoor, Israel
Chanan Rapaport, Israel
Yoshihiro Kogane, Japan
Pablo Gonzales Casanova, Mexico
Jan Drewnowski, The Netherlands
Siri Naess, Norway
Ibrahim H. Abdel Galil, Sudan
Sten Johansson, Sweden
John Hall, United Kingdom
Aubrey McKennell, United Kingdom
Frank M. Andrews, USA
G.E.Alan Dever, USA
Otis D. Duncan, USA
Abbott L. Ferriss, USA
Irving Horowitz, USA
Kenneth Land, USA
Mancur Olson, USA
Robert Parke, USA
Frank W. Young, USA

FRANK M. ANDREWS AND STEPHEN B. WITHEY

3. DEVELOPING MEASURES OF PERCEIVED LIFE QUALITY: RESULTS FROM SEVERAL NATIONAL SURVEYS*

(Received 3 May, 1973)

ABSTRACT. This report presents the current status of a series of studies oriented toward the assessment of perceived life quality. The conceptual model proposes that a person's overall sense of life quality is understandable as a combination of affective responses to life 'domains', which are of two types – role situations and values. Over 100 items used to measure a wide variety of domains and 28 items assessing perceived overall life quality are presented. Various subsets of these items were used in interviews with several representative samples of American adults. Based on these data the domain items were grouped into a smaller number of semi-independent clusters which were internally stable across 10 different subgroups of the respondents and whose inter-relationships were highly replicable in independent national samples. A series of analyses, some replicated in more than one survey showed: (1) an additive combination of 12 selected domains explained 50–60 % of the variance in an index of overall life quality, (2) neither other domains nor several social characteristic variables contributed additional explanatory power, (3) this level of explanation was achieved in each of 22 subgroups of the population, and (4) additive combinations of domains worked as well as more complicated combinations.

We are embarked on a major effort to develop measures of perceived life quality. The effort is part of the larger movement within the United States and a number of other countries to develop an expanded set of social indicators which can be monitored over time. It is hoped that through the generation and analysis of data from such indicators improvements can result in our understanding of the causes and directions of social changes, and in policymaking oriented toward efforts to improve the quality of life.

Social indicators can be classified into two broad types: (1) those based on reports about experiences and characteristics of the reporter's own personal life, and (2) those based on reports of events or situations which are not part of the reporter's own life. Sometimes these two types of indicators have been referred to as 'subjective' and 'objective' respectively, though it can be argued that certain experiential measures are at least as objective as many of the so-called 'objective' measures. Examples of the first class of social indicators would include reports by respondents of their sense of safety when they go out alone at night, or their sense of satis-

Alex C. Michalos (ed.), Citation Classics from Social Indicators Research, 75–100.
© 2005 *Springer. Printed in the Netherlands.*

faction with the amount of safety they perceive. Examples of the second class would include crime reports for a particular neighborhood or measures of street lighting and police patrols.

The social indicators movement currently includes efforts to develop and apply measures based on both the experiential and non-experiential types of reports. While our own work concentrates almost exclusively on experiential measures, there is no question about society's need for both. Only when both are concurrently measured will it be possible to know how demonstrable changes in living conditions are affecting people's sense of life quality, and – conversely – whether changes in people's sense of life quality can be attributed to changes in external conditions.[1]

I. RESEARCH GOALS

The basic orientation of our project is that of instrument development. We seek to construct a battery of items appropriate for inclusion in a survey questionnaire or interview which will be modest in number, broad in coverage, of substantial validity, and which will provide a statistically efficient means of assessing perceived life quality in the diverse domains most important for predicting people's general satisfaction with their lives. Among the specific goals are: (1) identifying and mapping relevant domains; (2) determining how (if at all) affective reactions to these domains combine to affect some more global sense of life quality; (3) assessing criteria people use in evaluating different aspects of their lives and the social contexts in which these evaluations are made; (4) linking feelings about life situations to reported behaviors, life conditions, and other attitudes; and (5) developing descriptive statements about the level of satisfaction Americans feel with respect to significant aspects of their lives. We are attempting to implement all of these goals while recognizing that people of different sub-cultures in the American population may respond differently and maintaining our concern that any measuring instrument be applicable to a wide range of such groups.

II. SCOPE OF THIS REPORT

This present report focuses mainly on the first two of the specific goals – namely, the mapping of domains and the determination of how reactions to them may be combined to predict people's sense of overall life quality. Discussion of these matters is preceded by a short description of our conceptual model.

It should be noted that this report discusses a research effort which is currently in progress. As of this writing, data designed to test the full complexity of the conceptual model are just being collected, and some previously collected data have not yet been fully analyzed. We feel some of the results to be reported are of much interest, but recognize the incompleteness of the analysis.

III. SOURCE OF DATA

The statistical results presented in this report are based on one of three national sample surveys of American adults – one conducted in May 1972 which contacted 1297 respondents, and two others each conducted in November 1972 which contacted 1072 and 1118 respondents.[2]

Two other data sources are occasionally mentioned – another national survey of American adults conducted in April 1973, and a group of 200 heterogeneous respondents who answered a lengthy questionnaire in the summer of 1973. Conclusions from the analysis of data from these two latter sources are not included here.

IV. CONCEPTUAL MODEL

The conceptual model underlying our work is reasonably straightforward. The basic concepts include the ideas of life-as-a-whole, of specific role-related situations within that life, and of evaluative criteria which we call 'values'. Furthermore, it is assumed that people implicitly – and sometimes explicitly – engage in a process of evaluation in which events occurring in a role-specific situation are evaluated according to a set of values to produce an affective response.

In addition to evaluation, the model includes another process – that of integration: It is assumed that the affective responses resulting from evaluating a particular role-situation in the light of particular values are integrated or combined to produce a general affective evaluation for that role situation. Integration is presumed also to occur across different role-situations to produce a global affective response to life-as-a-whole, what we will here refer to as 'perceived quality of life'. Of course, the integration may involve a differential weighting of the affective responses. At this level of elaboration, the conceptual model is basically two dimensional as shown in Exhibit 1.

Exhibit 1

Two dimensional conceptual model with examples of possible role-situations and values

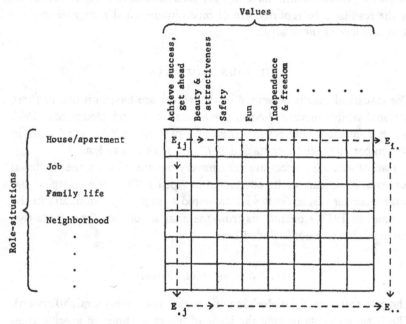

E_{ij} = Affective evaluative response to particular role-situation with respect to particular value
$E_{i.}$ = General affective evaluative response to role-situation (across values)
$E_{.j}$ = General affective evaluative response to value (across role-situations)
$E_{..}$ = General affective evaluative response to life-as-a-whole – i.e., perceived quality of life

As is suggested in Exhibit 1, some possible role-situations might include matters having to do with one's house or apartment, one's job, one's family, and the like. Possible values might include achieving success, having fun, experiencing beauty, and many others. One might then attempt to ascertain a person's level of satisfaction with the extent to which his house (say) helps him achieve success, promotes his standard of living, provides beauty, and the like. Combining across all relevant values (i.e., horizontally in Exhibit 1) would presumably produce a general affective response to the role-situation having to do with house. Similarly, combining across all relevant role-situations (i.e., vertically in Exhibit 1) would presumably produce a general affective response to a value, such as achieving success or having fun. Combining these general evaluations of either role-situations or values – the margins of the matrix shown in Exhibit 1 – produces a general evaluation of life-as-a-whole.

If one asks about the basic evaluation process by which an affective response comes to be associated with a particular role-situation in the light of a particular value, one essentially extends the model into additional dimensions to take explicit account of social contexts which are presumed to affect the evaluation process. Although we have made some initial explorations in these areas, these matters will not be treated further here.

The conceptual model just described has emerged as we have wrestled with the problems of designing instruments to assess perceived life quality and analyzed data resulting from those instruments. Our most recent instrument makes an explicit attempt to assess what are shown as E_{ij}'s in Exhibit 1, as well as the marginal E_i.'s and $E_{.j}$'s, and the E... This instrument is based on foundations laid by earlier work which focused on identifying relevant domains – role-situations and values, on assessing affective responses to them (the E_i.'s and $E_{.j}$'s), and on exploring appropriate combination systems to predict overall life satisfaction – the E... It is outcomes from this foundation building that are discussed here.

V. IDENTIFYING CONCERNS

The task of identifying appropriate domains – role-situations and values – took several forms. The starting point was an extensive list of items which, ideally, would include all the significant 'concerns' of people.

One source of such concerns was previous surveys which had included open questions about people's hopes, fears, worries, and the like. Eight different studies were examined.[3] Most were conducted on national samples of Americans (though data from 12 other countries were represented). Most were conducted within the preceding five years. All focused on substantive issues of high social, political, and/or psychological concern.

By scanning the coding categories developed for these studies a list of some 800 concerns was developed.

A second source was structured interviews, typically lasting an hour or two, with about a dozen people of heterogeneous backgrounds. These interviews, focused on the respondents' daily activities and their reactions to those activities, were conducted by project research staff (rather than field-staff interviewers), and were fully recorded on tape. These were useful in further expanding the list of concerns.

A third source, particularly useful for expanding our list of value-type domains, was previously published lists of values, including proposals by Rokeach (1973), White (1944), Allport and Vernon (1931), Morris (1955), Dodd (1951), Lepley (1957), and Kluckhohn (1953).

Finally, we checked to make sure that our domains included those receiving attention from official national and international bodies concerned with social indicators, and from certain other researchers known to be working on social indicators. Lists proposed by the U.S. Department of Health Education and Welfare, by the U.S. Office of Management and the Budget, by the organization for Economic Cooperation and Development, and by a half dozen other research groups in the United States were examined.

After some *ad hoc* clustering to combine concerns which were apparent duplicates, and after abstracting to capture what we believed was the essence of certain concerns, our list currently includes approximately 100 concerns. The 123 items we have used to assess these appear in Exhibit 2.

VI. MAPPING DOMAINS

Clearly, some of the 123 items shown in Exhibit 2 are closer (in the sense of statistical overlap) to some than to others, and a major analytic task has been to identify semi-independent subsets of these items. This is the mapping function.

One example of such a mapping is provided in Exhibit 3, which is based on a cluster analysis and on a Smallest Space Analysis (Guttman, 1968) of 62 items which were included in the May 1972 survey. Respondents indicated their affective response to each item using a seven-point scale ranging from 'Delighted' at the positive end to 'Terrible' at the negative end. Exhibit 4 shows the seven scale categories, plus three off-scale

Exhibit 2

Items used to assess affective responses to specific concerns

M = May 1972 national survey (N = 1297)
N¹ = November 1972 national survey Form 1 (N = 1118)
N" = November 1972 national survey Form 2 (N = 1072)
A = April 1973 national survey (N ≈ 1450)
J = July 1973 respondents (N ≈ 200)

How do you feel about . . .

1	Your children	M	J
2	Your wife/husband	M	J
3	Your marriage	M	J
4	Your own family life--your wife/husband, your marriage, your children, if any	N"	J
5	Close adult relatives--I mean people like parents, in-laws, brothers and sisters	M	J
6	The things you and your family do together	M N"	J
7	Your own health and physical condition	M N"	J
8	The extent to which your physical needs are met	A	J
9	The responsibilities you have for members of your family	M	J
10	How dependable and responsible you can be		J
11	Your opportunity to change things around you that you don't like	N"	J
12	Your chance of getting a good job if you went looking for one	N"	J
13	The extent to which you are tough and can take it	A	J
14	The way you handle the problems that come up in your life	M	J
15	The extent to which you can accept life as it comes and adapt to it		J
16	The extent to which you can adjust to changes in your life	A	J
17	The extent to which you get what you are entitled to--what is rightfully yours		J
18	The extent to which you are achieving success and getting ahead	A	J
19	The extent to which you compete and win at things		J
20	What you are accomplishing in your life	M N¹	J
21	Yourself--what you are accomplishing and how you handle problems	N"	J
22	Yourself	M	A J
23	How interesting your day to day life is		A J
24	The amount of beauty and attractiveness in your world		A J
25	The chance you have to enjoy pleasant or beautiful things	N"	J
26	Your sex life	N"	J
27	How much fun you are having	M N"	
28	The amount of fun and enjoyment you have		A J
29	The amount of physical work and exercise in your life		A J
30	The way you spend your spare time, your non-working activities	M N"	J
31	The amount of challenge in your life		J
32	The usefulness, for you personally, of your education	M	J
33	The extent to which you are developing yourself and broadening your life		A J
34	The variety and diversity in your life		J
35	The amount of imagination and fantasy in your life		J
36	How creative you can be	N"	J

37	The extent to which you maintain links to the past and to traditions			J
38	The amount of time you have for doing the things you want to do	M	N"	J
39	The amount of pressure you are under			AJ
40	The amount of relaxation in your life			J
41	Your chances for relaxation--even for a short time		N"	J
42	The sleep you get		N"	J .
43	The freedom you have from being bothered and annoyed			AJ
44	Your independence or freedom--the chance you have to do what you want			AJ
45	The privacy you have--being alone when you want to be		N"	J
46	The amount of friendship and love in your life			J
47	How much you are accepted and included by others			J
48	How sincere and honest you are			AJ
49	How sincere and honest other people are			AJ
50	How generous and kind you are			J
51	How generous and kind others are			J
52	The way other people treat you	M		J
53	The amount of respect you get from others			AJ
54	How fairly you get treated			AJ
55	How much you are admired or respected by other people		N"	J
56	The respect other people have for your rights		N"	J
57	The people who live in the houses/apartments near yours	M		J
58	People who live in this community	M		J
59	The people you see socially	M		J .
60	Your friends		N"	J
61	The things you do and the times you have with your friends	M		J
62	The chance you have to know people with whom you can really feel comfortable	M		J
63	How you get on with other people	M		J
64	How much you are accepted and included by others			AJ
65	The reliability of the people you depend on		N"	J
66	How dependable and responsible people around you are			J
67	The extent to which your world seems consistent and understandable			J
68	How much you are really contributing to other people's lives			AJ
69	Your religious faith	M		J
70	The religious fulfillment in your life			AJ
71	Things you do to help people or groups in this community	M		J
72	The organizations you belong to	M		J
73	How neat, tidy, and clean things are around you			AJ
74	Your housework--the work you need to do around your home	M	N"	J
75	Your job	M	N"	J
76	The people you work with--your co-workers	M		J
77	The work you do on your job--the work itself	M		J
78	The pay and fringe benefits you get, and security of your job	M		J
79	What it is like where you work--the physical surroundings, the hours, and the amount of work you are asked to do	M		J
80	What you have available for doing your job--I mean equipment, information, good supervision, and so on	M		J

81	How secure you are financially	AJ
82	How well your family agrees on how family income should be spent	N'' J
83	The income you (and your family) have	X N'' J
84	How comfortable and well-off you are	J
85	Your standard of living--the things you have like housing, car, furniture, recreation, and the like	M N'' J
86	Your car	M J
87	Your house/apartment	MN'N'' J
88	The outdoor space there is for you to use outside your home	M J
89	This particular neighborhood as a place to live	M J
90	This community as a place to live	M N'' J
91	The services you can get when you have to have someone come in to fix things around your home--like painting, repairs	M J
92	The services you get in this neighborhood--like garbage collection, street maintenance, fire and police protection	M J
93	The way the police and courts in this area are operating	M J
94	How safe you feel in this neighborhood	M J
95	Your safety	AJ
96	How secure you are from people who might steal or destroy your property	N'' J
97	The way you can get around to work, schools, shopping, etc.	M J
98	The schools in this area	M J
99	The doctors, clinics, and hospitals you would use in this area	M J
100	What you have to pay for basic necessities such as food, housing, and clothing	M N'' J
101	The goods and services you can get when you buy in this area--things like food, appliances, clothes	M N'' J
102	The taxes you pay--I mean the local, state, and national taxes all together	M J
103	The way your local government is operating	M
104	What your local government is doing	. N'' J
105	The way our national government is operating	M
106	What our national government is doing	N'N'' J
107	What our government is doing about the economy--jobs, prices, profits	M N'' J
108	Our national military activities	M J
109	The way our political leaders think and act	M N'' J
110	The condition of the natural environment--the air, land, and water in this area	M J
111	The weather in this part of the state	M J
112	Outdoor places you can go in your spare time	M J
113	Your closeness to nature	J
114	Nearby places you can use for recreation or sports	N'' J
115	The sports or recreation facilities you yourself use, or would like to use--I mean things like parks, bowling alleys, beaches	M J
116	The entertainment you get from TV, radio, movies, and local events and places	M J
117	The information you get from newspapers, magazines, TV, and radio	M J
118	The information and entertainment you get from TV, newspapers, radio, magazines	N'' J
119	How the United States stands in the eyes of the rest of the world	M J
120	Life in the United States today	M J
121	The standards and values of today's society	N'' J
122	The way people over 40 in this country are thinking and acting	M J
123	The way young people in this country are thinking and acting	M N'' J

Exhibit 3

Map of 62 items
Data source: 1297 respondents to May 1972 national survey

Key
single line: $r = 0.4000 - 0.4949$
double line: $r = 0.4950 - 0.5949$
triple line: $r = 0.5950 +$

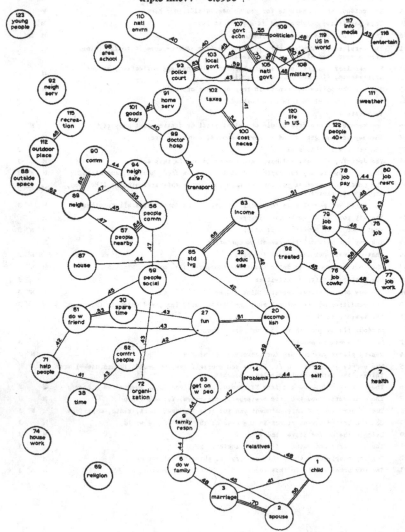

categories included to accommodate respondents who had never thought about the item or for whom it was irrelevant.

As is conventional in maps such as that in Exhibit 3, the closer two items are to each other, the higher was the correlation between them.[4] Of course, it would be surprising if 62 items as heterogeneous as these

Exhibit 4

Scale used in assessing affective responses

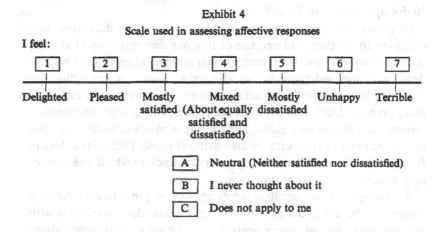

could be perfectly located with respect to each other in just two dimensions. Actually, four dimensions were required to meet the conventional goodness-of-fit criterion (alienation coefficient less than 0.15) of Smallest Space Analysis. However, the two-dimensional map shown in Exhibit 3 is a reasonably adequate representation of the actual relationships.

It is of interest to note that the highest correlations among these items tended to fall in the range 0.4 to 0.6. Of course, this degree of relationship was between items with short distances between them. The longest distances in Exhibit 3 are between items which correlated about zero with each other. Thus, based on Exhibit 3, one can see that a respondent who expressed an unusually positive reaction to his spouse was likely also to express an unusually positive reaction to his children. No prediction, however, could be made about his reactions to the national government based on knowledge of his feelings toward his spouse.

Although there is no need to attach conceptual meaning to the dimensions which emerge from Smallest Space Analysis, it is interesting to note that the most important dimension – the vertical dimension of Exhibit 3 –

arrays items according to social distance from the self: from concerns about self and family (at the bottom), through job and neighborhood concerns (in the middle), to governmental and media concerns (at the top).

These 62 items were reduced to 30 semi-independent domains by combining certain related items into clusters, eliminating others which were redundant, and leaving still others as single-item domains. (These 30 domains appear in Exhibit 7.)

Of course, the internal structure of a set of items may differ from one subgroup to another, and because of this our determination of clusters was based not only on the structure which resulted when all 1297 respondents were analyzed together, but also on separate analyses within ten different demographically defined subgroups. These subgroups included: men, women, blacks, four different age groups, two groups extreme with respect to socio-economic status, and a group of married, white, employed men in their middle years with children living at home. Each of the clusters formed from these 62 items had an internal structure which was reasonably similar in *all* of these subgroups.

An example of the result of applying such a procedure in defining clusters can be seen in our decision to form separate domains dealing with the local and national governments. Given the substantial interrelationships among local and national government items when all respondents were analyzed together, one might have assumed that all these items could be combined into a single cluster. The subgroup analysis, however, showed that men's affective responses to local government were unrelated to their responses to the national government. Consequently two separate domains were formed.

To explore the robustness of our clustering, several additional analyses were performed. A factor analysis with varimax rotation performed on the total set of 1297 respondents produced 14 factors, nearly all of which coincided well with our clusterings. Furthermore, an analysis based on ipsatized scores (which removed any overall differences between people which might be attributed to individual response bias and real differences in general life satisfaction) also showed a cluster structure highly consistent with that used in Exhibit 7.

Through such mapping and grouping of items semi-independent life domains can be identified, each of whose internal structures is known to be stable across a wide variety of population subgroups. These enter into the conceptual model discussed previously as role-situations or values. The affective responses to these domains constitute the margin entries – i.e., the E_i's and E_j's – of the model.

Shortly we shall report how these many domains, individually and in various combinations, relate to perceived overall quality of life (the $E..$ of the model). First, however, we report on the replicability of the basic domain structure and then turn to a short description of how we measured perceived quality of life.

Replicability of Domain Structures

Including some of the same items in two surveys of independent but equivalent national samples – the May 1972 and November 1972 (Form 2) surveys – provided an opportunity to assess the replicability of the basic domain structure portrayed in Exhibit 3. Eighteen identical (or nearly identical) items were included in both surveys.[5] These generated 153 relationships matchable from one survey to another. These relationships varied in strength from 0.0 to 0.7 (Pearson r's) in each survey, and correlated with one another 0.89 (Pearson r). This indicates that the relative magnitudes of the relationships in one survey were highly similar to those in the other and supports the notion that the basic structure used to identify domains – at least among these items – is itself highly replicable.

VII. MEASURES OF PERCEIVED OVERALL LIFE QUALITY

We have used about 30 different items to assess a person's affective response to his life as a whole. As shown in Exhibit 5, some have been straightforward questions asking "How do you feel about your life as a whole?" using several different response scales. Others have asked respondents to place themselves on a ladder-type scale. And still others asked the respondent to indicate whether certain specified affective experiences have actually occurred recently in his life.[6]

While it is our intention to explore the extent to which many of these can be predicted on the basis of affective responses to specific domains, the bulk of our analysis to date has focused on a scale which we have come to call 'Life #3'. This measure is computed as the arithmetic mean of the coded responses given by the respondent to the question "How do you feel about your life as a whole?" asked twice in the interview. These two items

Exhibit 5

Items used to assess affective responses to life as a whole

M   = May 1972 national survey (N = 1297)
N' = November 1972 national survey Form 1 (N = 1118)
N" = November 1972 national survey Form 2 (N = 1072)
A   = April 1973 national survey (N ≃ 1450)
J   = July 1973 respondents (N ≈ 200)

A   How do you feel about your life as a whole? (7-pt scale: Delighted . . .
    Terrible--see Exhibit 4) Short name: Life #1   MN'N"AJ

B   (Same as item A, asked later in interview) Short name: Life #2   M N"AJ

C   (Mean of coded answers to items A and B) Short name: Life #3   M N"AJ

D   How satisfied are you with your life as a whole these days? (7-pt scale:
    Completely satisfied . . . completely dissatisfied)   N'N" J

E   Where would you put your life as a whole on the feeling thermometer? (Graphic
    scale from very cold--negative to very warm--positive)   N'N"

F   Taking all things together, how would you say things are these days--would you
    say you're very happy, pretty happy, or not too happy these days? (3-pt scale)   M N" J

G   How do you feel about how happy you are? (7-pt scale: Delighted . . .
    Terrible--see Exhibit 4)   N" J

H   Considering how your life is going, would you like to continue much the same way,
    change some parts of it, or change many parts of it? (3-pt scale)   N" J

I   (Bradburn's Positive Affect Scale: number of five positive events experienced
    during past few weeks--e. g., "feeling on top of the world")   N" J

J   (Bradburn's Negative Affect Scale: number of five negative events experienced
    during past few weeks--e. g., "feeling depressed or very unhappy")   N" J

K   (Bradburn's Affect Balance Scale: Scale I minus Scale J plus five)   N" J

L   Most people worry more or less about somethings. Would you say you never worry,
    worry a little, worry sometimes, worry a lot, or worry all the time?   N'N" J

M   I think my life is Boring . . . Interesting (7-pt scale)   M   J

N   I think my life is Enjoyable . . . Miserable (7-pt scale)   M   J

O   I think my life is Useless . . . Worthwhile (7-pt scale)   M   J

P   I think my life is Friendly . . . Lonely (7-pt scale)   M   J

Q   I think my life is Full . . . Empty (7-pt scale)   M   J

R   I think my life is Discouraging . . . Hopeful (7-pt scale)   M   J

S   I think my life is Disappointing . . . Rewarding (7-pt scale)   M   J

T   I think my life Brings out the best in me . . . Doesn't give me much chance
    (7-pt scale)   M   J

U   Now, try and forget all the things in your life that annoy or worry you; how do
    you feel about the good and pleasant parts of your life? How do these nice aspects, N' J
    by themselves, make you feel? (7-pt scale: Delighted . . . Terrible--see Exhibit 4)

V   Now try and forget all the good and pleasant parts of your life; how do you feel
    about the things that annoy or worry you? How do these poor aspects, by themselves, N' J
    make you feel? (7-pt scale: Delighted . . . Terrible--see Exhibit 4)

W   Here are some circles that we can imagine represent the lives of different people.
    Circle eight has all plusses in it, to represent a person who has all good things
    in his life. Circle zero has all minuses in it, to represent a person who has   AJ
    all bad things in his life. Other circles are in between. Which circle do you
    think comes closest to matching your life? (Scale: row of nine circles with
    contents ranging from eight +'s to eight -'s)

X   Here is a picture of a ladder. At the bottom of the ladder is the worst life you might reasonably expect to have. At the top is the best life you might expect to have. Of course, life from week to week falls somewhere in between. Where on the ladder would you say was your <u>best week in the past year</u>--on which rung would you put it? (Scale: ladder with nine rungs extending from "Best life I could expect to have to "Worst life I could expect to have")   AJ

Y   Where on the ladder was your <u>worst week during the past year</u>--on which rung? (Same ladder scale as Item X)   AJ

Z   Where was your life <u>most of the time during the past year</u>? (Same ladder scale as Item X)   AJ

AA   Where was your life <u>five years ago</u>? (Same ladder scale as Item X)   AJ

AB   Where do you expect your life to be <u>five years from now</u>? (Same ladder scale as Item X)   AJ

Exhibit 6

Interrelationships among 12 measures of perceived overall life quality

Data sources: 1072 respondents to November 1972 (Form 2) national survey
1118 respondents to November 1972 (Form 1) national survey
1297 respondents to May 1972 national survey

Notes: Coefficients are product moment correlations
All coefficients based on November 1972 (Form 2) data unless otherwise noted
N' signifies November (Form 1) data
M signifies May data

	A	B	C	D	E	F	G	H	I	J	K	L	U
A Life #1													
B Life #2	.71												
	.61M												
C Life #3	.92	.93											
	.90M	.90M											
D 7-pt satisfaction	.64	.66	.70										
	.56N'												
E Thermometer	-.51	-.49	-.53	-.47									
	-.49N'			-.46N'									
F 3-pt happiness	.55	.54	.59	.49	-.39								
	.49M	.47M	.53M										
G 7-pt happiness	.68	.74	.77	.63	-.50	.57							
H Changes	.44	.39	.45	.44	-.36	.37	.37						
I Positive affect	-.33	-.34	-.36	-.30	.25	-.39	-.36	-.13					
J Negative affect	.30	.29	.32	.31	-.20	.31	.30	.36	.01				
K Affect balance	-.44	-.45	-.48	-.43	.32	-.50	-.47	-.35	.71	-.70			
L Worries	.24	.27	.28	.27	-.16	.24	.30	.22	-.12	.32	-.31		
	.21N'			.24N1	.13								
U Good parts	.37N'			.34N1	.25N'								.09N'
V Bad parts	.25N'			.27N1	.23N'								.27N1 .06N'

have typically been separated by about 8 to 12 minutes of intervening interview material, all of it focusing on quality-of-life issues.

We know that Life #3 has at least moderate reliability. Its two constituent parts typically correlate with each other in the range 0.6 to 0.7 – as can be seen in Exhibit 6. (Ninety-two percent of respondents to the May survey answered the two component items of Life #3 with answers that were either identical or in adjacent categories.) We also know that other global measures tend to correlate as well as or better with Life #3 than they do with other global measures – as is also shown in Exhibit 6. In the few comparative analyses we have run, Life #3 has been at least as predictable (sometimes more so) as other global measures when using affective responses to specific domains as predictors.

This index which we call Life #3 will play the role of dependent variable in the analyses reported next.

VIII. PREDICTING PERCEIVED QUALITY OF LIFE

Having identified a large number of specific life domains and several global measures of perceived life quality, the next step is to put the two sets together. What is an appropriate combination rule? Which domains are most important in predicting life quality? How well do the affective responses to different domains, taken together, explain a person's overall sense of life quality? Do prediction systems derived for one population subgroup work well in other subgroups? These are the questions which need answers.

Combination rule. After rather extensive analysis of the May 1972 data – which include the items needed to construct the Life #3 measure and the 30 domains shown in Exhibit 7, we came to the conclusion that a weighted additive combination of affective responses is adequate to capture virtually all the predictive power present in the domain clusters.[7] We had thought there might be substantial interactions in the data, but so far, none of marked effect has been found. We thought, for example, that if a person were in poor health this might dominate his sense of overall life quality, regardless of how he felt about the national government, his house, or his family. The data suggest, however, that this hypothesized interaction, and a large number of others which were checked, simply did not occur.[8]

Exhibit 7

Perceived quality of life (Life #3) predicted by affective responses to 30 domains

Data source: May 1972 national survey

		All respondents	Men	Women
N:		1297	547	750
Percent variance explained:		55%	64%	60%
Multiple correlation:		.74	.80	.77
Population estimate:		50%	51%	50%

		eta	beta	eta	beta	eta	beta
14+20+22	EFFICACY INDX	.55	.26	.53	.23	.57	.32
1+2+3	FAMILY INDX	.38	.19	.38	.20	.39	.16
83+85	MONEY INDX	.47	.15	.43	.15	.50	.14
27	AMOUNT OF FUN	.51	.15	.51	.19	.51	.17
87	HOUSE/APARTMENT	.36	.12	.40	.14	.35	.09
6	THINGS DO W FAMILY	.38	.11	.39	.12	.39	.13
38	TIME TO DO THINGS	.28	.09	.32	.16	.27	.10
123	YOUNG PEOPLE THINK	.15	.09	.11	.14	.23	.10
30	SPARE TIME ACTIVITES	.41	.09	.44	.09	.39	.08
112+115	RECREATION INDX	.22	.07	.26	.07	.22	.10
105+107+108+109	NATL GOVT INDX	.26	.07	.28	.09	.28	.10
97+99+101	CONSUMER INDX	.31	.07	.33	.11	.31	.11
93+103	LOCAL GOVT INDX	.23	.07	.31	.11	.18	.05
74	HOUSEWORK	.26	.07	.30	.12	.25	.06
116+117	MEDIA INDX	.15	.06	.22	.12	.12	.04
7	YOUR HEALTH	.29	.06	.29	.09	.30	.07
100+102	COST INDX	.26	.06	.26	.09	.29	.06
98	SCHOOLS IN AREA	.17	.06	.23	.09	.15	.08
92	SERVICES IN NGHBRHD	.20	.06	.26	.13	.18	.07
5	CLOSE ADULT RELATIVE	.22	.06	.25	.10	.22	.05
110	NATURAL ENVIRONMENT	.13	.05	.16	.09	.14	.05
62	COMFORTABLE PEOPLE	.31	.05	.35	.05	.30	.06
57+58+88+89+90+94	NEIGHBORHOOD INDX	.31	.04	.33	.07	.30	.04
122	PEOPLE OVER 40 THINK	.22	.04	.25	.10	.21	.04
72	ORGANIZATIONS BELONG	.21	.04	.22	.05	.21	.05
111	WEATHER	.12	.04	.19	.06	.10	.05
59+61	FRIENDS INDX	.34	.03	.36	.06	.34	.05
75+76+77+79+80	JOB INDX	.23	.03	.36	.11	.15	.02
69	RELIGIOUS FAITH	.24	.03	.28	.06	.24	.07
63	GETTING ON W PEOPLE	.31	.01	.35	.10	.30	.06

Predictive power. Exhibit 7 shows the results of using an additive model to predict Life #3 on the basis of the 30 domains identified in the May 1972 survey.[9] It shows results when all respondents were combined together, and also for men and women separately. The prediction scheme used in Exhibit 7 (and also in Exhibits 8–11) is that of Multiple Classification Analysis (Andrews, Morgan, Sonquist, 1967), a special form of multiple regression which does not assume that relationships are linear nor that predictor variables are intervally scaled.[10] One may note that in these data the 30 clusters explained 55% of the variance in Life #3 (multiple correlation = 0.74). When adjusted to produce an estimate for the population as a whole, this value was exactly 50%. Domains which made the largest independent contribution to this explanation (as shown by the beta coefficients in Exhibit 7) were those having to do with self-efficacy, family, money, fun, and housing. It is perhaps notable that all these domains refer to concerns close to self and home.

Exhibit 7 does not show the direction or form of the relationships between domains and Life #3. These are of considerable interest and can be summarized easily: Nearly all were close to linear and in the expected direction – i.e., positive affective responses to the domains tended to go with more positive evaluation of life-as-a-whole.

A look at the results when men and women were analyzed separately

Exhibit 8

Perceived quality of life (Life #3) predicted by subsets of the 30 domains of Exhibit 7

Data sources: May and November 1972 national surveys

Domain subset:		Best 16	Best 6	Selected 12	
Survey:		May	May	May	Nov
N:		1297	1297	1297	1072
Percent variance explained:		54%	49%	52%	62%
Multiple correlation:		.73	.70	.72	.79
Population estimate:		51%	48%	50%	59%
		beta	beta	beta	beta
14+20+22	EFFICACY INDX	.27	.28	.25	
21	YOURSELF				.17
1+2+3	FAMILY INDX	.18	.17	.19	
4	FAMILY				.19
83+85	MONEY INDX	.15	.20	.15	.18
27	AMOUNT OF FUN	.16	.21	.16	.23
87	HOUSE/APARTMENT	.12	.13	.11	.11
6	THINGS DO W FAMILY	.09	.10	.08	.09
38	TIME TO DO THINGS	.09		.07	.11
123	YOUNG PEOPLE THINK	.08			
30	SPARE TIME ACTIVITES	.08		.08	.07
112+115	RECREATION INDX	.06			
105+107+108+109	NATL GOVT INDX	.08		.09	
106+107+109	NATL GOVT INDX				.07
97+99+101	CONSUMER INDX	.06		.06	
101	GOODS & SERVICES				.06
93+103	LOCAL GOVT INDX	.06			
74	HOUSEWORK	.07			
116+117	MEDIA INDX	.05			
7	YOUR HEALTH	.06		.06	.09
75+76+77+79+80	JOB INDX			.02	
75	YOUR JOB				.10

Exhibit 9

Perceived quality of life (Life #3) predicted by affective responses to 28 domains
and by a subset of 12 domains

Data source: November 1972 national survey

Domain subset:		28 domains	Selected 12
N:		1072	1072
Percent variance explained:		67%	62%
Multiple correlation:		.82	.79
Population estimate:		61%	59%

		eta	beta	beta
21	YOURSELF	.54	.12	.17
4	FAMILY LIFE	.52	.12	.19
83+85	MONEY INDX	.57	.12	.18
27	AMOUNT OF FUN	.61	.15	.23
87	HOUSE/APARTMENT	.44	.13	.11
6	THINGS DO W FAMILY	.51	.08	.09
38	TIME TO DO THINGS	.31	.08	.11
30	SPARE TIME ACTIVITES	.47	.06	.07
106+107+109	NATL GOVT INDX	.25	.05	.07
101	GOODS & SERVICES	.25	.05	.06
7	YOUR HEALTH	.38	.09	.09
75	YOUR JOB	.37	.09	.10
55	ADMIRED BY OTHERS	.34	.07	
56	RESPECT FOR RIGHTS	.28	.04	
65	RELIABILITY OTHERS	.38	.10	
60	YOUR FRIENDS	.36	.06	
11	OPPORTUNITY CHANGES	.37	.04	
26	SEX LIFE	.40	.07	
96	SECURE FROM THEFT	.27	.05	
45	PRIVACY	.37	.07	
12	GETTING A GOOD JOB	.37	.07	
42	SLEEP	.31	.08	
121	SOCIETY'S STANDARDS	.26	.05	
114	RECREATIONAL PLACES	.27	.06	
36	CREATIVITY	.32	.02	
41	RELAXATION	.39	.06	
82	AGREEMENT SPENDING	.42	.06	
25	BEAUTIFUL THINGS	.55	.16	

shows a generally high similarity – both in total explanatory power, and
in the domains which made the biggest independent contributions – to the
results for the total population. One of the bigger discrepancies between
men and women occurred for a domain well down on the list – the job
index, which, perhaps not surprisingly, had a substantially higher beta for
men than for women.

Having discovered that these 30 domains explained about half the
variance in overall sense of life quality does not imply that all 30 were
in fact needed. Exhibit 8 records some of our explorations at reducing

Exhibit 10

Perceived quality of life (Life #3) predicted by 6 classification variables and affective
responses to 12 domains

		Data source:	May 1972 national survey	
Predictor set:		6 class + 12 domains	6 class	12 domains
N:		1297	1297	1297
Percent variance explained:		53%	8%	52%
Multiple correlation:		.73	.28	.72
Population estimate:		50%	5%	50%

		eta	beta	beta	beta
	INCOME FU	.18	.05	.16	
	SEX OF R	.04	.02	.01	
	RACE OF R	.03	.03	.03	
	FAMILY LIFE CYCLE	.20	.13	.19	
	R'S AGE-8PT	.09	.08	.12	
	EDUCATION R	.07	.03	.06	
87	HOUSE/APARTMENT	.36	.12		.11
30	SPARE TIME ACTIVITES	.41	.09		.08
6	THINGS DO W FAMILY	.38	.08		.08
7	YOUR HEALTH	.29	.05		.06
27	AMOUNT OF FUN	.51	.15		.16
38	TIME TO DO THINGS	.28	.07		.07
75+76+77+79+80	JOB INDX	.23	.03		.02
105+107+108+109	NATL GOVT INDX	.26	.09		.09
14+20+22	EFFICACY INDX	.55	.25		.25
1+2+3	FAMILY INDX	.38	.15		.19
97+99+101	CONSUMER INDX	.31	.07		.06
83+85	MONEY INDX	.47	.15		.15

the set – first to the 16 best predictors (which provided just as good an
explanation as the full set of 30), then to the six best (which did almost
as good a job), and finally to a selected set of 12. The 12 selected domains
were chosen with several criteria in mind: (1) demonstrated predictive
power (shown in Exhibit 7); (2) dispersion in the multi-dimensional space
(shown in Exhibit 3); and (3) potential policy relevance. Exhibit 8 includes
two columns of data for the 12 selected predictors – one showing results
from the May survey and one from the November (Form 2) survey.
While the explanatory power of these 12 was modestly higher in November
(a result we currently attribute to sampling fluctuations), the general
pattern of relationships is largely the same in the two surveys.

Exhibit 9 takes the 12 selected domains and combines them with other
domains measured in the November 1972 survey to see whether a further
increase in explanatory power can be achieved. While all of the 28 variables included in this analysis made their own contribution when others

Exhibit 11

Perceived quality of life (Life #3) as predicted by affective responses to 12 selected domains for all respondents and in 22 different population subgroups

Data source: May 1972 national survey

Population group	N	Percent variance explained	Multiple correlation	Population estimate
All respondents	1297	52%	.72	50%
Men	547	54%	.73	49%
Women	750	55%	.74	51%
16-29 years old	358	59%	.77	51%
16-29 years, head of household	276	63%	.79	53%
30-44 years old	356	69%	.83	63%
45-59 years old	275	61%	.78	51%
45-64 years old	363	56%	.75	48%
60-97 years old	305	53%	.73	42%
Low SES	337	57%	.75	48%
Mid SES	268	65%	.81	55%
High SES	408	60%	.77	54%
Employed men	413	58%	.76	51%
Low income	480	57%	.75	51%
Medium income	346	60%	.77	52%
High income	403	56%	.75	49%
Married	890	49%	.70	46%
Non-married	406	61%	.78	54%
0-11 grades of school	423	63%	.79	58%
High school graduate	307	64%	.80	55%
Some college education	330	58%	.76	49%
College degree	223	60%	.77	46%
Married and employed	512	55%	.74	50%

were held constant (i.e., all betas were greater than zero), the joint explanatory power of the set of 28 was about the same as that achieved using just the previously selected 12.

Thus in two surveys these 12 selected predictors proved to include all of the predictive power included in the larger sets of domains. Hence, we shall use these 12 in the analyses described next.

Predictive power of classification variables. In any attempt to explain perceived quality of life it is of interest to know to what extent it can be explained by conventional classification variables and how these variables compare in predictive power with affective responses to domains.

Exhibit 10 provides an answer. Here we see that six classification variables together explained only about five percent of the variance of Life #3, that the 12 selected domains together explained 50%, and that combining the classification variables with the domain scores produced no increase above the 50% level. In short, the classification variables alone related rather weakly to general sense of life satisfaction, and contributed nothing over and above the explanatory power of affective responses to these 12 domains.[11]

Application in subgroups of the population. Given the goal of constructing an instrument which will be usable in a wide variety of population subgroups, it is of interest to see how effective the 12 selected domains were at explaining variance in various subgroups. Exhibit 11 presents the results of 22 parallel analyses which begin to answer this question.

It is of considerable interest to note that these 12 domains explained about half of the variance in *each* of these groups, suggesting that these domains have a rather broad relevance to different subcultures in the United States. While it is true that the precise prediction formula by which these domains were optimally combined differed somewhat from group to group, it is our belief – based on exploratory analyses – that application of the formula derived for the total population will provide at least moderately good prediction even when applied to particular subgroups.

IX. SUMMARY AND DISCUSSION

This report presents the current status of a series of studies oriented toward the assessment of perceived life quality. Once developed and monitored over a period of years, it is our belief that such an assessment can make a significant contribution to the general goals of the social indicator movement – a better description and understanding of social change, and improved policy making.

Described here is a two-dimensional conceptual model which proposes that one's overall sense of quality of life is understandable in terms of a combination of affective responses (i.e., evaluations) of life 'domains'. Life domains are of two types: role-situations and values. Although not tested by results reported here, it is hypothesized that the role-situations are evaluated in terms of the values, and – conversely – that values are evaluated in the context of the role-situations. However, one of the important results which *is* reported is that additive combinations of affective responses to domains provided moderately good explanations of people's overall sense of life quality. The two-dimensional model can be easily expanded into additional dimensions to include social factors which may affect the evaluation process.

In an attempt to identify an appropriate set of domains, an extensive scan of several types of sources eventually led to the writing of 123 items to which people have been asked to give affective responses. (Data reported here come from several surveys of American adults. The surveys were each based on nationally representative probability samples which yielded between 1000 and 1500 respondents.) Through a variety of mapping and clustering techniques the 80-odd items from this total pool which had been included in surveys in May or November 1972 were grouped into a smaller number of semi-independent clusters. These 'clusters' (many of which include just a single item) constituted the domains of the model. Clusters were defined only when they were found to be internally stable in ten different demographic subgroups of the population. Replication in independent but equivalent national samples showed the interrelationships *between* domains also to be highly stable.

About thirty different measures of a person's sense of overall life quality are described, and of these one was selected for use as a dependent variable, to be predicted by the domains. A series of analyses, some of them replicated in more than one survey, showed that a particular subset of 12 domains could explain 50% to 60% of the variance in sense of overall life quality, that neither other domains nor standard classification variables contributed anything additional to this explanatory power, and that this level of explanation could be achieved in each of 22 different subgroups of the American population (defined in demographic terms) as well as in the population considered as a whole.

In its nature of a progress report, this document has necessarily left a number of important questions unexplored. Clearly, the reported results do not fully exploit the potential complexity of the conceptual model. This awaits further work. Also, one wonders how close to the actual upper limit is the achieved explanatory power of 50%–60%. Given the unreliability of the measures the upper limit is certainly not 100%. Further work will attempt to assess the reliability of the measures employed. It is also apparent that more domains have been identified than have been reported upon. Data pertaining to some domains have been collected only very recently, and await our attention. The roles of the various types of social contexts in the process of evaluating life quality also need exploration. These issues, and a number of others, will set the focus of our work in coming months.

While our work is far from complete, we believe the results reported here indicate a rational, empirical basis for measuring perceived quality of life, at any of several different levels of broadness, generality, and abstraction. Substantial data have been collected from representative national samples which can provide statistical baselines for any of a wide variety of possible quality-of-life measures which may ultimately seem most appropriate.

Institute for Social Research,
University of Michigan,
Ann Arbor

NOTES

* The research reported here has been funded through grant #GS3322 from the National Science Foundation, whose support is gratefully acknowledged. Results contained herein were presented to the 1973 Annual Convention of the American Sociological Association and to the 1973 Conference of the Urban and Regional Information Systems Association. We thank Kenneth Land for his comments on an earlier version of this report. Rick Crandall, Marita Di Lorenzi, William Murphy, and Elizabeth Taylor have assisted in the design and conduct of this project.

[1] Campbell (1972) has discussed this matter.

[2] The May 1972 survey was based on a sample of adults 18 years of age and older (but included married people of any age) living in non-institutional dwelling units in the 48 coterminous states. The response rate to this survey was 76 %. Several comparisons of the distributions of the survey respondents with distributions obtained from the Census lead us to believe these data are closely representative of the American adult population with respect to age, sex, and race.

The two November surveys were each the second wave of panel studies. The population from which the original samples were drawn was defined similarly to that for the May survey, except with the additional restriction that respondents had to be American citizens. Effective response rates for these two surveys are about 62 % each (i.e., number respondents to Wave 2 as a percent of number of sample selections for Wave 1). No comparisons of the respondents to the November surveys with Census distributions have yet been made. However, we have no reason to expect gross biases in the data.

[3] These surveys included: (1) A series of studies carried out by Cantril (1965) and his colleagues in 13 different nations which assessed human concerns; (2) a 1969 survey of the American population which focused on attitudes about the use of violence, subsequently reported in Blumenthal *et al.* (1972); (3) a 1969 national survey of Amer-

ican workers which assessed working conditions (Survey Research Center, 1971); (4) a recent national panel survey of American youth (Bachman et al., 1967); (5) several hundred interviews taken in low-income urban neighborhoods during 1970 (Lansing et al., 1971); (6) a 1971 national survey on issues relating to life quality conducted by our colleagues Campbell, Converse, and Rodgers (unpublished as yet); (7) a 1966 national survey conducted by our colleagues Miller, Converse, and Stokes dealing with political and election issues; and (8) a 1967 study of Detroit residents concerned with issues of race and civil disorder (Aberbach and Walker, 1973).

[4] For reasons of economy Pearson product moment correlations were used to assess relationships. Since the affective response scale achieved no more than ordinal measurement, one might argue that an ordinal-level statistic should have been used. A check on a subset of the relationships for which both types of statistics were computed showed that in these data the order of gammas correlated 0.95 with the order of the Pearson r's.

[5] The 16 identical items can be identified from information given in Exhibit 2. The nearly identical items were numbers 103–104 and 105–106, respectively.

[6] A number of these global measures have been used in previous studies. Items D, F, and M-T of Exhibit 5 were used by our colleagues Campbell, Converse, and Rodgers in their survey of quality of life (unpublished). Items used to produce the Positive Affect, Negative Affect, and Affect Balance scales were used previously by Bradburn (1969). Items F and L were previously used by Gurin et al. (1960). The items using a ladder-format response scale – X–Z, AA and AB – were adapted from Cantril (1965).

[7] The weight mentioned here is that derivable from fitting a least-squares regression model and is obtained from considering only the interrelationships among the domains and Life #3. No additional weighting variable is introduced. At an early stage in our work we thought it might be useful to introduce importance scores assigned to the domains by respondents as a weighting factor. However, extensive analysis of nationally representative data suitable for this purpose convinced us that no predictive gain could be achieved.

[8] This same conclusion that additive models were appropriate for combining domain satisfactions to predict a global measure of life satisfaction has also been reached by our colleagues Campbell, Converse and Rodgers from their analysis of another set of survey data on quality of life.

[9] Domains of Exhibit 7 consisting of a cluster of several items were measured by a single index score in this analysis. The index was computed as the mean of the coded responses to the indicated items.

[10] In addition to the several measures of joint predictive power indicated in Exhibit 7 (and subsequent exhibits), Multiple Classification Analysis (MCA) produces two other statistics of interest: eta and beta. Eta is the conventional measure of bivariate relationship between the dependent variable and the indicated predictor. Beta is a special measure unique to MCA (but analagous to the beta of multiple regression) which provides an indication of the strength of relationship between the dependent variable and the indicated predictor while statistically holding constant all other predictors.

[11] One might ask whether the low explanatory power of the classification variables could be attributed to the inappropriate use of an additive model in this analysis. A careful check showed that a routine which constructs an optimal model – including interaction effects if they are present (Morgan et al., 1971) – did no better than the simple additive model.

BIBLIOGRAPHY

Aberbach, J. and Walker, J., *Race in the City: Political Trust and Public Policy in the New Urban System*, Little, Brown, Boston, 1973.

Allport, F. H. and Vernon, P. E., *A Study of Values*, Houghton-Mifflin, Boston, 1931.

Andrews, F. M., Morgan, J. N., and Sonquist, J. A., *Multiple Classification Analysis*, Institute for Social Research, Ann Arbor, Mich., 1967.

Bachman, J. G., Kahn, R. L., Mednick, M. T., Davidson, T. N., and Johnston, L. D., *Youth in Transition*, Vol. I, Institute for Social Research, Ann Arbor, Mich., 1967.

Blumenthal, M. D., Kahn, R. L., Andrews, F. M., and Head, K. B., *Justifying Violence: Attitudes of American Men*, Institute for Social Research, Ann Arbor, Mich., 1972.

Bradburn, H. M., *The Structure of Psychological Well-Being*, Aldine, Chicago, 1969.

Campbell, A., 'Aspiration, Satisfaction, and Fulfillment', in A. Campbell and P. Converse (eds.), *The Human Meaning of Social Change*, Russell Sage Foundation, New York, 1972.

Cantril, H., *The Pattern of Human Concerns*, Rutgers University Press, New Brunswick, N. J., 1965.

Dodd, S. C., 'On Classifying Human Values: A Step in the Prediction of Human Valuing', *American Sociological Review* **16** (1951) 645–653.

Gurin, G., Veroff, J., and Feld, S., *Americans View their Mental Health*, Basic Books, New York, 1960.

Guttman, L., 'A General Non-Metric Technique for Finding the Smallest Euclidean Space for a Configuration of Points', *Psychometrika* **33** (1968) 469–506.

Kluckhohn, F. R., 'American Women and American Values', in L. Bryson (ed.). *Facing the Future's Risks*, Harper, New York, 1953.

Lansing, J. B., Withey, S. B., Wolfe, A. C., *Working Papers on Survey Research in Poverty Areas*, Institute for Social Research, Ann Arbor, Mich., 1971.

Lepley, R. (ed.), *The Language of Value*, Columbia University Press, New York, 1957.

Morgan, J. H., Baker, E., and Sonquist, J. A., *Searching for Structure*, Institute for Social Research, Ann Arbor, Mich., 1971.

Morris, C. and Jones, L. V., 'Value Scales and Dimensions', *Journal of Abnormal Social Psychology* **51** (1955) 523–535.

Rokeach, M., *The Nature of Human Values*, Free Press, New York, 1973.

Survey Research Center, University of Michigan, *Survey of Working Conditions, 1969*, U.S. Government Printing Office (No. 2916–0001), Washington, D.C., 1971.

White, R. K., 'Value Analysis: A Quantitative Method for Describing Qualitative Data', *Journal of Social Psychology* **19** (1944) 351–358.

MARK SCHNEIDER

4. THE QUALITY OF LIFE IN LARGE AMERICAN CITIES: OBJECTIVE AND SUBJECTIVE SOCIAL INDICATORS

(Received 2 December, 1974)

ABSTRACT. The concept of 'quality of life' as a tool of comparative social indicators research is analyzed. Inter-city comparisons of objective and subjective measures of well being are presented and the distinctiveness of these two dimensions of the quality of life is documented. The paper concludes with some observations on the implications that this distinctiveness has for the use of the concept 'quality of life' in future social indicators research.

One of the most important characteristics of social indicators is their ability to allow more detailed evaluation of social conditions than previously possible. Social indicators can provide scientifically accurate descriptions of the state of social entities. However, their major innovation in such descriptions has come not with their added accuracy but rather with their concern for evaluating the 'quality of life' of different communities. This use of social indicators to describe quality of life is a direct outgrowth of the normative connotations social indicators carry. In the overwhelming majority of social indicators research reports normative direction is assigned to each indicator employed, i.e., it is stated that the more of a measured condition the better (or vice-versa). Indeed, it has been argued that these normative implications are part of the very definition of social indicators (U.S. HEW, 1969:97).

This normative dimension of social indicators adds further depth to the types of description that can be presented. Not only can existing conditions and changes in these conditions be detailed, but normative statements can be made stating whether the conditions of life in society have improved or worsened, or, in other words, whether "things have gotten better, or people are 'better off'" (U.S. HEW, 1969:97).

Attempts to analyze quality of life have led to the development of essentially two major categories of social indicators. The first, and perhaps most commonly employed type of indicator, has sought to evaluate societal well being by utilizing objective measures of community con-

Alex C. Michalos (ed.), Citation Classics from Social Indicators Research, 101–115.
© 2005 Springer. Printed in the Netherlands.

ditions. Heavy reliance is placed on Census data and other governmental reports to assess the quality of life available to individuals in a given community. Measures of societal conditions in such areas as housing, health, and income are employed to describe the quality of life. Postulating 'consensus' that such conditions are inherent to the definition of the good life and that the direction of change in these conditions can be normatively evaluated (e.g., that higher income is better than lower income), comparisons of the quality of life of communities are made using these objective social indicators (see, for example, Sheldon and Moore, 1968; Flax, 1972; Smith, 1973). Conceptually, 'quality of life' becomes a function of the objective conditions of the community in which one lives.

On one level the equating of objective conditions and the quality of life is of course true. If we agree that less infant mortality, less substandard housing, less unemployment, etc. are desirable objective social conditions, are normatively 'good' for people to experience, and are part of the definition of the quality of life, then the distribution of these objective conditions across groups, between geographic units, or over time can be examined and comparisons made indicating improvement or retrogression in the quality of life *as measured by these specified and observed social conditions*. As long as the analysis of the quality of life using objective data is kept on this level there would appear to be no real problem. However, there is a strong tendency to use these specific social indicators data to generalize to more global quality of life statements and to equate the observed patterns in objectively measured conditions with actual differences in the life experiences of people.

The nature of problems caused by this tendency can best be seen in the broadness of the terms 'social well being' and 'quality of life' that are used in social indicators research. Comparisons of welfare between groups of people are being made based on the generated objective social indicators data. Yet it is arguable that actual individual welfare and the quality of life actually experienced by people is a much more highly subjective condition than implied by the social indicators research based on the objective data most frequently employed. It is certainly possible that individuals or social groups may be exposed to objectively better conditions of health care, environment, employment, etc. than other individuals or groups but subjectively feel that the quality of their personal life experiences are no better. Despite the often found assumption that objective social indicators data actually reflect the quality of life experienced by people, we have no reason to *a priori* assume that such a correlation exists. The connections between the 'quality of life' as measured by objective social indicators and the 'quality of life' subjectively experienced by people is really open to question (Campbell and Converse, 1972:9, passim).

This obvious point has led to the development of the second major class of quality of life measures – 'subjective social indicators'. This type of indicator is based not on the normative evaluation of objective social conditions but on survey research reports about life experiences and subjective evaluations of life conditions made by individuals. Subjective social indicators seek to *directly* tap the quality of life as experienced by people rather than imply a connection between objective social conditions and personal well being. And, as argued above, despite the implications of much of the work on objective social indicators, there is no *a priori* reason to believe that these two sets of conditions, i.e., objective life situations and subjective feelings of life quality, vary together. Yet the assumption of such correlations is intuitively appealing and has frequently been made. This in turn has led to confusion in the concept 'quality of life' as a tool of comparative research as well as a blurring of the distinction between the physical and psychological aspects of life quality. These ambiguities have produced a need to examine the extent (if any) of the intercorrelations between objective and subjective social indicators – a need that has been recognized by several researchers. For example, Stagner (1970) argues that:

objective indices are limited; inherent factors in (social) situations demand that subjective data... be considered. A set of psychological indicators would focus on the frequency and intensity of satisfaction (or dissatisfaction) with aspects of (life).... Effective use of these indicators will require that they be analyzed in relation to the objective (social indicators) data. (p. 59)

Andrews and Withey concur. They write:

Only when both (indicators of objective and subjective conditions) are concurrently measured will it be possible to know how demonstrable changes in living conditions are affecting people's sense of life quality, and -conversely- whether changes in people's sense of life quality can be attributed to changes in life conditions. (1973:2)

Smith (1973) similarly believes that attitudinal measures of life quality should be analyzed and compared to the patterns suggested by objective social indicators (p. 137). It would be at this juncture that social indicators could have their most significant impact on policy. If a set of objective conditions and indicators of those conditions could be identified that are strongly related to feelings of subjective life satisfaction, the significance of that finding for both policy makers as well as scholars is obvious.

The remainder of this paper will be an examination of this question of inter-correlations between the two types of social indicators we have identified.

I. DATA SOURCES

We have argued that social indicators are generally classifiable into two broad categories. The first type discussed, 'objective social indicators', are used to measure in a normative fashion the objective conditions of social aggregates. These measured conditions are not necessarily reflected in the life experiences of individuals (although that assumption is often found in social indicators research). The second type of social indicator, 'subjective social indicators', is based on direct reports of personal life experiences and life characteristics, and attempts to measure personal assessments of life quality. It was further suggested above that the extent to which objective and subjective 'quality of life' measures vary together was a question of both theoretical and, given the nature and meaning of social indicators, of practical importance. Fortunately, this correlation can be assessed empirically and the theoretical questions raised concerning the extent and nature of the inter-relationships investigated. The method used herein to accomplish this relies on the measurement of the degree to which variations in measured objective life conditions in fifteen of the largest cities in the United States correspond with variations in the level of subjective life satisfaction found in these same cities.[1]

The objective life conditions found in thirteen of these cities has been examined by the Urban Institute (Flax, 1972). In most instances, data from the U.S. Census and from other governmental agency reports are available to supplement the Urban Institute's work and provide data for the other two cities not previously analyzed. Measures of subjective life quality in these same cities are obtainable through reinterpretation of data included in the 1968 inter-city survey conducted by Campbell and Schuman for the National Advisory Commission on Civil Disorders.

Not only does the analysis of this data provide the opportunity to assess the question of the inter-correlation between the conditions measured by the two types of social indicators, but also taps in a direct fashion the need for inter-areal comparisons that is one of the major themes of current social indicators research (see, e.g., Gastil, 1970; Smith, 1973). It must be noted that the choice of indicators of both types is highly constrained by the availability of data. There is, however, considerable justification for the indicators chosen – justification that will be developed as this paper progresses.

II. SUBJECTIVE SOCIAL INDICATORS

While there is at this time no overwhelming consensus on actual measures of subjective life quality, there is a fairly widespread agreement that subjective life quality is related to such aspects of personal life as aspirations, expectations, happiness, and satisfaction. Moreover, recent research has tended to focus on satisfaction as the most useful indicator of subjective life quality (Stagner, 1970; Campbell et al., 1972; Rossi, 1972; Campbell, 1972; Andrews and Withey, 1973).

Given this, Andrews and Withey have probably progressed the furthest in the development of measures of subjective life quality. In their analysis, Andrews and Withey imply that subjective social indicators research should be concerned with measures of overall ('global') life satisfaction as well as measures of satisfaction with more specific aspects ('domains') of life. Further, they identify the domains that seem to be most important in structuring overall life satisfaction. They find that more than half of the variation in individual evaluations of general life satisfaction can be explained by an additive combination of affective responses across several specific life domains. These domains include the level of satisfaction with one's housing, one's family life, one's job, and one's income. In addition to the level of satisfaction with these specific aspects of life, feelings of personal efficacy, satisfaction with government operations, and satisfaction with the level of available services are also crucial to feelings of general life satisfaction (Andrews and Withey, 1973: Exhibits 7–11).

Comparisons of subjective life quality can be made using both the single summary measure of 'global' life satisfaction and those specific domains identified as important. In particular, given the concern for inter-areal analysis, comparisons of geographically defined social units using these measures would be particularly useful in analyzing subjective quality of life.

Measures of individual feelings across most the important life domains do exist in the attitudinal data gathered by Campbell and Schuman. This makes possible an analysis of city by city variation in subjective life experiences and life satisfaction with these specific conditions. Moreover, while an actual measure of global life satisfaction does not appear in the fifteen city survey, a general measure can be constructed by combining individual responses across the more specific measures that are available. The resulting 'standardized additive score' will hopefully approximate responses one would obtain from an actual measure of total perceived life quality.[2] Thus the survey data does provide a wide range of measures of subjective life satisfaction for fifteen cities.

Given this data, the first question to be asked is whether or not city residence has any impact at all on responses to these subjective social indicators, i.e., does it make sense to think of and investigate the differences between cities in the level of subjective life quality found among their residents. The amount of variance explained by city residence for blacks and whites separately across the subjective social indicators used in this study is reported in Table I. As can be seen, city residence has a small, but fairly constant, statistically significant effect on individual

TABLE I

Variance explained (omega, squared) in subjective quality of life measures by city residence (Fifteen cities)

Measure	White sample	Black sample
Satisfaction with Job	n.s.[a]	n.s.
Satisfaction with Home	1.8%	2.4%
Satisfaction with Money and Income	n.s.	3.4
Personal Efficacy	1.2	n.s.
Satisfaction with Level of Services	6.8	3.9
Citizen Competence	2.4	3.4
Government Distrust	3.2	11.5
Constructed Measure of Total Life Satisfaction	3.1	6.7

[a] n.s.: not significant at 0.05 level

feelings of life satisfaction across most of the specific measured life domains. While in general, city residence is more important in explaining the feelings of blacks than whites (especially with regard to feelings of government distrust), for neither race is city residence an especially strong determinant of subjective life satisfaction. This can also be seen by the fact that city residence explains only 6.7% of the variation in general life satisfaction of black respondents and only 3.1% of the variation in the general level of satisfaction of whites. It is apparent that cities are not characterized by large differences in the level of subjective life quality found among their citizens.

We do know, however, that these same cities are in fact characterized by large differences in the objective conditions found within their borders. For example, as measured by robbery rates, Milwaukee was about *20 times* safer in 1970 than was Washington, D.C. Moreover, the robbery rate in Washington was increasing at twice the speed of that in Milwaukee over the preceeding decade. In terms of infant mortality rates, a widely used indicator of community health, Philadelphia was *much* worse off than Cincinnati or Los Angeles. Other large differences between these cities across measures of objective conditions of wealth, social organization, health, safety, etc. are quite easily documented by Census data and the work of the Urban Institute (Flax, 1972).

If we are concerned with assessing the correlation between indicators of objective 'quality of life' and subjective evaluations of life quality, the above discussion immediately shows that *across these cities there is very little correlation between indicators of the two types of social conditions* in that major differences between cities in objective conditions are not at all reflected in similar differences in measures of subjective feelings of life satisfaction. We can support this conclusion with more specific data. However, this first requires the specification of indicators of objective social conditions that can then be correlated with the subjective evaluations obtained from the fifteen city survey.

III. OBJECTIVE SOCIAL INDICATORS

Just as disagreement exists concerning the measures that should be used as subjective measures of well being, disagreement also characterizes the selection of specific variables used as objective 'quality of life' indicators.

There is, however, considerable agreement on the broad categories from which these variables should be drawn. These broad categories include: (1) income, wealth and employment; (2) the environment (especially housing); (3) health (both physical and mental); (4) education; (5) social disorganization (crime, social pathologies such as alcoholism, drug

TABLE II

Objective social indicators employed

I. Income, wealth and employment.
    a. percent of labor force unemployed, 1968. (1)
       percent change in (a), 1967–1968.
    b. percent of households with income less than $3000. (2)
       percent change in (b), 1960–1970.
    c. per capita income adjusted for cost of living differences, 1968. (1)
       change in (c), 1967–1968.
II. Environment.
    a. percent substandard dwellings, 1970. (2)
       percent change in (a), 1960–1970.
    b. air quality (average yearly concentration of three air pollution components, 1968. (1)
       change in (b), 1968–1969.
    c. cost of transportation for a family of four, 1968. (1)
       percent change in (c), 1967–1969.
III. Health.
    a. infant (under 1 year) deaths per 1000 live births, 1968. (2)
       percent change in (a), 1962–1968.
    b. reported suicide rates per 100000, 1968. (2)
       percent change in (b), 1962–1967.
IV. Education.
    a. Median school years completed by adult population, 1967. (2)
       percent change in (a), 1960–1967.
V. Participation and alienation.
    a. percent of voting age population that voted in 1968 Presidential Election. (3)
       percent change in (a), 1964–1968.
    b. per capital contribution to United Fund Appeal, 1968. (1)
       percent change in (b), 1965–1970.
VI. Social disorganization.
    a. Reported robberies per 100000, 1968. (2)
       percent change in (a), 1964–1969.
    b. reported narcotics addiction rate, 1968. (1)
       percent change in (b), 1964–1969.

---

(1) Thirteen cities (no data on Gary and Newark)
(2) All fifteen cities
(3) Thirteen SMSAs (no data on Gary and Newark)

addiction, etc.); and, (6) alienation and participation (Smith, 1973:70). Any complete study of objective quality of life would have to include as least one 'key' variable from each of the above categories. Employing such key variables (Table II lists those employed in this study), each city with which we are concerned can be ranked according to its position relative to that of the other cities in our survey. The 'quality of life' rankings of the cities based on these objective social indicators can then be compared to rankings based on the indicators of subjective quality of life discussed above.[3] An empirical statement (Spearman's rho) of the intercorrelations of cities' positions across the measures of objective and subjective quality can be arrived at.

Inspection of the correlation coefficients (Table III) confirms our

TABLE IIIa

Correlations (Spearman's rho) between levels of objective and subjective measures of 'Life Quality'. (Level of significance 0.10). White sample.

Subjective measure	Objective measures	Coefficient
Satisfaction with job	No significant correlations	
Satisfaction with	percent low income households	0.61
Housing	change in percent low income households	0.53
	United fund contributions	−0.48
	Median school years	0.54
	change in air pollution	0.47
Satisfaction with money and income	No significant correlations	
Efficacy	percapita income	0.58
	city robbery rate	−0.54
	change in U.F. contributions	−0.60
	change in median school years	−0.81
	cost of transportation	−0.73
	change in cost of transportation	−0.49
	change in air pollution levels	0.47
Satisfaction with	change in low income households	0.54
Services	change in narcotics addiction rate	0.55
Citizen competence	unemployment rate	0.53
	change in unemployment rate	−0.74
	change in U.F. contribution	−0.49
Government distrust	percapita income	−0.47
	change in narcotics addiction rate	0.48
Constructed measure of Total life satisfaction	No significant correlations	

TABLE IIIb

Correlations (Spearman's rho) between levels of objective and subjective measures of 'Life Quality'. (Level of significance 0.10). Black sample.

Subjective measure	Objective measures	Coefficient
Satisfaction with job	No significant correlations	
Satisfaction with housing	United fund contributions	0.51
	change in air pollution levels	0.45
	change in unemployment rate	−0.51
	change in percent low income households	0.65
Satisfaction with money and income	No significant correlations	
Efficacy	unemployment rate	−0.45
	percent low income households	−0.46
	percent substandard housing	0.46
	infant mortality rate	−0.53
	change in suicide rate	0.64
Satisfaction with services	narcotics addiction rate	−0.50
	percapita income	0.47
	change in substandard housing	0.60
	robbery rate	−0.74
Citizen competence	change in robbery rate	−0.59
	percent low income households	−0.77
	substandard housing	0.57
	change in substandard housing	0.65
	change in infant mortality rate	0.49
	robbery rate	−0.70
Government distrust	change in robbery rate	−0.54
	robbery rate	−0.49
	change in narcotics addiction rate	−0.45
	change in low income households	−0.76
	change in substandard housing	0.48
	change in infant mortality rate	0.55
Constructed measure of	unemployment rate	−0.53
Total life satisfaction	robbery rate	−0.48

earlier impression – no consistent relationship is found. Of the total possible 416 correlations that can be computed for both racial groups, only 11% (9% for whites, 13% for blacks) are significant at the 0.10 level. Moreover, just about half of these are in the wrong direction! No objective measure is identifiable as more strongly related to feelings of subjective life quality than any other measure. Further, there are no consistent relationships between objective social indicators drawn from specific categories (e.g., participation and alienation) and the level of satisfaction in a similar category of subjective indicators (trust in government or political efficacy).

In short, there appears to be no evidence at all that, as measured by currently popular indicators, the objective social conditions of cities has any relationship with the levels of subjective life quality of their citizens. Changes over time in objective conditions similarly do not appear to have any correspondence with levels of subjective life quality. This lack of correspondence raises some important questions as to the meaning and interpretation of social indicators data and the directions that future social indicators research should take.

IV. CONCLUSIONS

We have found that no relationship exists between the level of well being found in a city as measured by a wide range of commonly used objective social indicators and the quality of life subjectively experienced by individuals in that city. Cities that are most well off as measured by objective indicators are not necessarily the same cities in which people are subjectively the most satisfied with their life situations. Conversely, cities that are worst off objectively are not necessarily the same cities where subjective dissatisfaction is highest. Moreover, while considerable differences in objective conditions between cities are readily apparent, city residence does not appear to be of any great importance in structuring individual evaluations of life experiences.

In short, the level of well being of cities, as described by objective social indicators alone, apparently tells us nothing about the 'welfare' or the 'life quality' actually experienced by individuals living in those cities. While inter-city comparisons of life conditions based on objective social indicators may alert us to inequalities or injustices in the distribution of an important aspect of well being (and, importantly, may alert decision makers about objective conditions that should be dealt with), this data tells us nothing about the levels of subjective life satisfaction of the individuals in those cities. Objective social indicators cannot be taken as direct measures of the welfare or the quality of life actually experienced by individuals.

This distinction must be carefully maintained in future social indicators research. Life satisfaction of individuals appears to be independent of the physical conditions of the cities in which they live. Therefore, inferences about experienced welfare cannot be made from the readily available objective social indicators of city wide conditions. The 'surrogate' measures of quality of life based on United States Census data or other such reports for large social aggregates (in this particular case, cities) are not really full measures of the phenomena that they have been employed to analyze.

In addition to this warning, these findings also point to avenues of future social indicators data collection and analysis that should be taken. First, one has to note the severe constraints on available social indicators data. While there has been recent large increases in the amount of social indicators research available, data is still limited. The choice of the cities actually examined as well as the choice of indicators employed to measure both objective conditions and the levels of subjective satisfaction were highly constrained. Much more important, however, is the fact that neither objective nor subjective social indicators for geographic units smaller than central cities are readily available. One major problem preventing the generation of such data remains the unresolved question of the characteristics that define communities and neighborhoods within cities. The data analyzed above certainly suggests that objective social conditions of the city as a whole do not relate to the subjective life evaluations of its citizens. But we do know that objective social conditions vary greatly between different geographic areas within cities. It remains a possibility that the objective conditions of sub-areas *within* cities, areas that individuals are more intimately familiar with, may impinge more fully on subjective evaluations of life than do the conditions of the city as a whole. As Rossi notes:

One of the main empirical issues in the social-psychological study of local communities is to ascertain whether the roles played by the local community in the lives of individuals are more in the way of a backdrop, providing a setting in which autochthonous processes are going on, or whether the local community characteristics are a significant input to the level of well being within areas, above and beyond the characteristics of individuals... (Rossi, 1972:84)

However, the answer to this important question must await both a workable definition of 'community' as well as the generation of good social indicators data for these smaller areas.

Similarly, just as the objective conditions of a city vary significantly among different geographic sub-areas of cities, so do they vary among different ethnic, racial, class and religious groups (to a large extent given the degree of segregation in American cities, these two facts are mutually supportive). Knowing a city-wide objective social indicator would, therefore, not tell us much about the nature of life conditions found in these different social groups. The available attitudinal data gives some evidence documenting the differences in the subjective evaluations of life quality of blacks and whites living in the same city. It has been noted elsewhere that blacks are uniformly more dissatisfied with the conditions of their lives than are whites (Schuman and Gruenberg, 1970). But more importantly for our purposes is the fact that there is no correspondence between the relative levels of subjective life quality of blacks and whites across cities. Taking the constructed measure of total life satisfaction as an example shows that across the cities surveyed no statistically significant correlation exists between the level of subjective life quality of whites and blacks in the same city. In particular, whites in Milwaukee were, overall, the most subjectively satisfied with their life conditions relative to whites in the other fourteen cities surveyed. Yet blacks in most other cities were, in general, more satisfied with their overall life conditions than were blacks in Milwaukee. On the other hand, while blacks in Pittsburgh were more satisfied overall than blacks in all other cities surveyed, whites in Pittsburgh were more dissatisfied with their conditions of life than in every other city but Saint Louis.

It would appear that aggregate objective social indicators must be refined along the dimensions suggested above. It is possible that once such relevant categories as neighborhood, race, ethnicity, etc. are taken into account the relationship between objective and subjective social indicators may increase. But this is just a possibility and must be researched further.

In essence, it becomes clear that there is a need for clarification of the terms employed in social indicators research and of the implications of statements made about social well being and the quality of life based on such research. We have documented the distinctiveness across cities of subjective and objective life conditions as measured by commonly employed social indicators. In particular, it is clear that these objective social indicators as now defined are highly limited tools in the investigation of life quality.

While the development of aggregate objective social indicators is still a valuable undertaking in its own right, it must constantly be remembered that the picture of the conditions of life they present is only one part of the totality of the quality of life experienced by people. The use of objective measures along as quality of life indicators is, therefore, highly suspect. Future developments and refinements may produce a greater correlation between objective and subjective social indicators for smaller, more carefully defined and more honogeneous groups. However, for the larger aggregates analyzed in this paper, no correspondence appears. At the current time, objective social indicators drawn heavily from government reports for large units, units defined more by political boundaries than by socio-psychological ones, do not appear to be very accurate measures of the total quality of life found therein.

SUNY, Stony Brook

NOTES

[1] The cities included in the survey are: Baltimore, Boston, Chicago, Cincinnati, Cleveland, Detroit, Gary, Milwaukee, New York, Brooklyn, Newark, Philadelphia, Pittsburgh, St. Louis, San Francisco, Washington, D.C. Of these cities, the objective social conditions of thirteen have been extensively examined by the Urban Institute (Gary and Newark are the other two cities).
[2] The standardized additive score representing general life satisfaction is constructed by transforming individual responses across the measures of each specific domain into standarized Z scores and then combining them additively into a single approximate measure of total subjective life quality.
[3] The ranking of cities on subjective social indicators is based on differences in the mean scores representing the 'average' level of satisfaction in a given city for a specific domain.

BIBLIOGRAPHY

Andrews, F. and Withey, S.: 1973, 'Developing Measures of Perceived Life Quality: Results from Several National Surveys', Institute for Social Research, Ann Arbor, Michigan.
Campbell, A.: 1972, 'Aspiration, Satisfaction and Fulfillment', in A. Campbell and P. Converse (eds.), *The Human Meaning of Social Change*, Russell Sage, New York, pp. 441–466.
Campbell, A., Converse, P., and Rodgers, L.: 1972, paper presented at the Conference on Subjective Measures of the Quality of Life, November 14, 15, 1972, Ann Arbor, Michigan.
Campbell, A. and Converse, P. (eds.): 1972, *The Human Meaning of Social Change*, Russell Sage, New York.

Cazes, B.: 1972, 'The Development of Social Indicators: A Survey', in A. Shonfield and
S. Shaw (eds.), *Social Indicators and Social Policy*, Heinemann Educational Books,
London, pp. 9–22.

Flax, M.: 1972, *A Study in Comparative Urban Indicators: Conditions in 18 Large
Metropolitan Areas*, Urban Institute, Washington, D.C.

Gastil, R.: 1970, 'Social Indicators and Quality of Life', *Public Administration Review*,
30, no. 6, pp. 596–601.

Henriot, P.: 1972, *Political Aspects of Social Indicators: Implications for Research*,
Russell Sage, New York.

Rossi, P.: 1972, 'Community Social Indicators', in A. Campbell and P. Converse,
op. cit., pp. 87–126.

Schuman, H. and Gruenberg, B.: 1970, 'The Impact of City on Racial Attitudes',
American Journal of Sociology 76, 213–261.

Sheldon, E. and Moore, W. (eds.): 1968, *Indicators of Social Change*, Russell Sage,
New York.

Smith, D.: 1973, *The Geography of Social Well Being in the United States: An Introduction to Territorial and Social Indicators*, McGraw-Hill Book Company, New York.

Springer, M.: 1970, 'Social Indicators, Reports and Accounts', *The Annals* 388, 1–13.

Stagner, R.: 1970, 'Perceptions, Aspirations, Frustrations and Satisfactions: An
Approach to Urban Indicators', *The Annals* 388, 59–68.

United States Department of Health, Education and Welfare: 1969, *Toward a Social
Report*, Government Printing Office Washington, D.C.

5. QUALITY OF LIFE

ABSTRACT. What is sought is a definition of Quality of Life (QOL). Other authors have defined QOL in terms of actual happiness or perceived satisfaction/dissatisfaction. The present paper defines it not as a summation of the individual happiness-states of all members of a society, but as the obtaining of the necessary conditions for happiness throughout a society. These conditions being necessary not sufficient, high QOL is compatible with actual unhappiness. The necessary conditions in question are identified with the availability of means for the satisfaction of human needs rather than human desires, and a Maslowian analysis of the former is proposed in default of any more satisfactory analysis. The paper concludes with a discussion of how maximizing need-satisfaction (as opposed to want-satisfaction) automatically guarantees fair distribution of needed goods. This ensures that in at least some respects high-QOL societies are societies characterized by justice.

Use of the phrase 'Quality of Life' seems to date back to 1964,[1] but no agreement yet exists as to what meaning it carries. In what follows we shall attempt to provide a definition.

Recent discussions on Quality of Life (henceforth QOL) have been motivated by two rather different concerns. The first of these represents a feeling on the part of many people that modern industrial society, despite impressive gains in affluence, ease of communication, and leisure, has not made any significant overall progress in improving man's lot. Mankind's prospects may, in fact, be less attractive now than they were 25 years ago.[2] Interest in QOL represents, therefore, under this interpretation, a desire for something better or a nostalgia for something lost.

The concept of *Quality of Life* has emerged in the last few years as an undefinable measure of society's determination and desire to improve or at least not permit a further degradation of its condition. Despite its current undefinability, it represents a yearning of people for something which they feel they have lost or are losing, or have been denied, and which to some extent they wish to regain or acquire.[3]

The second concern that has motivated research into QOL is the desire for an index of social well-being analogous to GNP and other measures of economic well-being. The emphasis here is on *measurability*, which has provided the thrust for recent intensive research on social indicators as a

Alex C. Michalos (ed.), Citation Classics from Social Indicators Research, 117–136.
© 2005 *Springer. Printed in the Netherlands.*

proper subset of social statistics. The ultimate aim (admittedly very far from realization now or in the foreseeable future) is to be able to aggregate all indicators into a master QOL index. Current interest in quality of life, then, stems from at least two distinct sources: one a popular concern and lack of satisfaction over what life has to offer, the other a desire on the part of social scientists to provide, for purposes of governmental decision-making as well as out of intellectual interest, measures of social progress.

Although the purpose of investigating QOL is clear enough, understanding of what exactly is being investigated is not. For example, is QOL something that pertains primarily to societies, to groups of people, or is it something that attaches basically to individuals, and is thence extended to societies or groups by a process of summation? Is QOL measured by collecting subjective reports of satisfaction/dissatisfaction, or of perceived well-being, on the part of individual members of society? Or is it measured by the number of schools and hospitals, by nutrition levels and command over goods and services, by crime rates and air quality? Is QOL one and the same for men and women, for Newfoundlanders and Albertans, for old and young, for Africa and Western Europe? Or is QOL a radically culture-bound concept, requiring that each segment of human society, each demographic group, seek out for itself an understanding of where it conceives life's quality to lie? None of these questions, as far as I know, has been answered. In the absence of at least rough agreement about answers, the concept of QOL can hardly be said to exist. Not only do we not know what it is, we don't even know what category it belongs to. What is needed, as a prerequisite to further work on QOL, is an understanding of what the expression 'quality of life' means.[4]

Let us begin with the word 'quality,' which is a slippery term because it has both an evaluative and a non-evaluative use. Used non-evaluatively, the word is similar in meaning to 'attribute' or 'character.' Thus if we say, "Life in Paris has a certain distinctive quality," we mean that it has a distinctive character. Furthermore, in the nonevaluative sense of the word, it is meaningless to ask whether QOL in Paris is greater or less than QOL in Rome. Instead, life in each of these cities has just the particular quality it has and no other. In its non-evaluative sense, the word 'quality' behaves somewhat like the word 'colour': every object has its own particular colour, and we cannot say that one colour is greater or less than another. But it is the evaluative rather than the non-evaluative sense of the word 'quality' that interests us here. Used in this sense, the word behaves more like 'weight,' which is a comparative term, than like 'colour.' Every object has a weight, and the weight of one object is always comparable in amount to the weight of another. However, in another respect, the word 'quality,' as used evaluatively, differs from both 'colour' and 'weight.' To say that something is of high quality is automatically to recommend it, to say that it is 'better' (in some sense) than something of low quality, whereas heavier things are not *per se* better than lighter ones. The notion of quality, as we shall henceforth understand it, not only differs from colour and resembles weight in being comparative, but also differs from weight in being evaluative. As used evaluatively, QOL admits of degrees, and it is meaningful to speak of QOL in Paris as being greater or less than QOL in Rome. QOL becomes, therefore, not a name for the particular character or savour of life in different regions of the globe, but for a property which characterizes different societies to different degrees, desirability being directly proportional to degree.[5]

The word 'quality' is sometimes confusingly employed in the sense of 'high degree of quality.'[6] For example, we sometimes speak of 'a quality wine,' meaning 'a wine of high quality,' or of 'losing the quality of life,' although strictly speaking life always has *some* degree of quality, whether high or low. These idioms are harmless, provided their literal meaning is recognized.

Merely saying that quality is an evaluative property admitting of degrees does not serve as a definition. As Baier points out, the quality of a thing is only one among many evaluative properties. Others include usefulness, efficiency, efficacy, worth, worthwhileness, value, merit, beauty. Specifying exactly what it is about something that constitutes its *quality*, as opposed to, say, its *usefulness* or its *beauty*, can be a complex matter. The extent of the complexity may be indicated by considering some examples. Good quality *wine* is distinguished by its body, colour, mellowness of taste, and aroma. A high quality *fabric* is generally one that wears well and is pleasing to the touch, although it may not be as useful as a drip-dry. *Air* quality is a function of the gaseous emissions and particulate matter it contains, together with ozone (at the seashore). Poor quality *restaurants* are those that are dingy, or dirty, or serve inferior meals, and are sometimes but not always characterized by low quality *service*. And so forth. In Baier's terminology, the quality of a thing is both *multi-criterial* and *type-dependent*. It is multi-criterial because the applicability of the word 'quality' depends on the presence or absence not of one but of a cluster of other properties.[7] It is type-dependent because the criteria which determine the quality of one type of thing (say wine) are not the same as those which determine the quality of another (say fabric). Now, what lessons can be learned from all this about quality of *life*?

To begin with, the word 'life' in the phrase 'quality of life' refers not to my life or your life or Bob Brown's life but to 'life in a certain society,' or 'life in a certain region of the earth's surface.'[8] Given that QOL applies to regions or societies, what are the criteria to be used in assessing it? This is, of course, the nub of the question. If we review the examples given above, those of quality of wine, fabric, air, restaurants, and service, we note that a common element runs through them all, namely, an intimate relation to human beings and their needs, wants, and desires. Without the human denominator, there *is* no such thing as quality of wine, fabric, air, restaurants, or service. Just as the proof of the pudding lies in the eating, so the proof of the quality of the wine lies in the drinking, or of the fabric in the wearing. And so it might be said, proof of the quality of life lies in the living. This would seem to indicate that regions of high QOL were regions where living was somehow enhanced, where people got more out of life, in some sense, than people did in other regions.

We are on the right track, but we must proceed carefully. We first need a name for the state of life-enhancement: let us borrow an old term and call it 'happiness.' There is much to be said about this term and only a tiny fraction of it can be said here, but the following will indicate broadly how we shall understand it.

(i) Unlike pleasure, happiness is not episodic. Feelings of pleasure and pain are episodes, and can occur both in the context of a happy life, and in the context of an unhappy life. We must distinguish 'feeling happy now' from 'being happy.'

(ii) Happiness is closely related to (may even be identical with) fulfillment. Each person has certain talents or capabilities or potentialities. Whether he is happy or not depends to a large extent on whether these capabilities are realized.

(iii) Plato argued long ago that the happy life was the good or virtuous life. There may well be a moral dimension to happiness but the state of the argument has not advanced much since Plato.

(iv) Happiness may best be found by not seeking it. In Mill's words: "Those only are happy... who have their minds fixed on some object other than their own happiness; on the happiness of others, on the improvement of mankind, even on some art or pursuit, followed not as a means but as itself an ideal end. Aiming thus at something else, they find happiness by the way."[9]

Given the notion of happiness, it might seem that we could proceed directly to define QOL in terms of the general or average happiness of the people in a region or society. But this would be, in the opinion of the author, a mistake. The reasons why it would be a mistake are rather complicated, and need to be considered carefully.

First, we already have a perfectly good measure of social welfare in terms of happiness, coming down to us from Bentham and Mill, as incorporated in the theory of utilitarianism. It is true that Mill defined happiness in terms of pleasure and the absence of pain rather than in terms of fulfillment. But, with this difference, to define QOL in terms of the general happiness, of 'the greatest happiness of the greatest number,' would be merely to repeat Mill's work.

A second and more important reason for not defining QOL in terms of the general happiness is this. Suppose we have a region R in which the general happiness is very high. People are fulfilled, gather together frequently for joyful communal activities, and subscribe passionately to certain common goals. An outsider X, who defines QOL in terms of happiness, decides that R is the place for him and moves in. Alas, he experiences nothing but frustration and anguish. Why? Because the people who inhabit R are a group of snobs or bigots who refuse to admit X. Alternatively, let S be a region of inutterable misery and deprivation (e.g., Bangladesh after a flood). Yet Y, who moves there, is sustained by an inner life of intense religious convictions and leads a dedicated and fulfilled existence. What these examples indicate is that QOL is independent of the general happiness. Region R may seem at first sight to be a high-QOL area but in fact is not, its happiness being based on inequity (we shall return to questions of justice and inequity later). Region S is a low-QOL area and remains so, no matter how many happy and fulfilled religious people move into it.

Consider a third example. Let T be a society with every conceivable amenity, both physical and social. T has good schools, full employment, excellent health care, very little crime, democratic government, incorruptible officials, clean air, a high level of affluence, and no poverty. And yet, for one reason or another, almost everyone in T is unhappy. A's mother has just died, B can't get along with his boss, C has an anxiety neurosis, D and E suffer the pangs of unrequited love, F is married to the wrong man, etc. Does this mean that QOL in T is low? It would if QOL were measured by summing the individual unhappinesses of A, B, C,.... But intuitively, one would think that the QOL of T were high, and to insist that it is low indicates only that we have chosen the wrong definition. Suppose now that the psychological atmosphere in T improves. A gets over his mother's death, B changes jobs, C goes to an analyst, D and E get married, and F gets divorced. Does QOL increase? No. The sum total of human happiness increases, but this is not QOL.

What then *is* QOL? Just as quality of wine is something that pertains to wine, and quality of a fabric something that pertains to a fabric, so QOL is something that pertains to a society or region. Just as quality of wine is different from the pleasureable taste that one gets from drinking it, but is in some way causally connected with it, so QOL is different from happiness, but is in some way causally connected with it. We shall say that QOL consists in the obtaining of the *necessary conditions* for happiness in a given society or region. The concept of a 'necessary condition for happiness' is vague, and needs to be elaborated

Nicholas Rescher, in a work which explores at some length the relationship between happiness and welfare, puts forward three factors that must be distinguished in any discussion of happiness:[10]

(1) *General happiness requisites.* What it requires for an arbitrary member of the human species to be happy. The general happiness requisites or requirements (GHR's) do not vary from person to person. Note that the GHR's are *necessary* conditions for happiness, not sufficient conditions.

(2) *Idiosyncratic happiness requisites.* What it requires for me to be happy, or for you to be happy, or for Bob Brown to be happy. The IHR's will in general differ from one person to another.

(3) *Happiness itself.*[11] The actual state of being happy.

Let us re-examine the case of society T, the society which had every conceivable amenity but whose members were unhappy, in the light of these distinctions. Plainly it is quite possible, in the case of any society, for the *general* happiness requirements to be satisfied although, for any individual member of that society, his *idiosyncratic* happiness requirements are not. This is the case in society T. The necessary conditions for happiness are satisfied, where by 'necessary conditions' we mean GHR's, i.e., what is necessary for a person (any person) to be happy. But the sum total of the GHR's do not constitute a sufficient condition for happiness. In addition, each person has certain idiosyncratic requirements, the IHR's, which if not met will frustrate the attainment of happiness. The IHR's, unlike the GHR's, are very much a matter of the individual differences and contingencies which separate one person from another: I may like tennis and you may like golf, with the result that I am miserable and you are happy in a region that has only golf courses. Or X's spirit may be broken by the loss of a loved one, while Y may be able to reconcile himself and rise above the loss. Whether people are happy, therefore, depends as much upon certain needs being met that are peculiar to them as individuals, as upon the satisfaction of needs they share with everyone else.

Quality of life, as we shall define it in this paper, consists in the satisfaction of the general happiness requirements. To the extent that the GHR's are met in a given society or region, what we shall understand by QOL is high in that society or region; to the extent that they are not met, QOL is low. In the next few paragraphs, I shall point out certain consequences of adopting this definition of QOL, and how the definition differs from other definitions that have previously been proposed. In the last part of the paper, I shall take up the extremely difficult question of what the general happiness requirements are.

The first and probably most important consequence of our definition is that QOL is not to be determined by questioning people about how satisfied or dissatisfied they are. Questions like: "Taken altogether, how would you say things are these days – would you say you are very happy, pretty happy, or not too happy?"[12] though no doubt interesting and important in their own right, have nothing to do with QOL. The approach to QOL taken here runs directly counter to all the proposed definitions of the concept which are to be found in the first and so far only published volume devoted explicitly to QOL.[13] Thus we find:

The premise on which the studies are based is that *quality of life* refers to human experience, and the criteria of *quality of life* are those dimensions of life by which people experience levels of satisfaction-dissatisfaction (pleasure-pain, happiness-unhappiness, etc.).[14]

And in another paper:

By *quality of life* we mean an individual's overall perceived satisfaction of his needs over a period of time.[15]

Finally, in reporting on the results of a QOL questionnaire, Dalkey and Rourke state:

In our instructions to the subjects *we defined the term 'Quality of Life' (QOL) to mean a person's sense of well-being, his satisfaction or dissatisfaction with life, or his happiness or unhappiness.*[16]

Each of these definitions of QOL represents what we may call a *subjectivist* approach to the matter. By contrast, the definition of QOL in terms of happiness requirements rather than happiness is an attempt to provide an *objective* definition.

The difference between the subjective and the objective approaches to QOL parallels a long-standing dispute in the field of social indicators, which we shall digress for a moment to explore. This is, whether to admit subjective indicators as measures of social welfare. At a seminar on social indicators in 1972, Dorothy Walters, of the Economic Council of Canada, spoke both of the need for such indicators and of the problems involved in obtaining them:

Part of our current dilemma arises out of the apparent paradox that measured improvements in objective conditions have not been associated with similar improvements in satisfactions. This whole 'subjective' area provides an opportunity for creative theoretical and operational research.... There is a large political content in this emphasis on attitudes and reactions. In view of the sensitive nature of these data, it is probably preferable that the major developments in subjective data take place in private agencies and institutions.[17]

Despite these difficulties, it seems now to be generally acknowledged that a complete social indicator program will of necessity have to admit subjective data. Thus, in its policy statement on social indicators, the OECD asserts:

The perceptions which individuals and groups have of fundamental aspects of their well-being are a necessary and important component of the social indicator program.

This type of information reveals another dimension of reality and may also show up objective factors which have not previously been recognized as significant. The well-being of individuals in many goal areas cannot be readily detected without recourse to the account of the individuals themselves.[18]

The two most recent compendia of socal indicators in the U.S. and Canada both profess an interest in subjective data, although in fact they contain mostly non-perceptual material.[19]

In view of the generally-accepted belief that subjective data are needed in any satisfactory social indicator program, and that what is indicated by social indicators, roughly and broadly, is social well-being or quality of life, would it not seem that we were over-hasty in rejecting a subjective definition of QOL in terms of perceived happiness or felt satisfaction? It might. But a closer examination of how subjective indicators behave, and how they relate to 'objective' data, shows that it is possible to combine, within a single conceptual or methodological framework, the notion of a subjective QOL *indicator* with that which is *constitutive* of QOL, the latter being wholly non-subjective.

Perhaps the most suggestive and interesting work done on subjective indicators is that of Stanley Seashore on job satisfaction.[20] Seashore argues that in assessing the quality of working life (QWL) we must take into account not only such objective measures as pay, hours of work, health conditions and pension plans, but such things as *satisfaction* with pay, *preference* for more or fewer hours of work, *need* for a vacation, *perception* of hazard, *expectation* of promotion.[21] Pay and satisfaction with pay are two very different things, and both, according to Seashore, are relevant to QWL. One might think that job satisfaction varied as widely or more widely than working conditions, but surprisingly this is not so. In the U.S. in 1969–70, 85% of the employed adults reported themselves as being at least 'somewhat' satisfied, and only 15% dissatisfied. Although adequate time series are not yet available, Seashore anticipates that these figures will remain fairly constant, for the following reason. Job dissatisfaction, on his analysis, represents an unstable and transitional state, which is sooner or later removed by man's capacity to adapt himself. 'Adaptation,' of course, may take many different forms, such as changing jobs, lowering expectations, cognitive distortion, aggression, and other more pathological ways of coping with the situation. But in one way or another, if Seashore's theory is correct, the large majority of working people will come round to being 'satisfied,' or at least to expressing themselves as 'satisfied.' Even Ivan Denisovitch, in his Siberian labour camp, meets and overcomes challenges in a way not too different from the way in which North American workers do, and at the end of the day goes to bed a 'satisfied' man.[22]

Now, if all this is so, what becomes of QWL? If both good working conditions and bad working conditions produce a more or less constant percentage of workers who describe themselves as 'satisfied,' will we not be forced to conclude that quality of working life is something that varies independently of job satisfaction? It won't do to say that QWL is constituted by some *combination* of objective and subjective factors. We might as well say that the quality of a fabric lies not in the fabric but consists in some esoteric combination of properties of the fabric together with pleasurable feelings on the part of the wearer. No, quality of a fabric lies in the fabric, and QWL lies in working conditions. The role played by job satisfaction indicators is to indicate *which* working conditions are important in determining QWL. At the moment, we have only rather imprecise ideas concerning this. Is good pay more or less important than good relations with one's supervisor? How important is the element of creativity in work? What leads to dissatisfaction with pay? These are questions that cannot be answered without talking to and observing people at work, and this is, in a sense, the job that subjective indicators do for us. Working conditions constitute QWL, while job satisfaction reports, sometimes in a rather oblique way, indicate it.

Let us leave the matter of whether QOL is objective or subjective and turn to another question. This is, whether what constitutes QOL varies from one region or society to another. This is not the question whether QOL varies in degree, but whether what counts as QOL varies. Is QOL a culture-bound or regional concept?

According to the definition of QOL proposed above, QOL consists in the satisfaction of the general happiness requirements in a given region. The general happiness requirements are those requirements which are necessary conditions of anyone's happiness – without which no member of the human race can be happy.[23] Since there is but one human species in all regions of the world, the criteria which determine QOL do not vary from one region to another. It is a consequence of our definition that what makes for high or low QOL in Alaska is exactly the same as what makes for high or low QOL in Tahiti. Therefore QOL, although it applies to regions, is not a region-relative or society-relative concept.[24]

Another question: if QOL, in a given region, consists of the satisfaction of certain requirements, in the absence of which no one can be happy, does this mean that if only one person in the region is happy, then the requirements are met and consequently QOL is maximized? No, this is not what is intended. What is intended, and what should be stated explicitly, is that QOL in a given region consists in the satisfaction of the GHR's *throughout the region*, i.e., for each inhabitant. The greater the percentage of people in the region for which the GHR's are satisfied, the higher the level of QOL. This is somewhat oversimplified, since it does not take into account structural inequities in a region. For example, if in a developing country there exist only a few hospitals, then a certain percentage of the population will be effectively denied health care and QOL may be increased by increasing the number of hospitals. But if all the new hospitals are built in the home area of the country's president, then even if no health care redundancy exists, QOL will suffer, since inequities have been introduced which are not simply the result of chance (i.e., how far one's home happens to be from a hospital). This example indicates that a principle of equity or justice plays some part in the specification of what constitutes QOL, and leads us to the last part of the paper, in which the nature of the general happiness requirements is discussed.

To specify what the GHR's are is not at all easy. What I have to say on the subject is tentative, and will raise more problems than it resolves. To begin with, are the general happiness requirements provided for by the satisfaction of human needs, or by the satisfaction of human wants and desires? This question is an important one, and to answer it we must briefly discuss the notion of what it is to need something, and how it differs from wanting or desiring.

The concept of a *need* is an extremely general one. Given any object O, whether animate or inanimate, and any state S of O, then what O needs (relative to the state S) is whatever is required for O to attain S, or, if O is already in S, to remain in S.[25] We often omit the qualifier, 'relative to the state S,' in speaking of needs. Thus we speak of an engine needing oil without normally mentioning that the engine needs oil in order to function smoothly. But these ellipses are common and, in most cases, well understood. Some philosophers and psychologists conceive of a need as a *lack*. But a need is not necessarily a lack, since it is perfectly possible to say that a person needs all his strength to lift something without suggesting that he lacks the strength.[26]

The notion of a want or desire is more restricted, since apart from archaic or colloquial uses of the word 'want,' as in 'This coat wants mending,' only animate subjects can want or desire anything. What a person wants, and what he needs, are in general quite independent of one another. I may want a cigarette, although I may not need one; I may need to go to the dentist, although I may not want to. Wants differ from needs in at least the following respects:

(i) Unlike the specification of a need, the full specification of a want does not necessarily involve reference to any end state which fulfillment of the want promotes. A man needs money in order to eat, but a miser may simply want or desire it, not as a means to something else, but for its own sake.

(ii) Wants are controllable in a way that needs are not. One can check one's desire for food, but not one's need for it. We can eagerly want things, but not eagerly need them. Furthermore, we can only want what is to some degree within our grasp, whereas what we need may be conceptually out of reach. To lead a happy life, for example, we may need to have had a happy childhood.

(iii) What we want bears a close relationship to what we believe. For example, whether or not mountain air is good for my health, I may want a holiday in the mountains because I believe it to be good for my health. In contrast, what I believe is strictly irrelevant to what I need.[27]

(iv) Generally speaking, people are the best judges of what they want, but not of what they need. What I may want is a large juicy steak, whereas all I may need for nutritional purposes is soup, raw carrots, and rice. So, if you want to know what I want, ask me, whereas if you want to know what I need, an expert's advice would be as good or better.

(v) Philosophers frequently distinguish between the 'intensional' character of wanting and desiring, as opposed to the 'extensional' character of needing. I may want to punch the next person I meet, and the next person I meet may be Muhammed Ali, but his does not entail that I want to punch Muhammed Ali. On the other hand, if I need to punch the next person I meet, and if the next person I meet is Muhammed Ali, then I need to punch Muhammed Ali.[28]

(vi) The satisfaction of a want or desire differs in an important way from the satisfaction of a need. Frequently, the satisfaction of a want or desire requires the occurrence of an event in the world of physical things, as when a person satisfies his desire for food by consuming a meal. However, *whether the desire is satisfied* is never settled by examining the physical world. Instead, it is settled by examining the person's mind (or, if we are materialists, the state of his brain). In the case of needs, on the other hand, the question of *whether a need is satisfied* is normally though not always settled by examining the physical world. Whether my need for food is is satisfied, for example, as opposed to my desire, is purely a matter of the quantity and the variety of the food I eat, and not of whether I feel content.

Summing up the differences described under (ii)–(vi), we might say that wanting and desiring are *psychological states*, whereas the state of needing something is not a psychological state. Combining this result with the one obtained earlier about the non-subjective character of QOL, we are able to infer something about the general happiness requirements. QOL, as we have defined it, consists in the fulfillment of the GHR's. Since the presence or absence of unsatisfied wants is a mental phenomenon, fulfillment of the GHR's cannot lie in the satisfaction of human wants. If anything, it must lie in the satisfaction of human needs.

An important consequence of focussing on needs rather than wants is that we avoid the escalation problem. Wants tend to escalate in the sense that if you give me what I want, I shall stop wanting it and want something else. This phenomenon, of rising expectations or rising aspirations, is sometimes appealed to in order to explain how it is that modern man, in the face of a steadily rising standard of living, continues to regard himself as less happy than his forebears.[29] The phenomenon was known to the Epicureans, who embodied it in the following proportion:[30]

$$\text{degree of satisfaction} = \frac{\text{attainment}}{\text{expectation}}$$

Unlike wants, however, needs do not escalate. There is no suggestion that if you give me what I need, then I immediately start to need something else. Hence if QOL is measured in terms of the satisfaction of needs, not wants, comparisons of QOL in societies at different times and places will be possible, whereas if QOL is measured in terms of wants we shall find, as Seashore did with job satisfaction, that in all societies QOL tends to seek a certain equilibrium level.

If satisfaction of the general happiness requirements is to be understood as consisting in the fulfillment of needs, it still remains to be said what human needs are. As we saw earlier, 'X needs Y' is always short for 'X needs Y in order to Z.' In the context of the general happiness requirements, we may interpret 'to Z' as 'to be happy.' But what is it that human beings need in order to be happy? This is an extremely difficult question. Perhaps the most ambitious and the most widely known attempt to answer it is that of Abraham Maslow, whose 'hierarchy of needs' is an ordered list with the property that higher needs cannot be met until the more basic ones have been. Maslow's hierarchy is as follows.[31]

(1) *Physiological needs.* The lowest category of needs, comprising the need for food, water, sleep, shelter, reproduction, etc. These needs are prepotent, and if they are not satisfied, dominate the individual's behaviour.

(2) *Safety or security needs.* Needs for protection from harm and for a life that is safe and secure, including assurances about the future satisfaction of physiological needs.

(3) *Belongingness needs.* The need for love and affection. These needs are of two kinds – the passive need to be loved and accepted, and the active need to love others.

(4) *Esteem needs.* People's need for a stable, firmly based, usually high evaluation of themselves. Like belongingness needs, esteem needs divide into a need for the esteem or respect of others, and for self-respect or self-esteem.

(5) *Self-actualization needs.* These needs, the highest in Maslow's hierarchy, are often said to differ from the others in being 'growth' rather than 'deficiency' needs, although the exact nature of the intended difference is unclear. The satisfaction of self-actualization needs is said to correspond roughly to "what some personality theorists call the 'fully mature' person, adding to the notions of emotional balance and of self-acceptance a notion of drive, of open-ended achievement in unfamiliar and challenging situations."

It will be noted that most of the needs in Maslow's hierarchy are what we may call 'psychological' needs, meaning that the purpose of meeting them is to achieve a psychological state of health or happiness. However, although the end state is psychological the means of achieving that state are in general not. For example, one way to satisfy belongingness needs is (in Africa at least) to be a member of an extended family, but being a member of an extended family is not a psychological state. The question of just what physical, interpersonal, or social institutions are causally related to what psychological end-states is one that admits of no simple answer. No doubt the answer is different in different societies. But if Maslow's theory, or some theory similar to it, is correct in asserting that a list of needs can be drawn up which holds for all men at all times and places, then the first step will have been made in laying down a set of objective criteria for QOL.

Against this, it has been objected that Maslow's need hierarchy is too abstract and general to be of any use in assessing QOL. Taking as an example the low-level need for shelter, Michalos remarks:

We get practically instant agreement that people need shelter. And then what? What do we do with that? What follows by way of research or policy from that? There's not much point in launching a search to find out what per cent of our people don't have shelter. Virtually everyone lives *in something*. We must go beyond mere shelter to do anything useful and then we are beyond Maslow on this basic need. We must talk about space per person, toilets and tubs, kitchens and windows, and so on to get anywhere talking about shelter.[32]

Michalos is, of course, right in implying that we cannot assess QOL in any very satisfactory way by merely counting 'shelters' (unless we are UNHCR people dealing with refugees). But Maslow's need hierarchy will take us a little farther than this. In a 'shelter,' is good insulation necessary? Yes, if it is needed to sustain body temperature. A bathroom? Yes, for health reasons, unless some equally convenient sanitary facility is available. Does each member of the family need to have his own room? Only if a case can be made for such an arrangement on the basis of esteem and self-actualization needs. Etc. Plainly, a lot of work needs to be done, but at the moment I know of no argument demonstrating that the need hierarchy (or something like it) is incapable of providing appropriate criteria for assessing QOL. And the need hierarchy possesses a sufficient degree of generality that we shall not be forced into culture-bound absurdities like asserting that QOL in Burma must be low because they don't have bathrooms or two-car garages.

The last matter I wish to take up is the question of equality or justice, which was discussed briefly earlier. The central problem is whether or not the way in which goods and amenities are distributed in a society is relevant to QOL. In our earlier discussion of the example of the distribution of hospitals in a developing country, we asserted that distribution was indeed relevant, and that an unjust or inequitable distribution would actually lower QOL. But our treatment of the matter was hasty, and it was not made clear *why* injustice should be incompatible with high QOL, or what relationship, if any, existed between quality of life and equality. So let us examine the matter a little more carefully.

Consider a society in which the general happiness requirements of a certain percentage of the population are met. Suppose that, in addition, there now exist means of providing for additional GHR's. There need be nothing very subtle about this; let us suppose that there is hunger, and that a certain amount of food becomes available. How shall the food be distributed? It could, of course, be given to those whose needs are already met, but no increase in QOL would result from this, since once a need is satisfied, any further attempt at satisfaction is redundant.[33] The only way of using the additional food to increase QOL, therefore, would be to give it to those whose needs were not met. (Recall that we defined QOL in a given region as consisting in satisfaction of the GHR's throughout the region, i.e., for each inhabitant.) QOL could be increased in this way until the needs of all members of the society were met, following which no further increase would be possible. Note that fair and equal distribution of the GHR's in a society where QOL is maximal is guaranteed, and that what guarantees it is the fact that each person's needs are finite, and their limits fixed. Furthermore, when we confine ourselves to the GHR's and exclude the IHR's, no person's needs differ from another's.

Several comments must be made. First, it is perhaps not strictly true that a person's needs are finite, and cannot be increased without limit. In particular, it might seem that Maslow's need hierarchy was quite open-ended about human needs. It is true that I need only a finite amount of food, clothing, and shelter, but is there any limit to the amount of love a person needs? Can an upper bound be placed on one's need for self-actualization? Perhaps not, but it is not clear that there is any limit on the amount of material available for the satisfaction of love needs and self-actualization needs either. Those needs for the satisfaction of which only limited resources are available, such as needs for food and shelter, are (fortunately) limited in extent.[34] And those which are not limited in extent seem capable of all being satisfied, without person X's needs conflicting with person Y's.

In a society in which resources are adequate to satisfy everybody's needs, the problem of distribution is solved automatically by going ahead and satisfying needs. But we have not yet solved the problem of when resources are inadequate, since it has not yet been shown that a society in which the needs of A, B and C are each partially met has a higher QOL than one in which A and B are fully satisfied and C's needs are met minimally if at all. A slave state, for example, might exhibit the latter structure, or a contemporary society in which women hoe, chop wood, cook, fetch water and look after the children, while the men drink beer, keep an eye on the cattle, and discuss important clan and village matters. If we think in terms of the need hierarchy, however, it will be seen that a more equitable distribution of labour and of amenities would actually increase need satisfaction, since love, esteem and self-actualization needs are all deprived in slave and quasi-slave conditions. If QOL is defined in terms of need satisfaction, therefore, societies with high QOL will in general exhibit juster and more equitable distribution patterns than those with low QOL, since the satisfaction of certain needs requires such patterns.

A final remark about wants, In our imaginary society where people were hungry and where extra food became available, the satisfying of needs automatically ensured fair distribution because the needs of individuals were limited. But suppose our society had been, not a society of unsatisfied needs, but a society of unsatisfied wants? Since what a man wants is potentially limitless, one possible distribution would be to give everything to one extremely concupiscent individual. This is, of course, an unjust distribution, but nothing rules it out as long as what we are concerned with is maximizing the satisfaction of wants. It *is* ruled out, however, if we are interested in satisfying needs rather than wants. It was doubtless the potentially limitless character of wants, together with the fact that wants conflict and that what one man wants may be to exploit other men, that led philosophers beginning with Hobbes to develop the notion of the social contract as a compromise on which civilized life could be built. In this connection it is interesting to note that if instead of trying to construct an optimal solution to the problem of satisfying human wants, we were to construct an optimal solution to the problem of satisfying human needs, then a principle of justice requiring fair distribution of needed goods would be derivable without the theoretical apparatus of a social contract.

Dept. of Philosophy, McGill University and
Advanced Concepts Centre, Environment Canada

NOTES

[1] "These goals cannot be measured by the size of our bank balances. They can only be measured in the quality of the lives that our people lead." (Lyndon B. Johnson, Madison Square Garden, 31 October 1964.)

[2] See for example Robert Heilbroner, *The Prospect for Man*, New York Review of Books, January 24, 1974.

[3] *The Quality of Life Concept*, Environmental Protection Agency, Washington, 1973, p.iii.

[4] It is an interesting question, to what extent we are describing an *already-established* meaning of the expression, and to what extent we are prescribing or recommending a meaning *for future adoption*. Obviously the situation with regard to the concept of QOL is very different from the situation with regard to, say, causation or freedom, for these latter notions have a long history in the philosophical literature. On the other hand, the notion of quality of life has some intuitive content, and is very far from being a neologism like 'quark' that we can define as we will. These facts lend QOL studies a certain charm of their own.

[5] It has been suggested that we identify 'quality in the evaluative sense' with 'value'. If this suggestion is to have any merit, we must carefully distinguish the many senses in which the word 'value' is used. Since it is perfectly possible to say of a high-quality rug in a shop that it is undervalued, plainly quality cannot be identified with market or exchange value. For similar reasons, it cannot be identified with any of the following: survival, nutritional, surprise, historical, decorative, or entertainment value. Could the quality of something be identified with its 'intrinsic' value? This might seem plausible in the case of a rug, but is much less plausible in the case of air or restaurant service. Is poor quality air, air which is of low intrinsic value? What is the intrinsic value of high quality service? These questions seem impossible to answer. For this reason, it appears preferable to keep the categories of 'quality' and 'value' separate. For an excellent discussion of the notion of value, including the slippery notion of 'intrinsic' value, see Kurt Baier, 'What is Value?', in *Values and the Future* (ed. by Baier and Rescher), New York 1969, especially pp. 49–50.

[6] See Kurt Baier, 'Towards a definition of "Quality of life"', in *Environmental Spectrum* (ed. by R. O. Clark and P. C. List), New York 1974, p. 63. Baier's paper contains an excellent discussion of many issues surrounding the notions of 'quality' and of 'life', although the definition of QOL given below represents a somewhat different approach from his.

[7] Multi-criteriality gives rise to indeterminancy, since it may be impossible to say whether a restaurant that serves good food badly is of higher or lower quality than one that serves bad food well.

[8] This point is made by Baier. It is I suppose possible to attach a meaning to the ex-

pression "quality of Bob Brown's life," but this would require a separate investigation, distinct from that of the present paper.

9 John Stuart Mill, *Autobiography*, Columbia University Press, 1924, p. 100.

10 Rescher, *Welfare*, Pittsburgh 1972, pp. 62–63. I have changed Rescher's terminology from 'Consensus happiness requisites' to 'General happiness requisites,' because I think it unlikely that any consensus exists on what these requisites are. Nor do I believe that one can arrive at what they are by interviewing people and trying to obtain a consensus of their opinions.

11 Rescher calls (3) 'Hedonic mood.' The difference between hedonic mood and happiness has already been indicated.

12 Norman Bradburn and David Caplovitz, *Reports on Happiness*, Chicago 1965.

13 *The Quality of Life Concept*, Environmental Protection Agency, Washington 1973 (henceforth cited as QOL-EPA).

14 Kenneth W. Terhune, 'Probing Policy-Relevant Questions on the *Quality of Life*', QOL-EPA p. II–22.

15 Arnold Michell, Thomas J. Logothetti, and Robert E. Kantor, 'An Approach to Measuring the *Quality of Life*', QOL-EPA, p. II–37.

16 Norman C. Dalkey and Daniel L. Rourke, 'The Delphi Procedure and Rating *Quality of Life* Factors', QOL-EPA p. II–210.

17 Dorothy Walters, 'Social Intelligence and Social Policy', in *Social Indicators*, (ed. by N. A. M. Carter), The Canadian Council on Social Development, Ottawa, 1972, p. 16. In 'On Looking before Leaping', in the same volume, Gail Stewart provides some extremely perceptive criticisms of the social indicator movement.

18 *The OECD Social Indicator Development Program*, OECD, Paris, 1973, p. 12. It is of interest to note that, among the OECD member delegations, Sweden objected to the inclusion of subjective indicators and presented a formal paper on the subject. See Alan H. Portigal (ed.) *Measuring the Quality of Working Life*, Department of Labour, Ottawa, 1974, p. 46.

19 See the introductory remarks in *Social Indicators 1973*, Office of Management and Budget, Washington 1973, p. xiii, and in *Perspective Canada*, Ottawa 1974, p. xxii. Subjective indicators, which are based upon people's reported attitudes, preferences and beliefs, must be distinguished from statistics which reflect the collecting agency's judgements and values. Almost all statistics fall into the latter category: what, for example, constitutes being 'unemployed'?

20 Stanley E. Seashore, 'Job Satisfaction as an Indicator of Quality of Employment', in the Portigal volume cited above, pp. 9–38, plus discussion, pp. 39–55. Reprinted (without the discussion) in *Social Indicators Research* 1 (1974), 135–168.

21 Seashore, p. 21.

22 A. Solzhenitzyn, *One Day in the Life of Ivan Denisovitch*; Seashore, p. 53.

23 There may be problems here. What of the abnormal individual who can walk barefoot through the snow and survive on 200 calories a day? I suppose we shall have to end up talking in terms of 'typical' or 'average' human beings – convenient fictions!

24 Again, quite different opinions are expressed in the EPA volume: "QOL is viewed by many as not applying to the nation as a whole. In their view, the only way QOL could be applied at the macro-level would be by homogenizing the country, forcing everyone to accept the same value standards." (QOL-EPA p. I–11) This difficulty is avoidable by not basing the definition of QOL on value standards.

25 See Alan R. White, 'Needs and wants', *Philosophy of Education Society Proceedings*, 1974; also to appear as a chapter in White's forthcoming book, *Modal Thinking*. I am

indebted to White's paper for most of what I say about the distinction between needs and wants.

[26] To suppose otherwise, as White remarks, would be interpret "You are never here when I need you", as railing against logical necessity.

[27] It may be, of course, that what I need is to believe something. Doctors and missionaries, to be effective, need to believe that their work is worthwhile. But if so, they do not merely *believe* that they need to believe, but they *in fact* need to believe.

[28] Care is necessary in dealing with these inferences. Because my fuel tank is low, I may need to stop at the next gas station, and the next gas station may be empty, but it doesn't follow that I need to stop at an empty gas station.

[29] Rescher, *op. cit.* p. 45, cites various studies between 1939 and 1963 which indicate that Americans, by a ratio of 2 to 1 or better, regard earlier generations as happier, but at the same time reject the idea of going back.

[30] Rescher, p. 43.

[31] A. H. Maslow, *Motivation and Personality*, New York, 1954, pp. 35–47. The characterization of the various levels in the hierarchy given here derives partly from that of Mitchell, Logothetti and Kantor in QOL-EPA, p. II–46 ff., and from G. Huizinga, *Maslow's Need Hierarchy in the Work Situation*, Groningen 1970, pp. 21–24.

[32] Alex C. Michalos, 'Strategies for Reducing Information Overload in Social Reports', *Social Indicators Research* 1 (1974), 124.

[33] It is true that the security needs of those who have food already might be met, but these needs are of lesser weight than the prepotent physiological needs, and the gains in satisfying security needs might be nullified by losses in love and esteem needs.

[34] Whether the fit between limited resources and limited needs in these cases is a happy coincidence, or a matter of logic, is a question I leave to others.

6. DOES MONEY BUY SATISFACTION?

(Received 10 September, 1975)

ABSTRACT. There was no change in the distribution of satisfaction with the standard of living among Detroit area wives between 1955 and 1971, although current-dollar median family income more than doubled and constant-dollar income increased by forty per cent. Cross-sectional variation in satisfaction is, however, related to income and, in particular, to relative position in the income distribution. Whereas regressions of satisfaction on income in current or constant dollars, or the logarithm thereof, suggest that at the same income there was less satisfaction in 1971 than in 1955, there is no significant year effect in the equation using the income-position variable. Easterlin's thesis that rising levels of income do not produce rises in the average subjective estimate of welfare is supported. The thesis raises difficult questions for students of subjective social indicators.

As proponents of subjective social indicators have recognized, it is imperative to understand how persons' ratings of their own well-being relate to objective measures of their circumstances. This paper contributes an item of evidence to the issue raised by Easterlin (1973), who reported, on the basis of studies of happiness in some 19 countries, "In all societies, more money for the individual typically means more individual happiness. However, raising the incomes of all does not increase the happiness of all." In explanation of this conclusion Easterlin observed that "Individuals assess their material well-being, not in terms of the absolute amount of goods they have, but relative to a social norm of what goods they ought to have." That the norm itself evolves has been documented by Rainwater (1974), who cited results of 18 Gallup Poll surveys, taken in the United States between 1946 and 1969, that asked the question, "What is the smallest amount of money a family of four needs to get along in this community?" According to Rainwater's figures, this amount, expressed in constant (1971) dollars, increased by a factor of 1.36 between 1954 and 1969 (about the same time period studied in this paper).

Whereas Easterlin's material relates to self-assessments of overall personal happiness and the data cited from Rainwater pertain to a hypothetical question about the income needed to maintain a minimum level of living, the data presented here concern ratings of the individual's

Alex C. Michalos (ed.), Citation Classics from Social Indicators Research, 137–144.
© 2005 *Springer. Printed in the Netherlands.*

own satisfaction or dissatisfaction specifically with her actual standard of living. The question used to elicit ratings of satisfaction, first asked of a sample of Detroit metropolitan area wives in 1955 (Blood and Wolfe, 1960), reads as follows:

Here is a card that lists some feelings you might have about certain aspects of marriage. Could you tell me the statement that best describes how you feel about each of the following? – For example, how do you feel about your standard of living... the kind of house, clothes, car, and so forth?
1. Pretty disappointed – I'm really missing out on that.
2. It would be nice to have more.
3. It's all right, I guess – I can't complain.
4. Quite satisfied – I'm lucky the way it is.
5. Enthusiastic – it couldn't be better.

(The remaining parts of the question, not considered here, asked about satisfaction with "understanding," "love and affection," and "companionship." The rating of the standard of living preceded these other items.) The same question was asked of a comparable sample of Detroit area wives in 1971 (Duncan, Schuman, and Duncan, 1973). The response distributions obtained in the two surveys are shown in Table I.

These data are consistent with the supposition that no aggregate change in satisfaction with the standard of living occurred over the 16-year period. The likelihood-ratio chi-square statistic for testing the hypothesis

TABLE I

Satisfaction of wives with the standard of living, Detroit area, 1955 and 1971

... how you feel about ... your standard of living – the kind of house, clothes, and so forth	Per cent distribution	
	1955	1971
(0) Pretty disappointed	2.6	1.3
(1) It would be nice to have more	19.2	20.0
(2) It's all right, I guess	18.4	16.0
(3) Quite satisfied	54.6	56.3
(4) Enthusiastic	5.2	6.3
	100.0	100.0
	(N=692)	(N=630)

Source: Detroit Area Study.

of independence of response and year is $X^2 = 5.6$, d.f. $= 4$, $P = .24$. Moreover, the portion of this chi-square value due to trend over the five satisfaction categories is $X^2 = 1.7$, d.f. $= 1$, $P = .19$, a similarly nonsignificant value. (See Simon, 1974, for the test used here.) Or, if we

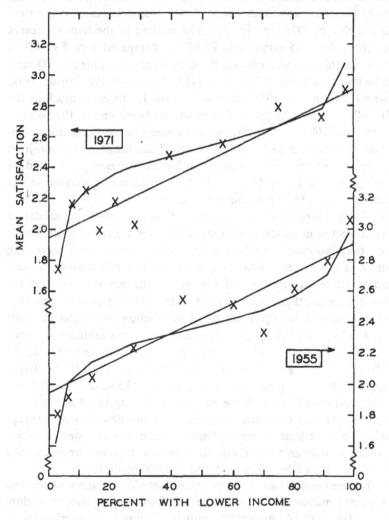

Fig. 1. Regression of satisfaction with standard of living on log of constant-dollar income (curved line) and on position in income distribution (straight line).

assign to the response categories the scores shown in parentheses in Table I, we find that the mean satisfaction score was 2.47 in 1971 and 2.41 in 1955; the difference of .06 produces a t-statistic of 1.20, $P=.23$, again a nonsignificant value.

This result is emphasized because data on income collected from the same respondents leave little doubt that material levels of living were in fact higher in 1971 than in 1955. The median of the family incomes reported in the 1955 survey was $5,827 as compared with $12,407 in 1971. Over this period, however, the consumer price index for Detroit (1967=100) rose from 82.2 to 121.7 (U.S. Bureau of the Census, 1974, Table 667); hence the 1955 dollar was worth 1.5 times as much as the 1971 dollar. Expressing the 1955 median family income in 1971 dollars we obtain $8,740, so that the median income in constant dollars increased by a factor of 1.42 over this period. Thus, the second proposition in Easterlin's conclusion is strongly confirmed: increasing the standard of living in 'real' terms does not lead to a subjective increase in the standard of living for the population as a whole.

We also find support for his first proposition, and, in a sense, validation of the subjective indicator, in the data depicted in Figure 1, which clearly shows that individual satisfaction typically increases with increasing incomes *in cross-section data*. In quantifying this relationship, we can entertain alternative methods of scaling the income variable, and the differences among them turn out to be instructive. Let us note, first, that the data points in the figure are mean satisfaction scores (on the scale 0, ..., 4 defined in Table I) for respondents in various arbitrary intervals of dollar income. The original data provide $1,000 intervals up to $8,000 in 1956 and $10,000 in 1971 and broader intervals for the larger incomes, with the open-end interval being $15,000 and over in 1955 and $25,000 and over in 1971. Some intervals were combined at the lower end of the scale so that each point on the figure describes the average satisfaction of at least 22 respondents. Income intervals were assigned the values of their midpoints, and the open-end intervals were assumed to have the values $24,000 in 1955 and $44,000 in 1971.

With these conventions, we may regress satisfaction score on income or a transformation thereof, using the ordinary least squares procedure and the test statistics associated with it. Estimates of coefficients in alternatively specified regression models are shown in Table II. We can quickly dismiss the models using dollar values, whether current or constant, i.e., Equations (2) and (4). These equations do not provide an adequate fit to the observed mean satisfaction scores, as shown by the fact that Equation (7) provides a significantly better fit. The fit is substantially improved by taking the logarithm of income, as in Equations (3) and (5). In using Equation (3), that is, using the logarithm of income in current dollars, we find that the equation must include a substantial negative year effect. At the same (current dollar) income, the 1971 respondent is substantially less satisfied, on the average, than her 1955 counterpart. Even after the adjustment for price change, as in Equation (5), the log-income specification leads to a negative estimate of the year effect. With a t-ratio of 1.61 ($P=.11$), this effect is not quite significant by the usual standard. Nevertheless, its occurrence provides motivation to investigate still a different transformation of the income variable.

TABLE II

Regressions of satisfaction on family income and year (with t-statistics in parentheses)

Equation	Definition of income variable	Intercept	Coefficient of – Income	Year	R^2
(1)	...	2.41	...	.059 (1.20)	.0010
(2)	Current dollars in 1,000's	2.17	.0340 (9.00)	−.189 (−3.30)	.0597
(3)	Log (base 10) of the above	1.63	1.03 (11.0)	−.263 (−4.56)	.0858
(4)	1971 dollars in 1,000's	2.08	.0317 (9.46)	−.064 (−1.23)	.0655
(5)	Log (base 10) of the above	1.44	1.03 (11.0)	−.082 (−1.61)	.0858
(6)	Per cent of families with lower income	1.93	.0095 (11.0)	.058 (1.19)	.0859
(7)	10 intervals for 1955 and 11 for 1971	...	...	...	.1030[a]

[a] Significantly larger, $F(18, 1301) \geqslant 1.6$, than R^2 for Equations (2) and (4) but not for Equations (3), (5), and (6).

In Equation (6) we substitute for income or its logarithm the position of the respondent in the income distribution. Here, the regressor is the percentage of wives in the sample (for each year) whose income is below the midpoint of the income interval in which the respondent falls (estimating that half the respondents within that interval fall below the midpoint). The measure of income, having been made completely relative, is one that cannot change over time in regard to its average or its distribution. It does, of course, describe variation between individuals at a point in time, although it transforms the scale along which that variation occurs. We find that Equation (6) fits as well as any of the other equations, if not better. The estimated year effect in this equation is necessarily the same (rounding errors and the like aside) as the estimate of gross change in the distribution of responses mentioned earlier and repeated as Equation (1). In Equation (6) as in Equation (1) the year effect is not significant.

Equations (5) and (6), then, are the two leading contenders. I know of no formal statistical test that could tell us that one should be preferred to the other. The difference between the R^2 statistics may seem trivial. It should be noted, however, that the upper bound of R^2 for any regression model is the value given for Equation (7). Moreover, if we delete the year effect from each equation, the R^2 for log of constant dollar income alone is .0840 and for the relative income measure alone it is .0850. Hence, the two variables do differ in regard to explained variation by almost one per cent of the explainable variation. (Incidentally, it is the practice of some researchers to report, not the R^2 values as given in Table II, but those values divided by the R^2 for Equation (7). Even though this enables them to take some satisfaction in high coefficients of determination, it would not change the facts of the present case, which include the fact that about 90% of variation in satisfaction scores occurs for respondents with the same income and only 10% is associated with differences between respondents in income.)

Comparison of the two equations may be facilitated by Figure 1. The straight line is the regression of satisfaction on position in the income distribution (ignoring year effect): $\hat{Y}=1.96+.0095\,X_6$. The curved line, while it plots values obtained from the linear regression of satisfaction on log of constant-dollar income ($\hat{Y}=1.44+.988\,X_5$), reveals the nature of the nonlinear transformation of income represented by X_6. (In fact, if the income distributions in these samples were exactly described by the lognormal distribution, we could straighten out the curves by applying the normal probability transformation to the percentages on the horizontal axis. But the proportions in the upper and lower tails of these distributions depart fairly markedly from those required to fit the lognormal.) Adoption of Equation (5), represented by the curved regression in the figure, would require comment on the cluster of three points, corresponding to percentages 16 through 28 (or incomes of $7,000 to $10,000), that fall well below the 1971 curve. A separate analysis, not reported here, does suggest that these points would have to be regarded as significant outliers from the point of view of Equation (5). Using Equation (6), however, they seem like part of the random scatter around the regression line.

Equation (6) is attractive as a model, therefore, because it fits well in the cross-section and because it does not require us to impute a downward net shift in satisfaction in the face of the observed gross stability of the satisfaction distribution. Of course, a model like Equation (6) cannot in principle explain a temporal shift in satisfaction, but that can be to its advantage if there is no such shift to explain.

If one is disposed to accept Equation (6) on these or other grounds, then a corollary must be accepted too: the relevant source of satisfaction with one's standard of living is having more income than someone else, not just having more income. And satisfaction measures as such cannot tell us whether a population with a higher average income is really 'better off' than a population with a lower one.

The same principle might be found to apply in other "domains of perceived life quality" (Andrews and Withey, 1974) besides the material level of living. To find out if this is so, we shall have to make overtime comparisons of comparable samples from the same population (whether 'same' is understood geographically or conceptually may become an awkward question) and employ not only absolute measures of the objective factors affecting perceptions of life quality but also measures of relative position in the cross-sectional distributions of those factors. It may even be necessary to develop an 'expectations index' for purposes of statistical deflation of subjective measures, much as we now use the consumer price index for a similar purpose.

ACKNOWLEDGMENTS

This paper is a report from a project on analysis of social trends supported by the Russell Sage Foundation. James A. McRae, Jr., and Bruce C. Rognlie assisted with computations.

Department of Sociology,
University of Arizona

BIBLIOGRAPHY

Andrews, F. M. and Withey, S. B., 'Developing Measures of Perceived Life Quality: Results from Several National Surveys', *Social Indicators Research* **1** (1974), 1–26.
Blood, R. O., Jr. and Wolfe, D. M., *Husbands and Wives*, Free Press, New York, 1960.
Duncan, O. D., Schuman, H., and Duncan, B., *Social Change in a Metropolitan Community*, Russell Sage Foundation, New York, 1973.
Easterlin, R. A., 'Does Money Buy Happiness?', *The Public Interest* **30** (1973), 3–10.
Easterlin, R. A., 'Does Economic Growth Improve the Human Lot? Some Empirical Evidence', in P. A. David and M. W. Reder (eds.), *Nations and Households in Economic Growth*, Academic Press, New York, 1974.
Rainwater, L., *What Money Buys*, Basic Books, New York, 1974.
Simon, G., 'Alternative Analyses for the Singly-Ordered Contingency Table', *Journal of the American Statistical Association* **69** (1974), 971–976.
U.S. Bureau of the Census, *Statistical Abstract of the United States: 1974* (95th ed.), U.S. Government Printing Office, Washington, D.C., 1974.

7. ON THE MULTIVARIATE STRUCTURE
OF WELLBEING

(Received 26 September, 1975)

Abstract. A mapping sentence is provided for defining the universe of observations of wellbeing. According to this, assessment of wellbeing is attitudinal. Data from several studies verify that the First Law of Attitude holds for wellbeing. These data also show the structure of the interrelationships among the variables to be that of intermeshing cylindrexes, in an SSA space of four dimensions. Areas of life play the role of polarizing facets, while self-versus-community and situation-versus-treatment serve as axial facets. Modulating facets include primary-to-secondary interaction, and generality-to-specificity.

1. INTRODUCTION

The concept of 'wellbeing' is widespread, but not technically defined in the social science literature. For example, it does not appear in English and English's (1958) *A Comprehensive Dictionary of Psychological and Psychoanalytical Terms* nor in the *International Encyclopedia of the Social Sciences* (1968). A description of the concept has been recently attempted by Andrews (1974, p. 280): "Wellbeing is broadly conceived to mean the 'level' of life quality – i.e., the extent to which pleasure and satisfaction characterize human existence and the extent to which people can avoid the various miseries which are potentially the lot of each of us".

Andrews' discussion is similar to that previously made by Bradburn and Caplovitz (1965, p. 1), where they make an explicit avowal of lack of definition: "The underlying assumption of this research is that there is a dimension variously called mental health, subjective adjustment, happiness, or psychological well-being, and that individuals can be meaningfully described as being relatively high or low on such a dimension. At present there is neither a generally agreed upon name for this dimension nor agreement as to the appropriate methods of deciding where a particular individual should be placed on it."

Psychological wellbeing may be regarded as an aspect of mental health, but this does not help clarify the definitional problem, since 'mental

Alex C. Michalos (ed.), Citation Classics from Social Indicators Research, 145–172.
© 2005 *Springer. Printed in the Netherlands.*

health' itself has no agreed-on definition (Jahoda, 1958). Furthermore, there are varieties of wellbeing other than psychological. Indeed, in related work, Allardt (1973, p. 1) emphasizes that the problem is not unidimensional: "Welfare is conceived as a multidimensional phenomenon composed of several dimensions of values" (p. 1).

Lack of a basic definition impedes both empirical research and theory development in any area, and this appears to have been true regarding 'wellbeing'. A proper definition here evidently must allow for multidimensionality. In the present paper we shall propose a formal definition for the universe of wellbeing items, and report on empirical multivariate research guided by this definition. We hope this will stimulate further systematic research in the area, and thus help fill an important lacuna in the social science literature.

In effect, we shall present a partial theory for the structure of intercorrelations among the varieties of wellbeing. By 'theory' we mean 'an hypothesis of a correspondence between a definitional system for a universe of observations and an aspect of the empirical structure of those observations, together with a rationale for such an hypothesis' (Gratch, 1973, p. 35). The aspect of the empirical observations on which we shall focus is the correlation matrix for wellbeing items for a population at a single point of time. (For an example of a dynamic theory – over several points of time – on a related topic, see Guttman and Levy, 1975.) The two sample correlation matrices which will serve as our main empirical data are given in Tables I and II below.

A clear framework for research on wellbeing, and the conduct of cumulative research made possible thereby, are especially important for the growing field of social problem indicators. The present development stems from our previous work on such indicators (Guttman, 1971; Guttman and Levy, 1975; Levy, 1976), and is part of current work on this broader topic. The empirical data come from the Continuing Survey (of the Israel urban adult population), conducted jointly by the Israel Institute of Applied Social Research and the Communications Institute of the Hebrew University. Two surveys – spring and summer of 1973 – provide the data for our main analysis. Further partial replication comes from data of a previous survey of spring 1971, as well as from some U.S. data of spring 1971.

2. DEFINITION OF THE UNIVERSE OF WELLBEING ITEMS

A preliminary definition for 'wellbeing' that may serve as a useful point of departure for social research is that given under 'welfare' in the *Concise Oxford Dictionary*:

Welfare. Satisfactory state, health and prosperity, wellbeing (usually of person, society, etc.; or with *my* etc.).

For the purposes of theory construction and research design, it has been found useful to define concepts through the universe of items with which the theory is concerned (Gratch, 1973; esp. pp. 36–7). This requires specifying facets both for the *domain* (question part) and the *range* (possible answers) of the items. The Oxford Dictionary definition implies at least two facets for the domain of the universe of items of wellbeing, as well as a common range for the items of this universe.

One facet for the domain is the subject whose wellbeing is being studied: an individual or a group. A second facet is the area of life in which the wellbeing is assessed: health, economic prosperity, and others.

The range implied by the definition is from 'very satisfactory' to 'very unsatisfactory'. We understand the concept of 'satisfactory' here to be normative. Accordingly, a further facet that may be considered is the referent who establishes the norm: the individual himself, his group, or some other individual or some other group (compare the definition of 'social problem' items in Guttman, 1971, pp. 45–6).

Clearly, the level of wellbeing of an individual or of a group may vary from one area of life to another – and within areas of life. As does any universe of items, that for wellbeing generates a multivariate distribution when observed for a given population. Different varieties of wellbeing items can have different sizes of correlations among themselves for the same population. Hence, it is of interest to ascertain the structure of interrelations among varieties of wellbeing: how do the differential correlations relate to the definitional system? Such an investigation is the main purpose of the present paper. We shall propose a theory for the structure of wellbeing and test it with empirical data.

The definitional system for wellbeing observations that we shall adopt is in terms of *facets*. Some of the facets have been mentioned above; the others were suggested in the course of designing actual items for the fieldwork.

3. THE UNIVERSE OF OBSERVATIONS

Defining a universe of *observations* requires specifying both the universe of items (content) and the population to be observed. The universe of items will be formally defined as follows:

An item belongs to the universe of wellbeing items if and only if its domain asks for $\left(\begin{array}{l}\text{cognitive}\\\text{affective}\\\text{instrumental}\end{array}\right)$ assessment of the $\left(\begin{array}{l}\text{level}\\\text{treatment}\end{array}\right)$ of the state of a social group in some life area, and the range is ordered from 'very satisfactory' to 'very unsatisfactory' according to the normative criterion of the respondent for that area of life.

As already noted, norms may vary from respondent to respondent. Generally, it is of interest to establish typologies of respondents by their norms. In the present study, it is assumed all respondents have essentially the same wellbeing norms on the life areas studied.

The population studied is that of adult Jews (20 years of age and over) residing in the larger cities of Israel: Jerusalem, Tel Aviv, Haifa, and Beersheva. The intention of the theory, of course, is to hold for any such social group in any country. Our main analysis is of the wellbeing items that were part of the spring and summer trimesters of 1973 of the Continuing Survey. The population samples consisted of 1940 respondents in the spring and 1830 in the summer, each of whom was interviewed in his home. As already remarked, supplementary data from an earlier trimester, and from the U.S., serve as partial replications for confirmation of the theory.

4. THE MAPPING SENTENCE FOR THE OBSERVATIONS

Observations are made by mapping the population into the categories of the items. Hence, design of observations implies design of the empirical mapping. A useful technique for expressing the design is that of the *mapping sentence*. This incorporates both the universe of items – such as defined above for 'wellbeing' – and the population studied.

Theory construction and development are facilitated by judicious construction of mapping sentences for the observations which are the concern of the theory. (For a general discussion of mapping sentences see Levy, 1976; also Elizur, 1970; Kernberg, *et al.*, 1972.) To this end, an optimal refinement of the facet design is sought. Our proposed mapping sentence for the observations on wellbeing is exhibited below. It contains more explicit facets than given above for the general definition for the universe of 'wellbeing' items.

Facets A and B appear in the item definition above, element a_2 indicat-

The Mapping Sentence

A

The $\begin{pmatrix} a_1 \text{ cognitive} \\ a_2 \text{ affective} \end{pmatrix}$ assessment by respondent (x) of the

B

$\begin{pmatrix} b_1 \text{ state of} \\ b_2 \text{ government's treatment for} \end{pmatrix}$ the wellbeing of his social (reference)

C $\qquad\qquad\qquad\qquad\qquad\qquad\qquad$ D

group $\begin{cases} c_1 \text{ self} \\ c_2 \text{ government} \\ c_3 \text{ State} \\ c_4 \text{ institution} \\ c_5 \text{ new immigrants} \\ c_6 \text{ poor} \\ c_7 \text{ other individuals} \\ c_8 \text{ on the whole} \end{cases}$ with respect to its $\begin{cases} d_1 \text{ primary internal} \\ d_2 \text{ primary social} \\ d_3 \text{ primary resource} \\ d_4 \text{ neighborhood} \\ d_5 \text{ town} \\ d_6 \text{ State} \\ d_7 \text{ World} \end{cases}$ secondary

E

environment, concerning a $\begin{Bmatrix} e_1 \text{ general} \\ e_2 \text{ specific} \end{Bmatrix}$ aspect of life area

F

$\begin{cases} f_1 \text{ recreation} \\ f_2 \text{ family} \\ f_3 \text{ on the whole} \\ f_4 \text{ security} \\ f_5 \text{ health} \\ f_6 \text{ economic} \\ f_7 \text{ education} \\ f_8 \text{ religion} \\ f_9 \text{ society} \\ f_{10} \text{ immigration} \\ f_{11} \text{ work} \\ f_{12} \text{ information} \\ f_{13} \text{ communication} \end{cases}$ according to his normative criterion for that life area

$\rightarrow \begin{pmatrix} \text{very satisfactory} \\ \text{to} \\ \text{very unsatisfactory} \end{pmatrix}$ in the sense of the element from facet B.

ing further who is administering the treatment. The further facets help delimit the subuniverse of wellbeing sampled in the present study.

The state or treatment is that of a certain group in a certain environmental framework. Accordingly, facet C classifies groups, and facet D environmental frameworks. For example, a respondent may evaluate his own state of wellbeing in terms of his internal primary environment (his mood, happiness, etc.) or his secondary environment (e.g. satisfaction from life in his town). Similarly, he may estimate the wellbeing of other social groups (new immigrants, the State, etc.) (To distinguish the political 'State' from 'state' meaning 'situation', the former is written throughout this paper with a capital 'S'.)

In this research, environmental facet D is treated as an ordered facet. The elements are ranked in terms of 'distance' from the respondent himself. For example the 'State' is defined to be a secondary framework for 'self' (of the respondent), and is more distant from 'self' than is a primary environment such as mood.

Facets E and F list the life areas for the various kinds of wellbeing. Facet F specifies the life area itself (family, recreation, economics, residence, etc.), and Facet E specifies whether assessment is being made for the life area as a whole or for some particular aspect of it (e.g. economic problems of the State vis-à-vis the particular economic problem of the poor).

The spring study contains a sample of 24 items from this universe of content. These are listed in the following table, along with the structuples which show how each fits into the Cartesian set $ABCDEF$ defined by the six facets. For example, question 3 has been assigned the structuple $a_1 b_1 c_1 d_2 e_1 f_2$. This means that the first struct, a_1, of this structuple is the first element of facet A, namely 'cognitive'. The second struct is b_1, indicating that it is the *state* of wellbeing being assessed. Indeed, all of the first twelve questions have the struct b_1; each of these deals with a state of wellbeing. The remaining questions include some with the struct b_1 and some with the struct b_2, the latter assessing *treatment*.

For convenience, we have included 'self' in the list of social groups; it is a group consisting of only one person. Question 3 has c_1 as its struct from facet C, since that question deals with the wellbeing of the respondent's self. The next struct, d_2, indicates that the primary social environment of c_1 is involved in the assessment. The last two structs, $e_1 f_2$, show that the family life area in general is being assessed.

The structuples for the other questions have parallel interpretations. Spelling out the whole Cartesian set $ABCDEF$ would provide a listing of some 5824 structuples ($2 \times 2 \times 8 \times 7 \times 2 \times 13$). To include one question of each kind in the study would require asking 5824 questions of each respondent. The necessity for selecting only a sample of questions for this study is apparent, as in most research projects which are well designed. No strictly systematic sampling design was attempted in the selection of the present 24 items; it was endeavored to have each life area represented, with about half the items dealing with 'state' and the other half with 'treatment'. Some further distinctions were between cognitive and affective assessments, and between personal wellbeing and that of the State as a whole.

The questions were put in closed form to the respondents: the categories of the ranges are indicated in the following table. In each case there are from four to five categories, and each range is ordered normatively from 'very satisfactory' to 'very unsatisfactory'.

List of Questions and their Structuples
Spring 1973 Survey

Question number	Contents	Structuple [a]
1	Generally speaking, are you happy these days? (very happy... very unhappy)	$a_2 b_1 c_1 d_1 e_1 f_3$
2	How is your mood these days? (very good all the time... not good almost all the time)	$a_2 b_1 c_1 d_1 e_1 f_4$
3	In general, how do you evaluate your family life? (very good... very bad)	$a_1 b_1 c_1 d_2 e_1 f_2$
4	In general are you satisfied with the way you spend your leisure time? (very satisfied... not at all satisfied)	$a_2 b_1 c_1 d_2 e_1 f_1$
5	In general, how do you evaluate your health these days? (very good... not at all good)	$a_1 b_1 c_1 d_3 e_1 f_4$
6	Is your family income today sufficient? (definitely sufficient... insufficient)	$a_1 b_1 c_1 d_3 e_1 f_6$
7	Are you satisfied with your education level? (very satisfied... very unsatisfied)	$a_2 b_1 c_1 d_3 e_1 f_7$

[a] Definition of the structs in the structuples is given in the mapping sentence above. The structs of the structuples here are elements of the facets in the mapping sentence.

List of Questions (continued)

Question number	Contents	Structuple
8	In general, are you satisfied with the apartment you live in? (very satisfied... very unsatisfied)	$a_2b_1c_1d_3e_1f_1$
9	In general, how do you evaluate the neighborhood you live in? (very good... not at all good)	$a_1b_1c_1d_4e_1f_1$
10	In general, are you satisfied with life in *your town* these days? (very satisfied... not at all satisfied)	$a_2b_1c_1d_5e_1f_1$
11	Do you want very much to continue living in this town? (definitely yes... definitely no)	$a_1b_1c_1d_5e_2f_1$
12	Do you want very much to move to another town? (definitely no... definitely yes)	$a_1b_1c_1d_5e_2f_1$
13	In general, how do you evaluate the current situation in the country with respect to work relations between employers and employees? (very good... not at all good)	$a_1b_1c_3d_6e_1f_{11}$
14	Do you think that now the relations between new immigrants and veterans are good? (very good... not at all good)	$a_1b_1c_3d_6e_2f_9$
15	When you watch Israeli TV, in general to what extent are you satisfied with the programs? (very satisfied... very unsatisfied)	$a_2b_1c_3d_6e_2f_{13}$
16	In general, how do you evaluate the existing situation in your (or your spouse's) place of work with respect to work relations between employees and employers? (very good... not at all good)	$a_1b_1c_1d_2e_1f_1$
17	In general, what in your opinion is the condition of new immigrants in the past 12 months? (very good... not at all good)	$a_1b_1c_5d_6e_1f_{10}$
18	What is your opinion of the way the government handles economic problems of the country? (very good... not at all good)	$a_1b_2c_2d_6e_1f_6$
19	Do you think the government is doing enough these days to explain its decisions? (very much... almost nothing)	$a_1b_2c_2d_6e_1f_{12}$
20	Are you satisfied with the way the government handles strikes? (very satisfied... not at all satisfied)	$a_2b_2c_2d_6e_2f_{11}$
21	Are you satisfied with the way the Histadrut handles strikes? (very satisfied... not at all satisfied)	$a_2b_2c_4d_6e_2f_{11}$

List of Questions (continued)

Question number	Contents	Structuple
22	What is your opinion of the way the authorities handle immigration problems? (very successfully... not at all successfully)	$a_1b_2c_2d_6e_2f_{10}$
23	In your opinion, is the government doing enough for the economically deprived to improve their condition? (much more than is necessary... much less than necessary)	$a_1b_2c_6d_6e_2f_9$
24	To what extent are you satisfied with the way the government handles problems related to terrorist activities against Israelis abroad? (very satisfied... not at all satisfied)	$a_2b_2c_2d_7e_2f_6$

The summer study contains a sample of 22 items which are also classified by the mapping sentence. Details will be omitted, but reference is made in appropriate places below on how the empirical findings replicate those of the spring survey.

5. ASSESSMENT OF WELLBEING IS ATTITUDINAL

The formal faceted definition above implies that the universe of wellbeing items is a subuniverse of attitudinal items: *all wellbeing items are attitudinal*. To prove this proposition, let us consider Guttman's definition of the universe of attitudinal items (Gratch, 1973, p. 36):

An item belongs to the universe of attitude items if and only if its domain asks about behavior in a $\begin{pmatrix} \text{cognitive} \\ \text{affective} \\ \text{instrumental} \end{pmatrix}$ modality toward an object, and its range is ordered from $\begin{pmatrix} \text{very positive} \\ \text{to} \\ \text{very negative} \end{pmatrix}$ towards that object.

The domain of wellbeing items does contain the facet of the three modalities of behavior toward an object. Furthermore, the wellbeing range of 'very satisfactory' to 'very unsatisfactory' is a special case of the attitudinal range 'very positive' to 'very negative'. Thus, each wellbeing item has its domain and its range conform to those necessary and sufficient for attitudinal items, which was to be shown.

It follows that general propositions about attitudes should hold in particular for assessment of wellbeing. We shall see that this is so for our data.

6. 'STATE OF SELF' AND 'GOVERNMENT'S TREATMENT' AS OBJECTS OF ASSESSMENT

An important point to be clarified is the nature of the *object* of the attitude for the case of wellbeing. What is it that is being assessed from positive to negative? This is a profound type of question which is basic to theory construction for attitudes. As the following discussion will show, the object need not always be 'obvious'; the discussion will illustrate a strategy to help pin down the object.

Technically, what is being immediately assessed is the domain of each variable in the observed set. In the present case, each domain is defined by a structuple of six structs-one from each of the six content facets. However, one or more of these facets may be specified to define the objects of the attitudes, and the others to be modifiers of these objects. The differential roles of the facets should have implications for the structure of the intercorrelations of the variables defined by them.

Inspection of the mapping sentence suggests that facet E is a modifier of facet F, facet F is a modifier of facet D and facet D is a modifier of facet C. Hence none of facets D, E, and F appears to be that of objects of the attitude; they are modifiers of the objects. Facet A modifies the act of assessment and hence also is not a candidate for being the object of the assessment. This leaves facets B and C for consideration.

Facet C presents a variety of social groups to which we have added the label 'reference' for one's self. This allows for the alternative variety of social groups which one does *not* consider to be his references, but which are not part of the present project. We interpret the concept of reference group here to be that of 'one's greater self', so that 'his social reference group' can be regarded as a collective noun. Accordingly, one kind of object can be specified to be the (wellbeing) state of one's greater self. This is being rated from high to low under the various qualifications made by facets C, D, E, and F. The specification of this collective object is made by the first element of facet B, together with the collective title of facet C.

Element b_2 here is more complicated than b_1. Treatment has at least three major facets of its own: treater, type of treatment, and treated. In the present study, only one treater was asked about – namely the government. Types of treatment were not differentiated. The treated are again enumerated by facet C. Hence the mapping sentence above condensed the treaters and treatments into the one element b_2: 'government's (unspecified) treatment', and the object being assessed can be specified by b_2 and the collective title of facet C.

Were the government part of each respondent's greater self – all Israelis identify with the government – then the two varieties of objects associated with b_1 and b_2 could be regarded as subvarieties of a single object again: one's greater self.

However, since we cannot assume such identification *a priori*, we regard the varieties as distinct from each other. This distinction is expressed by having the range of the mapping sentence refer back to facet B. Had we but a single collective object, the range would be with respect to this object and would not need qualification by a particular facet.

The fact that at least two distinct kinds of objects are involved in this wellbeing research turns out to have important implications for the structure of the observed correlation matrices.

Let us now go on to explore what kinds of empirical lawfulness hold within 'state' items and within 'treatment' items, as well as between both kinds of items, for the given population of respondents.

7. WELLBEING AND THE FIRST LAW OF ATTITUDE

In discussing the structure of interrelations among a set of variables, a first question that may be asked concerns the signs of the correlations. Are the regressions monotone? If so, are the correlations of one sign or are they not? It must be recognized, of course, that the question of sign of a correlation is meaningful only if the meaning of direction is specified in advance. The range of the mapping sentence serves this purpose of specifying a common direction *a priori* for each variety of object (b_1 and b_2). The ranges of the items have the common notion of discrepancy from a norm: 'more satisfactory' to 'less satisfactory'. Given a monotone relationship between two variables for the population being studied, a positive correlation means that respondents who give replies that are more 'satisfactory' on one variable tend to give more 'satisfactory' replies on the other. Study of the bivariate regressions between the 24 items showed that they are indeed monotone. The monotonicity coefficients of the items are presented in the matrix below.

Having a common range for a subset of items leads to the possibility

TABLE I

Interrelationships among 24 wellbeing variables (monotonicity coefficients) Spring 1973 survey

#	Variable	1	2	3	4	5	6	7	8	9	10	11	12	13	14	15	16	17	18	19	20	21	22	23	24
1.	Happiness	—	77	66	55	56	35	26	30	28	45	23	14	06	06	02	23	07	11	—00	01	—03	07	09	09
2.	Mood	77	—	51	51	60	35	31	26	26	36	12	05	03	03	—08	26	—07	11	—07	—04	—07	—04	05	04
3.	Good family life	66	51	—	49	44	32	27	35	34	38	26	24	01	—00	—00	22	02	—01	—08	—14	—10	04	02	—05
4.	Satisfied with leisure	55	51	49	—	38	39	42	38	29	37	27	29	16	11	09	24	—03	10	05	06	—02	04	10	08
5.	Good health	56	60	44	38	—	28	25	17	23	20	03	—02	—07	—05	00	26	—09	—03	—10	—05	—04	—17	—01	—02
6.	Sufficient income	35	35	32	39	28	—	28	26	22	32	32	24	23	17	15	18	—20	05	—03	—06	—17	—02	16	—04
7.	Satisfied with education	26	31	27	42	25	28	—	33	59	55	41	37	06	08	08	14	—10	17	10	16	06	05	16	10
8.	Satisfied with apartment	30	26	35	38	17	26	33	—	59	38	29	29	06	14	07	14	—11	06	06	—05	—08	19	19	08
9.	Good neighborhood	28	26	34	29	23	22	59	59	—	55	55	41	11	17	03	15	—07	10	04	01	19	09	08	09
10.	Satisfied with life in town	45	36	38	37	20	32	55	38	55	—	70	64	23	08	15	28	06	27	21	19	16	13	17	10
11.	Want continue live in town	23	12	26	27	03	32	41	29	55	70	—	88	12	16	08	28	07	16	15	13	08	08	08	07
12.	Not to move to another town	14	05	24	29	—02	24	37	29	41	64	88	—	06	10	16	22	04	05	07	08	10	05	05	05
13.	Good labor rel. in country	06	03	01	16	—07	23	06	06	11	23	12	06	—	34	17	31	07	39	33	47	45	25	24	04
14.	Immigrants-veterans relations	06	03	—00	11	—05	17	08	14	17	08	16	10	34	—	17	18	17	30	29	29	19	33	32	19
15.	Satisfied with tv programs	02	—08	—00	09	00	15	08	07	03	15	08	16	17	17	—	—05	—05	32	29	33	32	12	17	13
16.	Good labor rel. at work	23	26	22	24	26	18	14	14	15	28	28	22	31	18	—05	—	—05	22	04	15	04	10	10	10
17.	Immigrants' condition good	07	—07	02	—03	—09	—20	—10	—11	—07	06	07	04	07	17	—05	—05	—	03	—03	15	13	42	—00	10
18.	Gov. handling economic prob.	11	11	—01	10	—03	05	17	06	10	27	16	05	39	30	32	22	03	—	53	54	44	37	42	20
19.	Gov. explains its decisions	—00	—07	—08	05	—10	—03	10	06	04	21	15	07	33	29	29	04	—03	53	—	44	38	37	40	13
20.	Gov. handles strikes	01	—04	—14	06	—05	—06	16	—05	01	19	13	08	47	29	33	15	15	54	44	—	84	43	32	22
21.	Histadrut handles strikes	—03	—07	—10	—02	—04	—17	06	—08	19	16	08	10	45	19	32	04	13	44	38	84	—	35	22	15
22.	Gov. handles immigration	07	—04	04	04	—17	—02	05	19	09	13	08	05	25	33	12	10	42	37	37	43	35	—	18	18
23.	Gov. helps deprived	09	05	02	10	—01	16	16	19	08	17	08	05	24	32	17	02	—00	42	40	32	22	18	—	17
24.	Gov. handles terrorism abroad	09	04	—05	08	—02	—04	10	08	09	10	07	05	04	19	13	10	10	20	13	22	15	18	17	—

TABLE II

Interrelationships among 22 wellbeing variables (monotonicity coefficients) Summer 1973 survey

	1	2	3	4	5	6	7	8	9	10	11	12	13	14	15	16	17	18	19	20	21	22
1. Happiness	—	71	43	36	54	29	23	49	29	21	14	19	22	06	20	36	12	08	09	13	15	20
2. Mood	71	—	34	40	60	34	25	48	31	23	10	15	12	-07	25	39	07	08	10	04	20	12
3. Satisfied with social group	43	34	—	54	29	21	06	38	21	24	12	14	15	12	10	14	19	17	19	16	31	22
4. Success in acquiring friends	36	40	54	—	36	22	23	32	45	18	02	05	10	-04	20	15	-01	17	25	02	17	00
5. Health condition	54	60	29	36	—	34	24	41	37	36	01	-04	07	-10	27	12	-01	-01	25	05	14	-06
6. Sufficient income	29	34	21	22	34	—	65	35	21	28	-01	27	07	-02	09	19	06	05	03	05	17	22
7. Able to save	23	25	06	23	24	65	—	29	12	11	08	20	01	-04	03	13	10	04	-13	04	11	25
8. Satisfied with work	49	48	38	32	41	35	29	—	52	28	15	14	14	08	08	24	11	04	14	11	27	13
9. Success in performing job	29	31	21	45	37	21	12	52	—	17	09	07	14	-01	16	18	-00	-10	22	08	09	-04
10. Safe to walk at night	21	23	24	18	36	28	11	28	17	—	08	-06	04	-00	30	20	-13	-05	16	03	12	-08
11. Employer-worker relations	14	10	12	02	01	-01	08	15	09	-08	—	39	39	42	-01	37	45	51	15	30	30	48
12. Satisfied with economic situation	19	15	14	05	-04	27	20	14	07	-06	39	—	29	36	05	37	70	47	14	27	28	57
13. Ethnic relations	22	12	15	10	07	07	01	14	14	04	39	29	—	64	05	30	35	28	17	28	25	36
14. Country success in ethnic integ.	06	-07	12	-04	-10	-02	-04	08	-01	-00	42	36	64	—	-01	26	50	36	22	32	22	46
15. Security situation of Israel	20	25	10	20	27	09	03	08	16	30	-01	05	05	-01	—	40	-01	-08	35	-03	06	-04
16. General situation of Israel	36	39	14	15	12	19	13	24	18	20	37	37	30	26	40	—	-07	22	25	17	27	43
17. Gov. handling economic problems	12	07	19	-01	-01	06	10	11	-00	-13	45	70	35	50	-01	-07	—	51	23	44	34	67
18. Gov. handling strikes	08	08	17	17	-01	05	04	04	-10	-05	51	47	28	36	-08	22	51	—	16	31	27	54
19. Gov. handling security problems	09	10	19	25	25	03	-13	14	22	16	15	14	17	22	35	25	23	16	—	25	17	32
20. Health Min. handling health prob.	13	04	16	02	05	05	04	11	08	03	30	27	28	32	-03	17	44	31	25	—	67	33
21. Satisfied with medical services	15	20	31	17	14	17	11	27	09	12	30	28	25	22	06	27	34	27	17	67	—	33
22. Gov. handling current problems	20	12	22	00	-06	22	25	13	-04	-08	48	57	36	46	-04	43	67	54	32	33	33	—

that all their regressions will not merely be monotone but will also have the same sign, namely positive (or zero). This has been shown to be the case for intelligence (cf. Guttman, 1965) and for certain attitudes (cf. Guttman and Levy, 1975; Levy, 1976; Levy and Guttman, 1974). A special case for which nonnegative correlations are hypothesized has been called by Guttman the 'First Law of Attitude' (Gratch, 1973, p. 36). In this special case, the object of the behavior is constant: all the attitudes are towards the same object. Since wellbeing items are all attitudinal, it is important to specify whether a given set of wellbeing items is concerned with one or with more than one object. This is the motivation for the preceding discussion of facet B. In the light of that discussion, we shall deal here with the distinctions between three subuniverses: (1) wellbeing state of self, (2) wellbeing state of reference groups other than self, and (3) treatment by government.

7.1. *Wellbeing State of Self*

In the list of the 24 variables, the first twelve deal with the state of the respondent in different life areas of facet F. Regarding these as twelve modifications of a single object – state of the self – provides a rationale for the hypothesis that the First Law of Attitude should hold for this subset. And indeed the intercorrelations among these items in Table I are all positive or zero.

This replicates the findings of the data of a previous trimester of the Continuing Survey (March–April, 1971), with further crosscultural replication from data of the Quality of Life survey of the University of Michigan (Summer, 1971), as reported in Levy (1976).

7.2. *Wellbeing State of Reference Groups (Other than Self)*

Similarly, the next five items deal with the state of one's reference groups (apart from self). The correlations among these five items are again positive or virtually zero, conforming to the First Law.

The largest of the correlations here is only 0.34 which is much smaller than many of the correlations in the self's sector. The areas of life of these five items do not overlap those of the previous twelve items. There was an opportunity to replicate this aspect of wellbeing in the following trimester of the Continuing Survey. Six items were asked on the state of wellbeing of one's reference groups, five of which are not in the previous trimester. Their intercorrelations are shown in Table II, replicating the phenomenon of all being positive or zero. The First Law is sustained again.

The specification that the reference groups here are part of the one's greater self, so that both varieties of state refer to but a single object 'greater self', leads to the hypothesis that the intercorrelations between the first twelve items and the next five should conform to the First Law of Attitude. The 12×5 off-diagonal submatrix of Table I provides some support for this hypothesis. A rather systematic exception is the item on the state of new immigrants: while the correlations are small, they tend to be largely negative. This may be taken as providing indirect evidence that new immigrants are not yet regarded as part of one's greater self by a substantial part of the population.

Two further interesting negative correlations are between television on the one hand and mood and health on the other. These raise interesting questions about the relation between mass media of communication and one's greater self, which may deserve exploration on other occasions.

Replication of the findings on the greater self can be seen in the data of Table II (Summer 1973 survey). In the 9×6 off-diagonal submatrix of the correlations between state of self and state of other reference groups, the correlations are almost all positive or zero. Again the new immigrants provide an exception.

7.3. Treatment by Government

The last seven items in Table I are on the Israel government's treatment of the various reference groups. (One of these items is on the Histadrut rather than government; we have left it in because of the close association between the government and Histadrut in this matter.) The First Law of Attitude is well sustained for these items. In the lower right hand 7×7 submatrix of Table I the correlations are all positive, many of them substantially so. The population is indeed behaving as though the government's treatment were a single object of the several assessments.

The Summer 1973 survey again confirms the findings on treatment. The lower right hand corner of Table II contains only positive correlations.

We have not specified that the government necessarily be regarded as part of one's greater self, so that we do not hypothesize that the First Law

of Attitude hold between state of greater self and government's great-
ment. The relevant correlations are in the last seven rows of Table I. The
correlations here are all small and largely positive, but with a scattering
of negative correlations. This phenomenon is replicated in Table II.

Having discussed the signs of the correlations, we go on to the main
part of the theory to be proposed here, namely hypotheses on the relative
sizes of the correlations and not merely their signs.

8. THE HYPOTHESIS OF INTERPENETRATING CYLINDREXES

Great variation in size occurs among the correlations. For example, in
Table I, the largest coefficient is 0.88 while the smallest is −0.17. A next
task in analyzing the structure of the interrelationships is to explicate the
location of large and small correlation coefficients. This is facilitated by
the parsimonious geometrical portrayal of the matrix provided by smallest
space analysis, in particular SSA-I (cf., Guttman, 1968; Lingoes, 1973;
Loether and McTavish, 1974). Such a data analysis technique alone is
insufficient for theory testing. Data analysis remains barren unless a
correspondence is established with the definitional system of the observations.

The hypothesis we propose for a correspondence between the well-
being mapping sentence and the SSA is that of interpenetrating cylindrexes. A cylindrex is defined in terms of two concepts: a two-dimensional
radex and an axis orthogonal to it. A radex (cf., Guttman, 1954, 1964)
is a circular arrangement in the plane, so then an axis perpendicular to
it helps define a cylindrical configuration: the circular arrangement is
repeated at each segment – or stratum – of the axis.

To rationalize a cylindrex hypothesis requires facets playing at least
three roles. Two roles are needed for the radex: polarizing and modulating. The polarizer's elements correspond to different directions from an
origin in the plane, while the modulator's elements correspond to relative
distance from this origin. The third role is for specifying order along the
axis of the cylinder.

Empirical studies on various topics have found that the facet of areas
of life often plays a polarizing role (Adi and Kamen, 1971; Guttman and
Levy, 1975; Guttman et al., 1970; Levy, 1975, 1976; Levy and Guttman,
1971a, b). Our wellbeing data belong to this series of replications that

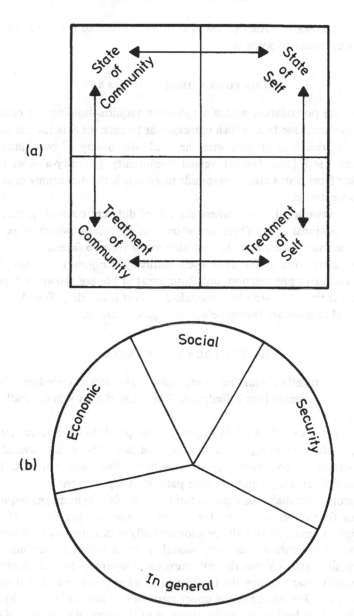

Fig. 1a–b. The four-dimensional duplex-radex of wellbeing. (a) Duplex of axes for cylinders. (b) Radex of strata of cylinders.

verify the radex hypothesis, and also provide evidence for the more inclusive cylindrex hypothesis.

9. THE FOUR CONDITIONAL AXES

To see the polarization within a cylindrex requires holding the central
axis constant. One facet which corresponds to such an axis for our data
is that of reference groups, with the crude dichotomy of two kinds of
elements: self (and family) versus community (country-as-a-whole).
Another facet which also corresponds to an axis is the dichotomy of state
versus treatment.

Having two axial facets, where each is of different content, generates
four conditional axes. These are shown in Figure 1a, which is essentially the fourfold table of the cartesian set of the two facets.

The polarization itself is shown schematically in Figure 1b. To simplify
the preliminary presentation, only four areas of life are shown in Figure
1b, and their subdivision by a modulating facet is omitted. Two detailed
empirical radexes are shown below in Figures 3 and 4.

10. THE FOUR CYLINDREXES

Each axis, together with the given radex, generates a cylindrex. Four
axes, then, generate four cylindrexes. These are shown schematically in
Figure 2.

The axis of cylindrex (a) in Figure 2 corresponds to state-versus-treat-
ment, holding wellbeing of community constant. The axis of cylindrex
(b) corresponds to community-versus-self, holding state constant. The
axes of cylindrexes (c) and (d) have parallel interpretations.

A proper simultaneous representation of the four cylindrexes requires
at least four dimensions, two for Figure 1a and two for Figure 1b. In
principle, Figures 1a and 1b are geometrically orthogonal to each other,
and hence generate a four dimensional space in which the cylindrexes
intermesh. Figure 2 shows the cylindrexes as if separated from each other,
but tilted to suggest how the intermeshing takes place in higher dimensional space. For example, the upper parts of cylindrexes (a) and (b) are
identical: they both contain the variables of the *state* of wellbeing of the
community. In the 4-space, these two parts of cylinders should be in

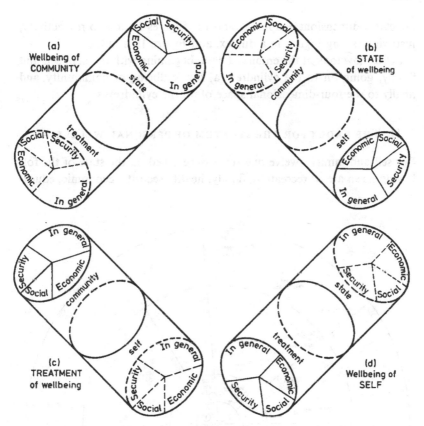

Fig. 2.   The four intermeshing cylindrexes of the duplex-radex of wellbeing.

exactly the same place. Similarly, the other three pairs of adjacent half cylinders should each be identically located in the 4-space.

The available data permit us to document only cylindrexes (a) and (b). No questions were asked about treatment of self in any of the studies, so there is no empirical evidence as yet about cylindrexes (c) and (d).

Both the Spring and Summer·surveys of 1973 support the hypothesis of cylindrexes (a) and (b). The Spring survey has the most detail for the radex, especially for self and family, so we shall discuss the radex in terms of those data. The Summer survey was designed more to fill in the overall picture suggested by the Spring results. Indeed, this second survey gives direct two-dimensional empirical plots for Figures 1a and 1b respectively, justifying calling Figure 1a a duplex, and Figure 1b a radex.

Let us now look at the empirical data, beginning with radex of self and family, going on to the cylindrex (a) for wellbeing of community, and finally to the four-dimensional space of all the cylindrexes.

11. THE RADEX FOR THE STRATUM OF PERSONAL WELLBEING

For self-and-family, twelve questions were asked on the state of the following seven areas: recreation, family, health, security, economic, educa-

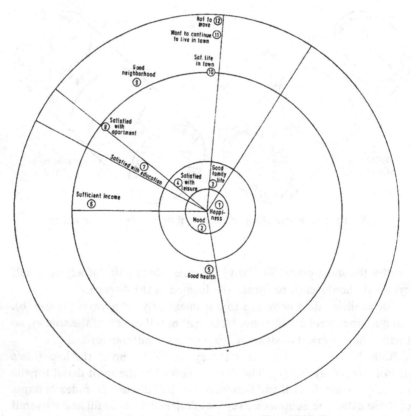

Fig. 3. Radex of personal wellbeing (from Table I).

tion, and in general. We had no *a priori* theory of order amongst the elements of this facet. A non-ordered facet is often to be hypothesized to be polarizing, since each element may be hypothesized to correspond to a different direction in the empirical space. Let us now go on to the data analysis to see at this stage what it means to have a correspondence between a polarizing facet and the structure of interrelationships among the data. Smallest space analysis of the submatrix of the interrelationships amongst the wellbeing variables for self-and-family shows that a two-dimensional space gives a rather good fit to the data. This approximate space is shown in Figure 3. Each of the first twelve wellbeing variables is represented as a point in this space. The distance between two points tends to increase as the coefficient between the two variables concerned decreases.

12. CIRCULAR ORDER OF REGIONS: AREAS OF LIFE

Figure 3 can be partitioned into regions emanating from an origin, where each region corresponds to an element from Facet *F*, namely some life area. There is a circular order of regions, since the six directions lie in a two-dimensional space. The order portrayed in Figure 3 is an empirical consequence of the data; it provides an empirical circular ordering of the elements of Facet *F*. Beginning at the upper part of the circle and going clockwise, the order is as follows: recreation (f_1), family (f_2), general (f_3), health (f_5), economic (f_6), education (f_7), and back to recreation (f_1).

The technical meaning of the geometric circularity is as follows. If we take points corresponding to two variables that lie at an equal distance from the origin but from different regions, then the correlation coefficients between them will increase as the regions are closer together in the circular order. For example: in Figure 3, variables 5, 6, and 8 are approximately equally distant from the origin, but in different regions. The region of income for variable 6, is the middle of the three. Accordingly, the distance from 8 to 5 is greater than that from 8 to 6 and from 6 to 5; the coefficients of correlation should have a corresponding order. Indeed, in Table I, $\mu_{56} = 0.28$ and $\mu_{68} = 0.44$, while smaller than both of these is $\mu_{56} = 0.17$. Items 8 and 5 do correlate less with each other than do the other pairings of items.

13. MODULATION OF DISTANCE FROM THE ORIGIN: ENVIRONMENT

If variables are not equidistant from the origin, then merely knowing in which regions they fall is not sufficient for reproducing the relative sizes of their correlation coefficients. Information is needed also about distance from the origin. Such further information corresponds to modulating facets.

Facet D proves to play the role of a modulator. The environmental framework of the respondent serves to partition Figure 1 into circular regions around the origin. Variables belonging to the *primary* environment are concentrated in the three innermost circles. The circle closest to the origin contains the intimate internal primary variables (d_1): happiness and mood (items 1, 2). Variables belonging to the social primary environment (d_2) are in the second circle: family life, and recreation (items 3 and 4). In the third circle are resources of the primary environment (d_3): health, income, education, and dwelling (items 5, 6, 7, 8).

The outlying circle corresponds to secondary environment variables. Here we find items which deal with the neighborhood and the city of the respondent $(d_4, d_5$: items 9, 10, 11, 12).

The transition from primary environment to secondary environment modulates the distance from the origin in the space of self's wellbeing (Figure 3). If we take two variables from the same region which lie approximately on the same radius in the region, the coefficient between them will increase as they become equally distant from the origin. For example, let us take three points from the recreation region: wanting to go on living in one's town (item 11), satisfaction with dwelling (item 8) and satisfaction with ways one spends leisure time (item 4). These three variables differ in degree of primacy, the most different being items 4 and 11. And indeed according to Table I, the coefficient between items 4 and 11 is lower than the coefficients between 8 and 11, and between items 8 and 4: 0.27 against 0.29 and 0.38.

Variables which are very close to the center will be very close to each other even if their directions in the map are different. This is because they are lying in a circle of small diameter.

14. THE DISTANCE FROM HAPPINESS

In the center of the circle lies the assessment of the respondent's feeling of happiness. Happiness is closest to variables which relate to the respondent's internal and social primary environment. The monotonicity coefficients between happiness (item 1) and between mood (internal primary environment) is 0.77. Similar to these are the coefficients between happiness and social primary environments (0.66 with family life, and 0.55 with satisfaction with ways of spending leisure time).

The resources (income, dwelling, education, health) – which are also a part of the individual's primary environment – tend to be less correlated to happiness. The monotonicity coefficients between happiness (item 1) and between the resources variables vary from 0.26 to 0.35, with the exception of health (0.56). That is, primary resources – excluding health which is crucial for survival – are less related to happiness than are variables of internal and social primary environment. The feeling of wellbeing in physical aspects of life cannot predict personal happiness as well as can socio-psychological aspects of life. Variables concerning secondary environment – like neighborhood and town – tend to be even less correlated with happiness (the coefficients do not exceed 0.28), with the exception of satisfaction with life in town in general (0.45) which is even closer to happiness than primary resources. Perhaps it is possible to regard this variable as a resource of a primary environment.

The origin, happiness, in Figure 3 is determined by the partitionings related to the two facets: area of life and primacy of the environment. This origin is *not* central to the *empirical* distribution of the points in the map. To the contrary, the variables of the central circle are in a corner of the empirical distribution of the points. Almost all remaining variables are in the upper left section of this origin, while the lower right region is empty. Indeed, the substantive origin is not surrounded by empirical points. This phenomenon is replicated in the Summer survey, for the stratum of personal wellbeing. However, for the stratum of community wellbeing, this region appears to correspond to the area of security. Questions on this were not asked for personal wellbeing.

15. SOME FURTHER FACETS

Facets A, B, C, and E are not mentioned in the analysis of Figure 3. Facet B is held constant in the sample of the questions about self's wellbeing: all these questions deal only with *situation* (b_1) and not with treatment (b_2). Therefore this facet cannot distinguish further lawfulness in Figure 3. The same applies to facet C, which is also held constant in the questions on the wellbeing of the self: all these questions relate to the respondent himself (c_1) and not to any other social group. As for facet A, there did not turn out to be separate empirical regions for cognitive and affective evaluations.

With regard to Facet E, there is a tendency for questions on specific aspects of life area to be farther away from the origin than more general questions on the same topic. For example: wanting to go on living in the same city is more distant than general satisfaction with life in the city. This facet presents a clearer systematic partition in the context of community wellbeing, to be discussed next.

16. THE CYLINDREX OF COMMUNITY WELLBEING

To study community wellbeing, twelve items were available: five on state and seven on treatment. Three items have such low correlation altogether amongst themselves and all the rest (items 16, 17, 24 in Table I), that they are known in advance to be geometrically remote and hence no further information about them is to be learned from the SSA. The nine remaining items – three of state and six of treatment – have a good technical fit in a two-dimensional space: coefficient of alienation 0.13. However, the theory of Figure 2a suggests going on to three dimensions, and indeed Figure 2a is confirmed thereby.

The six treatment items do show a circular order according to areas of life. This time the modulating facet is from *generality* to *specificity* of treatment. The two items asking about treatment in general (items 18 and 19) are in the center of the radex, while the four specific treatment items are towards the periphery. This same modulator also appears in the earlier 1971 radex.

The three state items lie in a stratum above the six treatment items. Altogether, then, the nine items provide a cylindrical configuration as hypothesized from their facets.

This cylindrex is replicated in the data of the Summer survey. The details will not be shown separately but are part of the overall four-dimensional picture to be presented next.

17. The four dimensional picture

SSA in four dimensions of Table II fortunately came out with a rotation of axes that directly approximates Figure 1. The plane of the first and third dimensions of the SSA approximates Figure 1a, while the plane of the second and fourth dimensions approximates Figure 1b. These two plane projections, as given by the computer, are shown in Figure 4.

In Figure 4a, the plane is partitioned into four regions according to the four elements of the cartesian set of Figure 1a. One region is empty of points. No questions were asked about treatment of self, and the data

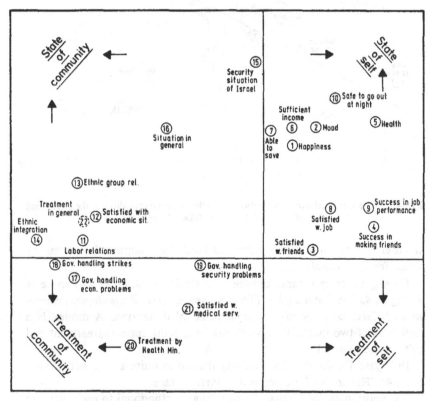

Fig. 4a. The empirical duplex projection of wellbeing corresponding to the axial facets self-vs-community and state-vs-treatment (from SSA of Table II).

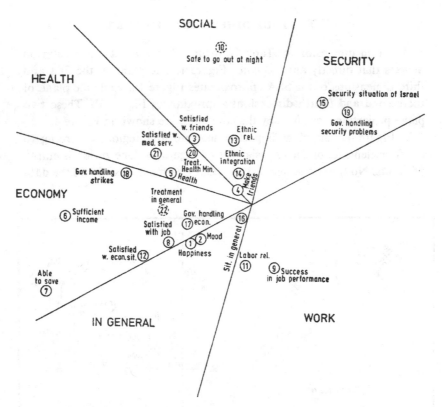

Fig. 4b. The empirical radex projection of wellbeing corresponding to the polarizing facet of areas of life (from SSA of Table II).

themselves act as if they recognize this fact! The computer left an empty space for such variables.

Having a correspondence between a cartesian set and the SSA space as in Figure 4a is called a *duplex*. (This is a special case of a *multiplex*, wherein each facet corresponds to an orthogonal dimension. A duplex is a multiplex of two facets, the two facets here being state-vs-treatment and self-vs-community.)

In Figure 4b, the variables are partitioned in quite a different fashion from 4a. The areas of life act as a polarizing facet.

The coordinates of Figures 4a and 4b are orthogonal to each other in the four-dimensional SSA space. Hence, the two figures together generate intermeshing cylindrexes as implied by Figure 2. Only two complete cylindrexes, (a) and (b), are discernable from the data, as well as the connection between the upper portions of (c) and (d). The lower portions of (c) and (d) are missing because of the blank region in Figure 4a, for treatment of self.

Regions subdivided by modulating facets are not shown explicitly in Figure 4b, since our variables turn out to have different modulators for different strata.

It is difficult to conclude the discussion of wellbeing without asking: what correlates most with personal happiness? We have already looked into this within the radex of Figure 3, for state of wellbeing of self. How about the relationship of personal happiness with one's assessment of the situation of one's community? According to Table II, the highest correlation between personal happiness [in the lower part of cylindrex (b)] and the variables in the upper part of cylindrex (b) is with the 'general situation of Israel' ($\mu_2 = 0.36$). This says something about the axis of the cylinder being long compared with the diameter of the radex. Wellbeing items tend to correlate more within the stratum of self than with the stratum of community.

To assess systematically the relative spreads along axes and diameters of the intermeshing cylindrexes of wellbeing requires more variables than available in the present data.

REFERENCES

Adi, P. and Kamen, C.: 1971, 'An Analysis of Developments in Wage Demands and Consumption Plans Owing to the New Taxation and Price Increases', Jerusalem: The Israel Institute of Applied Social Research, July 1971 (Hebrew).

Allardt, E.: 1973, *About Dimensions of Welfare*, Helsinki, Research Group for Comparative Sociology, Univ. of Helsinki.

Andrews, F. M.: 1974, 'Social Indicators of Perceived Life Quality', *Soc. Ind. Res.* 1, 279–299.

Bradburn, N. M. and Caplovitz, D.: 1965, *Reports on Happiness*, Chicago, Aldine Publishing Co.

Elizur, D.: 1970, *Adapting to Innovation*, Jerusalem, Jerusalem Academic Press.

Gratch, H. (ed.): 1973, *Twenty-Five Years of Social Research in Israel*, Jerusalem, Jerusalem Academic Press.

Guttman, L.: 1965, 'A Faceted Definition of Intelligence', in R. Eiferman (ed.), *Studies in Psychology*, Scripta Hierosolymitana, 14, 166–181.

Guttman, L.: 1971, 'Social Problem Indicators', *Ann. Am. Acad. Politic. Soc. Sci.* 393, 40–46.

172   S. LEVY AND L. GUTTMAN

Guttman, L.: 1968, 'A General Nonmetric Technique for Finding the Smallest Coordinate Space for a Configuration of Points', *Psychometrika* 33, 469–506.

Guttman, L.: 1954, 'A New Approach to Factor Analysis: the Radex', in P. F. Lazarsfeld (ed.), *Mathematical Thinking in the Social Sciences*, Glencoe, Ill., The Free Press.

Guttman, L.: 1964, 'The Structure of Interrelations Among Intelligence Tests', *Invitational Conference on Testing Problems*, Princeton, Educational Testing Service.

Guttman, L. and Levy, S.: 1975, 'Structure and Dynamics of Worries', *Sociometry*, in press.

Guttman, L., Levy, S., and Mann, K. J.: 1970, *Adjustment to Retirement*, Jerusalem, Israel Institute of Applied Social Research, (Hebrew).

Jahoda, M.: 1958, *Current Concepts of Positive Mental Health*, New York, Basic Books.

Kernberg, O. *et al.*: 1972, Psychotherapy and Psychoanalysis: Final report of the Menninger Foundation's Psychotherapy Research Project. *Bulletin of the Menninger Clinic*, The Menninger Foundation.

Levy, S.: 1975, *Political Involvement and Attitude*, Jerusalem, Israel Institute of Applied Social Research.

Levy, S.: 1976, 'Use of the Mapping Sentence for Coordinating Theory and Research: a Cross-Cultural Example', *Quality and Quantity* (in press).

Levy, S. and Guttman, L.: 1971a, *Zionism and the Jewish People as Viewed by Israelis*, Jerusalem, Israel Institute of Applied Social Research, (Hebrew).

Levy, S. and Guttman, L.: 1971b, *The Public's Reactions to Current Problems*, Jerusalem, Israel Institute of Applied Social Research, (Hebrew).

Levy, S. and Guttman, L.: 1974, *Values and Attitudes of Israel High School Youth*, Jerusalem, Israel Institute of Applied Social Research, (Hebrew, with English translation of Introduction and Summary).

Lingoes, J. C.: 1973, *The Guttman-Lingoes Nonmetric Program Series*, Ann Arbor, Michigan, Mathesis Press.

Loether, H. J. and McTavish, D.: 1974, *Descriptive Statistics for Sociologists*, Boston, Allyn and Bacon.

FRANK M. ANDREWS AND RONALD F. INGLEHART

8. THE STRUCTURE OF SUBJECTIVE WELL-BEING IN NINE WESTERN SOCIETIES*

ABSTRACT. The structure of subjective well-being is analyzed by multidimensional mapping of evaluations of life concerns. For example, one finds that evaluations of Income are close to (i.e., relatively strongly related to) evaluations of Standard of living, but remote from (weakly related to) evaluations of Health. These structures show how evaluations of life components fit together and hence illuminate the psychological meaning of life quality. They can be useful for determining the breadth of coverage and degree of redundancy of social indicators of perceived well-being. Analyzed here are data from representative sample surveys in Belgium, Denmark, France, Germany, Great Britain, Ireland, Italy, Netherlands, and the United States (each N ≈ 1000). Eleven life concerns are considered, including Income, Housing, Job, Health, Leisure, Neighborhood, Transportation, and Relations with other people. It is found that structures in all of these countries have a basic similarity and that the European countries tend to be more similar to one another than they are to USA. These results suggest that comparative research on subjective well-being is feasible within this group of nations.

1. INTRODUCTION

Interest in social indicators of life quality, including citizens' perceptions of their own well-being, has inspired a number of sample surveys in recent years.[1] Such surveys, particularly when done on a comparative and repetitive cross-national basis, have enormous potential for providing information about changing levels of social and economic development and about the processes and conditions that lead to or are associated with the 'good life'. However, the feasibility and usefulness of comparative research in this area — as in any area — are contingent upon the identification of an underlying phenomenon that is in fact *comparable* from one society to another. While a person's sense of happiness, satisfaction, etc. is of acknowledged importance, the cross-cultural comparability of the phenomenon of perceived well-being is largely unexplored. This paper reports an initial, and necessarily incomplete, examination of the comparability of psychological structures of subjective well-being in nine western societies.

This Introduction develops the conceptual framework for the analysis that follows, and describes some of the interests that motivate this presentation. Section 2, Data, describes the sample surveys from which reasonably comparable data from nine nations have been extracted and details the items

173

Alex C. Michalos (ed.), Citation Classics from Social Indicators Research, 173–190.
© 2005 *Springer. Printed in the Netherlands.*

and response scales used to measure perceived well-being. The section on analysis methods discusses the statistical techniques by which we identified the structures of perceived well-being and assessed their similarity across countries. There follows the main substantive results – first for USA and then for eight European nations. The final section of the paper provides some general conclusions, some cautions about interpretation, and some suggestions for further investigation of the issues.

Research on perceived well-being commonly distinguishes between evaluations of life-as-a-whole (sometimes referred to as general or global evaluations) and evaluations of specific life concerns, such as housing, job, relations with other people, safety, or fairness. When we refer to the "structure of subjective well-being" we refer to the way specific life concerns, and evaluations of them, fit together in people's thinking. For example, we ourselves have shown that among American adults evaluations of one's marriage are – quite reasonably – strongly related to evaluations of one's spouse, that evaluations of national political leaders are strongly related to evaluations of government economic programs, but that evaluations of the first pair are virtually independent of evaluations of the second pair. These statistical results suggest that Marriage and National government are distinct life concerns for most Americans. When one combines these results with numerous others, some of which will be described later in this paper, one can identify a psychological structure, or 'cognitive map', from which one can infer the relative positions of life concerns as they are perceived by a particular group of people.

Such structures are interesting for a number of reasons. In showing how well-being perceptions are organized in people's thinking, they indicate some fundamental aspects of what evaluations of life quality *mean* to these people. Such structures help to identify the distinct well-being concerns that particular groups have, and show the extent that evaluations of these different concerns overlap or intersect with one another. This suggests one of the important practical uses of such structures: They provide guides to the adequacy of coverage and statistical efficiency of indicators of perceived well-being. To the extent that people in different societies organize their thinking about well-being in basically similar ways, it is feasible and potentially productive to undertake cross-cultural research with standardized instruments and to make well-grounded comparative statements based on the results. However, if the basic phenomenon that is being investigated – well-being perceptions – shows markedly different structures in different societies, measurements and interpretations must be society-specific and any comparative statements must be advanced with extreme caution.[2]

The main substantive purpose of this paper is (a) to explore the structural similarity of well-being perceptions in nine western societies. In so doing, we shall have the opportunity to pursue two other matters of more didactic interest. (b) Our analysis is based on a set of national sample surveys that offer rich opportunities for secondary analysis, and our use of these data may increase analysts' awareness of their existence and accessibility. (c) This analysis involves use of some relatively new statistical methods for assessing similarities among configurations (i.e., structures) and illustrates the need for some further statistical developments; perhaps it will encourage statisticians to pursue these developments.

Before proceeding further, the reader should be cautioned that the analysis reported here is of a rather exploratory nature. The issue of crosscultural similarities in structures of perceived well-being is a fundamental one for those interested in comparative research or in social policies, but the data requirements for a fully adequate investigation are immense. While the data at our disposal are unusually extensive, they are not ideal, and they cannot provide a definitive estimate of the degree of cross-cultural similarity of structures. As will be seen, however, our results do suggest that the similarities may be substantial, and in so doing they suggest that further investigations along this line seem promising.

2. DATA

The data analyzed here come from representative national surveys of the non-institutionalized adult populations in the following nine countries: USA, France, Great Britain, Germany, Italy, Netherlands, Belgium, Denmark, and Ireland. The American data are those of Andrews and Withey (1976) and were collected in May 1972.[3] The European data come from a series of parallel surveys conducted by the European Economic Community and were collected in each of the EEC countries in May 1976.[4] The American survey includes 1297 respondents; each of the eight national European surveys includes approximately 1000 respondents (range 923 to 1047). All of the surveys were conducted by personal interviews using professional field staffs and methods such as to suggest that the data include no unusual quality problems. Interviews were conducted in the native language of the respondents.

In the American survey more than 60 questions asking for evaluations of various life concerns were answered by the respondents. The European data include fifteen such items, of which 11 are reasonably similar to those in the

EXHIBIT 1

Items Used to Assess Evaluations of Life Concerns in American and European Surveys

Reference	American wording	European wording
(Lead in)	In the next section of this interview we want to find out how you feel about parts of your life and life in this country as you see it. Please tell me the feelings you have now – taking into account what has happened in the last year and what you expect in the near future.	Now I would like you to indicate on this scale to what extent you are satisfied with your present situation in the following respects...
house	Your house/apartment	The house, flat or apartment where you live
neigh	This particular neighborhood as a place to live	The part of the town or village you live in
income	The income you (and your family) have	The income of you and your family
std lvg	Your standard of living – the things you have like housing, car, furniture, recreation and the like	Your standard of living; the things you have like furniture, household equipment, and so on
job	Your job	Your present work – in your job or as a housewife
spare time	The way you spend your spare time, your non-working activities	The way you spend your spare time
trnspt	The way you can get around to work, schools, shopping, etc.	Your means of transport – the way you can get to work, schools, shopping, etc.
health	Your own health and physical condition	Your present state of health
time	The amount of time you have for doing the things you want to do	The amount of time you have for doing the things you want to do
treated	The way other people treat you	The respect people give you
get on w peop	How you get on with other people	In general terms, your relations with other people

American data. Exhibit 1 presents the exact wording of these 11 items as presented to the American respondents and to English-speaking European respondents.

The American respondents recorded their feelings about these life concerns along a seven-point scale that ranged from 'Delighted' to 'Terrible,' or in one of several off-scale categories: 'Neutral (neither satisfied nor dissatisfied),' 'I never thought about it,' or 'Does not apply to me.'[5] The European ratings were along an eleven-point scale of satisfaction that ranged from 'Completely dissatisfied' to 'Very satisfied.' While the 7-point Delighted-Terrible and 11-point Satisfaction scales are not identical, previous research suggests that the substantive differences between them are likely to be rather small and that both offer effective means of measuring evaluations of life concerns (see Andrews & Withey, 1976, Chapters 3 and 6).

3. ANALYSIS METHODS

Our interests required the performance of two distinct analytic tasks: (a) identification of the structure of well-being assessments in each country and (b) determination of the similarities among these structures.

The structures were identified using Smallest Space Analysis,[6] one of the several forms of non-metric multidimensional scaling (Guttman, 1968; Shepard, Romney, and Nerlove, 1972). Within each country, associations (product-moment r's) between each pair of the well-being assessments were determined, and the resulting matrix of intercorrelations was used as input to Smallest Space Analysis. Smallest Space Analysis then iteratively approaches that configuration of points (i.e., of life concern assessments) in multidimensional space which maximizes the similarities of rank orderings of the distances between the pairs of points and the associations (correlations) between the respective life concern assessments. Thus, assessments that show strong positive associations with one another, suggesting that they tap the same life concern or highly related ones, are placed close to one another, and assessments that are statistically independent are placed far apart. Of course, given a large number of life concern assessments, there is no necessity that a perfect consistency can be achieved between the distances of the points in a small-dimensioned space and the sizes of the associations among the assessments; however several statistics are available for measuring this consistency.[7]

In the present analysis, structures of subjective well-being were identified by using *all* of the available well-being assessments — more than 60 assessments in the American data and all 15 items in the European data. Although only 11 assessments were similar between the American and European surveys, the placement of these 11 within each national structure could be more accurately determined within the context of a larger set of items than if only the associations among these 11 had been considered. After trial fittings in spaces of several different dimensionalities, it was determined that a three-dimensional space permitted an adequate portrayal of the structures.[8]

The second major analysis task was to determine the similarity between the various national structures, represented by the three-dimensional configurations of 11 items, as extracted from the larger structures. The rigid ('procrustean') approach proposed by Schönemann and Carroll (1970) was used to match the configurations, and then the degree of match was measured by the Lingoes-Schönemann S statistic (Lingoes and Schönemann, 1974).[9]

The technique of matching involves taking one configuration as the 'target' and then rotating, moving, and contracting or dilating another configuration so as to get the corresponding points in each configuration to match one another as closely as possible. Note that the right (90°) angles between the axes are kept rigid and that none of these several transformations changes the relative distances among the pairs of points within either of the configurations; the transformations merely serve to remove inconsequential differences in the original locations, orientations, and sizes of the configurations.

The Lingoes—Schönemann S statistic has two characteristics that make it well suited for assessing configurational similarities in our analysis: (a) It is a symmetric statistic — i.e., it has the same value regardless of which configuration is used as the target. (b) It is scale-invariant — i.e., the value of the statistic does not depend on the 'size' of the configurations. These two characteristics are particularly desirable in the present analysis, where our desire to measure the similarity among all possible pairs of nine configurations makes it impossible to use the same target for all comparisons.

Since the S statistic is not yet well known, it may be helpful to comment on its interpretation. Lingoes and Schönemann (1974, page 426) note that $S^{1/2}$ is the matrix analogue of a coefficient of alienation ($= (1-r^2)^{1/2}$). Thus low S values imply high similarity (low alienation) and high values imply low similarity. For example, an $S^{1/2} = 1.0$ implies a zero product-moment correlation between the dimensional locations of the points in the two configurations, and an $S^{1/2} = 0.0$ implies a perfect match (product-moment $r = 1.00$). As will be seen in the following section, values of $S^{1/2}$ of 0.5, 0.6, or 0.7 were typical for the configurations matched here, and these values of $S^{1/2}$ correspond to product-moment correlations between the dimensional locations of 0.87, 0.80, and 0.71, respectively.

So far as we are aware, there have not been, as yet, any statistical tests developed for the S statistic,[10] nor any explorations of how S is afffected by various types of measurement errors in the variables that define the configurations. With respect to tests of S, it seems likely that the Schönemann – Carroll transformations, which take advantage of whatever matchings that exist between two configurations, would act to *decrease* the expected value of S (e.g., pairs of perfectly random configurations would probably show mean values of S below the theoretical S value of 1.00). On the other hand, the impact of measurement errors on the variables probably acts to *increase* the value of S (e.g., two identical latent configurations, each represented by data containing different measurement errors, would probably not generate the theoretical $S = 0$). It is virtually certain that both of these effects have influenced the S values reported in the next section,[11] but the extent to which the two effects may have canceled each other is unknown.

4. RESULTS

It will be most convenient to begin the presentation of results with the configuration for the 60+ life concern evaluations by the American respondents and to note how the 11 items that are similar to those in the European data fit within this larger structure. Following this, we shall examine similarities in the structure for all possible pairs of countries. Finally, we present plots of the structures in selected European nations and of a derived combined configuration for all eight European nations, and compare these structures to that for the USA.

Structure for USA

Exhibit 2 shows the three-dimensional structure for evaluations of 63 life concerns by American respondents and indicates the 11 items from this set that are similar to those used in the European surveys. Several things are worth noting.

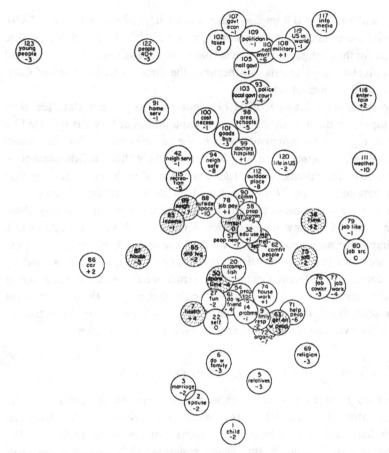

EXHIBIT 2. Three-dimensional structure of evaluations of 63 life concern items by American respondents.

Notes: Stippled items are those for which similar items exist in European surveys. Signed numbers indicate position on the third dimension. Data source: 1297 respondents to 1972 American national survey. Based on Exhibit 2.4 of Andrews and Withey (1976). For exact wording of all items see Exhibit 2.1 of Andrews and Withey (1976); wording of stippled items appears in Exhibit 1 of the present paper.

(a) One dimension, shown vertically in the exhibit, seems to array items according to the psychological immediacy of the life concern. The dimension ranges from items tapping family concerns (near the bottom of the exhibit), through items tapping concerns about one's relations with the immediate external environment — job, neighborhood, relations with other people, etc.

(in the middle of the exhibit), to items tapping concerns about the larger society — national government, mass media, etc. (near the top).[12]

(b) Items that, on the basis of their content, would seem to tap the same life concern do in fact tend to cluster together and thereby serve to locate the nature and approximate postion of the underlying concern. For example, note the cluster of job items at the right side of the exhibit, the cluster of family items at the bottom, the cluster of government items at the top, and many others.[13]

(c) The 11 items that are similar to items in the European data (stippled in Exhibit 2) represent a rather limited middle segment of the total structure identified for American respondents. The European data contain no items that are similar to items at the extremes of the vertical (the psychological immediacy) dimension: There are no items at all that tap concerns about marriage or family, and those that tap more remote societal concerns were substantially different from those used in the American survey. Thus what appears to be a major dimension of the American structure will be, of necessity, rather attenuated in the structural matches that follow.

(d) Despite the restricted structural differentiation of the 11 items that are similar to those in the European surveys, a careful examination shows some interesting locational differences. We shall pause to detail them here so that later we can compare them with the European structures. With respect to the first two dimensions of the exhibit (the vertical and horizontal dimensions), one can see that the more personally immediate items — assessments of health, of one's relations with other people, of how one spends one's spare time, and of the amount of time available — are in the lower or right-hand portions of the structure, while items assessing more psychologically remote economic or physical concerns — housing, neighborhood, income, standard of living, and transportation — are in the upper-left portion of the structure. On the third dimension (which runs from 'in front of' to 'in back of' the plane of the exhibit), the housing and neighborhood items are well 'back,' the income and standard of living items, the two items tapping relations with other people, and the spare time item are modestly 'back,' and the health item is somewhat in 'front'.

Similarity Among Nine Countries

Having examined the structure of subjective well-being assessments in some detail as derived for American respondents, we can now ask how similar it is to comparable structures for respondents in eight European countries. We can also ask how similar the European structures are to one another. Some initial answers appear in Exhibit 3, which presents values of $S^{1/2}$ for all possible comparisons among the nine countries.[14] Also shown in Exhibit 3 is the similarity of each national structure to a derived structure which represents the single best-fit approximation to the eight individual European structures.

EXHIBIT 3

Degree of dissimilarity between structures of life concern assessments in nine countries

	USA	FRA	GB	GER	ITA	NLD	BEL	DEN	IRE	(EC)
United States	–									
France	0.77	–								
Great Britain	0.78	0.44	–							
W. Germany	0.71	0.74	0.66	–						
Italy	0.70	0.66	0.67	0.72	–					
Netherlands	0.64	0.70	0.64	0.72	0.72	–				
Belgium	0.75	0.52	0.56	0.73	0.81	0.63	–			
Denmark	0.77	0.68	0.63	0.73	0.75	0.46	0.55	–		
Ireland	0.65	0.69	0.56	0.54	0.56	0.58	0.76	0.72	–	
(European centroid)	0.65	0.61	0.57	0.67	0.68	0.62	0.64	0.63	0.61	–

Notes: The measure of dissimilarity is $S^{1/2}$, a matrix alienation coefficient (Lingoes and Schönemann, 1974). Low values of $S^{1/2}$ indicate high configurational similarity.

The left-most column of the exhibit shows how the USA structure (of 11 items, as contained within the larger set of 63 items shown in Exhibit 2) matches each of the European national structures (of 11 items as contained within their own larger sets of 15). One can see that the coefficients vary only modestly – from 0.64 to 0.78. This suggests that Americans' structure of well-being perceptions is about as similar to the structure of one European country as it is to another. Within the limited range of the differences, however, the American structure is most similar to that of The Netherlands, closely followed by Ireland, and least similar to the structures in Great Britain, France, and Denmark.

The fact that the British structure is *least* similar to the American has interesting implications: It suggests that the cross-national differences we observe do not reflect artifacts of translation, for the wording of the British and American items was closely similar (in some cases identical), yet the differences between the American and British structures are greater than those between the American pattern and that resulting from questions posed in German, French, Dutch, Danish or Italian.

Probably more important than these modest differences, however, is the absolute level of the coefficients in the left-most column of the exhibit. With values approximating 0.7 (which, as noted in Section 3 of this paper, correspond to product moment r's of about 0.7), the data suggest a rather substantial configurational similarity between structures of well-being assessments in the United States and these European countries.

The value of 0.65 shown for the match between the American configuration and the European centroid configuration is also of interest. This figure suggests that the European *average* is somewhat closer to the USA structure than are most of the individual European countries. Thus while the European average structure is certainly not identical to the American structure, as the individual European national structures deviate away from their own average, they also tend to deviate away from the American structure rather than toward it. Or in still other terms, the American structure has (slightly) more in common with Europe-as-a-whole than with most of the individual European structures.

Exhibit 3 also provides interesting results on the similarities among the various European structures themselves. Here the coefficients vary from 0.44, for Great Britain and France (which are most similar to one another), to 0.81, for Belgium and Italy (which are least similar). Furthermore, if one computes some averages based on the data in Exhibit 3 one finds that of all the individual national structures, the British structure is most typical of the European structures (mean $S^{1/2} = 0.59$) and the Italian structures is most distinctive (mean $S^{1/2} = 0.70$). The same results can be seen in Exhibit 3 by comparing the individual European structures to the European centroid.

To summarize these various findings from Exhibit 3 we can observe that: (a) there seems to be a basic similarity in structures among all nine of these western societies; (b) within this basic similarity the European structures are distinct from the American structure; (c) even within Europe there is modest heterogeneity; and (d) if one averages out the differences among the individual European structures, the result is a structure that is closer to the American structure than are most of the individual European structures.[15]

Structures for EEC Countries

What *are* the European structures? Lack of space precludes a presentation of each one, but Exhibits 4 and 5 present the structures for the Netherlands and Great Britain, respectively.[16] The Dutch structure was selected because it is the individual structure most similar to the American one; and the British structure because, while still basically similar, it matches the USA least well.

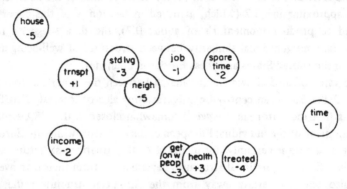

EXHIBIT 4. Three-dimensional structure of evaluations of 11 life concern items by Dutch respondents.

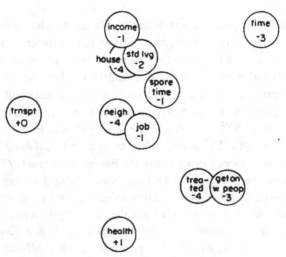

EXHIBIT 5. Three-dimensional structure of evaluations of 11 life concern items by British respondents.

As presented in Exhibits 4 and 5, the Dutch and British structures are oriented to agree with the presentation of the American structure in Exhibit 2.

In the case of both the Dutch and British structures one can see the same basic pattern among these 11 items that was identified previously in our discussion of the American structure. Note that all the personally immediate items (health, relations with other people, spare time activities and amount of time available) are located in the lower or right-hand portions of the structures, while the more psychologically remote economic or physical concerns fall in the upper left portions. Note also that, comparable with the American structure, housing and neighborhood are both well 'back' on the third dimension, that the two items that tap relations with other people, the income and standard of living items, and the spare time item are modestly 'back,' and that the health item is somewhat in 'front' of the plane of the exhibit.[17]

Another view of the similarities and differences between the American and European structures is presented in Exhibit 6. Plotted there is the United States structure (reproduced from Exhibit 2 and shown by the U's) and also

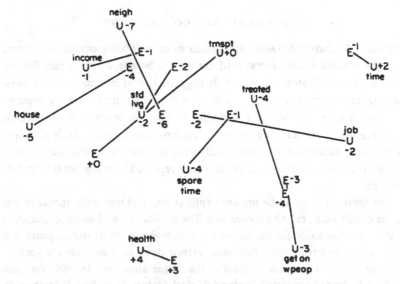

EXHIBIT 6. Match between three-dimensional structures of evaluations of life concern items by American and European respondents.

Key: U = location in United States structure; E = location in European centroid structure.

the best-fit average European structure (the European centroid configuration that was discussed previously and for which similarity measures were presented in Exhibit 3 – shown by the E's).

The basic similarity of the two configurations in the first two dimensions is indicated by the fact that most of the linkage lines are relatively short, and in the third dimension by the close similarity in values of the signed numbers.

With this exhibit it is easy to identify the modest differences that do exist. In the European centroid configuration, compared to the United States structure: the two items tapping relations with other people are much closer together; the job item is much closer to assessments of income and standard of living; and the transportation item moves out to a less central position while income, housing, and neighborhood evaluations move into more central positions. While one might speculate about the inter-cultural causes of these discrepancies, we feel such speculation is best avoided for the present. These differences may be at least partly real, but they are almost certainly at least partly the result of various methodological artifacts.[18] We believe that what is most important is the basic similarity of the structures.

5. COMMENTS AND CONCLUSIONS

The basic similarities between the structures of well-being assessments across the nine western societies examined here is, we believe, an important finding for the social indicators movement. It suggests that it is feasible to do cross-national comparative research – at least in these countries – on the topic of perceived well-being and that meaningful comparable results can be expected from the use of standardized survey instruments and methods. Only if people in different societies think about well-being in basically similar ways would this be the case, and the initial explorations reported here suggest that in fact they do.

The limited nature of the present explorations, and hence the tentativeness of the conclusions, must be recognized. The number of well-being assessments that were reasonably similar across the national surveys at our disposal was only eleven, and it happens that these eleven items represent only a portion of what previous research suggests is the larger structure. In addition, this analysis is limited by certain methodological factors, including differences in the times at which the American and European surveys were conducted (1972 versus 1976), differences in the response scales used by the two sets of respondents (7-point Delighted-Terrible versus 11-point Satisfaction) and differences in the wording and linguistic translations of the items. Some of these differences are endemic to any cross-national research and will always compete with the hypothesis that observed differences are attributable to cultural effects, but even within the limits of what is feasible in current cross-cultural research, one could design data better suited to address the issue of structural similarity.

Besides the restrictive nature of the data at our disposal, the definitiveness of the results is limited by the lack of statistics for testing the significance of similarities between configurations and the limitations of knowledge regarding how various types of measurement errors affect measures of configurational similarity.

Assuming that these data and statistical limitations may some day be removed, we would propose some promising extensions of this line of research. (a) Of course, we would wish to extend the descriptive data about similarity of structures beyond the nine western countries examined so far. Would other western countries show similar patterns? What about well-being perceptions in non-western countries? (b) To the extent that significant differences in structures of well-being assessments were identified, one would want to move beyond the descriptive phase and begin to ask what accounts for the structural differences and what impact they have on the behavior of people, governments, etc. Even within the range of the modest differences noted among the nine western societies investigated here, there are hints that similarity varies directly with geographical contiguity, with the comparability of the socio-economic systems, and/or with the general *level* of well-being.[19] Any conclusions along these lines, however, must be extremely tenuous with the present data and would have to be checked against results for a wider range of societies. (c) We have in this paper identified *national* structures (plus one *regional* structure — the European centroid configuration). While national structures are conceptually convenient and have an obvious interest, it is possible that other groups of persons should be considered. One can imagine cross-national groupings based on characteristics such as age, sex, occupation, socioeconomic status, cultural group, language, and others. (One can also imagine performing the analysis on certain sub-divisions *within* a given national grouping, but the research on this topic to data suggests that structural differences are modest.[20])

Institute for Social Research
University of Michigan

NOTES

* Prepared initially for presentation at the 1977 Annual Meeting of the American Statistical Association, Chicago, August 1977. We are grateful to Kai Hildebrant for his skillful processing of data for this paper and for many useful suggestions regarding the analysis. Ed Schneider and James Lingoes also provided helpful advice.
[1] See, for example, Abrams (1974); Allardt (1975); Andrews & Withey (1976); Campbell, Converse, and Rodgers (1976); Development Academy of the Philippines (1975); Hall (1976), Inglehart (1977); Rabier (1974); and Riffault and Rabier (1977).
[2] Structural similarity does not, of course, imply that all societies will be similarly satisfied – either in general or with respect to specific life concerns; rather, it means that the *relationships* among the well-being assessments will be similar.
[3] Collection of these American data was supported by grant GS3322 from the National Science Foundation. These data, together with four other sets of survey data on perceptions of well-being collected under the direction of Andrews and Withey, are available from the Social Science Archive of The Institute for Social Research, The University of Michigan, Ann Arbor, Michigan and also from the Inter-University Consortium for Political and Social Research.
[4] These European data are extracted from the May 1976 Euro-Barometer, a series of national surveys conducted semi-annually in the EEC countries and coordinated by the Commission of the European Community. For more details on these surveys and a report of results from earlier Euro-Barometers, see Inglehart (1977), Rabier (1974), and Riffault and Rabier (1977). These and other data from the series are available from the Belgian Archives for the Social Sciences, Catholic University, Louvain, and also from the Inter-University Consortium for Political and Social Research.
[5] The off-scale categories were rarely used (with obvious exceptions, such as inquiries about "job"), and were treated as missing data.
[6] The technique is implemented in a computer program called MINISSA (Roskam and Lingoes, 1970; Lingoes and Roskam, 1973; Lingoes, Guttman, and Roskam, 1977). Input to MINISSA was a matrix of Pearson correlation coefficients (computed with pairwise deletion of missing data).
[7] We have, above, likened the identification of psychological structures to 'cognitive mapping.' This analogy is legitimate: If one submits a matrix of distances between *geographic* points (e.g., cities) to Smallest Space Analysis, it will produce an acceptable geographic map of the region involved.
[8] Coefficients of alienation, a measure of the consistency between the interpoint distances in the multidimensional space and the intercorrelations among the life concern assessments, ranged from 0.10 to 0.13 for the eight European countries when 15 items were arrayed in three-dimensional space, and was 0.19 for USA when more than 60 items were arrayed in three-dimensional space. Comparable figures for two-dimensional space were 0.18–0.21 for the European countries and 0.26 for USA. When only the 11 items that are similar in the USA and European data were arrayed in three dimensions, the coefficient of alienation for the USA data was 0.10.
[9] Two computer programs were used to accomplish these tasks: PINDIS (Lingoes and Borg, 1976; Lingoes, Guttman, and Roskam, 1977), and SPACES (Computer Support Group of the Center for Political Studies, 1976).
[10] Neel, Rothhammer, and Lingoes (1974) report a Monte Carlo exploration of the stability of S in one application but do not provide statistical tests which are of general applicability.
[11] From previous analyses (Andrews and Withey, 1976, Chapter 6), we can estimate that the American data used in this paper has validity of about 0.7, reliability of about 0.8, and includes about 10 percent correlated measurement error and about 40 percent uncorrelated measurement error. A roughly similar composition is expected to characterize the European data.

[12] The two other dimensions of the space, while needed to locate items in correct relative position to one another, do not seem to show conceptually meaningful progressions. While such progressions are interesting if found, there is no necessity that they occur, and no requirement that one "interpret" the dimensions of a structure. (Note that the same applies to the 2 — or 3 — dimensions of geographic or celestial maps.)

[13] Andrews and Withy (1976, Chapter 3) identify 12 clusters among these items.

[14] Values of the square root of S (i.e., of $S^{1/2}$) rather than of S are presented because it is this statistic that Lingoes and Schönemann (1974) propose as the matrix analogue of a coefficient of alienation (and because these values are produced by the PINDIS and SPACES computer programs used for the present analysis).

[15] In an exploration going one step beyond the similarity analyses reported in this sub-section, we considered the possible effects of differential weighting of the dimensions of the configurations. (This is another capability of the PINDIS and SPACES computer programs referenced previously.) While differential weighting made it possible to more closely match most of the configurations, the differences were not large and the basic pattern of results just described for Exhibit 3 was maintained. In a related but as yet unpublished analysis, Russell Dalton has examined cross-national similarities in the structure of perceived well-being using 1973 and 1975 European data. His results are in general accord with those reported here and provide an approximate replication from an independent source.

[16] Configurations for the other six European countries will be provided upon request.

[17] Campbell, Converse, and Rodgers (1976, pg. 74-75) report a matching of American and British structures based on different and somewhat more limited data than those used for Exhibits 2 and 5. While some of the details of their matching differ from what we find here, their general conclusion — that "the correspondence is fairly close" — clearly agrees with ours. Levy (1976) has also reported a matching of well-being structures derived from American and Israeli respondents. Here, also, a conclusion of there being a substantial match was also put forward, though a numerical assessment of the degree of fit was not made.

[18] These include differences in item wordings (particularly for the job item), in the set of other items that were present when the original structures were determined, and in the error compositions of the measures.

[19] For example, we observed a correlation of about 0.3 between the similarity of structures of perceived well-being (shown in Exhibit 3) and the differences between the countries in mean satisfaction with "life in general." Given a more heterogeneous set of countries, this relationship might appear stronger and, if so, might be attributed to the operation of Maslovian principles.

[20] Andrews and Withey (1976, Chapter 2) and Campbell, Converse, and Rodgers (1976, Chapter 3) both report explorations of differences in such perceptual structures among subgroups of the American population. Both sets of investigators, using entirely independent sets of data, came to the same general conclusion: that while modest differences appeared among structures identified for the subgroups, the basic features of the structure identified at the national level remained evident. Andrews and Withey (1976, Chapter 4) also showed that the same prediction equation was about equally effective for a large number of different subgroups for predicting feelings about general well-being on the basis of evaluations of life concerns.

REFERENCES

Abrams, M. 'Subjective social indicators'. *Social Trends*, No. 4. London, Her Majesty's Stationary Office, 1973.

Allardt, E. 'Dimensions of welfare in a comparative Scandinavian study'. *Research Reports* No. 9. Helsinki, Research Group for Comparative Sociology, University of Helsinki, 1975.

Andrews, F. M. and Withey, S. B. *Social Indicators of Well-being: Americans' Perceptions of Life Quality*. New York, Plenum, 1976.

Campbell, A., Converse, P. E., and Rodgers, W. L. *The Quality of American Life: Perceptions, Evaluations, and Satisfactions*. New York, Russell Sage Foundation, 1976.

Computer Support Group of the Center for Political Studies. *SPACES*: Program Writeup. Ann Arbor, Michigan, Institute for Social Research, The University of Michigan, June 1976.

Development Academy of the Philippines. *Measuring the Quality of Life: Philippine Social Indicators*. Manila, Development Academy of the Philippines, 1975.

Guttman, L. 'A general nonmetric technique for finding the smallest coordinate space for a configuration of points'. *Psychometrika*, 1968, 33, 469–506.

Hall, J. 'Subjective measures of quality of life in Britain: 1971 to 1975; Some developments and trends'. *Social Trends*, No. 7. London, Her Majesty's Stationary Office, 1976.

Inglehart, R. F. *The Silent Revolution: Changing Values and Political Styles among Western Publics*. Princeton, Princeton University Press, 1977.

Levy, S. 'Use of the mapping sentence for coordinating theory and research: A cross cultural example'. *Quality and Quantity*, 1976, 10, 117–125.

Lingoes, J. C. and Borg, I. 'Procrustean individual difference scaling'. *Journal of Marketing Research*, 1976, 13, 406–407.

Lingoes, J. C., Guttman, L., and Roskam, E. E. *Geometric Representations of Relational Data*. Ann Arbor, Michigan, Mathesis Press, 1977.

Lingoes, J. C. and Roskam, E. 'A mathematical and empirical study of two multidemensional scaling algorithms'. *Psychometric Monographs*, 1973, 38.

Lingoes, J. C. and Schönemann, P. H. 'Alternative measures of fit for the Schönemann-Carrol matrix fitting algorithm'. *Psychometrika*, 1974, 39, 423–427.

Neel, J. V., Rothhammer, F., and Lingoes, J. C. 'The genetic structure of a tribal population, the Yanomamo Indians. X. Agreement between representations of village distances based on different sets of characteristics'. *American Journal of Human Genetics*, 1974, 26, 281–303.

Rabier, J. R. *Satisfaction et Insatisfaction Quant aux Conditions de Vie dans les Pays Membres de la Communaute Europeene*. Brussels, Commission of the European Communities, 1974.

Riffault, H. and Rabier, J. R. *The perception of poverty in Europe*. Brussels, Commission of the European Communities, 1977.

Roskam, E. and Lingoes, J. C. 'MINISSA-I: A FORTRAN IV (G) program for the smallest space analysis of square symmetric matrices'. *Behavioral Science*, 1970, 15, 204–205.

Schönemann, P. H. and Carroll, R. M. 'Fitting one matrix to another under choice of a central dilation and a rigid motion'. *Psychometrika*, 1970, 35, 245–255.

Shepard, R. M., Romney, A. K., and Nerlove, S. B. *Multidimensional Scaling*. New York, Seminar Press, 1972.

FRANK M. ANDREWS AND AUBREY C. MCKENNELL

9. MEASURES OF SELF-REPORTED WELL-BEING: THEIR AFFECTIVE, COGNITIVE, AND OTHER COMPONENTS*

(Received 24 April, 1979)

ABSTRACT. This investigation begins from the hypothesis that social indicators of perceived well-being – e.g., people's assessment of their own life quality – will, like other atttudes, reflect two basic types of influences: affect and cognition. In addition, the indicators were expected to include two other components: unique variance (mainly random measurement error) and correlated measurement error. These ideas are investigated using a structural modeling approach applied to 23 assessments of life-as-a-whole from a national survey of Americans ($N = 1072$) and/or a survey of urban residents in England ($N = 932$). In both sets of data, models that included affective and cognitive factors fit significantly better than more restricted models. Furthermore, as expected, measures of (a) 'happiness', 'fun', and 'enjoyment' tended to be relatively more loaded with affect than were measures of (b) 'satisfaction', 'success', and 'meeting needs'; and (c) measures designed to tap both affect and cognition tended to fall between the first two groups. In addition, the results suggest that measures employing relatively many scale points and direct assessments yield more valid indicators of people's evaluations of life-as-a-whole than do measures based on three-point scales or on explicit comparisons with other times or groups. These results contribute to basic knowledge about the nature of life quality assessments, help to explain some previously puzzling relationships with demographic factors such as age and education, and may be useful to designers of future studies of perceived well-being.

1. INTRODUCTION

Previous research on the nature of attitudes suggests that they include at least two fundamental components: *cognition* and *affect*. In figurative language, cognition refers to the rational, 'from-the-head', aspects of a person's response, while affect refers to the emotional, 'from-the-heart' (or 'from-the-gut') components.

Measures of perceived ('subjective') well-being – one type of social indicator – are fundamentally measures of attitudes, and hence can be expected to reflect cognitive and affective elements. Furthermore, different measures of perceived well-being can be expected to include different combinations of cognition and affect. In fact, this may explain why different measures of well-being sometimes show distinct patterns of relationships to other variables.

This article reports a series of explorations into the affective and cognitive

Alex C. Michalos (ed.), Citation Classics from Social Indicators Research, 191–219.
© 2005 *Springer. Printed in the Netherlands.*

components of some of the more widely used measures of perceived well-being. It is shown that the expected differences among the measures do indeed appear and that these differences replicate in independent social indicator surveys conducted in the United States and Great Britain.

From the standpoint of basic science, the research reported here represents an attempt to understand some of the fundamental types of influences that determine the responses people give when asked about their well-being. From a more applied perspective, this report may offer guidance to future investigators who face practical problems of selecting or constructing measures for use in studies of self-reported life quality.

In Sections 2 and 3 we briefly review the intellectual heritage out of which the present study arises – some recent studies on perception of well-being, and some of the relevant past research pertaining to the nature of attitudes, respectively. Section 4 describes the 23 measures of global well-being that will be the focus of attention here, the two major data sources that have been analysed, and the structural-equation methodology that has been employed. The statistical results, and certain checks on those results, are presented in Section 5. Section 6 summarizes the results and describes some needed further research.

2. CONNECTIONS TO SOME PREVIOUS RESEARCH ON PERCEIVED WELL-BEING

The past decade has witnessed an expanding worldwide interest in the compilation of various types of social indicators. Some of the work has taken the form of conducting sample surveys of national, regional or metropolitan populations to assess perceptions of well-being – i.e., of people's direct first-hand evaluations of the quality of their lives, both in general and with respect to numerous specific life concerns (for example, job, family, neighborhood, public services, sense of fairness, safety, and many more). Among the major recent quality-of-life surveys are those described by Allardt (1973) in Scandinavia, Andrews and Withey (1976) and Campbell, Converse, and Rodgers (1976) in USA, Abrams (1973) and Hall (1976) in England, and Blishen and Atkinson (1978) in Canada. Earlier surveys by Cantril (1966) in 13 countries and by Bradburn (1969) in USA should also be mentioned.

These surveys, and many others with similar objectives, have used a variety of different questions to elicit people's attitudes about their lives. A common way to obtain feelings at the most global level has been to ask the simple question, "How do you feel about your life as a whole?" and then to provide a set of answer categories that range from 'Delighted' to 'Terrible', or from 'Completely satisfied' to 'Completely dissatisfied', or from 'The best I could expect to have' to 'The worst I could expect to have'. There are numerous alternatives, however, and sometimes respondents have been asked about happiness ('How happy are you?'), about positive affect ('During the past few weeks did you ever feel on top of the world?'), about negative affect ('During the past few weeks did you ever feel depressed or very unhappy?'), about the frequency of worrying, about current mood, and many more. This list is not exhaustive, but serves to illustrate some of the approaches that have been tried. (For a list of more than 60 different measures of global well-being, a proposed typology for classifying these measures, and information on how most of the measures related to each other in one set of American data, see Andrews and Withey, 1976, Chapter 3.)

In the most general terms, it can be said that most of the different measures of perceived global well-being have shown broadly similar patterns of relationships to other variables. For example, richer people have expressed more positive sentiments than poorer people; blacks – at least in the United States – have rated their life quality lower than have whites; and most of the global measures that have been submitted to multivariate analysis have been reasonably predictable by additive combinations of evaluations of more specific life concerns.

Although the most basic patterns are broadly similar, closer examination reveals subtle but potentially important differences among the measures. There is no reason to assume that (1) all measures tap people's underlying feelings with the same sensitivity, or (2) that all measures tap the same set of underlying feelings. In fact, past research in psychometrics would lead one to expect that some answer formats would provide more precise measures than other formats, and that different question wordings (e.g., asking about 'happiness' versus 'satisfaction') would result in measures with different orientations. Indeed, the published work on social indicators includes some hints that these kinds of differences do in fact occur. For example, Campbell, Converse, and Rodgers (1976) report that feelings of happiness tended to be lower among older people, but that feelings of satisfaction tended to be higher. A partial replication is reported by Andrews and Withey (1976): They also found that happiness declined with age (but satisfaction showed no clear upward trend). In another example Smith (1978) reports that measures of happiness and affect show seasonal variations over the year but that measures of satisfaction remain constant.

The fact that different measures show somewhat different patterns of relationships raises the fundamental question, Why? It would seem reasonable to suppose that the measures are tapping different components of people's attitudes about their own well-being. Given that self-reports of well-being are reports about attitudes, and the well-established usefulness of analysing attitudes in terms of their affective and cognitive components, it seems reasonable to expect that these differences in the measures might be attributable to their comprising different combinations of affect and cognition. McKennell (1978) and McKennell and Andrews (1980) have presented extended theoretical discussions and some empirical data in support of this view.

3. CONNECTIONS TO SOME PREVIOUS RESEARCH ON THE NATURE OF ATTITUDES

Interest in the nature of attitudes has a long history in social psychology. After reviewing 16 previous definitions of *attitude*, Allport defined it as follows in 1935: "It is a mental and neural state of readiness to respond, organized through experience exerting a directive and/or dynamic influence on behavior." Forty years later, in another extensive review of the attitude literature, Fishbein and Ajzen (1975) defined *attitude* as: "a learned predisposition to respond in a consistently favorable or unfavorable manner with respect to a given object." It seems obvious that people's responses to questions about perceived well-being in quality-of-life surveys meet the above definitions and hence that knowledge about the nature of attitudes may have something to contribute to our understanding of self-reports of well-being.

The idea that mental states may include various conceptually distinct components has been around for thousands of years. According to McGuire (1968), philosophers have concluded that there are basically three perspectives from which the human condition can be viewed: *knowing*, *feeling*, and *acting*, and he cites both Hindu and classical Greek sources as proposing that attitudes include cognitive, affective, and conative (i.e., behavioral) components. A basically similar trilogy of components has been investigated by social psychologists for the past several decades. Ostrom (1969), for example, describes the situation as follows:

At the most global level, attitudes can be characterized as an evaluation of the attitude objective on a pro to con continuum. This generalized evaluation can be analyzed into three components: affective, behavioral, and cognitive.

The [affective] component includes... favorable to unfavorable feelings... [expressions of] like or dislike, feelings, and emotional and physiological reactions. Perhaps the phrase 'gut reaction' best conveys the spirit of this component.

The [behavioral] component includes... supportive to hostile actions... [reflecting] personal action tendencies,... past actions, future intentions, and predicted behavior in hypothetical situations.

The cognitive component includes... desirable to undesirable qualities... [reflecting] values and attributes assigned to the attitude object,... beliefs about the object, characteristics of the object, and relationships of the object with other objects (including self). Evaluative phrases which are not on the emotional continuum should also be included. (Ostrom, 1969, p. 16)

While the conceptual distinctions between the cognitive, affective, and behavioral aspects of attitudes seem reasonably clear, the statistical relationships among these components are of some debate. One could argue — as do Insko and Schopler (1967) for example — that a 'triadic consistency' should generally prevail among the three components. The investigation reported by Ostrom (1969) did indeed find high overlaps among the three components. Alternatively, one could *define* the components to be statistically independent of one another — arguing, for example, that cognitive components are those aspects which are different from (i.e., statistically unrelated to) affective components. For reasons of convenience, and because of the nature of the data that are available to us, we adopt this latter strategy, but we also show that the degree of presumed overlap between affect and cognition actually has little effect on the general conclusions that will be drawn about the nature of self-reports of well-being.

Although investigators of attitudes sometimes also consider a behavioral component as part of an attitude (and sometimes *intentions* are further distinguished from actual behavior), behavior will not be considered in the present report. The assessments of perceived well-being that are examined below are evaluations of life quality that have no direct behavioral referents, and hence a behavioral component seems of little relevance. This is not to say, however, that the measures of well-being are expected to be statistically independent from either actual behavior or behavior intentions: on the contrary, such links probably do exist, but seem not to be constituent parts of the particular survey measures that have been widely used to date. (Exploration of these links should be on the agenda for further research.)

4. DATA SOURCES, MEASURES, AND ESTIMATION METHODOLOGY

4.1 *Data sources*

The data analysed in this report come from two separate surveys.

One survey was designed to be representative of American adults and was based on a probability sample of all American citizens aged 18 and over (and married persons under 18) living in households in the continental United States (except households on military reservations). These data were collected under the direction of Andrews and Withey in November 1972 from 1072 respondents as part of a larger face-to-face personal interview study (see Andrews and Withey, 1976, Appendix B, for further details on sampling design, response rates, etc.). Data were collected by trained interviewers of the University of Michigan's Survey Research Center.

The second survey was of British adults. It was conducted in March 1975 under the direction of Abrams and Hall and was based on a representative sample of people aged 16 and over living in British metropolitan areas. The number of respondents to this survey was 932. Other analyses of these British data have been reported by Abrams (1976) and by Hall (1976).

4.2 *Measures of global well-being*

Although plans for the present analyses had not been formulated at the time the surveys were originally designed, the desirability of including a wide range of different measures of global well-being was clear. Thus it happens that the range of measures now at our disposal, while not ideal, is nevertheless rather well suited to our needs.

The analyses reported below focus on 23 different measures of global well-being. Of these, 10 were assessed in the American survey and 16 in the British survey (there are three measures that are identical in both surveys).[1] Exhibit 1 presents the exact wording of each question and response scale, a short code name for each measure, and the source(s) of the data. The heterogeneous character of these various ways of assessing people's feelings about their life-as-a-whole is immediately evident.

The order of presentation within Exhibit 1 is in accord with our initial expectations about the relative sensitivity of the measures to affective and cognitive elements. The measures can be divided into four groups:

EXHIBIT 1

Measures of global Well-being

Variable's group and name	Description	Suvey[a]
Group A		
Life 1	"How do you feel about your life as a whole?" Answered on scale with seven main categories: 'Delighted,' 'Pleased', 'Mostly satisfied', 'Mixed (about equally satisfied and dissatisfied)', 'Mostly dissatisfied', 'Unhappy', 'Terrible'; plus several off-scale categories – 'Neutral', and 'I never thought about it' – which were excluded in analysis.	A
Life 2	Same as Life 1 but asked later in the interview.	A
Group B		
Sat 11-pt	"All things considered, how satisfied or dissatisfied are you with your life as a whole these days?" Eleven point response scale (numbered 0–10) labelled at the ends with: 'Dissatisfied' and 'Satisfied'.	B
Sat 7-pt	"How satisfied are you with your life as a whole these days?" Seven point response scale, labelled at the ends with: 'Completely satisfied' and 'Completely dissatisfied'.	A
Sat 3-pt	"In general, how satisfying do you find the way you're spending your life these days? Would you call it completely satisfying, pretty satisfying, or not very satisfying?"	A
Make sat	"...how you feel about your present life": Seven point response scale labelled at the ends with 'Makes me completely dissatisfied' and 'Makes me completely satisfied'.	B
Doing well	"When you think of the things you want from life now, would you say you were doing very well, fairly well, or not too well?"	B
Successful	"...how you feel about your present life": Seven point response scale labelled at the ends with 'Unsuccessful' and 'Successful'.	B
Meets needs	"... how you feel about your present life": Seven point response scale labelled at the ends with 'Does not meet my needs in any way' and 'Meets my needs in every way'.	B
Bet th des	"...how you feel about your present life": Seven point response scale labelled at the ends with 'Is very much worse than I deserve' and 'Is very much better than I deserve'.	B
Group C		
Affect pos	Bradburn's Positive Affect Scale: the number of five positive events experienced. "During the past few weeks did you ever feel ...particularly excited or interested in something? ...proud because someone complimented you on something you had done? ...pleased about having accomplished something? ...on top of the world? ...that things were going your way?"	A, B

Exhibit 1 (continued)

Affect neg	Bradburn's Negative Affect Scale: the number of five negative events experienced. "During the past few weeks did you ever feel ...so restless that you couldn't sit long in a chair? ...very lonely or remote from other people? ...bored? ... depressed or very unhappy? ...upset because someone citicized you?"	A, B
Happy 7-pt	"...how you feel about your present life": Seven point response scale labelled at the ends with 'Un-happy' and 'Happy'.	B
Happy 3-pt	"Taking all things together, how would you say things are these days – would you say you're very happy, pretty happy, or not too happy these days?"	A, B
Make happy	"..how you feel about your present life": Seven point response scale labelled at the ends with 'Makes me extremely unhappy' and 'Makes me extremely happy'.	B
Happy D–T	"How do you feel about how happy you are?" (Same delighted-terrible response scale as Life 1)	A
Fun	"...how you feel about your present life": Seven point response scale labelled at the ends with 'Full of fun' and 'No fun at all'.	B
Enjoyable	"...how you feel about your present life": Seven point response scale labelled at the ends with 'Enjoyable' and 'Miserable'.	B

Group D

Change 11-pt	"Think of how your life is going now. How much would you like to change your life as it is now?" Eleven point response scale (numbered 0–10) labelled at the ends with 'Not at all' and 'A very great deal'.	B
Change 3-pt	"Considering how your life is going, would you like to continue much the same way, change some parts of it, or change many parts of it?"	A
Bet future	"...how you feel about your present life": Seven point response scale labelled at the ends with 'Will get very much worse in the future' and 'Will get very much better in the future'.	B
Worry	"In general, how much would you say you worry these days?" Same response scale as Change 11-pt.	B
Thermometer	"Where would you put your life as a whole these days on the feeling thermometer?" Vertical scale running from "100° – very warm or favorable feeling' to '0° – very cold or unfavorable feeling' with intermediate numbers and labels at 85°, 70°, 60°, 50°, 40°, 30°, and 15° (see Andrews & Withey, 1976, p. 367, for full wording of intermediate labels).	A

[a] Key to surveys: A = American data (Andrews & Withey, 1976)
B = British data (Abrams, 1976; Hall, 1976)

A. The first two measures, Life 1 and Life 2, were specifically designed to tap *both* affective and cognitive elements.

B. The second group consists of measures that were expected to be primarily sensitive to cognitive elements. The first four measures in Group B, all of which assess *satisfaction*, were expected to be more sensitive to cognitive than affective elements because of the notion that the concept of satisfaction requires some kind of comparison — either explicit or implicit — between a level of achievement and some standard (e.g., what one expects or aspires to) and hence involves the kind of judgmental thinking and knowledge that is the hallmark of cognition. The remaining four measures in Group B, although not phrased in terms of satisfaction, were also expected to be sensitive primarily to cognitive aspects because each of these items involves a comparison with certain implied or explicit criteria.

C. The third group consists of eight measures that were expected to be primarily affective in orientation. The first two of these measures — Bradburn's scales of Positive affect and Negative affect — were expected to come as close as any of these measures to representing 'pure' affect. These two scales, each consisting of five separate items, have been taken directly from Bradburn (1969). (His finding — surprising when it first emerged — that these measures were uncorrelated with each other replicated in both of the present surveys. The product-moment correlations between these two scales were 0.01 and 0.00 in the American and British data, respectively.) Next there follow four items in Group C that ask about *happiness*. The first three of these happiness items have simple answer scales that were expected to give the measure a heavily affective cast; the fourth happiness measure, which was answered on a more complex scale that includes ideas of satisfaction as well as affect, was expected to come closer to being 'balanced' with respect to affect and cognition than the other three, but still to be primarily affective. The final two measures in this group — those asking about fun and enjoyableness — were also expected to be predominantly sensitive to affective components.

D. The fourth group includes five items that clearly tap attitudes about global well-being, but for which we had no clear expectations regarding their relative sensitivity to affective and cognitive components. Included here are two measures that ask about desired changes in the future, another than asks about expected changes in the future, one that asks about worries, and a very general item about life-as-a-whole answered on a response scale (the feeling thermometer — widely used for assessing attitudes toward political candidates) which provided few clues regarding the likely affective-cognitive balance in the answers.

4.3 *Estimation methods*

General approach. To estimate the sensitivity of global measures of well-being to their presumed underlying affective and cognitive elements requires that these components be disentangled from each other, and from certain other components that will shortly be described. The new technology of structural equation modelling with unmeasured variables offers a powerful means for accomplishing this.

What one knows, on the basis of the observed data, is how the various measures relate to one another. Using this information jointly with a causal model — i.e., with some specific ideas about factors that might have influenced the measures and hence affected their covariation — one can seek a mutually consistent set of influence estimates that will account for the entire set of observed covariations. While one can never 'prove' — in an ultimate sense — that a particular causal model is correct, various pieces of evidence will determine the degree of confidence one may have in the model. Among the criteria are (1) the extent to which the model incorporates current thinking about relevant sources of influence, (2) the degree to which the model succeeds in accounting for the observed patterns in the data, and (3) the reasonableness of the parameter estimates produced by the model, considering other things already known or suspected about the measures.

The models used in the present analyses presume that there are four types of influences that may be present, in varying degrees, in measures of global well-being. These four are: (1) affective reactions a person has to his or her life-as-a-whole; (2) cognitive reactions to life-as-a-whole; (3) reactions that have nothing to do with life-as-a-whole but which influence two or more of the well-being measures because of the way they were assessed (i.e., 'correlated errors', or 'methods effects'); and (4) everything else that might influence a single measure but which has nothing to do with a person's reactions to global well-being (i.e., 'uncorrelated errors').

Exhibit 2 presents the model that was applied to the American data. A generally similar model was applied to the Britsh data and will be discussed later.

Parameter estimates for this and all other models were computed by

LISREL III, a computer program that estimates linear structural equation systems by maximum likelihood methods (Joreskog and Sorbom, 1976).

The basic model. The model portrayed in Exhibit 2 is a straightforward implementation of the causal hypotheses sketched previously. Within the rectangles on the left and right of Exhibit 2 are the actual measures being

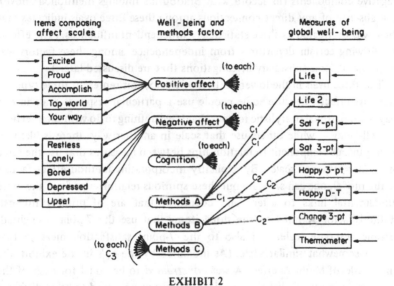

EXHIBIT 2
The structural model that was applied to American data.

analysed. The first block of five rectangles on the left contains the items that constitute Bradburn's Positive affect scale, and the second block of five contains the items of the Negative affect scale (see Exhibit 1). On the right are eight measures of global well-being. It is the interrelationships among these 18 items that this model seeks to explain. The model assumes that the relationships vary because the measures are differentially sensitive to some of the same underlying sources of influence.

The arrows going to each rectangle symbolize inputs from particular sources of influence. Although not shown in Exhibit 2, each arrow carries a number (a 'parameter estimate') which indicates *how much* influence enters along that path.

The three ovals in the upper center of Exhibit 2 represent the affective and cognitive reactions which we presume people have to their life-as-a-whole. Note that the affective reactions have been separated into positive and negative components (in accord with Bradburn's findings mentioned above). The absence of any direct connections among these three ovals indicates that they will be treated as three statistically independent influences. (The effects of allowing certain departures from independence among these factors was the topic of some subsidiary investigations that are discussed later.)

The three ovals in the lower portion of the exhibit represent three types of methods effects. Because some people use a particular response scale in one way — for personal or stylistic reasons that have nothing to do with their feelings of well-being — while others use that scale in another way, there is likely to be a spurious component to relationships between measures that use the same or similar response scales. By explicitly incorporating method effect factors in the model, one can separate out these spurious relationships from the more fundamental links to affect and cognition that are of primary interest. Method factor A links to the three items that use the 7-point Delighted-terrible response scale, and also to the 7-point satisfaction measure that used a somewhat similar scale. (As indicated by the c_1's in the exhibit, the magnitude of Methods effect A was *constrained* to be equal for each of the measures using the Delighted-terrible scale, but was allowed to be of different magnitude for the 7-point satisfaction measure.) Method factor B links to the three measures that have similar three-category response scales; the c_2's in the exhibit indicate that this method effect was constrained to be equal for each of these measures. Finally, Method factor C links to each of the 10 affect items, all of which were answered in a simple yes-no format; the c_3 in the exhibit indicates that all of these method effects were constrained to be equal.

In addition to the inputs from affect, cognition, and shared methods effects, each measure is presumed to include certain random (i.e., uncorrelated) errors. The short arrows entering each rectangle from the perimeter of the exhibit represent the influences of these random errors. (Because the Thermometer measure uses a response scale different from that of any other measure in this analysis, any effect attributable to that scale will be included in the uncorrelated error component of this measure.)

The substantive meaning of the unmeasured causal variables. A reasonable concern, when one examines a model such as that portrayed in Exhibit 2, is with the 'meaning' of the unmeasured variables indicated by the ovals. What leads one to believe that they operate in accord with the labels that have been placed on them? The answer lies in how the ovals are linked, or *not* linked, to each other and to the observed measures, and in how these linkages have been controlled (e.g., by constraining them to be equal) (Burt, 1976).

In the case of the factor labelled Positive affect, this factor was expected to act like pure positive affect because it is the *only* factor that can uniquely explain the covariation among the items of Bradburn's Positive affect scale, covariation which — as noted previously — was presumed to result from these items' common sensitivity to positive affect. (Note that the Methods factor C, because all its links are constrained to be equal, can represent only something that all five positive affect items and all five negative affect items have in common and to the same degree, and hence this factor will not pick up positive affect.)

Parallel comments explain why the Negative affect factor was expected to come reasonably close to representing pure negative affect.

Unfortunately, none of the available measures seemed even close to being an indicator of pure cognition. Accordingly, the cognitive factor has been defined through a process of residualization. The cognitive factor is what the global well-being measures share that is *not* affect (either positive or negative) and that is *not* attributable to common method effects. This approach to defining a cognition factor, despite its being indirect, seems well supported by both theory and analytic results. As noted in Section 3 of this paper, there is substantial evidence that some kind of cognitive mental process seems to be one of the underlying factors that influence attudes. And, as we have shown elsewhere (McKennell and Andrews, 1980), a cognitive factor residualized as here: (1) does make a useful contribution to explaining the pattern of covariations among global measures of well-being; (2) yields highly consistent factor loadings across a substantial variety of causal models; and (3) shows replicable cross-national results.

While the ability to estimate the parameters of structural equations incorporating unmeasured variables, as required by the model portrayed in Exhibit 2, represents a very important and quite recent technological development, it must be recognized that the values obtained are only *estimates* of what may go on in the real world. We believe the model appropriately incorporates past and current theorizing about the nature of attitudes and about likely sources of errors in observed measures, and, furthermore, the model does indeed explain the relationships among the measures rather well and on the basis of reasonable parameter estimates (as will be detailed in Section 5). Nevertheless, there is no direct way to 'prove' that results from applying this model are precisely correct. What seems important at this point is to observe that nothing to date has suggested a fundamental flaw in the model or its application, and that although the numerical values of some of the parameter estimates will vary according to certain assumptions made in specifying the model, the overall pattern of results, and hence the general conclusions to be derived from them, seem not to be heavily dependent on these assumptions.

5. RESULTS

This section begins by presenting the results from the analysis of measures in the American data. Then follows a description of results from the British data. Finally a series of subsidiary analyses designed to check the sensitivity of the conclusions to various assumptions made in the main analyses are presented.

5.1 *Measures in the American data*

Exhibit 3 presents the results of applying the model portrayed in Exhibit 2 to the well-being measures included in the American survey. Before turning to its 12 columns of information, however, it is important to report that the model performed quite satisfactorily in accounting for the variances and covariances among the measures.[2] There were a total of 171 such variance or covariance statistics to be 'explained', and the average predicted value of each was within ± 0.04 of the observed value and in no case was a prediction off by as much as 0.19.

In Exhibit 3, columns 3—9 indicate the sensitivity of the well-being measures to various components of attitudes about life-as-a-whole, columns 10 and 11 indicate sensitivity to other influences (correlated and random measurement errors), and column 12 is a total. Note that the figures under 'Other' components are subdivided into two types of components: Correlated measurement error variance attributable to a measure's sharing common response scales (shown in column 10), and unique variance (shown in column 11), most of which is probably random measurement error, but some of which might be a measure's valid reflection of attitudes that have nothing to do with feelings about life-as-a-whole. Note, also, that the figures for the totals in column 12 all come close to 100%, as one would expect. (The small discrepancies from 100% are primarily attributable to the model's not being able to account precisely for all the variance of each measure while simulta-neously having to account for all the other variances and covariances.)

The results shown in Exhibit 3 are generally in accord with our expecta-tions, sketched earlier, about the composition of these global measures. How-ever, there is one substantial surprise, and a few other results may call for adjustments in our expectations.

As noted in the initial discussion of the measures, the Group A measures — Life 1 and Life 2 — were expected to reflect substantial amounts of both affect and cognition. The affect-cognition ratios presented in column 7 show that the two types of components come close to being balanced in these measures. In the case of Life 1, the ratio of 0.8 is based on estimates that 26% of the variance reflects affective components and 33% reflects cognitive components (see columns 5 and 6). Furthermore, the affective component is itself evenly divided between positive and negative affect — 13% of the measure's variance being attributable to each, as is shown in columns 1 and 2. For Life 2, the affect-cognition ratio is nearly the same, at 0.7, as it is for Life 1, and none of the variance component estimates differ in a statistically significant way from those for Life 1.[3] For an indication of the extent to which the Life 1 and Life 2 measures are sensitive to feelings about life-as-a-whole, one may refer to column 8 of the exhibit, where it is shown that approximately 60% of the variance of these measures (59% and 61%, res-pectively) is estimated to tap either affect or cognition (column 8 is the

EXHIBIT 3

Estimated variance components for measures of global well-being in American data

Group	Measure	'True' variance							Other variance		Total
		Affect		Sum	Cognition	A:C ratio	Total L-A-W		Common methods	Unique	
		Pos.	Neg.				%	coef			
(1)	(2)	(3)	(4)	(5)	(6)	(7)	(8)	(9)	(10)	(11)	(12)
A	Life 1	13%	13%	26%	33%	0.8	59%	0.77	10%	31%	100%
	Life 2	15%	11%	26%	35%	0.7	61%	0.78	10%	26%	97%
B	Sat 7-pt	10%	14%	24%	32%	0.8	56%	0.75	3%	39%	98%
	Sat 3-pt	8%	15%	23%	19%	1.2	42%	0.65	5%	51%	98%
C	Happy 3-pt	19%	14%	33%	15%	2.2	48%	0.69	5%	45%	98%
	Happy D-T	18%	12%	30%	29%	1.0	59%	0.77	10%	29%	98%
D	Change 3-pt	2%	17%	19%	12%	1.6	31%	0.56	5%	64%	100%
	Thermometer	8%	6%	14%	26%	0.5	40%	0.63	0%	60%	100%

sum of columns 5 and 6). Since some readers will be accustomed to 'validity coefficients' as these are reported in the psychometric literature, column 9 reports the measure's estimated sensitivity to aspects of life-as-a-whole in this form — 0.77 and 0.78 for Life 1 and Life 2, respectively. (Column 9 is simply the square root of column 8.) Finally, the model indicates that about 10% of each measure's variance is attributable to common methods effects, and that another 25–31% is attributable to other unique sources (mainly random measurement error).

Thus the first part of Exhibit 3 contains no surprises, and in fact this characterization of the Life measures, while considerably more detailed than those available previously, is in excellent accord with previous analyses of these same data and with validity estimates for these measures when they were included in other data (e.g., Andrews and Withey, 1976, Chapter 6).

The surprises in Exhibit 3 come with respect to the Group B measures — the 7-point and 3-point satisfaction measures. It was expected that including the term 'satisfaction' in the question would make these measures somewhat more cognitive in orientation than the Life measures. That this seems not to be the case, however, can be seen by the affect-cognition ratios in column 7. The 7-point satisfaction measure has a ratio of 0.8, very similar to the Life measures, and the 3-point satisfaction measure has a ratio of 1.2, and hence is somewhat *more* affectively oriented than the Life measures. In fact, the 7-point satisfaction measure ' differs in only minor respects from the Life measures; it seems slightly less sensitive to both affect and cognition, and the balance of positive and negative affect tilts slightly toward negative affect.[4]

The 3-point satisfaction measure, besides having a surprisingly affective cast, seems notably less valid as an indicator of attitudes about life-as-a-whole (e.g., note columns 8 and 9). While the relatively affective cast of this measure was not expected, its lower overall sensitivity to attitudes about life-as-a-whole is just what one would expect on the basis of this measure's having only three response categories. There is substantial evidence that small numbers of answer categories (2–4) tend to reflect less true variance than larger numbers (5 or more) — see, for example, Cochran, 1968; Connor, 1972; Ramsay, 1973. The results in Exhibit 3 are consistent with this: Three of the four lowest validity coefficients (in column 9) are for measures using 3-point response scales.

The two happiness measures, Group C in Exhibit 3, are, as expected, relatively more affectively oriented than the Life measures (note their affect-cognition ratios of 2.2 and 1.0). Furthermore, again as expected, the Happy D-T measure is compositionally closer to the Life measures (which use the same D-T scale) than the 3-point happiness measure. The balance of positive and negative affect in both of these happiness measures (which is in favor of positive affect) is just opposite to that in the two satisfaction measures (where negative affect predominates). Finally, one may note that while the 3-point happiness measure has a high affect-cognition ratio, this ratio is high not because the measure is especially sensitive to affective components, but because it is especially *in*sensitive to cognitive components; unfortunately, the overall validity of this measure is only modest.[5]

The two measures in Group D — 3-point change and feelings about life-as-a-whole measured on the Thermometer scale — were ones about which we had no clear expectations regarding sensitivity to affect and cognition. In these data the affect-cognition ratios show the change measure to be weighted in favor of affect (and this is mainly *negative* affect — see columns 1 and 2), and the Thermometer measure to be weighted in favor of cognition. However, of all the measures in Exhibit 3, these two seem least sensitive to feelings about life-as-a-whole (note their low validities, in columns 8 and 9, and the large amounts of unique variance, in column 11).

Before describing some of the subsidiary analyses done to check the stability of these findings, or considering the implications these results have for people with practical concerns about measuring well-being, we present the results from the British survey, since in many ways they replicate and extend the pattern of the present findings.

5.2 *Measures in the British data*

The model that was applied to the British data was highly similar to that used for the American data and shown in Exhibit 2. There were only two modifications: (1) instead of including all 10 individual components of Bradburn's scales of Positive and Negative affect, the sclaes themselves were substituted,[6] and (2) because the measures used response scales that differed from the American survey, the methods factors had to be altered.[7]

The model applied to the British measures came even closer to reproducing their observed variances and covariances than did the model applied to the American data. The average (absolute) discrepancy between the observed and estimated values was only ± 0.02, and the highest discrepancy among all 136 was less than 0.12. As may be seen in column 12 of Exhibit 4, the model came reasonably close to accounting for 100% of the total variance of each measure.

Exhibit 4 presents the main statistical results for the British data and is laid out parallel with Exhibit 3. The British data included no measures in Group A, so the exhibit begins with the Group B measures — those that were expected to be relatively more sensitive to cognitive components than the measures included in Group C. A glance at the affect-cognition ratios in Exhibit 4 will confirm that this is indeed the case for most of the measures: The Group B measures tend to have lower ratios than the Group C measures. In fact, out of 30 comparisons between measures in Group B and C, only two comparisons run counter to the expected direction, and for neither of these is the discrepancy substantial.

Several of the Group C measures — Enjoyable, Fun, and Happy 7-point — appear very heavily loaded with affective components, as does one of the Group D measures. For these measures the affect-cognition ratios range from 4.0 up to 13.5. For example, Exhibit 4 estimates the Enjoyable measure as consisting of 27% affective variance, approximately evenly split between positive and negative affect, and only 2% cognitive variance, for an affect-cognition ratio of 13.5. The Worry measure also has a ratio at about the same level, but here nearly all of the affect is negative affect, a characteristic that seems intuitively reasonable. The Fun measure, in contrast, is estimated to be twice as sensitive to positive affect as to negative affect and (like Enjoyable and Worry) very little influenced by cognitive components. None of these measures with relatively heavy emphasis on affective components, however, shows more than mediocre validity (see columns 8 and 9 of Exhibit 4).

While the broad patterns evident in Exhibit 4 tend to be in accord with our initial expectations, and to replicate the major patterns in the American data, there are some interesting discrepancies between the U.S. and British results.

One can note, for example, that measures that ask about happiness in the British data tend to tilt in favor of negative affect, while the American data showed happiness items tending toward positive affect. (On the other hand, the satisfaction items tilt toward negative affect in both the British and American data sets). One can also observe that Change 11-point, a British measure, seems primarily sensitive to cognitive components, while the 3-point change measure, which occurs in the American data, was more sensitive to affective influences. One can also observe that the estimated validities (columns

EXHIBIT 4

Estimated variance components for measures of global well-being in British data

Group	Measure	'True' variance					Total L-A-W		Other variance		Total
		Affect		Sum	Cognition	A : C ratio	%	coef	Common methods	Unique	
		Pos.	Neg.								
(1)	(2)	(3)	(4)	(5)	(6)	(7)	(8)	(9)	(10)	(11)	(12)
	Sat 11-pt	11%	24%	35%	20%	1.8	55%	0.74	1%	45%	101%
	Make sat	13%	18%	31%	25%	1.2	56%	0.75	10%	35%	101%
	Doing well	8%	9%	17%	20%	0.9	37%	0.61	4%	60%	101%
	Successful	12%	14%	26%	16%	1.6	42%	0.65	10%	50%	102%
	Meets needs	9%	18%	27%	23%	1.2	50%	0.71	10%	42%	102%
	Bet than des	8%	7%	15%	8%	1.9	23%	0.48	10%	70%	103%
B	Happy 7-pt	10%	30%	40%	10%	4.0	50%	0.71	10%	40%	100%
	Happy 3-pt	12%	20%	32%	15%	2.1	47%	0.69	4%	49%	100%
C	Make happy	12%	20%	32%	19%	1.7	51%	0.71	10%	37%	98%
	Fun	20%	10%	30%	3%	10.0	33%	0.57	10%	57%	100%
	Enjoyable	12%	15%	27%	2%	13.5	29%	0.54	10%	62%	101%
D	Change 11-pt	1%	7%	8%	14%	0.6	22%	0.47	1%	77%	100%
	Bet future	11%	0%	11%	5%	2.2	16%	0.40	10%	76%	102%
	Worry	2%	24%	26%	2%	13.0	28%	0.53	1%	72%	101%

8 and 9) for measures in the American data tend to come out somewhat higher than in the British data. Whether these differences reflect true cultural differences, or result from different methodological contexts in which the data were collected and analysed, or both, cannot be immediately determined.

One difference between the British and American results that is immediately obvious, but which may be an artifact of assumptions made in specifying the model, is the fact that most measures that can be matched between the two surveys seem more sensitive to affective components in the British data. Note, for example, that the Group B measures in the American data have affect-cognition ratios of about 1.0, but that in the British data the ratios for measures in this group run from 0.9 up to 1.9. While this could reflect a cultural difference, we know from the experimentation described in note 7 that the size of the affect-cognition ratios is heavily dependent on assumptions made in specifying the model (but that these assumptions do not greatly influence the *rank order* of the ratios which are the primary focus of our attention).

5.3 *Further analyses*

In addition to the two main analyses just described, a number of additional analyses were performed to check the stability of the results under alternative assumptions and to see whether certain demographic variables would relate in expected ways to the factors of affect and cognition. One set of subsidiary analyses that checked the sensitivity of the British results to alternative assumptions about the validity of the affect scales has already been described in note 7 and needs only to be referenced here. Several other analyses, however, also merit attention.

Age and education related to affect and cognition. One of the empirical observations that suggested one consider separate factors that might underlie well-being measures was the finding that happiness and satisfaction showed different relationships to the age of respondents. (Happiness declined with age, satisfaction did not.) By adding age (and also education) to the model shown in Exhibit 2, we could examine the relationships of these variables to the unmeasured factors of affect and cognition that we presumed underlay the measures of global well-being.[8] The results for age were very much as expected: Age related negatively to both the positive and negative affect factors (−0.25 and −0.22, respectively), and positively to the cognition factor (+0.08). Education showed a different pattern: It related positively to positive affect (+0.28), and negatively to the negative affect and cognition factors (−0.07 and −0.12, respectively). Thus this analysis provided confirmation that the affect and cognition factors as operationalized in the model would relate differently to outside variables, and with patterns that seemed reasonable in the light of previous evidence. Since it was the differing patterns of relationships between well-being measures and age that had stimulated our initial interest in distinguishing affective and cognitive factors, being able to demonstrate that these factors as implemented in our model would indeed relate differently to outside variables was of considerable importance.

The relationship between positive affect and negative affect. One of the assumptions built into the model in Exhibit 2 is that the positive affect factor is statistically independent from the negative affect factor. While this assumption is in accord with Bradburn's findings that the two affect scales were statistically independent from each other and showed different patterns of relationships with other variables, the conclusion about the independence of positive and negative affect has been questioned by other investigators (Cherlin and Reeder, 1975; Brenner, 1975).

The implications of correlated error in the affect items for the observed zero correlation has not been considered in the literature. For example, it is entirely possible that the true underlying correlation between positive and negative affect could be negative but that measures tapping these affects could yield an observed correlation of zero because correlated errors would essentially cancel out the 'true' negative relationship, particularly after this had been attenuated by the effects of random error. This is a topic that needs further investigation.

In fact, tests with our model show that a good fit to the data could be achieved assuming *any* relationship ranging from 0 to −1.0 between the affect factors simply by allowing compensating changes in the impacts of Methods factor C. Thus it was important to see whether the basic conclusions described earlier regarding the order of the measures with respect to their relative sensitivity to affect and cognition would change if the positive and negative affect factors were allowed to be related to one another.

Accordingly two further models were run in which the affect factors were related to one another −0.50 and −0.88. The affect-cognition ratios continued to order the measures in essentially the same way as in Exhibit 3 (where the relationship between the affect factors was fixed at zero).[9] Hence our major conclusions are not dependent on the assumption of independence between the affect factors. Furthermore, not only does the order of the measures on the affect-cognition ratio stay about the same, but so also do the values of the ratios themselves. For example, the Life 1 measure has an affect-cognition ratio of 0.8 under the assumption of independence between affect factors (as shown in Exhibit 3) and 0.9 when we assume the affect factors correlate −0.88.

The relationship between the affect factors and the cognition factor. Another assumption incorporated in the model in Exhibit 2 is that cognition is appropriately defined as being statistically independent of affect. While such a definition for cognition has an appealing elegance and simplicity to it, one could imagine counter-arguments that would suggest that relationships might occur between cognition and the two affect factors. Are the results presented earlier sensitive to what one assumes about these relationships? Although we have not actually run versions of the basic model that incorporate this change, other modelling work we have performed is instructive on this point. In the basic model (Exhibit 2), cognition is essentially a correlated residual: Cognition is what well-being measures have in common that is not affect and not shared methods effects. If cognition were allowed to be related to the affect factors, the cognitive factor would no longer be a pure residual but would also provide an alternative linkage between measures of well-being and the items in the affect scales. The effect would be that the measures would be estimated to be relatively more sensitive to cognitive components and less sensitive to affective components. Although the affect-cognition ratios would tend to decrease, there is no reason to expect that the relative positions of the measures according to these ratios would change. In short, the basic pattern of results reported previously would remain stable.

6. SUMMARY AND CONCLUSIONS

Beginning from the observations that measures of perceived well-being are attitudes, and that prior research suggests that attitudes include affective and cognitive components, we have analysed a substantial set of evaluations of life-as-a-whole (23 measures in all) to try to determine the extent to which each reflects affective, cognitive, and other components.

We find that the measures do indeed differ in a number of interesting ways that are of potential importance both theoretically and practically. Most of these differences are in close accord with what a careful consideration of the content and form of the item and its response scale would lead one to expect. Furthermore, the patterns of differences are basically similar in two representative but independent sets of data – one collected in the United States, the other collected in Great Britain.

For most of the measures examined, the total variance has been apportioned among five different components by using a structural modelling approach. These components are: positive affect, negative affect, cognition, common methods effect (mainly correlated error), and unique effects (mainly random error). Except for the fact that together these components should account for 100% of a measure's variance, each of these components is free to vary in any amount, and the resulting range of possible 'mixtures' could be – and in fact was found to be – substantial.

The estimated composition of each measure, i.e., the extent to which each measure reflects each of the five components, has been fully described above, and here only three of the main trends will be summarized.

1. If one considers the *ratio of affective to cognitive components*, one finds that some measures are much more affectively oriented than others. This finding, replicated in both the British and American data, is one of the basic justifications for distinguishing these components. Doing so represents a conceptual and statistical refinement over a common past practice of considering that all global measures are simply reflections (perhaps to differing degrees) of a single underlying factor, feelings about life-as-a-whole. Measures that ask about happiness, fun, and enjoyableness (in addition to Bradburn's scales of positive and negative affect) fall in the group for which relatively high affect-cognition ratios were observed. On the other hand, items that employ the term 'satisfaction' and/or that involve comparisons with implicit or explicit criteria tend to have lower affect-cognition ratios.

2. One can also consider the *ratio of the two types of affect* – i.e., whether the measure tilts toward positive or negative affect, or is reasonably balanced between the two. The data suggest that satisfaction measures tend to tap more negative than positive affect and that in the United States (but

not in Great Britain) the reverse is true for happiness measures. In the British data, an item that asked about fun was much more sensitive to positive than negative affect, whereas an item that asked about worries was heavily loaded with negative affect.

3. Still another way measures can be compared is with regard to the *ratio of their estimated true variance to total variance* – i.e., the percentage of their total variance that is estimated to tap feelings about life-as-a-whole rather than reflecting common methods effects or unique sources, most of which would probably be random errors. In one sense, this is an examination of the internal validity of the measures. There was a rather consistent tendency for measures employing 3-point response scales to show lower validities than measures with scales having more response categories. It also appears that explicitly comparative measures, i.e., ones that involve comparisons over time or with other groups, are markedly less valid as reflectors of absolute evaluations of life-as-a-whole than are measures that call for a direct assessment.

Given that different measures are differentially sensitive to positive affect, negative affect, cognition, and other (mainly error) factors, as this analysis and others reported by McKennell (1978) and McKennell and Andrews (1980) have shown, it seems important that designers, analysers, and users of surveys that assess perceived well-being should be sensitive to some of the issues involved. If one wants to assess absolute evaluations of perceived well-being, then one should seek measures that do this well; these will be the measures with relatively high validity coefficients. However, one faces further decisions regarding the desired mixture of affects and cognition: mainly cognition, mainly positive affect, mainly negative affect, or some balance among the three. Unfortunately, the issues do not stop with making these choices, because the current portfolio of available measures is far from complete and the ideal measure for a particular purpose may not exist.

While we believe that a useful start has been made toward furthering knowledge about the nature and characteristics of well-being measures, there is much further research and development that needs to be undertaken. The list of activities would include at least the following: (1) The present paper deals exclusively with well-being measures at the global level, i.e., ones that assess life-as-a-whole. Theoretical considerations we have laid out elsewhere (McKennell and Andrews, 1980) strongly suggest that the separate influences of affect and cognition also need to be explored at the level of evaluations of specific life concerns ('domains'). So far as we know, no appropriate data for doing this now exist, but they could be developed. (2) As just noted above, even at the global level the portfolio of available measures is far from complete. Work needs to be done to develop valid measures that would have more purely cognitive orientations. (3) We believe that the question of what negative relationship, if any, exists between positive and negative affect needs investigation. As reported above, some initial analyses show that the surprising (but replicable) zero relationship between measures of these factors could be attributable to correlated methods effects. Further work on affect that makes due allowance for random and correlated errors in measurement and that examines how the affect *factors* relate to a variety of outside variables would be useful. (4) Finally, we feel that much additional work needs to be undertaken regarding the differential relationships of affect and cognition to a wide variety of outside variables: respondents' behaviors — past, current, and future, respondents' demographic characteristics, and respondents' social settings as assessed by 'objective' social indicators. As noted previously, hints of such differential relationships led to the present investigation, and we have reported above that our modelling analyses were responsive to such differences, but this topic has only been opened. This fourth undertaking seems a particularly promising approach both for suggesting how people come to evaluate their lives as they do (a basic *causal* question for research on social indicators) and for suggesting some of the implications of people's evaluations (a basic *effects* question).

Institute for Social Research,
University of Michigan, U.S.A.

Social Sciences Faculty,
University of Southampton, England

NOTES

* We are grateful to John Hall and Mark Abrams for providing us with a copy of their data, to Mary Grace Moore for data processing, and to Suzanne Gurney for typing assistance. Grant #SOC77–06525 from the National Science Foundation supported the analysis reported here. Some of these results were presented at the Annual Meeting of the American Psychological Association, New York, 1979.
[1] In this counting Bradburn's scales of positive and negative affect are treated as single measures. Each of these scales is based on five items (as shown in Exhibit 1), and in the

analysis of the American data these individual items, rather than the composite scales, were used.

[2] As is common practice in analyses of this type, all variables were standardized prior to being analysed – i.e., transformed to have means of zero and variances of 1.0. This transformation has no effect at all on the main substantive results presented here but makes many of the parameter estimates more immediately interpretable.

[3] The LISREL program computes standard errors for the model's parameter values, and none of the parameters involving Life 1 and Life 2 differ by even as much as one standard error.

[4] These comparisons between the Satisfaction and Life measures, as well as other comparisons to be discussed later, raise issues of the statistical significance of the observed differences. While theory as well as statistical significance needs to be considered in interpreting a set of results (Morrison and Henkel, 1970), we have performed about forty tests on selected differences shown in Exhibits 3 and 4 using a test described by McNemar (1972, p. 140). (This test compares two relationships computed for the same set of respondents and is relevant because the measurement model parameters used to derive Exhibits 3 and 4 may be thought of as factor loadings or correlation coefficients.) The overall pattern of results from these significance tests is clear: Given the sizes of our samples, most differences in Exhibits 3 and 4 of 8 percentage points or more meet conventional criteria for statistical significance (p. < 0.05), and most differences of 5 to 7 percentage points are at the margin of statistical significance ($0.05 < p < 0.1$).

[5] In addition to the Group C measures shown in Exhibit 3, the analysis included the 10 items that compose Bradburn's scales of positive and negative affect. Although these items are not the primary focus of this report, in order that all estimates from the model may be available, we here report the estimated variance components for these 10 measures. The percent of variance attributable to positive affect in the first five items (ordered as shown in Exhibit 2) was: 12%, 27%, 43%, 22%, and 34%; the percent of variance attributable to negative affect in the second five items was: 19%, 37%, 31%, 51%, and 11%; the percent of variance attributable to a common methods effect in all 10 items was 2%; and the percent of variance estimated to be unique in each item was: 86%, 70%, 55%, 76%, 64%, 78%, 61%, 67%, 47%, and 86%. Although Bradburn's positive and negative affect scales Themselves were not included in the analysis of the American data, by knowing the relationships between those scales and other global measures, and the estimated variance composition of the global measures (reported in Exhibit 3), we can estimate that both the Positive affect and Negative affect scales have validities of approximately 0.87 (i.e., that approximately 76% of each scale's variance represents the intended affect factor and that approximately 24% is error).

[6] The use of single multi-item affect scales to define the affect factors rather than five separate items required an a priori estimation of the validity of these scales. After examining the American data, where our results suggested the multi-item affect scales would each have had validity of about 0.87 (see note 6), and after finding somewhat lower relationships among the individual affect items in the British data, an estimated validity of 0.80 was used. Several alternative validity values (0.87, 0.70, 0.50) were also tried, and it was determined that while the assumed validities of the affect scales have a substantial effect on the estimated affect-cognition ratio for the measures (column 7 in Exhibit 4), and for the statistics on which this ratio depends (columns 3–6), the *rank order* of the measures with respect to this ratio tends not to change markedly. (Land and Felson (1978) discuss the rationale behind this kind of exploration of the sensitivity of results to assumptions made when specifying the model.)

[7] Three separate types of response scales are represented among the 14 measures of global well-being in the British data and shown in Exhibit 4. These are: 3-point scales (Doing well and Happy 3-point), 11-point scales (Sat 11-pt, Change 11-pt, and Worry), and 7-point scales (all 9 remaining measures). As in the model shown in Exhibit 2, a

separate methods factor was defined for each type of response scale and linked to all measures that employed that scale. All the links from any one methods factor were constrained to have equal parameter estimates. (In order for this equality constraint to work as intended, it was necessary that all measures be scored in the same direction, i.e., numerically higher scores had to imply more positive evaluations, and since four of the measures —Enjoyable, Fun, Worry, and Change 11-pt — had been presented to respondents in the opposite direction, their scores were reversed.)

[8] Incorporation of age and education into the model shown in Exhibit 2 was accomplished by adding age and education to the list of observed measures, by adding an age factor and an education factor to the set of unmeasured variables, by fixing the linkage of each of these two factors with its respective indicator at 1.0, and by estimating all the linkages involving these two new factors and the previous three substantive factors, positive affect, negative affect, and cognition. As the analysis was actually run, all previous free and constrained parameters were re-estimated, but most changed very little from what has already been reported in Exhibit 3.

[9] In the most extreme case (assuming a -0.88 relationship between the affect factors), the order of the measures on the affect-cognition ratio was: Thermometer, Life 1, Sat 7-pt, Life 2, Happy D-T, Sat 3-pt, Change, and Happy 3-pt. This sequence has a rank order correlation of $+0.9$ with the order shown in Exhibit 3.

BIBLIOGRAPHY

Abrams, M. A.: 1973, 'Subjective social indicators', Social Trends No. 4 (London, Her Majesty's Stationery Office).

Abrams, M. A.: 1976, A review of work on subjective social indicators: 1971–1975 (London, Social Science Research Council Survey Unit).

Allardt, E.: 1973, About dimensions of welfare: An exploratory analysis of a comparative Scandinavian survey (Helsinki, University of Helsinki Research Group for Comparative Sociology).

Allport, G. W.: 1935, 'Attitudes', in C. Murchison (ed.) Handbook of Social Psychology, (Worcester, Mass., Clark University Press), pp. 798–884.

Andrews, F. M. and S. B. Withey: 1976, Social Indicators of Well-being: Americans' Perceptions of Life Quality (New York, Plenum).

Blishen, B. and T. Atkinson: 1978, Anglophone and Francophone differences in perceptions of the quality of life in Canada (Paper presented to the 9th World Congress of Sociology, Uppsala, Sweden).

Bradburn, N. M.: 1969, The Structure of Psychological Well-being (Chicago, Aldine).

Brenner, B.: 1975, 'Quality of affect and self-evaluated happiness', Social Indicators Research 2, pp. 315–331.

Burt, R. S.: 1976, 'Interpretational confounding of unobserved variables in structural equation models', Sociological Methods and Research 5, pp. 3–52.

Campbell, A., P. E. Converse and W. L. Rodgers: 1976, The Quality of American Life: Perceptions, Evaluations, Satisfactions (New York, Russell Sage Foundation).

Cantril, H.: 1965, The Pattern of Human Concerns (New Brunswick N.J., Rutgers University Press).

Cherlin, A. and L. G. Reeder: 1975, 'The dimensions of psychological well-being', Sociological Methods and Research 4, pp. 189–214.

Cochran, W. G.: 1968, 'The effectiveness of adjustment by subclassifications in removing bias in observational studies', Biometrics 24, pp. 295–313.

Conner, R. J.: 1972, 'Grouping for testing trends in categorical data', Journal of the American Statistical Association 67, pp. 601–604.

Fishbein, M. and I. Ajzen: 1975, Belief, Attitude, Intention, and Behavior (Reading, Mass., Addison-Wesley).

Gable, R. K., A. D. Roberts and S. V. Owen: 1977, 'Affective and cognitive components of classroom achievement', Educational and Psychological Measurement 37, pp. 977–986.

Hall, J.: 1976, 'Subjective measures of quality of life in Britain: 1971 to 1975 – some developments and trends', Social Trends No. 7 (London, Her Majesty's Stationery Office).

Insko, C. A. and J. Schopler: 1967, 'Triadic consistency: A statement of affective-cognitive-conative consistency', Psychological Review 74, pp. 361–376.

Joreskog, K. G. and D. Sorbom: 1976, LISREL III: Estimation of Structural Equation Systems by Maximum Likelihood Methods (Chicago, National Educational Resources, Inc.).

Land, K. C. and M. Felson: 1978, 'Sensitivity analysis of arbitrarily identified simultaneous-equation models', Sociological Methods and Research 6, pp. 283–307.

McGuire, W. J.: 1968, 'The nature of attitudes and attitude change', in G. Lindzey, and E. Aronson, (eds.) The Handbook of Social Psychology (2nd edition), Vol. 3 Reading, Mass., Addison-Wesley).

McKennell, A. C.: 1978, 'Cognition and affect in perceptions of well-being', Social Indicators Research 5, pp. 389–426.

McKennell, A. C. and F. M. Andrews: 1980, 'Models for cognition and affect in the perception of well-being', Social Indicators Research, in press.

McNemar, Q.: 1962, Psychological Statistics, Third Edition (New York, Wiley).

Morrison, D. E. and R. E. Henkel (eds.): 1970, The Significance Test Controversy (Chicago, Aldine).

Ostrom, T. M.: 1969, 'The relationship between the affective, behavioral and cognitive components of attitude', Journal of Experimental Social Psychology 5, pp. 12–30.

Ramsay, J. O.: 1973, 'The effect of number of categories in rating scales on precision of estimation of scale values', Psychometrika 38, pp. 513–532.

Smith, T. W.: 1978, Happiness: Time trends, seasonal variations, inter-survey differences and other matters. (Unpublished GSS Technical Report No. 6. Chicago, National Opinion Research Center).

10. SATISFACTION AND HAPPINESS*

(Received 28 November, 1979)

ABSTRACT. I review the recent literature on satisfaction and happiness, identify some plausible next steps to take at the frontiers of the research field and offer some suggestions to facilitate those steps. Using partial correlation techniques, substantial levels of covariation are found among the variables that are used in predictions of satisfaction and happiness with life as a whole from satisfaction with specific domains (e.g. family life, health). Using path analysis, confirmation is found in a dozen domains for a model which has satisfaction as a function of a perceived goal-achievement gap, and the latter as a function of comparisons with previous best experience and the status of average folks. Using discriminant analysis, satisfaction with family life is found to be a powerful and predominant discriminator among three groups, identified as Frustrated (dissatisfied and unhappy), Resigned (satisfied and unhappy) and Achievers (satisfied and happy).

1. INTRODUCTION

The structure of this paper is as follows. There is a review of some of the anomalies that have been encountered by social indicators researchers (section 2), and an overview of studies exploring various explanatory hypotheses of the anomalies (3). Plausible next steps are considered in the fourth section (4). Beginning with section (5), I report the results of a small survey undertaken at Guelph to at least prepare the way for others to take the important next steps on a grander scale. The methods and sample are described (5) and some basic statistics are provided (6). Substantial intercorrelations among domain satisfaction scores and life as a whole satisfaction and happiness scores are shown (7). A path model of satisfaction and happiness, called simply the Michigan model, is examined in relation to a dozen domains (8). Types of satisfaction are distinguished (9), and there is a brief conclusion (10).

2. ANOMALIES AS PRODS TO RESEARCH

Nobody ever needed social indicators to learn that different people often have different feelings about the same things. That, after all, is what makes a horse race. Nevertheless, it is precisely this commonplace phenomenon that

221

Alex C. Michalos (ed.), Citation Classics from Social Indicators Research, 221–258.
© 2005 *Springer. Printed in the Netherlands.*

has stimulated much of the current research on so-called subjective or perceptual social indicators. We want to know *why* different people often have different feelings about the same things. If one asks oneself why this question
seems so pressing, I think the answer must be because much more often, most
of the time, most people feel practically the same way about most things. For
very good physical, biological and social reasons most people are more similar
than dissimilar to each other. If it were not so, then within any society the
habits of communication, entertainment, transportation, eating, working, and
so on would be unmanageable. Without plenty of uniformity, we would have
plenty of chaos. We expect and in more or less subtle ways we cultivate and
construct uniformity. Consequently, non-uniform, unexpected, unplanned
phenomena confront us as anomalies. Moreover, perceived anomalies are
necessary conditions of scientific research. When nothing is regarded as
strange and unaccounted for, nothing is regarded as in need of explanation.
The perceived need for an explanation of something is the threshold of scientific investigation, and probably magic, religion and philosophy for that
matter. (This is basically Kuhn's (1962, 1977) view.)

The social indicators movement has generated its own anomalies. For
example, although Cantril (1965, p. 194) reported a rank order correlation of
0.67 between his socioeconomic index and people's ratings of their present
life on the Self-Anchoring Striving Scale, he also found that

the rank order correlation between the index and personal economic concerns was 0.01,
with national economic concerns, −0.05; and with national social concerns, −0.01 − all
indicating a complete lack of any relationship.

(Cantril, 1965, p. 201) Campbell (1972) reported that nearly half of the relatively poor white American respondents in a 'large-scale urban survey'
described themselves as 'very satisfied' with their housing. Schneider (1975)
reported significant differences between American cities when appraised
using objective versus subjective indicators. Duncan (1975a) noticed that
although there was an increase in the standard of living of respondents in
Detroit from 1955 to 1971, there was no increase in the reported satisfaction
with the standard of living. Allardt (1976) found that material level of living
and reported satisfaction were independent. Hankiss *et al.* (1978) reported
similar levels of perceived quality of life for people living in countries with
dissimilar scores on a developmental index. Michalos (1980b) reported that
although Americans were over five times as vulnerable to violent crimes as
Canadians, national surveys in 1973 and 1974 revealed that roughly 40 per-

cent of respondents in both countries expressed some fear of walking alone at night in their own areas. It was anomalies such as these that prompted Campbell *et al.* (1976, p. 115) to speak of the 'dilemma' of social indicators research, namely, that

We become most suspicious of bias or measurement inadequacy when subjective assessment come into conflict with objective situations, although such discrepancies taken substantively are almost the principal reason for the conduct of the study [of subjective indicators].

Most of the research on subjective social indicators has centred around problems involved in the measurement of satisfaction or happiness with particular domains (e.g., housing, family relations and health) and with life as a whole. Measures of life as a whole are referred to as *global* measures, in contrast to more limited *domain* measures. In the next two sections I will briefly review some of the most salient literature in this field from the twentieth century. For a thorough and extremely thought-provoking historical review of the literature on satisfaction and happiness beginning in about the seventh century B.C., one should read Tatarkiewicz (1976). The next section is on the theories, models or hypotheses that have been proposed in order to explain perceived anomalies, e.g., hypotheses about the role of expectations, aspirations and so on in the determination of feelings of satisfaction. In the section following this review I present some ideas on plausible next steps to take in order to increase our understanding at key points in the current stage of the discussion.

3. OVERVIEW OF PREVIOUS RESEARCH

One of the first things that occurs to researchers interested in explaining anomalies in this field is that expectations have a lot to do with the way people feel about their objective circumstances. The hypothesis that reported satisfaction is a function of the perceived difference between achievement and expectations has been tested in a variety of experimental situations with mixed results. Confirming evidence has been reported by Spector (1956), Foa (1957), Hulin and Smith (1965), Ilgen (1969, 1971), Locke *et al.* (1970), Ilgen and Hamstra (1972), Greenstein (1972), Lewis (1973), Space (1974), Gelwick (1975), Al-Hoory (1976), and Campbell *et al.* (1976). Unsuccessful attempts to confirm the hypothesis have been reported by Kawakami (1967), Buckley (1969), Berkey (1971), Carey (1974), Weston (1974), Hibbs (1975), Newton (1976), Wantz (1976), and Morgan (1976).

Although some people (e.g., Pelz and Andrews, 1976) use the terms 'expectations' and 'aspirations' as synonyms, there are good logical and experimental reasons for avoiding such usage. This was recognized clearly in the early studies of Lewin et al. (1944). Logically or conceptually there is a difference between what one aspires, hopes, wants or would like to achieve and what one expects to achieve. For example, underdog candidates for all sorts of positions may have high aspirations but very moderate expectations. They need not, of course, but it is logically possible and it often happens. Aspiration implies a conative element that is lacking in expectation. One has an emotional or affective stake in aspirations that may be entirely missing from expectations. (Edwards and Tversky (1967) is a good place to begin exploring studies of the impact of desirability on probability assessments.)

The fundamental logical distinction between expectations and aspirations is supported by the experimental literature. While we have just seen that the hypothesis regarding satisfaction as a function of the gap between *expectation* and achievement has had at best equivocal success, the hypothesis regarding satisfaction as a function of the gap between *aspiration* and achievement has been almost uniformly successful. Using the same computerized bibliographic search procedures that uncovered the mixed reports about expectation and achievement, I found only a single unsuccessful attempt to link satisfaction to an aspiration-achievement gap, namely, Carpenter (1973). Successful attempts to find an association were reported by Thibaut and Kelly (1959), Patchen (1961a, 1961b), Cook (1968), Bharadwaj and Wilkening (1974), Thompson (1975), Warr and Wall (1975), Campbell et al. (1976), Danielson (1977), Dorsett (1977) and Mason and Faulkenberry (1978).

Hamner and Harnett (1974) found that satisfaction in a competitive situation was a function of two comparisons which interacted, namely, the perceived achievement-aspiration difference mentioned above and the difference between one's own perceived achievement and that of one's selected reference person. The idea that satisfaction might be a function of the perceived difference between one's own status and that of a reference person or group has received indirect support from Davies (1962), Feierabend et al. (1969), Gurr (1970), Easterlin (1973, 1974), and Scott (1979). Duncan (1975a, p. 273) claimed that "the relevant source of satisfaction with one's standard of living is having more income than someone else, not just having more income". Gurr (1970, p. 52) cited a passage from Aristotle's *Politics* suggesting the antiquity of the hypothesis.

Cambell *et al.* (1976) tested the hypothesis directly using three reference groups (typical Americans, most close relatives and most close friends) and satisfaction with two particular domains (housing and neighbourhoods). In each case they found a positive association between reported satisfaction with the domain, and the gap between respondents' present status and the status of the reference groups as perceived by the respondents. In their most sophisticated model of satisfaction with particular domains of life, these authors have such social comparisons feeding directly into aspirations (as in Lewin *et al.* (1944, pp. 340–341)), with the aspiration-achievement comparison directly related to satisfaction. Exhibit 1 illustrates their model. The most influential comparisons respondents made were not with other people, but with the most liked previous experiences they had had. (See Exhibit 1.)

EXHIBIT 1.
Campbell *et al.* (1976) model
of satisfaction with particular domains as
a function of comparisons and an aspiration-
achievement gap.

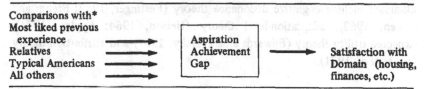

| Comparisons with*
Most liked previous
  experience
Relatives
Typical Americans
All others | → → → → | Aspiration
Achievement
Gap | → | Satisfaction with
Domain (housing,
finances, etc.) |

* Comparisons are listed in order of their influence on aspirations.

Andrews and Withey (1976) also tested the social comparison hypothesis directly for one reference group (most people) and three domains (self-accomplishments, housing and national government). In each case they found the anticipated positive association.

Equity theory might be regarded as a particular species of Aristotle's old hypothesis insofar as it is based on a perceived difference between what one gets and what one thinks one is entitled to get, *given* what some reference person or group gets. As the theory has been developed since Adams (1963, 1965), it has led to mixed results.That, at any rate, is the conclusion reached by three reviewers of the literature, namely, Lawler (1968), Pritchard (1969), and Burgess and Nielsen (1974). Abrams (1972) and Strumpel (1972) both claimed that the reported satisfaction of their respondents was partly a function of the perceived equity of their situations. Andrews and Withey (1976) used an item that required respondents to make a judgment about the appropriateness or fairness of their housing, self-accomplishments and national government without necessarily making a comparison to any reference group. That seems to be another species of equity theory, and it at least yielded results consistent with the hypothesis that such judgments do influence reports of satisfaction concerning the three relevant domains.

Some researchers have found a positive association between goal setting and job satisfaction, even if the goals were not achieved, e.g., Latham and Kinne (1974), Kim and Hamner (1976), and Umstot et al. (1976). Others have found that it is not merely the presence of goals that contributes to job satisfaction (whether the goals are achieved or not), but it is participation in the goal setting process that is satisfying. (Arvey et al., 1976). According to Umstot et al. (1976, p. 381), "A conservative weighing of the evidence suggests that goal setting has a strong, positive effect on productivity but an unknown effect on job satisfaction".

Some other theories that have a fairly direct relation to the ideas already discussed include cognitive dissonance theory (Festinger, 1957; Brehm and Cohen, 1962), adaptation-level theory (Helson, 1964; Appley, 1971), expected utility theory (Edwards and Tversky, 1967) and attribution theory (Jones et al, 1971).

4. NEXT STEPS

As the preceding brief overview suggests, there is no shortage of plausible models and more or less developed theories available to account for anomalies of reported satisfaction with various domains and with life as a whole. There are many more models and theories, and there is more experimental evidence than anyone could review in anything less than a long book. Campbell et al. (1976, p. 287) remarked that by 1972 there were over 3 000 articles, books and dissertations written on job satisfaction alone! Nevertheless, these authors concluded (correctly, I think) that "However worthy generic explanatory constructs like tastes or aspirations may be, they fall far short of providing any very elaborated theory." (Campbell et al., 1976, p. 483).

Apart from constructing a 'very elaborated theory', there are still some important developmental steps that can be taken. In the first place there is a question of the effects of intercorrelations among measures of satisfaction in particular domains and for life as a whole. Weaver (1978) reported several significant intercorrelations among domain satisfaction scores. He concluded that

The considerable interdependence among domain variables suggests that happiness is based on satisfaction in a number of different parts of life, that the employee whose happiness is significantly related to job satisfaction is also likely to experience satisfaction in other parts of life as well (Weaver, 1978, pp. 838–839).

Although Weaver worked with a global measure of happiness with life as a whole rather than of satisfaction with life as a whole, the scores from the two measures generally correlate with Pearson r's around 0.6 to 0.7 (McKennell, 1978). Atkinson (1979, p. 14) reported that age and income were so highly intercorrelated that "any analysis of one of these factors must proceed with the effects of the other held constant". A systematic search for intercorrelation effects among domain satisfaction scores and life as a whole satisfaction and happiness scores would improve our understanding of such scores, and their change over time.

A second important question concerns the role of an aspiration-achievement gap in the explanation of satisfaction with particular domains and life as a whole. I have already noted that such a gap was found to be influential in reported satisfaction measures for housing, neighbourhoods, self-accomplishments and national government. Mason and Faulkenberry (1978) also found it influential in assessments of satisfaction with income and public safety. As Campbell et al. (1976) pointed out, so far no one has been able to design a questionnaire item that lends itself to repeated use across a variety of domains and that captures respondents' feelings about aspiration-achievement gaps. Consequently, different researchers focus on certain domains and invest the additional resources required to explore the relevant gaps in the limited areas. Thus, Campbell et al. (1976, p. 484) concluded that

it remains quite conceivable that the general structuring of standards of comparison and aspiration levels might take quite a different form in other more disparate domains such as financial situation or marriage.

A similar suggestion was made by Duncan (1975a, p. 273). In other words, the model illustrated in Exhibit I may be appropriate for some domains and inappropriate for others. Clearly, what is required is the design and testing of a new efficient questionnaire item for a variety of domains and for life as a whole. Such an item is introduced and used in the following sections of this paper.

All previous tests of the hypothesis concerning the influence of an aspiration-achievement gap on reported satisfaction have involved the calculation of the gap from separate measures of aspiration and achievement. These procedures presume that the calculations researchers make are roughly identical to the calculations respondents make. The fact that relatively strong connections have been found between gap measures thus calculated and reported satisfaction measures suggests that the presumption is not entirely unfounded. Nevertheless, from the point of view of the basic assumption behind the study of perceptual or subjective indicators, the *perceived* gap between one's aspirations and achievements should be more closely related to reported satisfaction than the calculated gap. The gap we calculate for respondents may be significantly different from the gap they perceive on the basis of their own calculations and intuitions. The new efficient questionnaire item mentioned in the previous paragraph should allow us to capture the perceived gap between aspirations and achievements.

5. METHOD AND SAMPLE

In April 1979 I set out to try to pave the way for the important next steps described in the previous section. A campus mail questionnaire was distributed to the 867 members of the University of Guelph's Staff Association. This is the local union representing our office, clerical and technical staff. After three follow-up requests, a total of 357 or 41 percent of the questionnaires were recieved. Exhibit 2 summarizes the sample.

According to our personnel department, the office, clerical and technical staff is 70 percent female and 30 percent male. Sixty-six percent are married and 34 percent are not. As you can see, then, the sample has more women and married folks than the population from which it was drawn. Moreover, the sample is nowhere near demographically representative of Guelph, Ontario or Canada. My guess would be that it is roughly representative of office, clerical and technical staffs in most universities in Canada and probably the United States. Whether one looks at the demographic characteristics (sex, age, marital status, education and family income) of university faculties, staffs or students, I suspect one would find considerable homogeneity. I imagine, for example, that our staff is more like the staff at York University or the University of Waterloo than it is like the staff at Canadian General Electric (which is also located in Guelph). Nevertheless, it is not necessary to speculate about what bigger group our 357 people might plausibly represent. It is a partially

EXHIBIT 2
Sample Composition

		N	Percent		N	Percent
Sex:	Male	80	22	*Education*		
	Female	277	78	Completed grade 8 or less	4	1
		357	100	Completed 13 or less to 9	123	35
				Completed some college,		
Age:	18–34	249	69	university, trade school	108	30
	35–44	42	12	Degree, college or univ.	122	34
	45–64	64	18		357	100
	65–up	2	1			
		357	100	*Total Family Income*		
				0–$ 4 999	5	1
Marital Status				$ 5 000–$ 9 999	70	20
Single		112	31	$ 10 000–$ 14 999	94	27
Married		206	58	$ 15 000–$ 19 999	55	16
Separated		16	5	$ 20 000–$ 24 999	50	14
Divorced		15	4	$ 25 000 and over	76	22
Widowed		8	2		330	100
		357	100			

self-selected group with the composition specified in Exhibit 2, and I'm not making any inferences about any other group. I should add, however, that there are some remarkable similarities in the results reported here and elsewhere in North America.

The questionnaires had 64 items in five pages and took about 20 minutes to fill out. Besides the opening demographic page, there were four pages with 13 items covering 12 domains and life as a whole. The four pages covered perceived satisfaction, the goal-achievement gap, life compared to average folks the same age and life compared to the best previous experience. (To save space and shorten sentences I don't always put 'perceived' or 'reported' in front of 'satisfaction', 'goal-achievment gap' and so on. Similarly, I usually shorten phrases like 'satisfaction with free time activity' to 'free time activity'. In context these abbreviations should not be misleading.)

All of the 53 substantive items called for a single checkmark on a seven point rating scale, with one off scale option called 'No opinion'. The instructions and format of my satisfaction items were adapted from Andrews and Withey (1976) with small changes. In particular, their scale has 'pleasant' and 'unhappy' where mine has 'very satisfying' and 'very dissatisfying.' My instructions were as followes.

Below are some words and phrases that people use to identify various features of their lives. Each feature title has a scale beside it that runs from 'Terrible' to 'Delightful' in seven steps. In general we think of the numbers correlated with words such as the following:

1	2	3	4	5	6	7
Terrible	Very Dissatisfying	Dissatisfying	Mixed	Satisfying	Very Satisfying	Delightful

Please check the number on the scale beside each feature that comes closest to describing how you feel about that particular aspect of *your life these days*.

Twelve domain titles followed these instructions, namely, health, financial security, family life, friendship, housing, job, free time activity, education, self-esteem, area you live in, ability to get around and secure from crime. These were followed by the global question "How do you feel about your life as a whole?" Because my questionnaire was designed with one eye on using it in rural settings, I used 'area you live in' instead of the more common 'neighbourhood'. I considered 'transportation' and 'mobility', but finally settled for 'ability to get around'. In future studies other domains may be added or substituted.

The instructions and format of my goal-achievement gap items run thus:

Some people have certain goals or aspirations for various aspects of their lives. They aim for a particular sort of home, income, family life style and so on. Compared to your own aims or goals, for each of the features below, would you say that your life measures up perfectly now, fairly well, about half as well, fairly poorly or just not at all. Please check the percentage that best describes how closely your life now seems to approach *your own goals*.

Not at at	Fairly poorly	Half as well as your goal	Fairly well	Matches your goal	No opinion
0%	20% 30%	50%	70%	80% 100%	
1	2 3	4	5	6 7	8

The same twelve domain titles followed these instructions and were in turn followed by the global question "Now, considering your life as a whole, how does it measure up to your general aspirations or goals?"

The instructions and format of my average folks comparison items ran thus:

So far we have asked you to appraise several features of your life itself and in relation to your goals. Now we would like you to compare your life with that of other folks of your own age. Compared to average people of your age, for each of the features listed below, would you say that your life is a perfect fit (average), a bit better or worse, or far better or worse. Please check the number on the scale that comes closest to comparing your life to *the average*.

Far below average	Worse than average	Average	Better than average	Far above average	No opinion
1	2	3	4	5	6	7	8

Following the twelve domain titles, there was the global question "Now, considering your life as a whole, how does it measure up to the average for people your age?"

The instructions and format of my previous best comparison items ran thus:

Our final request is to have you compare your life now to your all time high. Compared to your own previous best experience, for each of the features listed below, would you say that your life now is far below the best it has been, worse than the best, matches the best, is better than your previous best, or far above the best it has ever been before. Please check the number on the scale that comes closest to comparing your life to *your previous best*.

Far below the best	Worse than best	Matches the best	Better than best	Far above the best	No opinion
1	2	3	4	5	6	7	8

Following the twelve domain titles, there was the global question "Now, considering your life as a whole, how does it measure up to the best in your previous experience?"
After this question, there was the following:

Finally, considering your life as a whole, would you describe it as very unhappy, unhappy, an even mixture of unhappiness and happiness, happy, or very happy?

Very unhappy	Unhappy	Mixed	Happy	Very happy	No opinion
1	2	3	4	5	6	7	8

Notice that, with the exception of the satisfaction scale, two scale numbers but only one verbal description is provided for the areas between the midpoints and the extremes, e.g., '$_2$unhappy$_3$'. The aim was to eliminate 'noise' from disparate verbal cues (e.g., Andrews and Withey's insertion of 'unhappy' in a satisfaction scale), and to stay to a single scale-length.

6. MEANS, STANDARD DEVIATIONS AND SKEWS

Exhibit 3 summarizes some of the basic statistics of our diverse measures. The entries in the first four rows are arithmetic means of the means, standard deviations and skewness measures of the 12 domain scores taken collectively.

The skewness measures are those of the SPSS manual (Nie, *et al.*, 1975). Symmetric distributions have a zero value, while positive and negative values indicate clustering of values to the left and right of the mean, respectively. Thus, the top row of Exhibit 3 tells us that the mean of the means of the 12 domain satisfaction scores was 5.18, the average standard deviation for these 12 scores was 1.20 and the average skew was −0.67 (i.e., the values were clustered to the right of the mean). The entries in the last five rows are for each of the five global items described earlier (i.e., life as a whole satisfaction, goal-achievement gap, average folks comparisons, previous best comparisons and happiness).

From Exhibit 3 it's easy to see that, taken collectively, goal-achievement gap scores had the highest mean and the most skew, with rightside clustering. The average standard deviation for these scores was just barely bigger than that of the domain satisfaction scores, which was the smallest of the lot. The most variable set of scores of the four was that of average folks comparisons, which practically had a symmetric distribution. Insofar as Andrews and Withey (1976, pp. 206−210) are right about the virtues of symmetric distributions from the point of view of statistical operations, the average folks comparisons measures have some advantage over domain satisfaction measures.

Turning to the global measures, satisfaction with life as a whole had the highest mean, the lowest standard deviation and the greatest skew. As indicated earlier, this item was adapted from Andrews and Withey (1976). Although our samples were not comparable, they reported a mean of 5.30, a standard deviation of 1.05 and a skew of 1.05 for their comparable item.

EXHIBIT 3
Means, Standard Deviations and Skews

Average for 12 domains	Mean	Standard Deviation	Skew
Satisfaction	5.18	1.20	−0.67
Goal-achievement	5.21	1.23	−0.81
Average folks	4.86	1.52	0.06
Previous best	4.51	1.37	−0.14
Global items			
Satisfaction	5.45	1.06	−1.02
Goal-achievement	5.19	1.06	−0.90
Average folks	5.06	1.12	−0.55
Previous best	4.81	1.28	−0.29
Happiness	5.36	1.28	−0.60

EXHIBIT 4
Domain means, standard deviations and skews*

	Means				Standard Deviations				Skews			
	SAT	GOAL	AVE	BEST	SAT	GOAL	AVE	BEST	SAT	GOAL	AVE	BEST
Health	5.50	5.61	5.05	4.12	0.97	1.06	1.23	1.37	-0.51	-1.20	-0.23	0.26
Financial security	4.56	4.73	4.64	4.63	1.30	1.19	1.25	1.51	-0.58	-0.63	0.03	-0.39
Family life	5.51	5.47	5.24	4.76	1.34	1.40	1.37	1.43	-1.07	-1.18	-0.48	-0.08
Friendships	5.34	5.27	4.83	4.36	1.22	1.23	1.27	1.36	-0.61	-0.68	0.06	0.16
Housing	5.25	5.01	4.87	4.58	1.21	1.29	1.19	1.50	-0.72	-0.53	0.17	-0.08
Job	4.74	4.62	4.61	4.40	1.36	1.39	1.20	1.53	-0.48	-0.61	-0.15	0.00
Free time activity	5.09	5.02	4.75	4.40	1.32	1.25	1.18	1.30	-0.54	-0.76	0.15	0.18
Education	4.70	4.96	4.71	4.56	1.04	1.15	1.00	1.20	-0.49	-0.55	0.55	0.73
Self-esteem	5.02	5.24	4.74	4.57	1.07	1.09	1.15	1.15	-0.72	-0.81	-0.10	0.21
Area you live in	5.37	5.33	4.89	4.47	1.22	1.23	1.12	1.40	-0.63	-0.77	0.37	0.23
Ability to get around	5.58	5.57	4.98	4.74	1.21	1.28	1.19	1.37	-1.05	-1.18	-0.06	0.04
Secure from crime	5.53	5.69	5.01	4.57	1.14	1.14	1.21	1.27	-0.68	-0.84	0.36	0.47

* SAT is short for satisfaction, GOAL for goal-achievement, AVE for average folks comparison and BEST for previous best comparison.

(Their skewness measure is positive for rightside clustering.) In terms of standard deviation and skew, my global goal-achievement gap measure was most similar to that of life satisfaction. However, the mean of the global happiness scores was most similar to the mean of life satisfaction scores.

Exhibit 4 summarizes some of the basic statistics for the 12 domains and the four different kinds of indicators. In terms of satisfaction, highest mean ratings went to the ability to get around, security from crime, family life and health. These same four domains obtained highest mean rating for goal-achievement and comparisons with average folks, although the order of the four changed. For comparisons with the best of previous experience, the domains of health and security from crime were replaced in the top four by financial security and housing.

In terms of satisfaction, financial security had the lowest mean rating, followed by education and job. Since all of the respondents were employees of the university and probably realised that the results of my study would find their way to the powers that be, they may have been sending the powers a message. The rest of that message shows up nicely in two other measures. Job had the lowest mean rating for goal-achievement and for comparisons with average folks of the same age as these respondents. Clearly, although these respondents are satisfied with their jobs, they are just barely satisfied. A score of 5 is labled 'satisfying' and the mean score was 4.74. Moreover, their current jobs seem to take them half to two-thirds of the way toward their occupational goals, and to leave them slightly better off than they perceive average folks their age to be. In terms of their best previous experience with the 12 domains, the lowest mean rating went to health.

7. INTERCORRELATION

As indicated earlier, some researchers have found significant intercorrelation or covariation among domain and global indicators. Exhibits 5 and 6 summarize a series of partial correlations undertaken in order to find out how much of particular zero-order relationships might remain if conceptually distinct but relevant variables are controlled. For example, given that satisfaction with one's job and family life are each associated with one's satisfaction with life as a whole, how much of the associations remain if one of the domain variables is partialled out? In other words, how much of the associations are package deals in which several aspects of the quality of one's life are tied together?

EXHIBIT 5
Correlations of domain, demographic
and happiness scores with satisfaction scores[a]

	(1)	(2)	(3)	(4)	(5)	(6)	(7)	(8)	(9)	(10)	(11)
Health	0.359	0.373	0.014	0.137	0.007	0.070	NS	0.132	0.011	0.062	NS
Financial security	0.400	0.409	0.009	0.212	0.001	0.196	0.001	0.226	0.001	0.220	0.001
Family life	0.602	0.661	0.059	0.393	0.001	0.257	0.001	0.380	0.001	0.245	0.001
Friendships	0.538	0.543	0.005	0.208	0.001	0.131	0.010	0.237	0.001	0.152	0.004
Housing	0.267	0.297	0.030	-0.089	0.05	-0.097	0.042	-0.056	NS	-0.062	NS
Job	0.343	0.355	0.012	0.133	0.008	0.133	0.009	0.156	0.003	0.161	0.003
Free time activity	0.413	0.448	0.035	0.131	0.009	0.122	0.015	0.093	0.052	0.074	NS
Education	0.359	0.376	0.017	-0.071	NS	-0.045	NS	-0.074	NS	0.050	NS
Self-esteeem	0.454	0.477	0.023	0.172	0.001	0.139	0.007	0.152	0.004	0.132	0.011
Area you live in	0.283	0.347	0.064	0.049	NS	0.064	NS	0.058	NS	0.079	NS
Ability to get around	0.330	0.387	0.057	0.119	0.017	0.112	0.023	0.098	0.044	0.093	0.053
Secure from crime	0.135[b]	0.220	0.085	0.028	NS	0.053	NS	0.026	NS	0.052	NS

[a] *Explanations column code:*
(1) Pierson r, P = .0001.
(2) Eta.
(3) Col. 2 minus Col.1.
(4) Correlation of domain listed at left with S, partialling out all other domain effects.
(5) Significance levels of partial correlations in Col. 4, 319 degrees of freedom.
(6) Correlation of domain with S, partialling out all other domain effects plus global happiness effects.
(7) Significance levels of partial correlations in Col. 6, 316 degrees of freedom.

(8) Correlation of domain with S, partialling out other domain effects plus five demographic variables (sex, age, marital status, education, family income).
(9) Significance levels of partial correlations in Col. 8, 303 degrees of freedom.
(10) Correlation of domain with S, partialling out all other domain, happiness and demographic effects.
(11) Significant levels of partial correlations in Col. 10, 300 degrees of freedom.
Significant levels less than 0.05 were uniformly labeled 'NS' for 'not statistically significant'
[b] P = 0.005

Generally speaking, such analyses run the risk of being either unnecessary or misleading. Suppose, for example, that A, B and C represent any three variables. If A and B are completely unrelated, then partial correlations of either variable with C while controlling the other will yield results identical to zero-order correlations. Nothing in A is related to anything in B; so partialling is unnecessary. At the other extreme, if $A = B$ then partial correlations of either with C while controlling for the other will yield results of zero, because one is merely partialling a 'relationship out of itself'. (Gordon, 1968) In such cases, whatever A and B designate may be strongly associated with whatever C designates, and the partial correlation coefficient of zero may be misleading.

In Exhibit 5 the dependent variable is my global measure of satisfaction with life as a whole, which hereafter will be abbreviated S. Column (1) gives the Pearson product moment coefficient r of each domain variable with S. Except for secure from crime, each domain variable is positively correlated with S above 0.27 with $P = 0.0001$ or better. Secure from crime correlates with S at 0.14 with $P = 0.005$.

Since Pearson's r measures only the linear association between variables and there was a possibility of curvilinear association, the same correlations were measured using the correlation ratio *eta*. (Guilford and Fruchter, 1978, pp. 296–300). The *eta* coefficients are listed in Column (2). The difference between r and *eta* values is a measure of the curvilinearity of the association between two variables. (Guilford and Fruchter, 1978). As Column (3) shows, with the exception of secure from crime, the difference between r and *eta* values never rose above 0.06, indicating practically no curvilinear association.

Column (4) shows the results of partialling out (statistically controlling) all other domain variables. In every case there was a fairly dramatic decrease in the correlation with S, indicating substantial covariation. Ignoring the three statistically insignificant correlations, the covariation ran from a maximum of 68 percent for free time activity to a minimum of 35 percent for family life. That is, 68 percent of the correlation coefficient measuring the linear association between satisfaction with free time activity and satisfaction with life as a whole represents shared covariation with the eleven other domain variables. Controlling the other eleven variables, the correlation between free time activity and S drops from 0.413 to 0.131. In the case of job satisfaction, when the covariation with all other domains is eliminated, the correlation with S drops from 0.343 to 0.133, a 61 percent decrease. The domain of family life has the highest correlation with S, $r = 0.602$, and also the least covariation with other domains, 35 percent. It would be a mistake, however, to infer uniqueness from strength of association. Friendship has a 0.538 correlation with S, 61 percent of which covaries with the eleven other domains. In general, the mean covariation of the eleven other domains with any particular domain-S correlation was 59 percent. In other words, an average of nearly 60 percent of the association between satisfaction with any domain and satisfaction with life as a whole represents a package deal in which several aspects of the quality of one's life are tied together.

Column (6) of Exhibit 5 shows the results of partialling out all other domains plus global happiness, which hereafter will be abbreviated H. I will have much more to say about relations between S and H later. Here it is sufficient to notice that the Pearson r association between S and H is 0.68 ($P = 0.0001$) and that following Andrews and Withey (1976) and McKennell (1978), I'm assuming H is a purer measure of affect than S. Thus, the point of partialling out H is to try to eliminate some of the affective component from S, leaving a purer cognitive component. Ignoring the four statistically insignificant correlations, in seven of the eight remaining partial correlations, the removal of H decreased the domain-S association still farther. Only the job-S association remained unchanged. The family life-S association, for example, dropped from 0.393 to 0.257.

Column (8) shows the results of partialling out all other domains plus five demographic variables (sex, age, marital status, education and family income). Ignoring the four insignificant correlations, comparison with Column (4) reveals that in five cases there was a further decrease in the domain-S association and in three cases there was an increase. The average change brought about by the partialling out of demographic variables was 0.02, hardly worth the bother. I suppose the demographic variables are relatively unimportant because of the homogeneity of the sample.

Column (10) represents the bottom line of this sort of statistical striptease. Here we have domain-S associations with all other domains, five demographic variables and happiness partialled out. So we're looking at domain-S associations in about as pure a form as anyone has ever looked at them. Comparison of Columns (10) and (1) are startling. First, only half of the associations are statistically significant in Column (10). Second, the remaining significant associations are all severely diminished from Column (1). The average decrease in the domain-S associations from (1) to (10) is 62 percent.

As interesting as the preceding exercise may have been, it is worthwhile to

EXHIBIT 6
Correlations of domain, demographic and satisfaction scores with happiness scores[a]

	(1)	(2)	(3)	(4)	(5)	(6)	(7)	(8)	(9)	(10)	(11)
Health	0.330	0.349	0.019	0.175	0.001	0.139	0.007	0.184	0.001	0.151	0.004
Financial security	0.310	0.329	0.019	0.084	NS	-0.003	NS	0.060	NS	-0.033	NS
Family life	0.585	0.607	0.022	0.376	0.001	0.234	0.001	0.373	0.001	0.239	0.001
Friendships	0.509	0.528	0.019	0.228	0.001	0.153	0.003	0.257	0.001	0.172	0.001
Housing	0.246	0.306	0.060	0.015	NS						
Job	0.243	0.271	0.028	0.027	NS						
Free time activity	0.335	0.370	0.035	0.032	NS						
Education	0.292	0.325	0.033	-0.071	NS						
Self-esteem	0.364	0.378	0.014	0.111	0.023						
Area you live in	0.229	0.270	0.041	-0.018	NS						
Ability to get around	0.246	0.273	0.027	-0.042	NS						
Secure from crime	0.078[b]	0.191	0.113	-0.067	NS						

a Explanations column code:
(1) Pearson r, P = .0001
(2) Eta
(3) Col. 2 minus Col. 1.
(4) Correlation of domain listed at left with H, partialling out all other domain effects.
(5) Significance levels of partial correlations in Col. 4, 319 degrees of freedom.
(6) Correlation of domain with H, partialling out other domains plus S effects.
(7) Significance levels of partial correlations in Col. 6, 316 degrees of freedom.
(8) Correlation of domain with H, partialling out other domain effects plus five demographic variables.

(9) Significance levels of partial correlations in Col. 8, 303 degrees of freedom.
(10) Correlation of domain with H, partialling out all other domain, demographic and S effects.
(11) Significance levels of partial correlations in Col. 10, 300 degrees of freedom.
'NS' is short for 'not statistically significant'.
The last 8 rows of columns (6) to (11) were omitted because there were no statistically significant associations.
b NS

remember the caveats introduced in the second paragraph of this section, and to recall Campbell, Converse and Rodgers's (1976, p. 122) warning of the danger of 'overcontrol'. "To overcontrol" they said, "is to adjust from view some contour of the data which is actually relevant in a substantive way to the more precise question being asked about reality." A case in point, for example, is the removal of H effects from domain-S associations. Technically, as we saw, the amputation is possible. But is the resulting satisfaction measure somehow purer or more valid, or just more artifact? Is it more frank or more Frankenstein? At this point, I suspect it is the latter.

Exhibit 6 summarizes a series of analyses that were patterned after those reviewed in Exhibit 5. The basic difference is that the dependent variable in these analyses is H, the global measure of happiness. Inspection of the first columns of Exhibits 5 and 6 reveals immediately that S is more closely related than H to domain satisfaction. In every case the domain-S association is stronger than the domain-H association. There is one statistically insignificant domain-H association, for secure from crime (which was an oddball earlier too). The *eta* minus r values in Column (3) again indicate the absence of any significant curvilinearity. The average *eta-r* difference is only 0.03. When we move to Column (4), in which all other domains are partialled out, we are left with only four statistically significant correlations (health, family life, friendships and self-esteem). In fact, with the exception of the self esteem-H association, we could just as well have omitted the last eight rows of every column from (4) to (11). To make a potentially long story short, it seems to me that the associations in Exhibit 6 suggest that H is not going to be as analytically useful as S as a basic dependent variable for quality of life studies.

8. PATH MODELS OF SATISFACTION

Campbell's *et al.* (1976) model of satisfaction was introduced earlier and illustrated in Exhibit 1. Because other researchers at the University of Michigan have worked with this model (Andrews and Withey (1976) for example), and in order to save space, I will hereafter refer to it as the 'Michigan model'. Given the brief literature review presented earlier and the historical antecedents documented in Tatarkiewicz (1976), there is no doubt that the Michigan model has very deep roots in Western civilization. To test the model directly for satisfaction and happiness with life as a whole, and for satisfaction with a dozen domains, I undertook a series of path analyses. Formal models similar to those employed here are discussed in detail in Kerlinger and Pedhazur (1973, pp. 307–314, 322–327), and Duncan (1975b, pp. 42–44). So interested readers can consult those texts for detailed analyses of the formal features of path analysis generally and the Michigan model in particular.

All of the path models considered here have the form of those in Exhibit 7.1. In all of the diagrams S and H are interpreted as usual, while G is short for the goal-achievement gap, P for comparisons with the best previous experience and A for comparisons with average folks of the same age. The arrows in the diagrams indicate proposed (hypothesized, theorized, imagined, etc.) causal relations, with effects named at the arrowheads and causes named at the end

EXHIBIT 7.1   SATISFACTION WITH LIFE AS A WHOLE

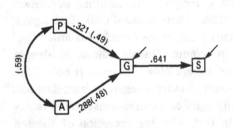 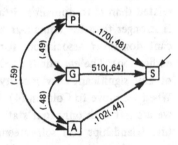

EXHIBIT 7.2   HAPPINESS WITH LIFE AS A WHOLE

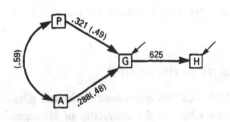 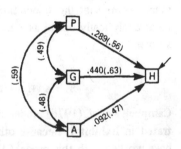

S   SATISFACTION WITH LIFE AS A WHOLE
H   HAPPINESS WITH LIFE AS A WHOLE
P   COMPARISONS WITH BEST PREVIOUS EXPERIENCE
G   GOAL-ACHIEVEMENT GAP
A   COMPARISONS WITH AVERAGE FOLKS

of the shafts. The small arrows without names at the end of their shafts represent error terms on the endogenous variables. The model on the left is the Michigan model and the model on the right is its most plausible competitor. Thus, in the Michigan model, S is supposed to be caused directly by G which is in turn directly caused by P and A. In its competitor, S is directly caused by P, G and A. The numbers in parentheses along the shafts are the zero-order correlation coefficients between the variables named at either end of the shafts, while the other numbers are standardized regression coefficients (betas) or path coefficients. In the Michigan model, the path coefficient connecting G to S is obtained by regressing S on G, and a multiple regression of G on P and A gives the path coefficients connecting these variables. The betas of the competitor are obtained from a multiple regression of S on P, G and A. For example, then, in the Michigan model of Exhibit 7.1, the numbers above the arrow from P to G indicate that the Pearson r between these variables is 0.49, and that there will be an average change of 0.32 in G for every unit change in P (when both P and G are standardized to have means of zero and standard deviations of one). The path coefficient is analogous to a partial correlation coefficient in that it indicates a relation between two variables with the effects of all others in the system held constant.

Testing the Michigan model means, in the present context, comparing its features to those of its competitor and answering the following question: Are all of the path coefficients in the Michigan model bigger than their alternatives in its competitor? In other words, does the Michigan model represent a system or structure of relationships that is stronger or tighter than the system represented by its competitor? A second question of interest concerns the relative strength of the connections from P to G, and A to G. Campbell *et al.* (1976) and Andrews and Withey (1976) found that the former (P to G) was uniformly stronger than the latter (A to G). So, the question is: Will the relative strength of these connections be duplicated here?

For a number of reasons that need not detain us, it is obviously possible to have data consistent or inconsistent with a hypothesis without the hypothesis being true or false, respectively. Since, if all other things are equal, beta values are liable to be lowered as the number of covarying predictor variables increases in a multiple regression, one must be especially cautious about assessing apparently supporting evidence for our models. (Gordon, 1968) Nevertheless, hypotheses should at least be regarded as live options as long as the results of tests are consistent with them. Thus, affirmative answers to the fundamental question raised above represent some support for the Michigan model as a relatively good explanatory account of reported satisfaction and happiness.

Inspection of Exhibits 7.1 and 7.2 reveals that our basic question has an affirmative answer. In 7.1, for example, P and A are stronger predictors of G than of S, as hypothesized in the Michigan model. G to S connections (betas) are the strongest in the systems whether one adopts the Michigan model or not. Similar remarks apply to Exhibit 7.2, with H substituted for S. Moreover, in both exhibits, the P to G connection is stronger than the A to G connection, as reported by Campbell et al. (1976).

Exhibits 8.1–8.12 summarize the results of testing the Michigan model in twelve domains. In these cases, S, P, G and A have to be interpreted as *domain specific*. For example, in Exhibit 8.1, S is short for satisfaction with one's own health, P for comparisons with the best previous experience of one's own health, A for comparisons of one's own health with that of average folks of one's age, and G for the gap between one's health goals and one's achievement of those goals. In all twelve domains the Michigan model looks superior to its competitor. In every domain P and A are better predictors of G than of S, and G is always the strongest predictor of S. With the single exception of free time activity, in every domain the path coefficient connecting A to G is bigger than that connecting P to G, *contrary* to hypothesis and to results obtained by Campbell et al. (1976) and Andrews and Withey (1976) for their domains of housing, neighborhood and self-accomplishment. (My 'area you live in' is analogous to the 'neighborhood' of Campbell et al. and 'self-esteem' is very roughly related (I guess) to Andrews and Withey's 'self-accomplishments'.)

I don't know how to account for the discrepancy with respect to the relative relations between comparisons with the best previous experience and average folks. Maybe it's peculiar to this sample; maybe it's peculiar to Canadians. As indicated earlier, one of the motives behind this investigation was the suspicion that other domains may involve psychological processes different from those proposed in the Michigan model. Maybe they do.

The implications of confirmation of most of the postulated relations in the Michigan model are profound. Insofar as this type of model can be substantiated, human satisfaction is not just a brute fact to be accommodated like the wind and rain. It is to some extent manageable in the best sense and manipulable in the worst sense. By providing relevant experiences and

EXHIBIT 8.1 SATISFACTION WITH HEALTH

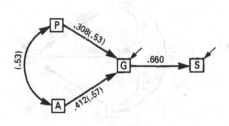

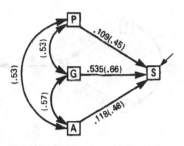

EXHIBIT 8.2 SATISFACTION WITH FINANCIAL SECURITY

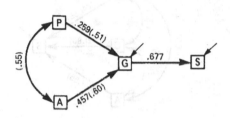

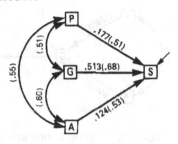

EXHIBIT 8.3 SATISFACTION WITH FAMILY LIFE

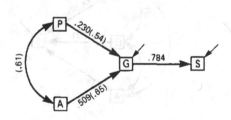

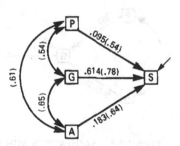

EXHIBIT 8.4 SATISFACTION WITH FRIENDSHIPS

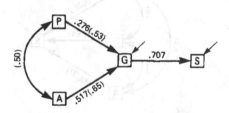

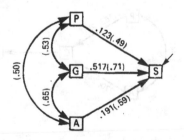

244   ALEX C. MICHALOS

EXHIBIT 8.5   SATISFACTION WITH HOUSING

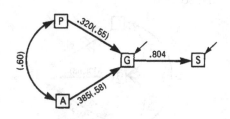
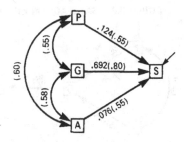

EXHIBIT 8.6   SATISFACTION WITH JOB

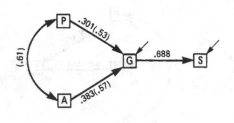
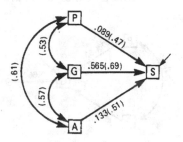

EXHIBIT 8.7   SATISFACTION WITH FREE TIME ACTIVITY

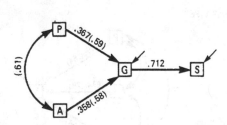
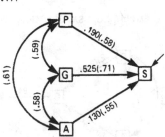

EXHIBIT 8.8   SATISFACTION WITH EDUCATION

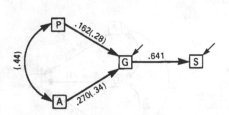
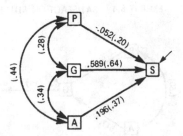

EXHIBIT 8.9 SATISFACTION WITH SELF-ESTEEM

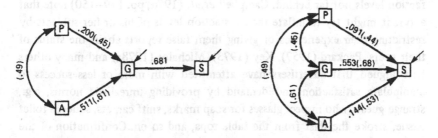

EXHIBIT 8.10 SATISFACTION WITH AREA YOU LIVE IN

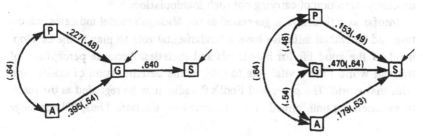

EXHIBIT 8.11 SATISFACTION WITH ABILITY TO GET AROUND

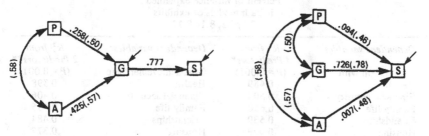

EXHIBIT 8.12 SATISFACTION WITH SECURITY FROM CRIME

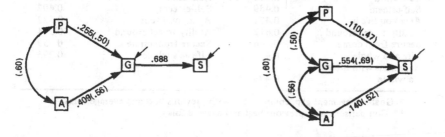

information, people's goal-achievement gaps may be altered, with their satisfaction levels not far behind. Campbell *et al*. (1976, pp. 149–150) note that a tyrant might try to inflate the satisfaction levels of his or her subjects by restricting their experiences or giving them false reports about the status of their peers. Packard (1957), Key (1973), Michalos (1978a) and many others have argued that advertisers have attempted with more or less success to manipulate satisfaction and demand by providing unrealistic norms, e.g., strange guests who inspect glasses for soap marks, sniff carpets, squeeze toilet tissue, stroke the dust from the table tops, and so on. Confirmation of the Michigan model provides a picture of the psychology of satisfaction that is a necessary condition of carrying out such manipulation.

Insofar as satisfaction is generated as the Michigan model indicates, education and individual initiative have a fundamental role to play in the development of the good life for individuals and societies. Accurate perceptions of the real world have a vital role to play in the determination of satisfaction with that world. The proverbial Fool's Paradise may be regarded as the result of experiencing uninformed or misinformed satisfaction. Thus, if knowledge

EXHIBIT 9
Percent of variance explained
in path models of exhibits
7.1, 7.2, 8.1–8.12

Dependent variables:	R^2 from 3 Predictors* ($P = 0.001$)	Dependent variables:	R^2 from 2 Predictors** ($P = 0.001$)
Satisfaction with		Goal-achievement gap	
Health	0.459	Health	0.398
Financial security	0.503	Financial security	0.406
Family life	0.650	Family life	0.455
Friendships	0.539	Friendships	0.484
Housing	0.499	Housing	0.377
Job	0.667	Job	0.397
Free time activity	0.556	Free time activity	0.423
Education	0.440	Education	0.137
Self-esteem	0.489	Self-esteem	0.402
Area you live in	0.471	Area you live in	0.322
Ability to get around	0.612	Ability to get around	0.374
Secure from crime	0.506	Secure from crime	0.359
Life as a whole	0.453	Life as a whole	0.295
Happiness with life as a whole	0.479		

* Goal-achievement gap, comparisons with previous best and average folks.
** Comparisons with previous best and average folks.

is a reasonable thing (i.e. something to which principles of sound reasoning are applicable), then so is satisfaction, taste, etc. Here the dreams of all naturalistic value theorists loom large. Values may be psychologically connected to facts roughly as theoreticians have held they ought to be logically connected. Again, unfortunately, this is not the place to examine these implications, though one ought to be aware of them. (Michalos, 1976; 1980a Chapter 1 address some of the issues.)

Exhibit 9 records the various percents of variance explained in the multiple regressions used to construct the paths in Exhibits 8.1–8.12. Some of these coefficients of determination (R^2) are fairly substantial, e.g. job (0.667), family life (0.650) and ability to get around (0.612). The percent of variance explained in S by P, A and G is, relative to the preceding figures, unimpressive (0.453). I did a bit better accounting for the variance in H (0.479). Allowing

EXHIBIT 10
Multiple regression of satisfaction with life as a whole on
domain satisfaction and demographic variables

	Predictors used		
	Six demographic variables	Ten domains[b]	Demographic & eleven domains[c]
Percent of variance explained	0.068	0.548	0.566 $(P = 0.001)$
Predictors:			
Demographic variables	*Beta*	*Beta*	*Beta*
Marital status	−0.135	a	0.014
Family income	0.109	a	−0.028
Age	−0.153	a	−0.128
Sex	−0.115	a	−0.096
Education	−0.030	a	−0.013
Work status	−0.026	a	0.044
Satisfaction variables			
Family life	a	0.348	0.351
Friendships	a	0.195	0.202
Financial security	a	0.152	0.184
Self-esteem	a	0.131	0.105
Job	a	0.100	0.109
Health	a	0.107	0.101
Ability to get around	a	0.088	0.082
Free time activity	a	0.083	0.062
Housing	a	−0.049	−0.019
Education	a	−0.026	−0.041
Secure from crime	a	–	−0.005

[a] predictor omitted.
[b] 'area you live in' and 'secure from crime' had F-levels too low to enter equation.
[c] 'area you live in' F-level was too low for admission.

for some attenuation due to measurement error, it is safe to say that I am able to account for well over fifty percent of the explainable variance in all of my dependent variables, (See Andrews and Withey, 1976, pp. 142–144, and Cochran (1970).)

As Exhibit 10 shows, best predictive results were obtained from eleven domains and six demographic variables to S, namely, $R^2 = 0.566$. Attempting to predict H in the same way (Exhibit 11), I was only able to reach an R^2 of 0.462, and even so a couple domains failed to be included in the equation due to unacceptably low F-levels.

EXHIBIT 11
Multiple regression of happiness with life as a whole on domain satisfaction and demographic variables

	Predictors used		
	Five Demographic variables	Eleven domains[b]	Demographic & ten domains[c]
Percent of variance explained	0.050	0.451	0.462 ($P = 0.001$)
Predictors:			
Demographic variables	*Beta*	*Beta*	*Beta*
Family income	0.167	a	0.065
Marital status	−0.126	a	−0.033
Age	−0.078	a	−0.016
Sex	−0.060	a	−0.055
Education	−0.039	a	−0.023
Satisfaction variables			
Family life	a	0.384	0.391
Friendships	a	0.225	0.238
Health	a	0.121	0.124
Financial security	a	0.092	0.073
Self-esteem	a	0.070	0.066
Ability to get around	a	0.050	0.039
Secure from crime	a	−0.048	−0.048
Job	a	0.033	0.034
Education	a	−0.033	−0.039
Free time activity	a	0.027	0.023
Housing	a	0.005	–

a Predictor omitted.
b 'Area you live in' F-level was too low to enter equation.
c 'housing' and 'area you live in' F-levels were too low for admission.

9. TYPES OF SATISFACTION

Campbell *et al.* (1976, p. 10) wrote that

It may be necessary to distinguish between a satisfaction which is associated with an experience of rising expectations and one which is associated with declining expectations. An individual who has achieved an aspiration toward which he has been moving may be said to experience the satisfaction of success. Another person may have lowered his aspiration level to the point which he can achieve, and he might be said to experience the satisfaction of resignation. The two individuals might be equally satisfied in the sense of fulfilled needs, but the affective content associated with success and resignation may well differ. In experiences of dissatisfaction, we might expect the affective content of disappointment and frustration to accompany any failure to achieve one's expectations.

This passage is instructive in a number of ways. In the first place, it may be noticed that the authors seem to use the terms 'aspiration' and 'expectation' as synonyms, a practice that ought to be discouraged. Second, the passage contains a hint of another assumption that is probably unwarranted. The basic view of these authors seems to be that satisfaction may be thought of as essentially a matter of need fulfillment, insofar as aspirations are somehow generated by needs. I suppose they would recognize some difference logically and psychologically between wanting something and needing something, but if they do, they never seem to allow the difference to emerge in their remarks about fulfillment. I have discussed these issues at length in Michalos (1978b), but here I only want to say that from the point of view of theorizing about and occasionally even managing satisfactions, it may be worthwhile to be scrupulously attentive to the difference between want and need fulfillment.

The third lesson to be learned from the quotation above is central to my purposes. That is the suggestion that one might begin to distinguish types of satisfaction on the basis of the significance of its affective component. McKennell (1978), Andrews and McKennell (1980), and McKennell and Andrews (1980), have explored this posibility with some success. McKennell (1978) suggested the following Boolean classification of people.

Subgroup	Interpretation	Short name
1. Satisfied – Happy	Satisfaction of achievement	Achievers
2. Satisfied – Unhappy	Satisfaction of resignation	Resigned
3. Dissatisfied – Happy	Satisfaction of aspiration	Aspirers
4. Dissatisfied – Unhappy	Satisfaction of frustration	Frustrated

Using this scheme, my sample was divided into the four groups illustrated in Exhibit 12. Achievers had scores of 5–7 on S and H; Resigned had 5–7 S and 1–4 on H; Aspirers had 1–4 on S and 5–7 on H; Frustrated had 1–4 on

EXHIBIT 12
Achievers, resigned, aspirers and frustrated

HAPPINESS	SATISFACTION	
	Terrible-Mixed (1–4)	Satisfied-Delighted (5–7)
Very unhappy	Frustrated	Resigned
Mixed (1–4)	$N = 46, 13.2\%$	$N = 52, 14.9\%$
	Group 4	Group 2
Happy	Aspirers	Achievers
Very happy (5–7)	$N = 2, 0.6\%$	$N = 248, 71.3\%$
	Group 3	Group 1

S and H. Curiously and unfortunately only two people out of 348 classifiable respondents (0.6%) fell into the Aspirers group. Campbell *et al.* (1976, pp. 36, 165–168) and McKennell (1978, pp. 401–403) found the dissatisfied-happy combination (Aspirers) to be especially characteristic of youth, and the Guelph sample is relatively youthful. Seventy percent of the respondents are 18 to 34 years old. Besides, you recall that in section 6 it was pointed out that, so far as their jobs are concerned, these respondents are only half to two-thirds along the way to their goals. So, I expected to find more Aspirers in the group. It's worth mentioning, however, that the global goal-achievement gap mean (5.19) is higher than the job goal-achievement gap mean (4.62) for the total sample (Exhibits 3 and 4), which indicates that there is globally a smaller goal-achievement gap than one would suspect from considering only the job domain. At any rate, it would have been pointless to try to perform a statistical analysis with a two-membered Aspirers group. So I confined the discriminant analysis to the three remaining groups.

Discriminant analysis has not been especially popular with social indicators researchers, although it is available in *SPSS* and there are some nice discussions of it in Kleinbaum and Kupper (1978) and Thorndike (1978). Without such a procedure we might discriminate our three groups (Achievers, Resigned and Frustrated) by selecting, say, some demographic variables and inspecting the means and variances of these variables for each of the three groups. With the procedure we simply form composite scores based on some selected set of variables and discriminate the groups on the basis of these scores. Technically speaking, a linear combination or function of variables is

EXHIBIT 13
Standardized discriminant
function coefficients

	Function 1	Function 2
Relative percent of variance explained in 12 variables	97.84	2.16
Canonical correlation	0.712 ($P = 0.0001$)	0.149 (NS)
Discriminators:		
Satisfaction with		
Health	−0.117	0.198
Financial security	−0.108	−0.416
Family life	−0.610	0.276
Friendships	−0.219	0.093
Free time activity	−0.099	−0.451
Education	0.154	0.042
Self-esteem	−0.196	0.444
Ability to get around	−0.103	−0.417
Demography		
Sex	0.115	0.126
Marital status	0.147	−0.216
Work status	−0.175	0.363
Education	−0.103	−0.607

constructed such that the variation of its values *between* any two groups will be greater than the variation of its values *within* the groups.

Exhibits 13–15 summarize the results of a discriminant analysis of the three groups (Achievers, Resigned and Frustrated) on the basis of 12 domain satisfaction and 6 demographic scores. Exhibit 13 lists the standardized discriminant function coefficients for the discriminating variables that had F levels sufficient to keep them in the equation. A single function accounted for 98 percent of all the variance in these variables, and the canonical correlation between this set of variables and the two variables (S and H) used to define the three groups was 0.712 (P = 0.0001). The second function was relatively worthless given the amount of variance left to be accounted for in the 12 variables and the statistically insignificant canonical correlation between it and H and S.

Inspection of the column under 'Function 1' reveals that family life is three times as important as its nearest rival, friendships, in determining the values of the function. Insofar as any single name would accurately describe what is captured by Funciton 1, one would have to say it is satisfaction with family life. Thus, given the question "Which domain satisfaction and demographic scores provide the maximum discrimination among Achievers,

EXHIBIT 14
Mean scores on variables
in the discriminant function for three groups

	Dissatisfied + unhappy = frustrated (N = 42)	Satisfied + unhappy = resigned (N = 49)	Satisfied + happy = achievers (N = 224) Total = 315
Satisfaction with			
Health	4.83	5.31	5.69
Financial security	3.50	4.47	4.79
Family life	3.71	5.14	5.99
Friendships	3.93	5.00	5.68
Free time activity	3.91	5.00	5.39
Education (Sat.)	3.98	4.61	4.92
Self-esteem	4.02	4.74	5.32
Ability to get around	4.67	5.55	5.80
Sex*	1.91	1.78	1.76
Marital status*	2.26	1.98	1.79
Work status*	1.12	1.02	1.06
Education*	2.79	3.12	3.02

* Demographic variables.

Resigned and Frustrated?", the answer is "Satisfaction with one's family life".

Exhibit 14 lists the mean scores of each of the 12 variables of the discriminant functions for each of the 3 groups. The domain satisfaction means provide a splendid summary of the difference among the groups. Indeed, given the predominance of satisfaction with family life as a discriminating variable, one can practically imagine the three groups distinguished along that single axis. Visually speaking, the plots of the means of this variable for the three groups are very similar to the plots of the group centroids, i.e. similar to roughly the means of the means of the scores of each individual on each variable for each group.

In an earlier study of the quality of life in a rural township in Ontario, Michalos (1978c) reported that satisfaction with family life was the strongest predictor of personal life satisfaction. A pilot survey in Guelph in the fall of 1977 revealed the same thing. (No report was written on that study.) Accordingly, I'm beginning to suspect that satisfaction with family life really is the primary determinant of satisfaction with life as a whole for Canadians. Campbell *et al.* (1976, p. 85) reported that family life satisfaction was the

EXHIBIT 15
Results of predicting
group membership from discriminant functions

Actual groups	Predicted groups		
	Frustrated	Resigned	Achievers
Frustrated (N = 42, 13%)	32 (76%)	4 (10%)	6 (14%)
Resigned (N = 49, 16%)	4 (8%)	9 (18%)	36 (74%)
Achievers (N = 224, 71%)	2 (1%)	3 (1%)	219 (98%)

Total N = 315
83 percent of grouped cases correctly classified.

strongest predictor of global well-being in their sample, and Andrews and Withey (1976, p. 169) had it in second place behind 'amount of fun'.

Exhibit 15 summarizes the results of using the discriminant functions to predict group membership. Eighty-three percent of the cases were correctly classified. Perfect accuracy of classification would have given 100% figures along the left to right diagonal in Exhibit 15. So it's apparent that the discriminant functions were strongest for predicting Achievers (98%) weakest for Resigned (18%), and pretty good for Frustrated (76%).

Several other discriminant analyses were undertaken with results similar to those just reported. When the three global predictors were used (goal-achievement gap, comparisons with previous best and average folks), two significant functions were obtained. The first function captured 95 percent of the variance in the three predictors and was dominated by the goal-achievement gap. The second function was led by comparisons with best previous experience.

10. CONCLUSION

I set out to review the recent literature on satisfaction and happiness, to identify some plausible next steps to take along the frontiers of this area of research and to offer some suggestions to facilitate those steps. Using partial correlation techniques, substantial levels of covariation were found among all the variables that were used in predictions of satisfaction and happiness with life as a whole from satisfaction with specific domains (e.g. family life, health). Using path analysis, confirmation was found in a dozen domains for a model which has satisfaction as a fuction of a perceived goal-achievement gap, and the latter as a function of comparisons with previous best experience and the status of average folks. Using discriminant analysis, satisfaction with family life was found to be a powerful and predominant discriminator among three groups, identified as Frustrated (dissatisfied and unhappy), Resigned (satisfied and unhappy) and Achievers (satisfied and happy).

University of Guelph,
Ontario, Canada

NOTE

* I am grateful for the help of A. M. Blanchet, L. Ferraro, R. A. Logan, S. McNeill, J. Tofflemire and the generous members of our university Staff Association who gave up their time to fill out yet another questionnaire. F. M. Andrews. O. D. Duncan, J. J. Hubert, K. C. Land, S. Swaminathan and F. W. Young gave me plenty of good advice, for which I am also grateful. Of course, I alone am responsible for this final version of the paper.

REFERENCES

Abrams, M.: 1972, 'Social indicators and social equity', New Society 22, 454–455.

Adams, J. S.: 1963, 'Toward an understanding of inequity', Journal of Abnormal and Social Psychology 67, 422–436.

Adams, J. S.: 1965, 'Inequity in social exchange', Advances in Experimental Social Psychology. (ed.) L. Berkowitz. (New York, Academic Press) pp. 267–299.

Al-Hoory, M. T.: 1976, Campsite Selection as a Decision-Making Process: A Behavioral Approach. (Logan, Utah, Utah State University) doctoral dissertation.

Allardt, E.: 1976, 'Dimensions of welfare in the comparative Scandinavian study', Acta Sociologica 19, 227–239.

Andrews, F. M. and Inglehart, R. F.: 1979, 'The structure of subjective well-being in nine western societies', Social Indicators Research 6, 73–90.

Andrews, F. M. and McKennell, A. C.: 1980, 'Measures of self-reported well-being: Their affective, cognitive, and other components', Social Indicators Research 8, 127–155.

Andrews, F. M. and Withey, S. B.: 1974, 'Developing measures of perceived life quality: Results from several national surveys', Social Indicators Research 1, 1–26.

Andrews, F. M. and Withey, S. B.: 1976, Social Indicators of Well-Being (New York, Plenum Press).

Appley, M. H.: 1971, (ed.) Adaptation-Level Theory (New York, Academic Press).

Arvey, R. D., Dewhirst, H. D. and Boling, J. C.: 1976, 'Relationships between goal clarity, participation in goal setting, and personality-characteristics on job satisfaction in a scientific organization', Journal of Applied Psychology 61, 103–105.

Atkinson, T. H.: 1979, Trends in Life Satisfaction Among Canadians 1968–1977. (Montreal, Quebec, Institute for Research on Public Policy).

Bharadwaj, L. K. and Wilkening, E. A.: 1974, 'Occupational satisfaction of farm husbands and wives', Human Relations 27, 739–753.

Bradburn, N. M. and Caplovitz, D.: 1965, Reports on Happiness (Chicago, Illinois: Aldine Pub. Co.).

Brehm, J. W. and Cohen, A. R.: 1962, Explorations in Cognitive Dissonance (New York, John Wiley and Sons, Inc.).

Buckley, H. D.: 1969, The Relationship of Achievement and Satisfaction to Anticipated Environmental Stress of Transfer Students in the State University of New York (Syracuse, New York, Syracuse University), doctoral dissertation.

Burgess, R. L. and Nielson, J. M.: 1974, 'Distributive justice and the balance of power', American Sociological Review 39, 427–443.

Burkey, R. E.: 1971, Effect of Discrepancy Between Expected and Actual Supervisory Behavior on Worker Performance and Job Satisfaction: An Empirical Study (Columbus, Ohio, Ohio State University), doctoral dissertation.

Campbell. A.: 1972, 'Aspiration, satisfaction and fulfillment', The Human Meaning of Social Change (ed.) A. Campbell and P. E. Converse. (New York, Russell Sage Foundation), pp. 441–466.

Campbell, A., Converse, P. E. and Rodgers, W. L.: 1976, The Quality of American Life (New York, Russell Sage Foundation).

Cantril, H.: 1965, The Pattern of Human Concerns (New Brunswick, New Jersey, Rutgers University Press).

Carey, J. F.: 1974, A Study of Dissonance in the Classroom Setting: Its Relationship to Teacher Job Satisfaction, Student Achievement and School Satisfaction (College Park, Maryland, University of Maryland), doctoral dissertation.

Carpenter, S. S.: 1973, User Satisfaction with a Planned Physical Environment (San Diego, California, United States International University), doctoral dissertation.

Cochran, W. G.: 1970, 'Some effects of errors of measurement on multiple correlation', Journal of the American Statistical Association 65, 22–34.

Cook, D. M.: 1968, The Psychological Impact on Management of Selected Procedures in Managerial Accounting (Austin, Texas: University of Texas), doctoral dissertation.

Danielson, L. C.: 1977, Effects of Success and Failure on Aspiration Level, Problem-Solving Performance, and Satisfaction with Performance (University Park, Pennsylvania, Pennsylvania State University), doctoral dissertation.

Davies, J. C.: 1962, 'Toward a theory of revolution', American Sociological Review 27, 5–18.

Dorsett, K. G.: 1977, A study of Levels of Job Satisfaction and Job Aspiration among Black Clerical Employees in City and County Governments of Greensboro, Guilford County, North Carolina (Greensboro, North Carolina, University of North Carolina), doctoral dissertation.

Duncan, O. D.: 1975a, 'Does money buy satisfaction?', Social Indicators Research 2, 267–274.

Duncan, O. D.: 1975b, Introduction to Structural Equation Models (New York, Academic Press).

Easterlin, R. A.: 1973, 'Does money buy happiness?', The Public Interest 30, 3–10.

Easterlin, R. A.: 1974, 'Does Economic Growth Improve the Human Lot? Some Empirical Evidence', Nations and Households in Economic Growth. (ed.) P. A. David and M. W. Reder. (New York, Academic Press), pp. 89–125.

Edwards, W. and Tversky, A.: 1967, (ed.) Decision Making (Middlesex, England, Penguin Books Ltd.).

Feierabend, I, K., Feierabend, R. L. and Nesvold, B. A.: 1969, 'Social change and political violence: Cross-national patterns'. Violence in America Volume II. (ed.) H. D. Graham and T. R. Gurr (Washington, D. C., U.S. Government Printed Office), pp. 498–509.

Festinger, L.: 1957, A Theory of Cognitive Dissonance (Stanford, California, Stanford University Press).

Foa, V. G.: 1957, 'Relation of worker's expectation to satisfaction with the supervisor', Personnel Psychology 10, 161–168.

Gelwick, B. P.: 1975, The Adult Woman Student and Her Perceptions and Expectations of the University Environment (Columbia, Missouri, University of Missouri), doctoral dissertation.

Gordon, R. A.: 1968, Issues in multiple regression', The American Journal of Sociology 73, 592–616.

Greenstein, G.: 1972, A Study of the Relationships Between Teachers' Feelings of General Satisfaction and the Needs and Expections Fulfillment Qualities of Their Organizational Press (Syracuse, New York, Syracuse University), doctoral dissertation.

Gurr, T. R.: 1970, Why Men Rebel (Princeton, New Jersey, Princeton University Press).

Hamner, W. C. and Harnett, D. L.: 1974, 'Goal setting, performance and satisfaction in an interdependent task', Organizational Behavior and Human Performance 12, 217–230.

Hankiss, E., Manchin, R and Füstës: 1978, Cross-Cultural Quality of Life Research: An Outline for a Conceptual Framework and Some Methodological Issues (Budapest, Center for Quality of Life Research, Hungarian Academy of Sciences).

Helson, H.: 1964, Adaption-Level Theory: An Experimental and Systematic Approach to Behavior (New York, Harper and Row, Inc.).

Hibbs, C. W.: 1975, Selected Factors Affecting Client Satisfaction in a University Counselling Center (Iowa City, University of Iowa), doctoral dissertation.

Hulin, C. L. and Smith, P. C.: 1965, 'A linear model of job satisfaction', Journal of Applied Psychology 49, 206–216.

Ilgen, D. R.: 1969, Satisfaction with Performance as a Function of the Initial Level of Expected Performance and the Deviation from Expectation (Urbana, Illinois, University of Illinois), doctoral dissertation.

Ilgen, D. R.: 1971, 'Satisfaction with performance as a function of the initial level of expected performance and the deviations from expectations', Organizational Behavior and Human Performance 6, 345–361.

Ilgen, D. R. and Hamstra, B. W.: 1972, 'Performance satisfaction as a function of the difference between expected and reported performance at five levels of reported performance', Organizational Behavior and Human Performance 7, 359–370.

Jones, E. E. et al. 1971, Attribution: Perceiving the Causes of Behavior (Morristown, New Jersey, General Learning Press).

Kawakami, D. T.: 1967, Changes in Self-Evaluation and Expression of Satisfaction with Vocational Decision (New York, Columbia University), doctoral dissertation.

Kerlinger, F. N. and Pedhazur, E. J.: 1973, Multiple Regression in Behavioral Research (New York, Holt, Rinehart and Winston, Inc.).

Key, B. W.: 1973, Subliminal Seduction (New York, The New American Library).

Kim, J. S. and Hamner, W. C.: 1976, 'Effect of performance feedback and goal setting on productivity and satisfaction in an organizational setting', Journal of Applied Psychology 61, 48–57.

Kleinbaum, D. G. and Kupper, L. L.: 1978, Applied Regression Analysis and Other Multivariable Methods (North Scituate, Massachusetts, Duxbury Press).

Kuhn, T. S.: 1962, The Structure of Scientific Revolutions (Chicago, University of Chicago Press).

Kuhn, T. S.: 1977, The Essential Tension (Chicago, University of Chicago Press).

Larson, R.: 1978, 'Thirty years of research on the subjective well-being of older americans', Journal of Gerontology 33, 109–125.

Latham, G. P. and Kinne, S. B.: 1974, 'Improving job performance through training in goal setting', Journal of Applied Psychology, 59, 187–191.

Lawler, E. E.: 1968, 'Equity theory as a predictor of productivity and work quality', Psychological Bulletin 70, 596–610.

Lewin, K. et al.: 1944, 'Level of Aspiration', Personality and the Behavior Disorders. (ed.) J. McV. Hunt (New York, Ronald Press Co.), 333–378.

Lewis, S. A.: 1973, Perceived Competence, Success-Failure, and Performance Feedback in Outcome Satisfaction and Expectancy Behavior (Buffalo, New York, State University of New York), doctoral dissertation.

Locke, E. A., Cartledge, N. and Knerr, C. S.: 1970, 'Studies of the relationships between satisfaction, goal setting and performance', Organizational Behavior and Human Performance 5, 135–158.

Mason, R. and Faulkenberry, G. D.: 1978, 'Aspirations, achievements and life satisfactions', Social Indicators Research 5, 133–150.

McKennell, A. C.: 1978, 'Cognition and affect in perception of well-being', Social Indicators Research 5, 389–426.

McKennell, A. C. and Andrews, F. M.: 1980, 'Models of cognition and affect in perceptions of well-being, Social Indicators Research 8, 257–298.

Michalos, A. C.: 1976, 'The morality of cognitive decision-making', The Winnipeg Conference on Action Theory. (ed.) M. Brand and D. Walton. (Dordrecht, D. Reidel Pub. Co.), pp. 325–340.

Michalos, A. C.: 1978a, 'Advertising: its logic, ethics and economics', A paper read at the Informal Logic Conference at the University of Windsor, Ontario, June 26–28, 1978.

Michalos, A. C.: 1978b, Foundations of Decision-Making (Ottawa, Canadian Library of Philosophy).

Michalos, A. C.: 1978c, 'Satisfaction with life and housing in rural Ontario', A paper presented at the Rural Sociological Society meeting in San Francisco, August 31, 1978.

Michalos, A. C.: 1980a, Foundations, Population and Health; North American Social Report, Volume One. (Dordrecht, D. Reidel Pub. Co.).

Michalos, A. C.: 1980b, Crime, Justice and Politics; North American Social Report, Volume Two (Dordrecht, D. Reidel Pub. Co.).

Morgan, S. M.: 1976, The Relationship Between Congruent Student and Supervisor Expectations, Student Performance, and Student Satisfaction in Counselling Practica (Knoxville, Tennessee, University of Tennessee), doctoral dissertation.

Nie, N. H. et al. 1975, Statistical Package for the Social Sciences (New York, McGraw-Hill Book Co.).

Newton, R. M.: 1976, Supervisor Expectations and Behavior: Effects of Consistent-Inconsistent Supervisory Pairings on Supervisee Satisfaction with Supervision, Perceptions of Supervisory Relationships and Rated Counsellor Competency (Columbia, Missouri, University of Missouri), doctoral dissertation.

Packard, V.: 1957, The Hidden Persuaders (New York, David McKay Co.).

Patchen, M.: 1961a, The Choice of Wage Comparisons (Englewood Cliffs, New Jersey, Prentice-Hall, Inc.).

Patchen, M.: 1961b, 'A conceptual framework and some empirical data regarding comparisons of social rewards', Sociometry 24, 136–156.

Pelz, D. C. and Andrews, F. M.: 1976, Scientists in Organizations (Ann Arbor, Michigan, Institute for Social Research).

Pritchard, R. D.: 1969, 'Equity theory: A review and critique', Organizational Behavior and Human Performance 4, 176–211.

Rescher, N.: 1972, Welfare (Pittsburgh, Pennsylvania, University of Pittsburgh Press).

Schneider, M.: 1975, 'The Quality of life in large American cities: Objective and subjective social indicators', Social Indicators Research 1, 495–509.

Scott, J. P.: 1979, 'Single rural elders', Alternative Lifestyles 2, 359–378.

Space, M. A.: 1974, Vocational Role Image, Perceptions of Employers' Expectations, and Job Satisfaction in Novice Nurses (New York, Columbia University), doctoral dissertation.

Spector, A. J.: 1956, 'Expectations fulfillment and morale', Journal of Abnormal and Social Psychology 52, 51–56.

Strumpel, B.: 1972, 'Economic well-being as an object of social measurement', Subjective Elements of Well-Being. (ed.) B. Strumpel. Paris: OECD, 75—122.
Tatarkiewicz, W.: 1976, Analysis of Happiness (The Hague, Martinus Nijhoff).
Thibaut, J. W. and Kelley, H. H.: 1959, The Social Psychology of Groups (New York, John Wiley and Sons).
Thompson, A. P.: 1975, Subjective Expectations and Job Facet Predictability in Job Satisfaction (London, Ontario, University of Western Ontario), doctoral dissertation.
Thorndike, R. M.: 1978, Correlational Procedures For Research (New York, Gardner Press, Inc.).
Umstot, D. D., Bell, C. H. and Mitchell, T. R.: 1976' 'Effects of job enrichment and task goals on satisfaction and productivity: Implications for job design', Journal of Applied Psychology 61, 379—394.
Wantz, R. A.: 1976, A Multivariate Analysis of Client Expectation, Client Satisfaction, and Client Personality Characteristics at the Ball State University Counselling Practicum Clinic (Muncie, Indiana, Ball State University), doctoral dissertation.
Warr, P. and Wall, T.: 1975, Work at Well-Being (Middlesex, England, Penguin Books, Ltd.).
Weaver, P. J.: 1974, A Person-Environment Analysis of Performance, Satisfaction, and Expectancies of Job Trainees (Ann Arbor, Michigan: University of Michigan), doctoral dissertation.

TOM ATKINSON

11. THE STABILITY AND VALIDITY OF QUALITY OF LIFE MEASURES*

(Received 6 February, 1981)

ABSTRACT. Effective social indicators must be stable when individual or societal characteristics are unchanged and dynamic when circumstances alter. Highly reliable measures may be poor indicators because they are insensitive to change. Little evidence is available on the sensitivity or validity of objective and subjective indicators. A lack of panel data has restricted the assessment of the stability of subjective measures.

This paper examines longitudinal data on a representative sample of 2162 Canadians interviewed in 1977 and again in 1979. Test-retest correlations of approximately 0.50 were obtained for satisfaction and self-anchoring ladder measures among respondents who reported no significant changes in their lives during the past two years. Correlations were substantially lower, as expected, for those reporting life changes. Comparisons of the absolute values of these subjective indicators show that very little change in quality of life measures occurs when stable circumstances are reported but the indicators rise or fall significantly when situations change with downward adjustments being more dramatic than upward modifications. Positive and negative life events had little effect on overall evaluations of life quality.

In general, these findings provide very strong evidence for the stability and validity of subjective indicators over time. These measures, with one exception, were constant in unchanging situations and sensitive to change when it occurred.

INTRODUCTION

Measurement issues have provided a central focus of social indicators research over the last decade. Those interested in developing objective quality of life (QOL) measures have puzzled over which subset of the plethora of available statistics should be included in their models, and how to combine them into general indexes comparable to popular aggregate economic measures such as the Gross National Product and Consumer Price Index. Students of subjective or perceptual indicators have been no less concerned with the selection of conceptually suitable measures but have not had to wrestle with the question of how to combine them into a general index. Global measures of perceived well-being can be easily obtained through direct measurement, and previous research has demonstrated that evaluations of specific areas of experience such as work, marriage, etc. combine in a linear fashion to produce general QOL perceptions (Campbell *et al.*, 1976; Andrews and Withey, 1976).

259

Instead, research on subjective indicators, particularly in North America, has been greatly concerned with the reliability and validity of these measures. Subjective social indicators have been exposed to closer methodological scrutiny than any other attitudinal or value measure with the possible exception of the *F*-scale. Several factors are responsible for this concern. First, social indicators, whether objective or subjective, are intended to enlighten many areas of social policy and the consequences of poor measurement extend far beyond the confines of disciplinary interests. Second, those surveying QOL perceptions of the general public have had to rebut attacks that argue that most people are incapable of making consistent and honest evaluations of their own lives. Third, because subjective measures are designed and utilized directly by the researchers, they can be easily modified if proven inadequate, while objective indicators are based on data gathered by various government agencies for administrative purposes and the measurement process is beyond the control of those developing indicators. Finally, most researchers working on subjective measures have been trained as psychologists and are very familiar with the assessment of reliability and validity. Sociologists and economists who develop objective measures are more adept in the construction of statistical models which delineate causal influences and tend to ignore questions about the quality of their measures.

Assessments of the reliability and validity of subjective indicators have, with one major exception, been limited to analyses of cross-sectional surveys. Published studies provide substantial evidence that several QOL measures correlate well with each other, are relatively free of method effects and are not significantly affected by response biases such as social desirability. However, the absence of panel data on large representative samples has prohibited the evaluation of the stability of QOL measures over time and their sensitivity to the changing circumstances of people's lives. Indicators which are very stable over time may be poor candidates for systems meant to monitor change.

This paper presents an analysis of a representative sample of over 2000 Canadians interviewed in 1977 and again in 1979 about perceptions of their lives in general and specific areas or domains of them. Data is presented on the stability of several QOL measures and on their behaviour when individuals experience change in their lives during the two year period. The effects of several types of significant events on QOL assessments are briefly examined.

A. Previous Research

North American research on subjective indicators has made significant contributions to our understanding of the reliability and validity of several QOL measures. With the exception of one study, the methodological research on these measures have involved cross-sectional rather than panel data and have often included Frank Andrews as an investigator.

First, with associates at the Institute for Social Research (Andrews and Withey, 1976; Andrews and Crandall, 1976), and more recently with Aubrey McKennell and this author (Andrews and McKennell, 1980; McKennel, Atkinson and Andrews, forthcoming), he has examined reliability and validity using a methodology based on a multi-method, multi-trait matrix approach (Campbell and Fiske, 1959). A software package (LISREL) developed by Joreskog and Sorbom (1978) identifies the elements of an item score which result from trait variance, from method variance and from unique or random variation. Validity is the trait coefficient and reliability is the summed square of the trait and method effects.

Since reliability computed in this fashion roughly approximates standard reliability coefficients, it is possible to compile the following summary of item reliabilities from national surveys in Canada and the United States (exact question formats appear in Appendix A):

Measures	U.S.	Canada
Satisfaction		
7-point	0.59	0.68[a], 0.63
11-point		
Self-anchoring Ladder	0.54	0.56
Happiness (3-point)	0.52	
Delighted-Terrible	0.67[a], 0.70	

[a] Test-retest computation.

All estimates are fairly high with the classical test-retest cofficients suggesting reliabilities of about 0.70. Of the variance accounted for by method and trait factors, e.g. the reliability, 15 to 20% appears to result from method factors, the remainder from trait factors. These analyses indicate fairly high reliability and convergent validity for QOL measures and demonstrate that the correlations result primarily from trait, not method, variance.

Follow-up interviews with a small subset (*N* = 285) of a national sample in the United States have produced the only published data on the stability of

QOL measures over time (Campbell *et al.*, 1976; Rodgers and Converse, 1976). In brief, the test-retest correlations over an eight month period were as follows:

Index of Domain Satisfaction	0.76
Index of General Well-Being	0.53
Average Domain Satisfaction	0.53
General Life Satisfaction	0.42
Happiness	0.38

Although the stability of the two indexes and the specific domain satisfaction measures were high given the fairly long time lapse between interviews, the correlations for the life satisfaction and happiness items are cause for concern. Campbell and his colleagues point out, however, that these estimates provide the lower bounds of stability over time. Given the passage of eight months between interviews, it is likely that changes occurred in the lives of many individuals thus reducing the size of the correlation. From this perspective, a very high stability coefficient, e.g. the Domain Satisfaction Index, may disqualify a measure as a social indicator because of its insensitivity to change.

The present research continues the investigation of the performance of QOL measures over time begun by Campbell, Converse and Rodgers. A large panel survey allows the stability of QOL measures to be examined over a two year period for those reporting changes in their lives and those who do not report changed circumstances. The correlation of measures in the No Change condition provides a fair test of the stability of these indicators. In addition, comparisons of the difference and mean scores for Change and No Change groups will indicate the stability of measures in absolute terms and their sensitivity to changing conditions. Both attributes must be demonstrated if these measures are to be useful indicators of well-being.

Although this analysis does not fit the hypothesis-testing mold, three results are expected:

(a) the stability correlations will be higher for the No Change than the Change respondents;

(b) the No Change group will show little mean change in QOL measures over the two year period; and,

(c) those reporting changed circumstances will experience significant changes between 1977 and 1979 QOL indicators — increases for those in improved circumstances and declines for those in deteriorating conditions.

II. METHOD

A. Subjects

In 1977, a multi-stage probability sample of Canadian dwelling units yielded a sample of 3288 respondents. The response rate for the national sample was 70%. When weighted to compensate for over-sampling in some urban areas and response rate biases, the sample is representative of the non-institutionalized, adult (age 18 and older) population (Murray and Atkinson, forthcoming). The second wave of the study was launched in 1979 with a sample design which called for reinterviews of all 1977 respondents and new interviews in all dwellings from which the previous respondents had moved. Two thousand one hundred and sixty-two of the 1977 respondents (66%) were reinterviewed. Of this number, 1669 (77%) resided in the same location while 493 (23%) had moved. Of the 34% who were lost from the original sample, 16% were located but refused the interview, 7% had moved and could not be located and 6% were ill, aged or had died, and 5% were temporarily absent or unavailable for other reasons.

B. Measures

All interviews were conducted by trained interviewers of the Survey Research Centre at York University and sessions lasted an average of two hours. The interview was divided into sections which obtained information on the 'facts' of the respondents circumstances in each of twelve domains, e.g. work, leisure, housing, and included several questions requiring evaluations of that domain or specific aspects of it. A separate section dealt with assessments of life in general.

Three evaluations of general well-being were included in both interviews (See Appendix A for complete question text). They were:

(a) A life satisfaction measure which was similar but not identical to that used by Campbell et al. in their 1971 survey. The two questions were identically worded, but the Canadian survey used an eleven-point response scale while the U.S. version was restricted to seven points. The Canadian measure is identical to that used in Great Britain and in the European Community surveys.

(b) A self-anchoring ladder scale which was a modification of Cantril's

(1965) measure. The major difference between this measure and Cantril's is that his was anchored by the phrase 'the best possible life for you' allowing the interpretation that the imagined conditions must be obtainable by the respondent. The use of the 'ideal or perfect life' as an anchor in the current survey eliminates that ambiguity and permits personal definitions of the desired conditions without suggesting that such a life must be obtainable.

(c) A general happiness scale which has been used by the Gallup organization for several decades and has been used in several academically-based surveys including Bradburn (1969), Campbell *et al.* and the General Social Survey in the United States.

In each domain, respondents were asked to indicate their level of satisfaction using the same format as the general life measure.

Two indexes are computed from the QOL measures. The General Quality of Life Index combines responses from the life satisfaction, ladder and happiness measures while the Domain Satisfaction Index is an average of responses to the job, financial, housing, health and marriage/romance domains. These indexes are comparable to those developed by Campbell *et al.* which were more stable over time than individual items.

In addition to these evaluation questions, each section in the 1979 questionnaire included items requiring a comparison between respondent's current situation and that two years previous. The questions asked whether the current situation, e.g. their job, was better, worse or the same as two years ago. These items provide a summary measure of change in several areas of life and allow the respondent to interpret the impact of changes.

Finally, in 1979 each person was asked whether any of sixteen events had occurred in their lives during the past five years. Seven events are assumed to be negative — divorce/separation, romantic breakup, death of a family member, death of a close friend, serious injury of illness, lose touch with a close friend and a large decrease in income — while the other nine were positive — recent marriage, having children, a romance, new friends, new job, job promotion, on honour or award, changing residences and having a large income increase. If an event had taken place, they were asked to provide the date of the most recent occurrence and to indicate its effect on their lives. In this analysis, the effects of events occurring within the last two years i.e. since the 1977 interview, on repeated QOL measures is examined. Events which had occurred in the twelve months prior to the 1979 survey (labelled

78–79) are distinguished from those which took place between one and two years ago (labelled 77–78).

III. RESULTS

Any analysis of panel data must be cognizant of the effects of sample mortality. While the use of individual differences scores in these analyses eliminates the possibility that over time changes may result from differential dropout rates, sample mortality may reduce the representative nature of the panel if it is not randomly distributed. Table 1 compares the unweighted characteristics of the entire 1977 sample with those of the panel which was reinterviewed in 1979.

TABLE I

National sample and panel demographic characteristics

		1977 National sample	1977–79 panel
Gender –	Male	41%	41%
	Female	59	59
Family income –	Under $8000	22	19
	8000–13 999	24	24
	14 000–19 999	23	23
	20 000–up	31	34
Education –	Primary School or less	21	20
	Some Secondary	25	23
	Completed Secondary	30	31
	Some University	13	14
	Completed University	11	12
Employment status –	Working Full-time	46	46
	Working Part-time	10	11
	Not-Working	44	43
Marital status –	Married	67	68
	Widowed	8	8
	Divorced/Separated	7	7
	Never married	18	17
Age– 18–19		4	4
20–29		25	24
30–39		22	23
40–49		16	17
50–59		14	15
60–69		11	11
70+		7	6

Distributions shown in Table I indicate a high degree of similarity between the original sample and the 66% which was reinterviewed in 1979. The two samples are virtually identical on all attributes except family income where the panel has a slightly higher average income than the original sample ($17 950 to $17050). It is surprising that the age distributions are so similar given that younger persons are more mobile and harder to recontact while the aged are more likely to die or be incapacitated. Similarities between the two samples assure that, when weighted, both are representative of the Canadian population.

The stability of QOL measures is mot stringently tested by the zero-order correlations presented in Table II. Correlations were computed for the entire sample and separately for those who reported some changes in their circumstances and those whose situations did not change. Stability is indicated by the correlations for the latter group because these measures, if they are valid, should not correlate as highly for the change group.

TABLE II

Correlations of QOL measures repeated after two years

	Total sample	No change group	Change group	Z-score difference
Evaluations of Life in general				
Satisfaction scale	0.41	0.43	0.39	1.19
Self anchoring ladder	0.40	0.47	0.36	3.09[b]
Happiness scale	0.39	0.34	0.41	−1.91
General QOL index	0.53	0.55	0.52	0.98
Domain evaluations				
Job satisfaction	0.42	0.48	0.37	2.11[a]
Financial satisfaction	0.49	0.49	0.50	−0.34
Housing satisfaction	0.38	0.51	0.09	8.76[b]
Health satisfaction	0.53	0.56	0.45	2.96[b]
Marriage/Romance satisfaction	0.45	0.50	0.27	4.61[b]
Domain satisfaction index	0.58	0.60	0.56	1.40

[a] $p < 0.05$.
[b] $p < 0.01$.

Table II indicates that the stability of all general measures, except the happiness scale, is high — between 0.40 and 0.55 — for the sample as a whole. Domain measures were in the same range except for housing where the greatest amount of actual change occurred. Correlations for the No Change group were usually higher than those who experienced changes. These differences are very much in evidence among the domain specific measures suggesting that such indicators are more sensitive to change than terms requiring evaluations of very general conditions such as 'your life as a whole'.

Comparisons of these results with those reported by Campbell *et al.* show that the general assessments performed in virtually identical ways in the Canadian study even though the span between surveys was two years rather than eight months as in the earlier work. Our domain measures were less strongly correlated than those in the smaller U.S. study. Average correlations for the five areas were 0.58 in the U.S. versus 0.45 for the total sample and 0.51 for the No Change group in Canada.

This patterning of correlations in the current study supports the contention that domain ratings are more firmly rooted in the specific circumstances of the individual's life. As a result, stability coefficients for such measures decline more quickly than general indicators as the time period between observations increases. Rather than reducing the attractiveness of specific measures, this feature, and the marked differences between Change and No Change groups, recommends them as reliable and sensitive measures. The two indexes were more stable than the individual terms but may not be the best measurement tools if detecting change is a major objective of the research.

The weakest item assessed here is the happiness measure – it has the lowest stability correlations of the general measures and the No Change group had lower correlation than those whose lives had changed. The poor performance of this scale may result from a methodological fault or from differences between affective measures such as happiness and primarily cognitive scales like satisfaction. While affect may not be as good a social indicator as cognition, it is more likely that the item's problems stem from the use of a three-point response scale. Future research should utilize lengthier continuums with this measure rather than replicate the short scale because of its long history. A poor measure used twenty times in twenty times a poor measure.

In general, these stability coefficients, except the happiness item, are very encouraging given the lengthy period between the two administrations. These figures represent conservative estimates of stability because, although we attempted to eliminate persons who were experiencing changed circumstances, most peoples' lives changed during a two year period if for no other reason than they, their children, their houses, etc. have aged two years. Those using this type of satisfaction scale or ladder measure, i.e. ten or eleven-point scales, can be assured that they are fairly stable over long periods of time. Items which employ more abbreviated response continuums such as Campbell's *et al.* satisfaction measure and the Andrews/Withey Delighted-Terrible, probably enjoy similar reliability but may not share their sensitivity to change.

As suggested earlier, candidates for social indicator systems must not only be proven reliable by correlational tests but must have demonstrated stability and sensitivity in *absolute* terms. In Table III individual difference scores for the general QOL measures are analyzed by two measures of change – self-report change and the occurance of positive and negative events. The hypothesis that the No Change group would have more stable QOL scores than those reporting change is supported when the perceptual indicator of change is used as the independent variable but not when the event measures are involved. In most of the cases, however, the events produce difference patterns which are in the expected direction and approach statistical significance.

Differences in general life satisfaction fit the expected pattern almost perfectly with virtually identical scores for the No Change group. The negative change group suffered a larger drop in satisfaction than the gain experienced by the positive change group – a pattern which reappears throughout the following analysis. This finding in conjunction with the large proportion of persons who felt that their lives had improved over the two year period, suggests that people anticipate at least small improvements in life quality and that a deterioration produces a sharp drop in satisfaction, while improvements result in more modest increases.

It is also noteworthy that the positive change group had higher levels of satisfaction in 1977 and exceeded the average to a greater degree in 1979. Similarly the negative change group began below the mean and declined from there. The same pattern holds for all general Quality of Life assessment – the group reporting improvement between 1977 and 1979 were above average in the first survey and the margin increased during the two years. Apparently very high or low quality of life levels are the product of trends covering years rather than short term reversals of fortune. Future surveys should indicate the length of these cycles and identify the life events responsible for them.

The self-anchoring ladder scale shows the same difference patterns except

TABLE III

General QOL measures by perceived life change and significant events

	N	Means 1977	Means 1979	Differ- ence	Eta
GENERAL LIFE SATISFACTION					
Perceived change in life					
Better	1129	8.85	9.07	0.22	0.12[b]
Same	845	8.57	8.58	0.01	
Worse	155	7.68	7.05	−0.63	
Positive events					
0	557	8.67	8.69	0.02	
1 or 2	1113	8.69	8.73	0.04	0.06
3 or 4	374	8.58	8.75	0.17	
5+	86	8.29	8.86	0.57	
Negative events					
0	808	8.83	8.84	0.01	
1	741	8.65	8.79	0.14	
2	406	8.52	8.60	0.08	0.03
3+	175	8.12	8.22	0.10	
SELF-ANCHORING LADDER					
Perceived change in life					
Better	1129	7.29	7.73	0.44	
Same	845	7.12	7.45	0.33	0.17[b]
Worse	155	6.69	5.97	−0.72	
Positive events					
0	557	7.19	7.53	0.34	
1 or 2	1113	7.23	7.52	0.29	
3 or 4	374	7.06	7.40	0.34	0.02
5+	86	6.97	7.35	0.38	
Negative events					
0	808	7.28	7.66	0.38	
1	741	7.20	7.56	0.36	0.05
2	406	7.11	7.28	0.17	
3+	175	6.78	6.94	0.16	
HAPPINESS (3-POINT)					
Perceived change in life					
Better	1129	2.55	2.53	−0.02	
Same	845	2.43	2.29	−0.14	0.12[b]
Worse	155	2.24	1.98	−0.26	
Positive events					
0	557	2.51	2.37	−0.14	
1 or 2	1113	2.48	2.41	−0.07	0.05
3 or 4	374	2.46	2.38	−0.08	
5+	86	2.33	2.36	0.03	
Negative events					
0	808	2.52	2.45	−0.07	
1	741	2.47	2.41	−0.06	0.06
2	406	2.46	2.31	−0.15	
3+	175	2.37	2.24	−0.13	

Table III (continued)

	N	Means 1977	1979	Difference	Eta
GENERAL QUALITY OF LIFE INDEX					
Perceived change in life					
Better	1129	8.26	8.46	0.20	
Same	845	7.99	7.96	−0.03	0.18[b]
Worse	155	7.37	6.66	−0.71	
Positive events					
0	557	8.13	8.11	−0.02	
1 or 2	1113	8.12	8.15	0.03	
3 or 4	374	8.01	8.10	0.09	0.06
5+	86	7.74	8.16	0.42	
Negative events					
0	808	8.23	8.28	0.05	
1	741	8.08	8.19	0.10	0.05
2	406	8.00	7.94	−0.07	
3+	175	7.67	7.66	−0.01	

[a] $p < 0.01$.
[b] $p < 0.001$.

that the No Change group has significantly higher scores in 1979. Again the expectation of natural improvements in life quality may lead those who experience small increments to view their lives as substantially unchanged. While they recognize that they may have moved closer to some ideal life, they are not more satisfied because as much was expected.

Finally, the happiness measure presents the hypothesized pattern but the means decline for all three groups. The decline in happiness with increased age has been noted in several national studies but these drops are too large to result from a two year increase in the sample's average age. It may be that happiness levels in the population as a whole are declining while other QOL indicators remain steady or increase slightly.

Such divergent trends for the affective and cognitive indicators might account for an apparent paradox which often threatens this type of survey research. Most QOL surveys show relatively high levels of satisfaction in the face of the image of troubled, and perhaps declining, societies presented by the North American and Western European media and social critics. The general public also reflects a feeling that somehow the quality of life has declined. It may be that in cognitive terms 'we never had it so good' − higher standard of living, better health and education, etc. − but our affective morale has declined. We, as individuals, may not be as happy as we used to be. Put differently, we are better off now but enjoying it less. These speculations are based on the supposition of a trend which requires more than two surveys to confirm, but they argue for the maintenance of improved affective measures in QOL surveys.

TABLE IV

Satisfaction with job, finances, housing and health by perceived change and significant events

	N	Means 1977	1979	Difference	Eta
JOB					
Perceived change in job					
Better	377	8.40	8.59	0.19	
Same	533	8.49	8.30	−0.19	0.18[b]
Worse	70	7.77	6.59	−1.28	
Job promotion					
Did not occur	754	8.32	8.25	−0.07	
77–78	70	8.68	8.36	−0.32	0.03
78–79	156	8.66	8.41	−0.25	
FINANCIAL SITUATION					
Perceived change in income					
Large increase	390	7.37	8.03	0.66	
No major changes	1614	7.41	7.51	0.10	0.12[b]
Large decrease	145	6.81	6.48	−0.33	
Family income change					
Increase of 40% +	479	6.98	7.39	0.42	
Up to 40% increase	907	7.55	7.62	0.07	0.08[a]
Decline in income	477	7.49	7.42	−0.07	
HOUSING					
Perceived changes in housing					
Better	375	7.58	8.64	1.06	
Same	1718	8.47	8.39	−0.08	0.25[b]
Worse	60	7.97	6.17	−1.80	
Changed dwellings					
Did not occur	1667	8.54	8.41	−0.13	
77–78	172	7.27	8.20	0.93	0.17[b]
78–79	316	7.63	8.27	0.64	
HEALTH					
Perceived change in health					
Much better	84	6.62	7.99	1.37	
Somewhat better	137	7.16	7.24	0.08	
Same	1626	8.10	8.11	0.01	0.23[b]
Somewhat worse	256	7.12	6.17	−1.02	
Much worse	50	6.14	4.99	−1.15	

Table IV (continued)

	N	Means 1977	1979	Difference	Eta
Serious illness or injury					
Did not occur	1918	7.93	7.86	−0.07	
77−78	93	6.90	6.46	−0.44	0.04[a]
78−79	142	7.07	6.99	−0.08	
DOMAIN SATISFACTION INDEX					
Perceived change					
Better	1129	8.18	8.37	0.19	0.11[b]
Same	845	8.08	8.11	0.03	
Worse	155	7.32	6.99	−0.33	
Positive Events					
0	557	8.15	8.14	−0.01	0.11[b]
1 or 2	1113	8.15	8.17	0.02	
3 or 4	374	7.89	8.19	0.30	
5+	86	7.52	8.06	0.54	
Negative events					
0	808	8.22	8.34	0.12	0.07[a]
1	741	8.09	8.25	0.16	
2	406	7.98	7.89	−0.09	
3+	175	7.61	7.63	0.02	

[a] $p < 0.01$.
[b] $p < 0.001$.

Turning to difference patterns in satisfaction with job, financial situation, housing and health, Table IV presents group means.

Several characteristics are shared by results from each domain.

(1) As expected, the self-report domain change measure is always significantly related to changes in satisfaction levels.

(2) The reported No Change group has remarkably steady satisfaction means in all domains.

(3) Negative change groups usually differ from the No Change groups to a greater extent than positive change groups.

(4) Relationships between self-reported change and satisfaction levels are always higher than between events and changes in satisfaction.

Events related to the housing and financial domains were associated with satisfaction changes but promotions did not increase job satisfaction nor did serious illness produce the expected large drop in health satisfaction. Since those experiencing negative health events during the past two years had low satisfaction levels in 1977, the illness or injuries are probably recurring ones

TABLE V

Satisfaction with marriage and romantic relationships by perceived change and significant events

	N	Means 1977	1979	Difference	Eta
Perceived change in relationship					
Much better	172	8.55	9.28	0.73	
Somewhat better	134	8.29	7.97	−0.33	
Same	1503	8.94	8.69	−0.25	0.24[b]
Somewhat worse	42	7.09	5.02	−2.07	
Much worse	17	8.11	3.94	−4.17	
Got married					
Did not occur	1828	8.80	8.54	−0.26	
77–78	34	8.69	8.56	−0.13	0.07[a]
78–79	31	8.28	9.30	1.02	
Got divorced/separated					
Did not occur	1836	8.82	8.58	−0.24	
77–78	21	6.88	8.73	1.85	0.09[b]
78–79	36	8.13	7.15	−0.98	
Started romance					
Did not occur	1753	8.90	8.56	−0.34	
77–78	63	6.52	8.15	1.63	0.17[b]
78–79	77	8.09	8.72	0.63	
Ended romance					
Did not occur	1780	8.74	8.63	−0.11	
77–78	39	6.84	7.27	0.44	0.05
78–79	74	7.89	7.32	−0.57	

[a] $p < 0.01$.
[b] $p < 0.001$.

which had their major impact prior to the 1977 survey. In the work domain, promotions have a negative impact on job satisfaction although they are viewed as a positive event by most employees. Income changes have a significant but hardly overwhelming effect but the dependent measure is satisfaction with financial situation which is defined as involving income and expenditures. Improvement in income may be balanced by increased expenditures resulting in no real advancement.

Change in satisfaction with marriage and romantic relationships are presented separately in Table V because of the centrality of this domain to most individuals' quality of life and the amount of research published on the stressful nature of events involving status changes. Since each respondent was asked to indicate his or her satisfaction with whichever form of romantic relationship they had at the time, it is possible to compare individuals whose marital status has changed during the two year period.

Patterns observed in Table V are similar to those evidenced in other domains. One remarkable difference is the catastrophic effect of deteriorating relationships on satisfaction levels. Although the number of persons affected is small, the significance of these changes on quality of life is evident. However, the effects of the four events measure here, while usually significant, are not large. The events do not account for the large drops in satisfaction for those with deteriorating relationships. Most of the observed decline seems to be taking place within legally defined statuses. As suggested below changes in marital status come toward the end of a down trend most of which occurs without major events.

The pattern observed for those getting divorced or separated and those who have concluded a close romantic relationship is mot intriguing. In both cases, the immediate impact of the event is negative while the longer term effects, i.e. one to two years, are positive. To determine whether the apparent improvement after the first year resulted from the establishment of new romantic relationships, those who had formed new liaisons were excluded from the analysis. Persons who did not establish new relationships showed the same gains in satisfaction as those who did. Reseachers and others who view these events as inherently stressful and destructive have apparently overlooked the possibility that a bad marriage or relationship may be very stressful and release from it a positive step.

IV. DISCUSSION

These results provide considerable assurance that subjective measures possess the two attributes required of good social indicators — stability in unchanging situations and sensitivity to changing circumstances. While the endorsement does not apply to all subjective measures, this analysis demonstrates the validity of satisfaction measures for general quality of life and more specific domain evaluations. The self-anchoring ladder scale also appears to be a good indicator of general life quality and it would serve as well for domain assessments. Some doubts are in order for the happiness measure used here and it did not receive as much support as the other two indicators.

Opinions have been expressed in some quarters that subjective measures such as satisfaction are poor social indicators because they were so conditioned by expectations and restricted awareness as to be insensitive to changing circumstances. It is also argued that expectations and aspirations adjust very quickly to new situations and that satisfaction and other measures revert to their original levels immediately. This position would have led to predictions that (a) very few individuals would indicate any change in their situation, and/or (b) virtually no adjustment in subjective indicators would occur when changes did occur.

Our findings contradict both hypotheses in that significant numbers of respondents perceive changes in their lives and those changes were reflected, for better or worse, in their satisfaction levels. The fact that these changes took place over a two year period indicates that, while adaptation probably does occur, it is not instantaneous and will be detected by an indicator series which utilizes fairly frequent measurements. Future waves of this study should cast some light on the extent and rate of accomodation to new circumstances.

Both indexes of QOL had higher stability than the individual items suggesting their usefulness as indicators. In particular, the General QOL Index was more sensitive to personal change than its composite items. The Domain Satisfaction Index, however, adds little to the portrait obtained from the General Index and separate domain evaluations and is not crucial.

Finally, the relationships between actual changes in the QOL measures and perceived change was always higher than their association with specific events. It is often the case that low correlations between objective variables, in this case events, and subjective measures lead some users of social statistics to question the validity of the latter. This analysis suggests that it is the objective measure which may be insufficient. A case in point is the impact of promotions on job satisfaction. While advancement is usually viewed as a positive event, its effect on satisfaction is, if anything, negative. Many factors may explain this finding – more responsibility, longer hours, etc. – but the central point is that the objective event is too gross a measure to lead to a prediction of its effects. Additional information about changes in other job characteristics are required to understand personal reactions to work changes.

A second difficulty with objective measures is that the short-term consequences of objective changes may be in one direction and the long-term effects in the other. Divorce and separation appear to have neutral or negative short term impacts followed by a positive long-term consequence. Most analyses of the impact of changing conditions have not considered the possibility of time dependent effects and have assumed that the impact of change is constant, or at least in the same direction, over time.

Those who expect objective changes to produce large aggregate changes in subjective indicators also assume that the impact of events is the same for most individuals. Although not reported here, our analysis showed that the immediate impact of separation and divorce is either very negative or very positive. In aggregate, these opposite responses to the same event produced a modest, but significant, decline in sátisfaction. The assumption that most objective changes will produce the same effects ignores individual differences in values and judgement standards. It leads to the mistaken conclusion that the oft-reported lack of correlation between objective and subjective indicators results from the inadequacies of the latter.

V. CONCLUSIONS

In sum, this analysis should dispell several doubts about the utility of subjective social indicators. The measures used here, with the possible exception of the happiness scale, were shown to be stable in unchanging conditions and sensitive to change when it occurs. Given this evidence of the methodological soundness of these measures, two types of questions can now be raised. First, what is the extent and rate of adaptation to changing circumstances; and, second, what combinations of changing objective conditions lead to the judgement that one's situation is improving or deteriorating and cause changes in subjective indicators? An understanding of the dynamics of quality of life perceptions requires answers to both questions and panel studies are a more productive way of pursuing them than single corss sectional surveys.

Finally, although primarily methodological in focus, this analysis uncovered evidence of two trends which require examination. At the aggregate level, it appears that the trend in affective variables such as happiness may be down while satisfaction and other cognitive measures remain constant. If confirmed this divergence may lead to a better understanding of the way in which current quality of life experiences seem less rewarding than in 'the good old days'. At the individual level, these data suggest that low levels of perceived Quality of Life result from the cumulation of experiences which may require several years to amass. It is apparent that major life events make only a small contribution to this downward spiral and questions arise about the other depressants which gradually take their toll. A clear picture of the scenarios which result in low QOL conditions could lead to a better notion of how to intervene to preserve mental health.

Institute for Behavioural Research,
York University, Toronto

NOTE

* An earlier version of this paper was presented at the meetings of the American Psychological Association, Montreal, 1980. The research reported here was supported by the Social Sciences and Humanities Research Council of Canada (grant number S75–0332). The author would like to thank Michael Murray for his assistance in analyzing these data.

BIBLIOGRAPHY

Andrews, F. M. and Crandall, R.: 'The validity of measures of self-reported well-being', Social Indicators Research 3 (1976), pp. 1–20.

Andrews, F. M. and McKennel, A. C.: 'Measures of self-reported well-being: Their affective, cognitive and other components', Social Indicators Research 8 (1980), pp. 127–155.

Andrews, F. M. and Withey, S. B.: Social Indicators of Well-Being: American's Perceptions of Life Quality (Plenum, New York, 1976).

Bradburn, N.: The Structure of Psychological Well-Being (Aldine, Chicago, 1969).

Campbell, A., Converse, P. E., and Rodgers, W. L.: The Quality of American Life: Perceptions, Evaluations, Satisfactions (Russel Sage Foundation, New York, 1976).

Campbell, D. T. and Fiske, D. W.: 'Convergent and discriminant validities by the multitrait-multimethod matrix', Psychological Bulletin 56 (1959), pp. 81–105.

Cantril, H.: The Pattern of Human Concerns (Rutgers University Press, New Brunswick, N.J., 1965).

Joreskog, K. G. and Sorbom, B.: 'LISREL IV: Analysis of linear structural relationships by the method of maximum likelihood' (National Education Resources, Chicago, 1978).

McKennell, A. C., Atkinson, T., and Andrews, F. M.: 'Structural constancies in surveys of perceived well-being', in Szalia, A. and Andrews, F. M. (eds.), Comparative Studies on the Quality of Life (Sage Publications, London, forthcoming).

Murray, M. and Atkinson T.: 'Gender differences in correlates of job satisfaction', Canadian Journal of Behavioural Science (forthcoming).

Rodgers, W. L. and Converse, P. E.: 'Measures of the perceived overall quality of life', Social Indicators Research 2 (1976), pp. 127–152.

APPENDIX A: SUBJECTIVE QUALITY OF LIFE MEASURES

Satisfaction scale

All things considered, how satisfied or dissatisfied are you with your life as a whole? Which number comes the closest to how you feel?

```
 1   2   3   4   5   6   7   8   9  10  11
Completely            Neutral       Completely
dissatisfied                        satisfied
```

Self-anchoring ladder scale

Here is a picture of a ladder. At the top of the ladder is the best life you can imagine – the ideal life. At the bottom of the ladder is the worst life you can imagine – a life that is terrible. Using a number on this card, where on the ladder would you place your life at this time?

10	THE BEST
9	YOU CAN
8	IMAGINE
7	
6	
5	
4	
3	
2	
1	
0	THE WORST
	YOU CAN

IMAGINE

Happiness item

Generally speaking, how happy would you day you are – very happy, fairly happy, or not too happy?

Delighted-terrible scale

We want to find out how you feel about your life as a whole. Please tell me the feelings you have now – taking into account what has happened in the last year and what you expect in the near future.

I feel:

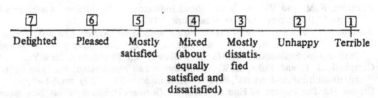

7	6	5	4	3	2	1
Delighted	Pleased	Mostly satisfied	Mixed (about equally satisfied and dissatisfied)	Mostly dissatisfied	Unhappy	Terrible

† RICHARD KAMMANN,* MARCELLE FARRY AND PETER HERB

12. THE ANALYSIS AND MEASUREMENT OF HAPPINESS AS A SENSE OF WELL-BEING

(Received 7 December, 1983)

ABSTRACT. General happiness is philosophically construed as a sense of well-being which in turn has been defined either as a complete and lasting satisfaction with life-as-a-whole or as a preponderance of positive over negative feelings. A factor analysis of thirteen well-being scales shows that these two definitions coalesce into a single general well-being factor which is distinguishable only from an independent stress/worries factor. Further evidence shows that familiar scales of neuroticism, depression and trait anxiety measure the same well-being dimension if only in the negative half-range. So does a list of somatic complaints. Various two-factor models of well-being that treat positive and negative affect as independent processes, or that distinguish between affective and cognitive components, are challenged on the grounds that they depend on the properties of Bradburn's affect scales which are found to be highly dependent on methodological parameters. Attention is drawn here to the role of test method effects and curvilinearities as factors influencing inter-scale correlations and structural models. It is concluded that well-being is a robust, primary dimension of human experience and that happiness research is alive and well in psychology.

Concepts of happiness and well-being are widely used in everyday parlance — people wish happiness to their family and friends and search for strategies to sustain it for themselves. William James remarked that it is the "secret motive" of all that people do and are willing to endure. Indeed many philosophers, from leading names among the classical schools of Greek thought to the Utilitarians and several contemporary philosophers, have considered happiness to be a central concept in the definition of the good life or the highest good, and the ultimate signpost to correct morality and social policy. (See Barrow, 1980, for a brief overview of happiness in ancient and modern philosophy.)

It is somewhat puzzling to notice that this ubiquitous quality of experience, either by the name of happiness or any recognizable synonym, has traditionally been a total "non-concept" in psychology and the social sciences. This neglect must surely be traced in large part to the rise of the behavioristic paradigm and the temporary ban on all aspects of self-reported human experience. However, it has recently re-entered the field under the concept of psychological or subjective well-being. As will be shown in this

Alex C. Michalos (ed.), Citation Classics from Social Indicators Research, 279–303.
© 2005 *Springer. Printed in the Netherlands.*

paper, aspects of unhappiness have in fact been under continuous study in clinical and personality psychology, but under other names.

POSSIBLE MEASURES OF WELL-BEING

Since our basic purpose is to look at the correlations among plausible measures of happiness and well-being, it is necessary to develop a list. Such measures could be classified at several different levels such as: area of psychology (clinical, personality, social), the theoretical paradigm of the researchers (such as disease model, factor analysis, social indicators), choice of item semantics, and choice of questionnaire technique. We shall use the first two levels jointly as our basic taxonomy, and take up items and test formats as needed to make basic distinctions.

The concept of *anxiety* and *depression* have long histories in clinical psychology, anxiety as a possible explanatory variable, and depression as a specific type of mental illness. Anxiety as concious experience was probably rescued from psychodynamic theory by need among experimental psychologists for a measure of chronic drive or activation level to use as a mediating variable in studies of human learning. Following the arrival of the Taylor *Manifest Anxiety Scale* in 1953, a number of trait and state scales of anxiety have been developed and put into use in many areas of psychological research.

Depression has a converging history, being initially a broad category of neurotic illness, but one that has failed so far to produce the required pattern of objective signs in observable behaviors or physiological indices. In recent years, the measurement of depression has shifted rapidly to self-report depression scales, including a subscale of the *MMPI*, various mood adjective checklists, the *Beck Depression Inventory* and graphic rating scales such as the visual analog technique applied to self or others. It is interesting to note that self-report scales of anxiety and depression are often as well correlated between these two constructs as they are among scales within the same construct, so that it is not even clear that these are two distinct modes of experience.

Meanwhile, a number of personality theorists have attempted to describe the basic structure of personality by the factor analysis of hundreds of personality test items. The single most reliable factor to emerge from a variety of studies using different methodologies for different purposes is a neuroticism-adjustment factor. This is the first of two basic factors in the

Eysenck Personality Iventory (EPI) (Eysenck and Eysenck, 1964), and is also a prominent second-order factor under the name Anxiety-Adjustment for the Cattell *16 PF* test of personality (Cattell *et al.*, 1970). In Coan's (1974) attempt to expand the Cattell model, adjustment again emerged as the number-one factor in the basic factor analysis, and reappeared in second place at the second-order level.

The items that measure neuroticism are concerned with a variety of negative feelings such as being easily hurt, irritable, highly strung, worrying a lot, being nervous, lacking social confidence, low self-esteem, and having bodily signs of stress such as lack of energy, trouble sleeping, aches and pain, thumping heart and trembling. It therefore seems reasonable to suppose that tests of neuroticism along with anxiety and depression scales measure subjective ill-being or recurring unhappiness, names which describe the same experience without the nuances of mental illness.

Gurin *et al* (1960) turned a corner on clinical theory when they set out to assess the overall level of mental health in the American population by means of the public survey technique. Among their items were questions about worries, fears of a nervous breakdown, satisfaction with life, a happiness rating, and optimism for future happiness. This important study paved the way towards the use of survey techniques to measure the quality of life.

In constructing the first true well-being inventory, Bradburn and Caplovitz (1965) and Bradburn (1969) thoroughly rejected the health-illness framework and all other remnants of the medical model in re-defining the focus of research as psychological well-being. According to Bradburn's model, well-being is a quality of experience (not of behaviors) that arises from the relative prevalence of good and bad feelings or positive or negative affect (PA and NA). It is a subjective experience, and unless we have reason to believe that people are lying, we can do nought else but to take their word for what they feel. The *Affect Balance Scale* asked subjects which of five positive feelings and which of five negative feelings have occurred in the past few weeks, and took the directional difference (PA score minus NA score) as the overall well-being score, which could thus range from −5 through 0 to +5.

A more debatable part of Bradburn's model is the claim of independence between the levels of positive and negative affect. This is based on the near-zero correlation between the two subscales but this finding, although well-replicated, may be limited to the particular 10 items format presented in the *Affect Balance Scale*.

Further information on the independence of positive and negative affect is made possible by the development of a well-being scale that, like Bradburn's, has separate items for positive and negative affect and uses the balance or net scoring formula to obtain the overall well-being score. This scale, called *Affectometer 1* in its 96-item format (Kammann et al., 1979) has now been condensed by further validation studies (Kammann & Flett, 1983a) to form the 40-item *Affectometer 2* for which a detailed user's manual is available (Kammann and Flett, 1983b).

The affectometers differ from the *Affect Balance Scale* first by using a completely new set of items that have been culled by empirical validation from an original pool of 435 potential items, and secondly in replacing the yes/no response format with a five-step graded scale for how often each feeling has been present over the past few weeks: not at all/occasionally/some of the time/often/all the time.

Although the affectometer items were selected on the basis of their correlations with a 6-step or 7-step happiness rating scale, other investigators have usually used a more widely known 3-step rating scale consisting the choices *very happy*, *pretty happy*, or *not too happy* as a check on the validity of their scales and inventories. Three-step happiness is also important because it has also been widely used in opinion surveys for over two decades, and has been used to assess trends in the quality of American life over time (e.g., Campbell et al., 1976; Smith, 1979).

Dupuy (1978) considered that an overall index of psychological well-being should reflect six basic qualities: freedom from health worry, high energy level, satisfyign-interesting life, cheerful mood, relaxed living, and a sense of control over own emotions and behavior. This framework led to the construction of an 18-item *General Well-Being (GWB) schedule*, some of the properties if which have been explored by Fazio (1977). Unfortunately, the *GWB* inventory was not available for our first study comparing well-being measures, but we were able to include it in Study 3.

This brings us to the measures developed by *social-indicators* researchers to assess the quality of life. Campbell et al (1976) obtained two fairly distinct factors from a factor analysis of several possible well-being items, the first factor leading to their *Index of Affect*, and the second to their *Index of Stress*. The *Index of Affect* is a set of eight scales for rating life-as-a-whole. These are 7-step scales represented by such adjective pairs is: 'boring-interesting', 'enjoyable-miserable', 'friendly-lonely', and others — these together constitute a single dimension of affect that should, in principle, agree well with the *Affect Balance Scale*, or an affectometer.

The *Index of Stress* has items focussing on general and financial worries, on feeling rushed, tied down and frightened, and fearing a nervous break-down. While it may seem odd that this does not correlate well with a measure of affect, Andrews and Withey (1976) also found that an item concerned with worries was not well correlated wirh measures of global well-being.

Another type of measure that is expected in the social indicators model to predict well-being is the *Sum of Satisfactions* score obtained by adding up a subject's satisfaction ratings across a well-chosen set of life domains or concern-areas, such as: family, friends, health, income, education, housing, neighborhood, work, recreation, and so on. An index of this type correlated rather better with the *Index of Affect* (0.57) than did the *Index of Stress* (0.40) (Campbell (et al., 1976)

More than any other group, Andrews and Withey (1976) have system-atically explored the measurement of concern-area satisfactions and also the statistical behavior of 68 possible questions about a person's global sense of well-being. Among the latter group of measures, the most prefered by several criteria were the assessment of life-as-a-whole on a 7-step *Delighted-Terrible* rating scale, or on graphic scaled called *Ladder, Circles,* or *Faces* (a sequency of line-drawing faces stepping down from a big smile to a big frown).

It is important to note that for Andrews and Withey, a global sense of well-being is defined by the judgment a person makes about his or her *life* as *a whole* – this may or may not agree with measures of *affect balance*. Indeed, their factor analysis placed the life-as-a-whole scales on a first factor, while Bradburn's positive and negative affect subscales each required a separate factor of its own (Andrews and Withey, p. 89). Again, it must be asked if this factor structure is a true property of good and bad feelings, or is a property of Bradburn's selection of items and the yes/no response format.

Two other measures of interest must be added to the list. As part of their pioneering study on mood and personality, Wessman and Ricks (1966) developed a 10-step *Elation-Depression* rating scale that has received consider-able use as measure of mood quality and some use as a happiness rating scale. This cale moves in labelled steps from 'Complete elation – rapturous joy and soaring ecstasy' to 'Utter depression and gloom – completely down – all is black and leaden.'

Fordyce has been interested in measuring happiness and preparing programs to help people attain that state. He has used both a simplified version of the elation-depression rating scale and a three-part question that asks people what percent of the time they have been happy, have been unhappy, and have been neutral (Fordyce, 1977). For purposes of the present study on well-being measures, we have converted this into a happiness balance scale by subtracting the reported percent of time unhappy from the reported percent happy; this is called *Net Time Happy*.

METHODOLOGICAL ASPECTS

In their comparison of alternative scales for use as social indicators, Andrews and Withney (1976) have called attention to a test's "method effect". This shows up as a portion of the reliable variance that arises from the format or structure of a test, rather than its content. Generalizing from their results, items which are presented in the same test format will usually gain an increment of intercorrelation for that reason, while items appearing in different formats will lack this source of covariance, or may even be negatively correlated regarding the methods factor. Thus items coming from the same test will usually have inflated intercorrelations while items coming from different tests will have deflated correlations by comparison.

It is not always clear which aspects of a test's format or structure contributes to a test method effect, but there are some obvious distinctions to be made among different measures of well-being. The first split is between multiple-item inventories and single-item ratings scales which tend to be of the 7-step variety, often in the semantic differential format, although the 3-step happiness scale also belongs here. These single-item rating scales are important historically as the simple and obvious measures to use in the first instance, and have been further developed for social indicators monitoring, even though the longer inventories are demonstrably more reliable.

Among the multi-item inventories, some use bipolar items with the full range of affect running from a highly positive feeling through neutral to a highly negative and ostensibly opposite feeling. Other scales have unipolar items that go only from neutral or no feeling to a high level of either a good or bad feeling, considered by itself. Where a scale, such as a measure of anxiety, depression or neuroticism has only items for negative affect, we may consider it a half-range well-being scale, or a measure of ill-being. The *Affect Balance Scale* and the affectometers are a departure from this tradition by including an equal number of items of positive affect which are taken into account in arriving at an overall score. Inventories using bipolar ratings scales, such as the *Index of Affect* use the full range for each item.

An aspect of the instructions for every well-being measure is the time frame the subject keeps in mind while answering. Most commonly this has been 'these days' or 'over the past few weeks' which may be roughly equivalent. These differ, however, from the unspecified time-frame or asking people what they 'usually do' that has been traditionally used with scales of neuroticism, depression and trait anxiety. There is evidence from Kammann *et al.* (1979) that people are sensitive to the time frame presented in the instructions. This might also account for Eysenck and Eysenck's (1964) observation of one-year retest stability coefficients of 0.81 and 0.84 for neuroticism which are very much higher than other well-being stability coefficients obtained under the instructions "these days" or "the past few weeks" which are in the vicinity of 0.50 to 0.55 (Kammann and Flett, 1983a).

Instructions combine with response options to define what the respondent is being asked to report. For example, Bradburn's items ask the subject to state *whether or not* (yes/no) the stated feeling has ever occurred during the past few weeks, while the affectometers ask the subject *how often* a feeling has been present on a graded scale: not at all/occasionally/some of the time/ often/all the time. Although this is sometimes referred to as a judgment of 'frequency' a more apt name would be 'prevalence' since feelings to not usually occur in brief repetitive bursts but commonly develop and persist over some time, and are thus available to the person even if not being consciously attended to all the time.

A common alternative to scaling the prevalence of feelings is to scale their intensity or some total quantity in answer to *how strongly* a feeling has existed, or simply *how* the person has been feeling, which is the question used commonly with the bipolar rating scales. In the latter case it is not really clear how the respondent weighs up the intensity of a feeling and its prevalence when deciding which step to choose on a 7-step rating scale between two opposite states such as rewarding-disappointing.

It is now possible to consider the psychometric properties of well-being scales. Where reported, most scales appear to have good reliabilities. *Affectometer 1*, *Affectometer 2*, the *GWB* schedule and the *Index of Affect* have produced alpha coefficients of 0.96, 0.95, 0.93 and 0.89, respectively. Eysenck and Eysenck (1964) report an alternate form reliability of 0.81 for

EPI Neuroticism. No consistency measure has been reported for Bradburn's *Affect Balance Scale*. Although item consistency cannot be calculated for single rating scales, Andrews and Withey (1976, p. 77) have established an average test-retest correlation of 0.66 for the Delighted-Terrible scale given twice in the same interview. This gives a best estimate of the 'immediate reliability' for that and other comparable rating scales that use at least seven steps. Since Andrews and Withey often use the average of both scores in the interview, the estimated reliability rises to 0.80 by the Spearman-Brown formula.

Response artifacts have not presented a significant problem in well-being scales. Simple response acquiescence is removed from the *Affect Balance Scale* and from *Affectometer 1* by the use of an equal number of positive and negative items. The role of acquiescence in bipolar rating scales is not known, but should logically not be very great. Social desirability on a short version of the Crowne-Marlowe (1964) *Social Desirability Scale* produced an inconsequential correlation with the Index of Affect (Campbell *et al.*, 1976, pp. 107–111) while the *EPI Lie* scale has correlated at 0.30 with *Affectometer 1* (Kammann *et al.*, 1979). Similarly, "mood right now" was not found to be an appreciable artifact in *Affectometer 1* scores (Kammann *et al.*, 1979).

While these findings are reassuring, the role of artifacts in self-reports deserves continuing scrutiny. Toward this end, the Wessman and Ricks *Elation-Depression* scale was used to measure "mood right now" at the beginning and end (Pre-Mood, Post-Mood) of the questionnaire used in the following study. Social desirability was also measured by the EPI Lie Scale, and by the Crowne-Marlowe *Social Desirability Scale*. However, before the study began it was noted that seven of the Crowne-Marlowe items were hardly distinguishable from valid well-being items and were therefore deleted in advance.

Although the scales reviewed above are all plausible measures of well-being, the intercorrelations among most of these measures are unknown. In addition to the two correlations already noted among the Campbell *et al.* inventories, the four Andrews and Withey sclaes (Delighted-Terrible, Ladder, Circles, Faces all applied to life-as-a-whole) have produced intercorrelations in the range 0.40 to 0.60 and correlate with Bradburn's *Affect Balance Scale* in the range 0.40 to 0.50 (Andrews and Withey, 1976, Chapter 3). A few correlations have also been reported between well-being and scales of anxiety or depression, but these will be reviewed in Study 3 where they become more relevant.

Thus there are pockets of modest intercorrelation among the whole array of measures, but many more correlations are untested than are known. In terms of factor analyses, Campbell *et al.* separated two factors for affect and stress (Campbell *et al.*, 1976) while Andrews and Withey (1976, p. 89) found a general well-being factor for their verbal rating scales as a group, plus two extra factors required for each of Bradburn's positive affect and negative affect (PA, NA) subscales. Andrews and McKennell (1980) elaborated on that factor structure to propose a *cognitive* component and an *affective* component (consisting itself of two independent components for positive and negative affect) as a more general two-factor model of well-being. The robustness of such models can be assessed by the factor analysis of a new and broader set of well-being measures.

STUDY 1: WELL-BEING SCALES

The purpose of the first study was to examine the intercorrelations and factor structure of 13 well-being scales, and the degree of bias that might be associated with mood-right-now and social desirability.

A list of 13 well-being scales is given in Table I with the number of items on each scale, the number of rating steps per item, wether the items are bi-

TABLE I

Thirteen well-being scales

Scale	N items	Item steps	Bi/Uni-polar	Reli-ability	Source
7-Step happiness	1	7	B		(e.g. Kammann, 1979)
3-Step happiness	1	3	B		Gurin, *et al.* (1960)
Elation-depression	1	10	B		Wessman and Ricks (1966)
Delighted-terrible	1	7	B	0.65	Andrews and Withey (1976)
Circles	1	9	B		Andrews and Withey (1976)
Faces	1	7	B		Andrews and Withey (1976)
Net time happy	2	100	U		Fordyce (1977)
EPI neuroticism	24	Y/N	U	0.81	Eysenck and Eysenck (1964)
Affect balance	10	Y/N	U	0.76	Bradburn (1969)
Index of affect	8	7	B	0.89	Campbell *et al.* (1976)
Index of stress	6	var.	U		Campbell *et al.* (1976)
Sum of satisfactions	34	7	B		Andrews and Withey (1976)
Affectometer 1	96	5	U	0.96	Kammann (1979)

polar or unipolar, reliability (or very short term stability) where known, and a source reference.

Two of the inventories will also appear in Study 2 because they provide separate scores for positive affect (PA) and negative affect (NA) items. These are Bradburn's *Affect Balance Scale* and *Affectometer*. Although these scales use unipolar items, response acquiescence is removed from the overall score when the subscales are combined by the formula, PA – NA.

Method

Scales. The *Elation-Depression* mood scale was adapted for this study by changing the instructions to elicit a rating of general happiness. For the *Sum of Satisfactions* measure, 34 satisfaction items were carefully selected from Andrews and Withey (1976) and presented with the usual 7-step Delighted-Terrible rating scale. The items referred to specific life areas such as husband/wife, friends, income, health, education, yourself, neighborhood, and the taxes you pay (Kammann, 1983). Otherwise, the *Delighted-Terrible, Circles* and *Faces* scales referred to life-as-a-whole these days. *Net time Happy* was defined as the "percent of time happy" minus the "percent of time unhappy".

Several scales were also used to measure response biases. The subject's mood-right-now was taken on the Elation-Depression scale both at the start of filling the packet of questionnaires and again at the end. Social desirability was measured on the *EPI Lie* scale and on the Crowne-and-Marlowe (1964) *Social Desirability Scale*. The latter scale, however, was reduced from 33 to 26 items by deletion of seven items that were indistinguishable from valid well-being items. These were items 3, 5, 10, 16, 21, 23 and 31. They were removed prior to the data analysis.

Subjects. The subjects were 44 males and 74 females ($N = 118$) representing a 39.4% voluntary participation rate from a nationwide telephone-book sample of adult New Zealanders to whom a questionnaire package was mailed in March, 1980.

Results

Sample Bias. Aside from the obvious sex bias which is standard in well-being surveys even with high participation rates (e.g., Andrews and Withey, 1976, p. 431), the sample represents a fair cross-section of the population. The median age was 36.8 years old with 5th and 95th percentile ranks at 18.5 and 68.4 years respectively. Median family income in 1979 was $11 800 (N.Z.) with 5th and 95th percentile ranks of $4500 and $41 000 respectively. The median education level was two years of high school (4th Form in New Zealand) with 5th and 95th percentiles equivalent to eighth grade and a university Bachelor's degree, respectively. These points agree reasonably well with 1980 census data for New Zealand. Exact agreement is not needed because these demographics have only trivial relevance to levels of well-being (Campbell et al., 1976; Kammann, 1983; Kammann and Campbell, 1983).

More germane are the sample's distributions on well-being measures. If we observe a substantial difference between the present mean (or SD) and that of a normative sample from another country, it could either mean that our sample is biased through self-selection or that New Zealanders in 1980 differ from other people at other times. It might also mean both. If, however, the present distribution agrees with overseas data, then it is more likely that neither sampling bias nor cultural difference is operating than it is likely that both are operating but are equal and opposite in magnitude and thus cancel each other out.

The present response distributions actually agree well with those of previous U.S. and U.K. random samples on the *Delight-Terrible, Circles*, and *Faces* scales for life-as-a-whole, and on the *Index of Affect, EPI Neuroticism* and the *Sum of 34 Satisfactions*. The means of the N.Z. distributions averaged 0.12 SDs (using US/UK SDs) below the overseas means, and the SDs averaged 12% smaller. The individual distributions for the 34 satisfaction items also agreed well with American norms, and produced an r of 0.94 between the N.Z. and the U.S. item means (Kammann, 1983b). Therefore, there seems to be no relevant bias in the present sample.

Factor analyses. The first factor analysis covered the 13 primary scales, the 4 PA and NA subscales, and the 2 mood scales. An orthogonal varimax rotation produced the most sensible interpretation and is shown in Table II.

There is no doubt that Factor I (53% of the variance) is a general well-being factor, being loaded with both PA and NA affectometer scales as well as bipolar scales. Factor II (7%) is a 'Bradburn factor' and is best distin-

TABLE II

Factor analysis and selected scale intercorrelations (with affectometer 1, index of affect, delighted-terrible and EPI neuroticism)

	Factors[a]				Correlations (*rs*)			
	I	II	III	IV	Afr	IA	D–T	EPI
7-Step hap	60	36	54	10	74	63	67	−58
3-Step hap	34	38	57	−08	54	57	62	−33
Ela-dep	45	05	65	18	52	43	56	−33
Del-ter (D–T)	52	42	52	10	66	70		−48
Circles	62	37	38	27	75	71	74	−63
Faces	22	27	33	69	53	49	47	−41
Net time hap	42	60	33	49	68	66	70	−50
EPI neur (EPI)	−80	−06	03	36	−70	−49	−48	
Bradburn ABS	48	81	07	01	63	61	56	−48
Ind affect (IA)	61	47	34	−03	74		70	−49
Ind stress	−07	24	04	−76	00	16	−02	22
Sum sats	69	−07	−31	−11	69	57	54	−53
Afctmtr (Afr)	83	24	36	15		74	66	−70
Afctmtr NA	−84	−19	−25	−18	−68	−58	−46	50
Afctmtr PA	73	22	45	10	66	37	42	−44
Bradburn NA	−70	−53	09	−06	−63	−55	−54	62
Bradburn PA	03	83	25	−05	36	41	33	−11
Pre-mood	02	08	82	07	27	19	24	−08
Post-mood	21	16	60	19	49	42	42	−35

Note: Decimals are omitted.

guished by Bradburn PA which fails to load appreciably on the first factor. Factor III (7%) is dominated by pre-mood, but also picks up modest loadings from the other single-item verbal (but not graphic) scales. This appears to reflect a small test-method or format effect shared among these scales. Factor IV (6%) reflects a compromise between *Index of Stress* and *Faces* which otherwise seem to have little in common ($r = -0.24$).

In the second factor analysis (not shown) the PA and NA subscales were omitted with the consequence that Factor II (the "Bradburn factor") disappeared, while the other three factors remained as before. Scale loadings on the general well-being factor generally increased, with some re-ordering as follows: *Affectometer* (0.88), *Circles* (0.77), *Index of Affect* (0.77), *EPI Neuroticism* (−0.76), *Affect Balance Scale* (0.73), *7-Step Happiness* (0.71), *Delighted-Terrible* (0.63). Since these become the scales of practical interest, they will be used to assess the effects of response artifacts.

Intercorrelations. Four of the seven best scales were chosen as benchmark variables to illustrate the size of the intercorrelations. These are shown in the right-hand section of Table II. In general, these rs confirm the pattern of factor loadings.

Artifacts. Against the seven best scales selected above, the median r with pre-mood was 0.26, and the median r with post-mood was 0.42; the difference between these two values having a $p < 0.10$. In subsequent studies not reported here we have not replicated this pre-post shift in the r level. We have found, however, that mood well-being correlations are nearly as high when mood is taken a week before or after as when it is taken simultaneously with well-being.

The median well-being rs for the *Lie* scale and *Social Desirability Scale* were 0.07 and 0.30, respectively. Although the latter value is significant at the 0.01 level, it is not large enough to make a practical difference. For example, when SDS is partialled out of the 0.74 r between *Affectometer 1* and *Index of Affect*, the resulting partial r is 0.71.

Discussion

Several well-being scales clearly measure a common dimension of experience traditionally measured only in its negative half-range by *EPI Neuroticism*. It is disappointing to note, in Table II, the modest validity of 3-step happiness which has been so widely used in opinion surveys.

The simple correlations among the longer inventories are consistently less than their scale reliabilities would permit. (This will be seen again in Study 3 for the correlation between the *GWB Schedule and Affectometer 1*.)

Although it is possible that each inventory taps a different facet of well-being it seems more probable that each inventory carries a significant test method effect. Andrews and Withey have demonstrated these effects are present among single item-rating scales, and our factor analysis also suggests a difference between single-item and multi-item scales. Since an inspection of the longer inventories reveals no obvious systematic differences in the semantic contents of their items, it seems likely that differences in task instructions or item formats may be significant in this group as well.

The present results for the Bradburn subscales do not completely agree with a previous factor analysis by Andrews and Withey (1976, p. 89) in which

PA and NA each required an extra factor of its own. In the present data, only PA really requires a separate factor. It is likely that PA and NA both emerged as unique for Andrews and Withey becauce their other measures were all single-item rating scales. Against the more varied scales and inventories in the present study, NA overlaps with the general well-being factor. The two studies agree, however, on the independence of Bradburn PA.

On the other hand, affectometer PA and NA both load highly on the first general well-being factor. Consequently, arguments or models based on the distinctive properties of Bradburn's PA and NA scales must be reconsidered. Consider again Andrews and McKennell's (1980) proposal that well-being may be divided into two separate components cognition and affect. The cognitive factor is a quasi-rational assessment of one's life situation, while the affective factor is more like a set of gut-level feelings. This model is certainly plausible, but the data offered in its support begin with the assumption that Bradburn's PA and NA subscales are more or less pure measures of affect, and that whatever they do not measure is the other, cognitive factor. However, the affectometer is just as plausibly a measure of pure affect and yet its subscales do not behave at all like Bradburn's. The next study will demonstrate this point more vividly.

STUDY 2: POSITIVE AND NEGATIVE AFFECT

On the basis of data arising from the *Affect Balance Scale*, Bradburn (1969) advanced the interesting thesis that positive and negative affect are two separate and independent modes of response. The evidence consists not only of the near-zero correlation between Bradburn NA and Bradburn PA, but also the finding that PA is better predicted by social participation and novel activity, while NA is better predicted by anxiety, worries, and somatic complaints. Further support comes from Costa and McCrae (1980) who observed that Bradburn NA tended to be uniquely associated with *EPI neuroticism*, while PA was distinctively associated with *EPI extraversion*. (The latter *r* was only 0.20 but with a large *N* it was highly 'significant'.)

On the other hand, it may be objected that Bradburn's 5 PA and 5 NA items are not necessarily good representatives of their corresponding affective domains. For one thing, some of Bradburn's items depend on the occurence of an event such as being complimented, accomplishing something, or being criticized. Furthermore, Bradburn's scale is unique in asking subjects if they 'have ever' (yes/no) over the past few weeks experienced the feeling described by each item. Recent studies of mood states have found that previously unipolar and independent feelings have formed into bipolar contrasts when the yes/no format was replaced by scales of graded response, and response acquiescence has been used as a correction factor (Lorr and Shea, 1979; Russell, 1979).

Brenner (1975) and Warr *et al.* (1983) have demonstrated that 4-step prevalence scaling, for example, ranging from 'rarely or never' to 'very often', tends to produce substantial negative correlations between positive and negative affect, although their items were not identical to the Bradburn items. Andrew and Withey (1976, p. 87, fn. 18) on the other hand, replicated Bradburn's essentially zero correlation when using a two stage procedure in which subjects first made a yes/no decision on each Bradburn item and then scaled all yes response into three prevalence levels. Whether this should be classified as a yes/no or prevalence scaling method is not clear and the issue remains open.

The argument that PA and NA correlate with different predictors of well-being also deserves close scrutiny. In Bradburn's (1969) data the association of NA with anxiety and physical syptoms could reflect a common test method effect based on negative items in a yes/no format. Similarly, the correlation between PA and social participation or novelty seems to depend primarily on positive items in a yes/no format.

In the same way, Costa and McCrae's observation of a correlation between NA and *EPI neuroticism*, or PA and *EPI Extraversion* could reflect negative items in a yes/no format (all of the neuroticism scale) and positive items in the yes/no format (the majority of the extraversion scale). In general, it must also be noted that most of the correlational distinctions made between PA and NA are based on rather low *r* values (or *gammas* or *O*s) that could be influenced by incidental features of methodology.

An alternative test fo the PA-NA hypothesis is made possible by *Affectometer 1* or *Affectometer 2*. *Affectometer 1* consists of 48 PA and 48 NA selected from a larger pool of 435 items on the basis of their correlations with *7-Step Happiness* (Kammann et al., 1979). For each item the subject chooses one of five graded response choices ranging from not-at-all to all-the-time for how often that feeling had been present over the past few weeks. *Affectometer 2* is a shortened version consisting of 20 PA and 20 NA items (Kammann and Flett, 1983a, b).

TABLE III

Correlations between positive and negative affect: Bradburn's
ABS versus affectometer 1, 2

Sample	N	r
Bradburn's PA by NA		
Bradburn (1969)	2735	0.08
Andrews and Withey (1976)	1072	0.01
Study 1 here	118	−0.25
Mean [a]	(3925)	0.05
Affectometer 1 PA by NA		
Irwin	78	−0.71
Dixon	193	−0.45
Blackman	55	−0.68
Farry	57	−0.69
Study 1 here	118	−0.70
Mean [a]	(501)	−0.66
Affectometer 2 PA by NA		
Flett-Power	112	−0.66

[a] *N*-weighted *Z*-transformed mean *r*.

Data on the PA-NA correlation are available not only from Study 1 above, but from five other samples of Dunedin adults. Of these, the Irwin sample was recruited by an acquaintance network, while the Dixon, Farry, and Blackman studies all used random samples, as did Flett and Power in their joint studies with *Affectometer 2*.

Table III shows the PA-NA correlations for these six samples as compared with three representative findings on Bradburn's *Affect Balance Scale*. It is clear that PA and NA as measured by the affectometers are highly negatively correlated with a mean *r* of −0.66. It is also worth noting that the lowest *r* of −0.45 in the Dixon study occurred in an early version of the affectometer that used only a three-step response scale (rarely or not at all, some of the time, often or much of the time) instead of the usual five-step affectometer response scale. Bradburn's is, of course, a two-step scale.

In Table IV, data from the Study 1 sample show that affectometer NA and PA are correlated with *neuroticism*, and are not correlated with *extraversion*, in contrast to the Costa and McCrae results, but in agreement with Warr *et al.* (1983). The affectometer results, then, are consistent with the bipolarity of pleasant and unpleasant affect observed by Russell (1979) and Lorr and Shea (1979) when graded response scales are used in mood studies.

TABLE IV

Correlations (rs) of PA and NA subscales with EPI extraversion and neuroticism

Scale	Neuroticism	Extraversion
(Data from Costa and McCrae, N = 559)		
Bradburn PA	−0.13 [a]	0.20
Bradburn NA	0.39	−0.03
Bradburn ABS	−0.34 [b]	0.16 [c]
(Data from Study 1, N = 118)		
Affectometer PA	−0.44 [a]	0.02
Affectometer NA	0.50	0.17
Affectometer 1	−0.70 [b]	−0.11 [c]

[a] Difference between −0.13 and −0.44 has $p < 0.001$.
[b] Difference between −0.34 and −0.70 has $p < 0.001$.
[c] Difference between 0.16 and −0.11 has $p < 0.05$.

Note: The rs shown for Costa and McCrae are the simple means of 4 rs from 4 repeated testings.

It is still true that a correlation of −0.66 is far less than could be achieved for PA and NA scales with known alpha reliabilities in the 0.90s. Some of the reliable variance on each subscale remains unpredicted by the other. This could be residual evidence in favor of Bradburn's two-factor model, but it is not necessarily so. On a full-range dimension of well-being from very happy to very unhappy, PA scales should most accurately discriminate in the upper half of the spectrum, while NA should sort out the lower half, giving the two subscales offset ranges of convenience. The PA subscale has too high a 'floor' while the NA subscale has too low a 'ceiling'.

STUDY 3. CLINICAL ASPECTS

The proposed overlaps between well-being and anxiety, depression and psychosomatic stress signs have yet to be tested. (The overlap with neuroticism was confirmed in Study 1.)

Insofar as these clinical aspects of well-being are measured on half-range scales with only negative items, their observed relationship with a full-range well-being scale should be underestimated by Pearson rs. A person with little or no depression may have any several degrees of positive well-being. Since most people place themselves somewhere in the positive region, above the midpoint, of a well-being scale, it is not surprising that scores on scales of depression and anxiety are often severely bunched up near the zero end of the scale. For these reasons Kammann and Flett (1983a) predicted and confirmed a curvilinear relationship between *Affectometer 2* and the *Beck Depression Inventory*. Although the *r* itself was −0.69, the *eta* was −0.84. As expected, the NA subscale by itself could predict depression as accurately as the total score, and more accurately than the PA subscale.

Nevertheless, even the known *r* values place depression and anxiety (along with neuroticism) squarely in the centre of well-being measurement. Previous studies at the University of Otago established *r*s close to −0.70 between the affectometer and *EPI Neuroticism* (Kammann *et al.*, 1979) and the *Beck Depression Inventory* (Lichter *et al.*, 1980).

Fazio (1977) correlated the *GWB Schedule* with six standardized scales of depression to observe *r*s ranging from −0.53 to −0.80 with a median *r* of −0.70. A similar analysis with three commonly used anxiety scales yielded *r*s of −0.52, −0.63 and −0.76. As expected, the depression and anxiety scales also correlated substantially with each other, yielding a median *r* of 0.64. To complete the argument it is only necessary to show that the *GWB Schedule* is itself a measure of well-being. This is the first goal of the present study.

The second goal is an exploration of a list of somatic complaints that have been interpreted by one psychologist or another as signs of stress or anxiety. An early study in New Zealand by Brian Dixon used the *Cornell Medical Index* to discover the link between health and well-being on a mixed sample of healthy and hospitalized adults. On the whole there was little evidence of a direct link between a medically defined disease or disability and score on the affectometer, a finding which was subsequently supported by Campbell *et al.* (1976) and Krupinski and MacKenzie (1979). It did seem, however, that health subscales correlated with the affectometer to the degree that they were stocked with items often associated with anxiety and stress. This suggested the need for a general exploration of somatic complaints.

Method

The first author surveyed a variety of sources listing psychosomatic symptoms, and generated a list of 41 somatic complaints supplemented by four complaints specific to men, and five complaints specific to women. The resulting items were then structured into a "Health Questionnaire" grouped in areas of bodily function such as lungs, heart and blood, skin and so on. The four response choices were never/rarely/sometimes/often scored as an interval scale.

The Health Questionnaire was then offered, along with *Affectometer 1* and *GWB Schedule* to a geographically random sample of one hundred Dunedin adults of whom 57 agreed to participate.

Results

The two well-being scales were intercorrelated with an *r* of 0.74. The total somatic complaint score correlated at −0.62 with the *Affectometer* and at −0.68 with the *GWBS*. Table V presents the individual item correlations with well-being (average of two *r*s) for the 27 items that reached the 0.05 level or beyond.

Discussion

The high correlation between the *GWB Schedule* and the affectometer, comparable to the highest *r*s in Study 1, confirms that the *GWB Schedule* is at least an acceptable measure of well-being and probably belongs in the list of preferred scales. The theoretical result is that Fazio's correlational data on the *GWB Schedule* may now be included toward the conclusion that depression and trait anxiety scales are measures of well-being in the negative half-range, that is, are measures of ill-being. Fazio's data take on even more significance in light of the possible curvilinearity not accounted for in his reported *r* values.

This clinical picture is further enriched by the correlations between the two well-being scales and many of the stress-related somatic complaints. Indeed, the total score on somatic complaints almost seems to provide a substitute for a well-being score, but our sample size is not large enough to specify the true *r* accurately. But it is true that items of this type are included in *EPI neuroticism*.

It is not implied here that all occurrences of somatic complaints in the list are purely 'psychological'. Some of the problems reported may have had an organic or 'medical' basis. Nevertheless, the absence of a correlation between medical conditions and well-being noted above suggests this is probably not the primary explanation. Brenner (1979) has also found suggestive evidence that depressed affect is more likely to lead to somatic disturbance at a later

TABLE V

Somatic complaints: mean correlations with affectometer 1 and GWBS

Complaint (abbr.)	Mean r	Complaint (abbr.)	Mean r
Wake up tired	-0.53	(F) Sex without pleasure	-0.43
Feel tired	-0.51	(M) Trouble keeping erection	-0.39
Spells of fatigue	-0.45	Painful urination	-0.38
Trouble staying asleep	-0.46	(M) Sex painful to penis	-0.28
Trouble getting to sleep	-0.38		
		Spells of dizziness	-0.41
Nausea	-0.48	Feel weak and faint	-0.27
Indigestion	-0.38		
Diarrhoea (the runs)	-0.35	General aches and pains	-0.39
No appetite	-0.29	Ordinary headaches	-0.33
		Neck pains	-0.28
Chest cramps	-0.43	Migraine headaches	-0.27
Breathing very fast	-0.39		
Trouble breathing	-0.38	Hands clammy and sweaty	-0.39
Attacks of hay fever	-0.28	Severe itching	-0.33
Tight chest	-0.27	Numbness of skin	-0.30

Note: N = 57 (females = 37; males = 20).

date than the reverse is true, while Vaillant's (1979) evidence indicates that psychological disturbance in middle-aged men contributes over time to physical health deterioration. Undoubtedly, there are circular loops in the mind-body system so that any assumption of one-way causation is bound to be inadequate. What especially needs to be doubted is the glib explanation that illness or disability directly leads to unhappiness.

This study has brought together a number of previous and present findings concerning "clinical" processes to show that these may now be subsumed under the more comprehensive concept of psychological well-being. In light of the available data, neuroticism, depression and trait anxiety may be seen as alternative technical names for a common condition of psychological ill-being or general unhappiness. This does not mean that no sub-types of ill-being or well-being can ever be discovered. It means that these different names do not now demonstrate different psychological phenoma. It also means that scales designed to measure neuroticism, depression and trait anxiety are measuring half a dimension when scales for the whole dimension are now available. Figure I is offered to help make this point.

GENERAL DISCUSSION

The concept of happiness that is so interesting and real in the lives of people is now taking its rightful place in scientific psychology. Although the word 'happy' may be used with many meanings in common language, its most important meaning philosophically is a complete and lasting sense of satisfaction with life as a whole (Tatarkiewicz, 1962/1976). Psychologically, however, we must expand or enrich the sense of satisfaction into the experience of really enjoying life, as having a high preponderance of positive feelings and few if any negative ones. In fact, our data suggest that global life satisfaction and the balance of affect come very close to an identity of meaning and that both of these interpret the phrase 'sense of well-being'. At the same time, we recognize that well-being is a degree word and that people may experience any number of gradations between the extremes of well-being, between complete happiness and total misery.

Our investigations show that there are many plausible scales available but that some of these are better than others in measuring the general well-being factor. The most important finding, however, is that this dimension of well-being overlaps strongly with the well-known dimension of neuroticism that

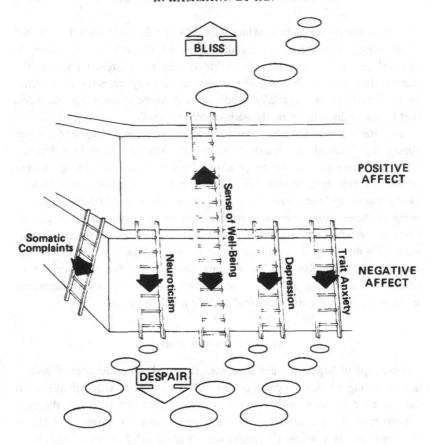

Fig. 1. Four short ladders for climbing down and one long ladder for climbing up. This proves for all time that scales for neuroticism, depression and trait anxiety are only half-asked well-being questionnaires.

regularly arises as a primary factor in the factor analysis of personality items. To this it may be added that scales of depression and trait anxiety also seem to be measuring the negative region of an overall well-being spectrum.

On the other hand, there are many loose ends that need to be clarified in further research, and these efforts must pay attention to certain methodological considerations. For example, studies relating positive affect to negative affect (by that name or any other such as depression and anxiety), must take into account the offset ranges of convenience of these two types of measures, and the impact of opposite skewness in their distributions which may create curvilinearities that are not detected by linear regression techniques. Also, much more attention needs to be given to the role of test method effects in inflating the correlations between two variables that are surveyed in a common test format, or deflating correlations when they are in disparate formats.

The hypothesis that positive and negative affect are two independent processes is now shown to be less than a universal structure for well-being. As an empirical result this orthogonality may depend very closely on the particular ten items and test format used in Bradburn's method; on the other hand, the general incompatibility of PA and NA reported here *could* be a peculiarity of the affectometer technique.

An obvious reconciliation would be to say that people can have very different feelings arising from separate episodes of life events, but since opposite feelings cannot usually occur at the same time, a general prevalence of one class of feelings precludes an equal prevalence of the opposite class. Unfortunately, the data are equivocal about this hypothesis. But as appealing as it may be as counter-intuitive model, there seems little excuse for continuing the claim that positive and negative affect are *in general* two independent processes. In fact, there is good reason to suspect that it is a methodological oddity. Furthermore, the alleged association between positive affect and extraversion, trivial to begin with, fades rapidly toward zero under the affectometer method, while positive affect sensibly emerges with a substantial negative correlation (-0.44) with (not extraversion but) neuroticism. Researchers who wish to defend the model of independence of positive and negative affect should now demonstrate that independence can be demonstrated by methods other than Bradburn's original procedure.**

NOTE

** Study 1 was supported by the New Zealand University Grants Committee (grant 77–166) and by the Department of Preventive and Social Medicine, University of Otago. Studies 2 and 3 were supported by Otago Research Committee Grant 37–671. Appreciation is due to Robyn Irwin, Graeme Dixon, Katharine Blackman, Ross Flett and Ann Power for use of their data in Study 2. Thanks are also due to Frank Andrews, Peter Bradshaw, Philip Brickman, Angus Campbell and Harold Dupuy for their encouragement, and in some cases their critical comments. Reprint requests to Richard Kammann, Department of Psychology, University of Otago, Dunedin, New Zealand.

BIBLIOGRAPHY

Andrews, F. M. and A. McKennel: 1980, 'Measures of self-reported well-being', Social Indicators Research 8, pp. 257–298.
Andrews, F. and S. R. Withey: 1976, Social indicators of well-being (Plenum Press, New York).
Barrow, R.: 1980, Happiness, 2nd ed. (Martin Robertson, Oxford).
Bradburn, N. M.: 1969, The structure of psychological well-being (Aldine, Chicago).
Bradburn, N. M. and D. Caplovitz: 1965, Reports of happiness: A Pilot Study of Behavior Related to Mental Health (Aldine, Chicago).
Brenner, B.: 1975, 'Quality of affect and self-evaluated happiness', Social Indicators Research 2, pp. 315–331.
Brenner, B.: 1979, 'Depressed affect as a cause of associated somatic problems', Psychological Medicine 9, pp. 737–746.
Campbell. A., P. E. Converse and W. L. Rogers: 1976, The Quality of American life (Russel Sage Foundation, New York).
Coan, R. W.: 1974, The Optical Personality (Columbia University Press, New York).
Costa, P. T. and R. R. McCrae: 1980, 'Influence of extraversion and neuroticism on subjective wellbeing: happy and unhappy people', Journal of Personality and Social Psychology 38, pp. 668–678.
Crowne, D. and D. Marlow: 1964, The Approval Motive (Wiley, New York).
Dupuy, H. J.: 1978, Self-representations of general psychological well-being of American adults (National Center for Health Statistics, Hyattsville, MD.).
Eysenck, H. J. and S. B. G. Eysenck: 1964, Manual of the Eysenck Personality Inventory (University of London Press, London).
Fazio, A. F.: 1977, 'A concurrent validational study of the *NCHS general well-being schedule*', DHEW Publication No. (HRA) 78–1347 (National Center for Health Statistics, Hyattsville, MD.).
Fordyce, M. W.: 1977, 'Development of a program to increase personal happiness', Journal of Counselling Psychology 24, pp. 511–521.
Gurin, G., J. Veroff and S. Feld: 1960, Americans View Their Mental Health (Basic Books, New York).
Kammann, R.: 1979, *Sourcebook for Affectometer 1* (Why not? Press, Dunedin, New Zealand).
Kammann, R.: 1983, 'Objective circumstances, life satisfactions and sense of well-being: consistencies across time and place', New Zealand Journal of Psychology 12, pp. 14–22.
Kammann, R. and K. Campbell: 1983, Illusory correlation in popular beliefs about the causes of happiness', New Zealand Psychologist 11, pp. 52–63.
Kammann, R., D. Christie, R. Irwin and G. Dixon: 1979, 'Properties of an inventory to measure happiness (and psychological health)', New Zealand Psychologist 8, pp. 1–2.
Kammann, R. and R. Flett: 1983a, 'Affectometer 2: a scale to measure current level of happiness', Australian Journal of Psychology 35, pp. 259–265.
Kammann, R. and R. Flett: 1983b, Sourcebook for measuring Well-Being with Affectometer 2 (Why not? Press, Dunedin, New Zealand).
Krupinski, J. and A. Mackenzie: 1979, The Health and Social Survey of the North West Region of Melbourne (Special publication No. 17), (Institute of Mental Health Research and Postgraduate Training, Health Commission of Victoria, Australia).
Lichter, S., K. Haye and R. Kammann: 1980 'Increasing happiness through cognitive retraining', New Zealand Psychologist, 9, pp. 57–64.
Lorr, M. and T. M. Shea: 1979, 'Are mood states bipolar?', Journal of Personality Assessment 43, pp. 468–472.

Nunnally, J. C.: 1978, Psychometric Theory (2nd ed.) McGraw-Hill, New York).
Russell, J. A.: 1979, 'Affective space is bipolar', Journal of Personality and Social Psychology 37, pp. 345–356.
Smith, T. W.: 1979, 'Happiness: Time trends, seasonal variations, intersurvey differences and other mysteries', Social Psychology Quarter 42, pp. 18–30.
Tatarkiewicz, W.: 1976, Analysis of Happiness (Martinus Nijhoff, The Hague) (originally published 1962).
Vaillant, G. E.: 1979, 'Natural history of male psychologic health: effects of mental health', The New England Journal of Medicine 301, pp. 1249–1254.
Warr, P., J. Barter and G. Brownbridge: 1983, 'On the independence of positive and negative affect', Journal of Personality and Social Psychology 44, pp. 644–651.
Wessman, A. E. and D. F. Ricks: 1966, Mood and personality, (Holt, Rinehart and Winston, New York).

* *University of Otago,*
Box 56,
Dunedin,
New Zealand

ALEX C. MICHALOS

13. MULTIPLE DISCREPANCIES THEORY (MDT)

(Received 13 February, 1985)

ABSTRACT. A fairly thorough account of multiple discrepancies theory (MDT) is presented, with a review of its historical antecedents and an examination of its strength in accounting for the happiness (H) and satisfaction (S) of nearly 700 university undergraduates. Basically, MDT asserts that H and S are functions of perceived gaps between what one has and wants, relevant others have, the best one has had in the past, expected to have 3 years ago, expects to have after 5 years, deserves and needs. MDT explained 49% of the variance in H, 53% in global S and 50% or more in 7 out of 12 domain S scores. The domains studied were health, finances, family, job, friendships, housing, area, recreation, religion, self-esteem, transportation and education.

INTRODUCTION

The aim of this paper is to present a fairly thorough and rigorous account of multiple discrepancies theory (MDT), review its historical antecedents and submit it to some empirical tests. The basic hypotheses of the theory are given in the next section, which is followed by a section reviewing the supporting evidence for its several hypotheses taken individually or in groups. The hypotheses are illustrated graphically and algebraically in the next section. Following the illustrative section, there is a section describing the sample of 700 University of Guelph undergraduates on whom the theory was tested, and the methods used. Then there is a section reviewing general results and comparing these to some results of earlier studies, followed by a review of results for MDT and a discussion.

BASIC HYPOTHESES

The basic hypotheses of MDT are as follows:

H1: Reported net satisfaction is a function of perceived discrepancies between what one has and wants, relevant others have, the best one has had in the past, expected to have 3 years ago, expects to have after 5 years, deserves and needs.

H2: ᴵAll perceived discrepancies, except that between what one has

305

and wants, are functions of objectively measurable discrepancies, which also have direct effects on satisfaction and actions.

H3:   The perceived discrepancy between what one has and wants is a mediating variable between all other perceived discrepancies and reported net satisfaction.

H4:   The pursuit and maintenance of net satisfaction motivates human action in direct proportion to the perceived expected levels of net satisfaction.

H5:   All discrepancies, satisfaction and actions are directly and indirectly affected by age, sex, education, ethnicity, income, self-esteem and social support.

H6:   Objectively measurable discrepancies are functions of human action and conditioners.

SUPPORTING EVIDENCE

Since I have already written an extensive review of the literature related to MDT in Michalos (1985), I will not undertake that task again here. However, it will be worthwhile to briefly indicate the variety of insights from several well-known theories that are incorporated into MDT.

Although nobody has bound together as many hypotheses or articulated a theory of multiple discrepancies as systematically as I have here, a number of people have worked with two or more discrepancy hypotheses in conjunction. As I have mentioned in all my earlier publications, I originally followed Campbell, Converse and Rodgers (1976) and Andrews and Withey (1976) fairly directly. Crosby (1982) used several gap hypotheses in conjunction, and cited seven other people who had also used multiple discrepancies, namely, Davis (1959), Runciman (1966), Gurr (1970), Williams (1975), Berkowitz (1968), Adams (1965) and Patchen (1961). Goodman (1974) and Oldham, *et al.* (1982) should also be listed as labourers in the same vineyard.

H1 refers to seven different perceived discrepancies. The idea that net satisfaction is a function of the perceived discrepancy or gap between what one has and wants is at least as old as the stoic philosophy of Zeno of Citium around 300 B.C. In the form of aspiration theory, Lewin *et al.* (1944) gave the idea a new start. More recent confirmations of the basic hypothesis have been reported by Bledsoe, Mullen and Hobbes (1980); Canter and Rees (1982); Cherrington and England (1980); Campbell, Converse and Rodgers

(1976); Andrews and Withey (1976); Michalos (1980a, 1982a, 1983a); and Crosby (1976, 1982).

The idea that net satisfaction is a function of the perceived discrepancy between what one has and relevant others have can also be found before the birth of Jesus Christ, namely, in Aristotle's *Politics* in the fourth century B.C. In the form of reference group theory, Merton and Kitt (1950) gave the hypothesis a provocative new start. Recent confirmations have come from Oldham and Miller (1979); Appelgryn and Plug (1981); Hatfield and Huseman (1982); Duncan (1975); Campbell, Converse and Rodgers (1976); Andrews and Withey (1976); Crosby (1976, 1982); Oldham, *et al.* (1982); Goodman (1974); and Michalos (1980a, 1982a, 1983a). Wills (1981, 1983) considers this sort of theory (by its other popular name, "social comparison theory") from the point of view of its usefulness in explaining people's behaviour and attitudes regarding help-seeking decisions, self-evaluation and self-enhancement.

Confirmations of the hypothesis that net satisfaction is a function of the perceived gap between what one has now and the best one has ever had in the past have been reported by Campbell, Converse and Rodgers (1976) and Michalos (1980a, 1982a, 1983a). Suls and Sanders (1982) present evidence supporting a developmental model in which evaluations based on this sort of perceived discrepancy occur in children around the ages of 4 to 5, while "social comparisons with similar others" occur a bit later around the age of 9.

Equity theorists have found considerable support for the hypothesis that net satisfaction is a function of the perceived gap between what one has and what one deserves. For examples, see Hatfield, Greenberger, Traupman and Lambert (1982); Walster, Berscheid and Walster (1976); Adams and Freedman (1976); and Goodman and Friedman (1971). In ordinary English one may distinguish an equitable distribution in which each person gets whatever is due to him or her from an equal distribution in which each person gets the same as every other person. (See Michalos (1982b) for more on this). However, equity theorists usually ignore this distinction and define equitable relationships as those in which "all participants are receiving equal relative outcomes" (Walster, Berscheid and Walster, 1976, pp. 2, 7). Cook (1975, p. 376) took a third and more relativistic view, asserting that "a state of equity is said to exist if the actual allocation of outcomes coincides with *p*'s beliefs about how they should be distributed... ."

The hypothesis that net satisfaction is a function of the perceived discrep-

ancy between what one has and expected to have was given a fairly systematic treatment by Festinger (1957). As indicated by several authors in Abelson
et al. (1968), Festinger's theory of cognitive dissonance mixed several kinds
of discrepancies together, although there was a tendency to emphasize the
gap between expected and actual states of affairs. Support for this hypothesis
has been reported by Campbell, Converse and Rodgers (1976); Weintraub
(1980); Oliver (1980); Ross, Mirowski and Duff (1982); and many others
cited in Abelson *et al.* (1968).

Person-environment fit theorists have hypothesized that, among other
things, net satisfaction is a function of the perceived fit between what a
person has (resources, abilities) and what a person needs. Considerable
support for this hypothesis has been reported in excellent review articles
by Harrison (1978, 1983) and Caplan (1979, 1983). Kurella (1979) and
Booth, McNally and Berry (1979) have also reported support for a similar
sort of hypothesis.

The seventh gap hypothesis incorporated into H1 involves the perceived
discrepancy between what one has now and expects to have in the future
(after five years). One would expect that optimism about the future would
bring satisfaction, and there is some experimental evidence supporting this
idea, e.g., Goodman (1966).

H1 refers to reported satisfaction because the survey research procedures
used to test MDT rely on personal reports. Although I usually omit the word
"reported", strictly speaking it is essential. Usually, I think, things are regarded
and reported as satisfying if and only if on balance they are satisfying. So,
typically, "satisfaction" has the force of "net satisfaction", and "dissatisfaction" has the force of "net dissatisfaction", Scales running from "very satisfied" to "very dissatisfied" presuppose that respondents are reporting net
assessments.

H2 affirms ontological realist or objectivist assumptions, namely, that
there is a world relatively independent of this or that person, containing
things with more or less objectively measurable properties, which are more or
less objectively comparable. (Festinger (1957) and Crosby (1982) emphasize
a similar point.) For example, according to H2, the perceived discrepancy
between what one earns and some relevant other person earns is to some
extent a function of a real or objectively measurable discrepancy; the perceived discrepancies between needs for nourishment or warmth and their
attainment are to some extent functions of real or objectively measurable

discrepancies; and so on. While I strongly suspect and there is some evidence that the mixture of objectively measurable and perceived discrepancies is a bit like a horse and rabbit stew, with perceived discrepancies represented by the horse, I will have little more to say on the matter here. The only exception to this realist assumption is in the case of perceived gaps between what one has and wants. In Michalos (1978) I gave a dispositional analysis of wanting which might allow one to distinguish objectively measurable from perceived wants. After performing many thought experiments on this view, I am still not persuaded that one could operationalize the two kinds of wanting in distinct ways. Moreover, I suspect that one could always regard dispositional wants as particularistic or adventitious needs as defined in Michalos (1978). If the latter is true, then it would be redundant to introduce objectively measurable wants as a partial determinant of perceived wants. These considerations led me to treat perceived wants as an exception in H2. H2 also affirms that objectively measurable discrepancies have a direct impact on net satisfaction and human action, as will become clearer shortly.

H3 is relatively straightforward, saying that the perceived gap between what one has and wants serves as a mediator between all other perceived gaps and net satisfaction. This hypothesis was confirmed by Campbell, Converse and Rodgers (1976) and Michalos (1980a, 1982a, 1983a). H1 and H3 taken together imply that perceived discrepancies have both direct and indirect (mediated) effects on reported net satisfaction. In Michalos 1980a, 1982a, 1983a, I compared two models, one with and one without a mediating variable, and I recommended the former. I was unable to see the obvious, namely, that a combination of the two models would provide a more accurate account of the dynamics of satisfaction than either model could provide separately. Here I have tried to articulate this insight.

H4 connects net satisfaction to human action in a fairly traditional utilitarian way. (For examples, see Kauder (1965), Luce and Raiffa (1957) Festinger (1957), Edwards and Tversky (1967), Kuhn (1974), and Harsanyi (1982).) The main difference between what is going on here and what has traditionally gone on in utilitarian discussions is that here we do not begin with utility, happiness, satisfaction or even preferences. From the crude utilitarianism of Shaftesbury (1711) to the most recent sophisticated utilitarianism of Harsanyi (1982), this view always begins with some sort of a given affect-laden attitude or interest, e.g., preferences. It is precisely this foundation, this given element in all utilitarian theories, that MDT is designed to break through and explain.

By the time H4 arrives on the scene, the most important innovative and explanatory work of MDT is virtually complete. At this point, one might go the way of a variety of utilitarians or naturalistic value theorists.

According to H5, discrepancies are directly and indirectly affected by certain demographic elements and/or conditioners. Although such elements have not been found to be relatively powerful predictors of satisfaction, they do have some impact. On average, perhaps as much as 10% of the variance in reported net satisfaction can be explained by demographic varia-bles. Generally speaking, the best and most recent literature reviews regarding the impact of demographic elements on satisfaction and happiness are in Diener (1984) and Veenhoven (1984). Examples of studies showing that age, sex, education, ethnicity and income have an impact on satisfaction and/or happiness include Campbell, Converse and Rodgers (1976); and Andrews and Withey (1976). A variety of researchers have found one or more of these variables related to satisfaction with life as a whole or to satisfaction with some domain of life. For example, Weaver (1980) found job satisfaction and age positively associated; Rhyne (1981) and Glenn (1981) found that sex had a differential affect on marital satisfaction. Barnett and Nietzel (1979) reported that personal self-esteem had an impact on marital satisfaction, and Diener (1984, p. 558) cited eleven studies indicating that "high self-esteem is one of the strongest predictors of [subjective well-being]". The importance of a variety of species of social support, measured in a variety of ways, is thor-oughly documented in excellent articles by Caplan (1979); Turner, Frankel and Levin (1983); Abbey and Andrews (1985); and Gottlieb (1984). La Rocco, House and French (1980) review several studies and provide a careful analysis of data on the moderating effects of social support on job strain (dissatisfaction). Their conclusion is that social support has greater direct than indirect effects.

The point of H6 is primarily to indicate that human action, including especially one's own, has a direct effect on the objectively measurable dis-crepancies of one's life, as do the previously mentioned demographic and/or conditioning elements. It is assumed, of course, that there is some time lag and directionality involved, and that events and actions are not their own causes or motives.

The basic hypotheses of MDT refer to functions without specifying them as linear or nonlinear. Equity theorists (e.g., Walster, Berscheid and Walster, 1976) and person-environment fit theorists (e.g., Harrison, 1978, 1983) have tended to predict and find U-shaped relationships between reported net satisfaction and their independent variables. There is evidence that people who get more or less than they think they deserve are dissatisfied, with those who get more being less dissatisfied than those who get less. There is also some evidence that people in a work environment that is too complex or too simple for their particular needs or wants are relatively less satisfied than people whose work environment fits their needs or wants fairly closely. At this point, we don't know if U-shaped relationships obtain between perceived discrepancies between what one has and deserves, and has and needs on the one hand, and what one has and wants on the other. It strikes me as likely that human agents alter their wants (wittingly or not) so as to maintain a minimum level of net satisfaction, which is essentially what aspiration theorists have always said. So, rather than expecting a nonlinear relationship between the perceived gap between what one has and wants and the other gaps, I would expect internal adjustments to be made that would tend to keep the relationship linear.

HYPOTHESES ILLUSTRATED

Exhibit 1 illustrates the relationships postulated in the basic hypotheses. In this Exhibit, capital letters stand for items in boxes (e.g., A stands for objectively measurable discrepancies) and numbers following letters stand for paths connecting items in boxes (e.g., A1 stands for the path connecting objectively measurable discrepancies to perceived discrepancies). Thus, our basic hypotheses H1-H6 yield the following derived hypotheses expressed in terms of Exhibit 1.

DH1.   Objectively measurable discrepancies (A) are a function of an agent's own action along the path E1 and conditioners along the path F1. Briefly, this may be expressed
$A = f(E1, F1)$ (From H6)

DH2.   Perceived discrepancies (B) are a function of objectively measurable discrepancies along the path A1 and the conditioners along the path F2. Briefly, this is
$B = f(A1, F2)$ (From H2, 5)

DH3.   The perceived discrepancy between what one has and wants (C) is a function of all other perceived discrepancies along the path

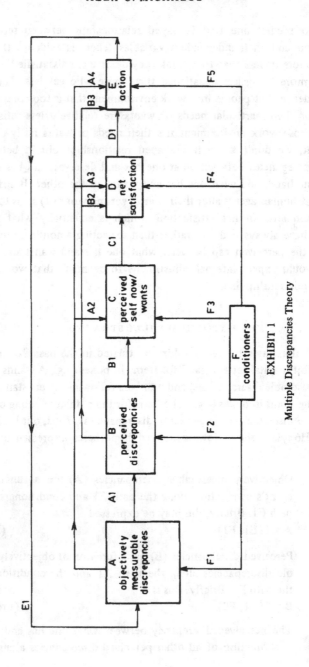

EXHIBIT 1
Multiple Discrepancies Theory

B1, objectively measurable discrepancies along the path A2, and the conditioners along the path F3. Briefly,

C = f (B1, A2, F3)   (From H1, 3, 5)

DH4.   Reported net satisfaction (D) is a function of the perceived discrepancy between what one has and wants along the path C1, objectively measurable discrepancies along the path A3, all other perceived discrepancies directly along the path B2, and the conditioners along the path F4. Briefly,

D = f (C1, A3, B2, F4)   (From H1, 3, 5)

DH5.   An agent's action (E) is a function of reported net satisfaction along the path D1, objectively measurable discrepancies along the path A4, all other perceived discrepancies directly along the path B3, and the conditioners along the path F5. Briefly,

E = f (D1, A4, B3, F5)   (From H2, 4, 5)

The general idea expressed in H4 is that people tend to try to maximize net satisfaction. DH5 provides a bit more information about the sources of resources and restrictions that help and hinder people from achieving their aims. Exactly which aspect of an agent's situation will become the focus of attention depends on the perceived relative expected net satisfaction attached to action directed to that aspect. For example, if one perceives greater expected net satisfaction connected to action designed to alter objectively measurable conditions of one's life rather than to action designed to alter one's own desires, one would tend to perform the former rather than the latter. Thus, if it is likely to be more satisfying to earn more money relative to one's peers than to try to want fewer material goods, one would tend to pursue a course of action designed to earn more money. If the prospects for closing the income gap between relevant others and oneself are practically hopeless, one would tend to focus on a more profitable course of action, such as trying to limit one's own desires. (Compare Corollaries IV.1 and 1.2 in Walster, Berscheid and Walster (1976), and Festinger (1957, pp. 6, 31 and 182).)

DH5 provides a number of potential avenues of intervention for those interested in altering people's net satisfaction. By noticing the relative impact (statistically, the beta value) of each relevant variable on net satisfaction, one can identify the place to intervene to get the biggest bang for one's buck.

For example, if it turns out that, say, perceived social comparisons have relatively less impact on net satisfaction than perceived inequities, then one might be wise to focus one's interventions on altering the latter rather than the former.

Exhibit 2 illustrates in greater detail the central core of relationships expressed in Exhibit 1, ignoring all references to objectively measurable discrepancies. In Exhibit 2, each perceived discrepancy in box B has an abbreviation, namely Ba for "the perceived discrepancy between what one has now and relevant others have", Bb for "the perceived discrepancy between what one has now and the best one has had in the past", and so on to Bf. Similarly, each conditioner in box F has an abbreviation, namely, Fa for "age", Fb for "sex", and so on to Fg. The path labeled B1 in Exhibit 1 is unpacked into its six constituents B1a–B1f in Exhibit 2. To keep the Exhibit relatively simple, the seven items in box F are not unpacked. Strictly speaking, as will be shown below, every path labeled with an F should be unpacked into seven constituents labeled, for example, F4a, F4b and so on. Thus, the derived hypotheses DH3 and DH4 yield the following expanded derived hypotheses expressed in terms of Exhibit 2.

EDH3. $C = f(B1a \ldots B1f, F3a \ldots F3g)$

EDH3 says that the perceived discrepancy between what one has and wants is a function of 6 other perceived discrepancies and 7 conditioners. Exactly how many and which of the elements of EDH3 will survive empirical testing is at present unknown. Much of what is known about these elements was briefly reviewed above and in Michalos 1980a, 1982a, 1983a, 1985.

From DH4, one may derive the following expanded derived hypothesis in terms of Exhibit 2.

EDH4. $D = f(C1, B2a \ldots B2f, F3a \ldots F3g, F4a \ldots F4g)$

EDH4 says that reported net satisfaction is a function directly of 7 perceived discrepancies, indirectly of 6 of these mediated by the discrepancy between what one has and wants, and directly and indirectly of age, sex, education, ethnicity, income, self-esteem and social support. Exhibit 2 and EDH4 are alternative representations of the perceptual core of MDT that will be our primary focus of attention in following sections.

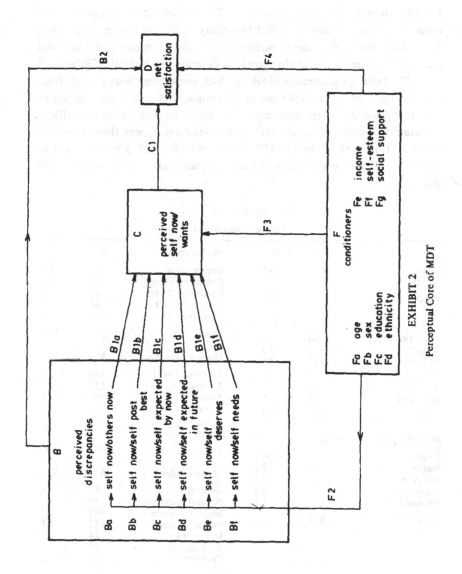

EXHIBIT 2

Perceptual Core of MDT

SAMPLE AND METHODS

In order to test the current version of MDT articulated in the previous sections, a convenience sample of 700 University of Guelph undergraduates was drawn from the 3130 students enrolled in the 1984 summer term (May and June). The composition of the sample is described in Exhibit 3. Briefly, of the 683 usable questionnaires obtained, 54% came from females, 70% from students aged 20 to 25, 84% from single people, 76% had 3 years or less of university, and 51% were majoring in biological or social sciences. Official registration statistics indicated that in the total enrollment there were 57% females, 71% aged 20 to 25, 85% single, and 78% had 3 years or less of university. So the sample was in fact fairly representative of the student body that term.

EXHIBIT 3
Sample composition

Sex	N	%	Work status	N	%
Males	314	46	Unemployed	471	69
Females	368	54	Employed 10 hrs.	68	10
Total	682	100	Employed 20 hrs.	55	8
			Employed 30 hrs.	34	5
Age	N	%	Employed 40 hrs.	54	8
17 to 19	60	9	Total	682	100
20 to 22	345	50			
23 to 25	135	20	Formal education	N	%
26 to 30	75	11	1 year or less	150	22
31 to 35	34	5	2 years	177	26
36 and up	33	5	3 years	191	28
Total	682	100	4 years	89	13
			5 years	14	2
Marital Status	N	%	Diploma/degree	61	9
Single	571	84.0	Total	682	100
Married	83	12.0			
Widowed	1	0.1	Major studies	N	%
Separated	15	2.0	General	57	8
Divorced	12	1.9	Natural sciences	30	4
Total	682	100.0	Biological sciences	161	24
			Social Sciences	182	27
			Humanities	24	3
			Engineering	21	3
			Commerce	35	5
			Other	172	26
			Total	682	100

The questionnaire was an extended version of those described in Michalos 1980a, 1982a, and 1983a. It had a demographic page with 7 questions yielding the information in Exhibit 3, an instruction page, a page defining the terms designating the 12 domains (Appendix B), and 8 pages containing items involving the assessment of domain and global satisfaction from 8 different perspectives. A 7-point Likert-type scale was provided on each of these pages to obtain data relevant to the 7 discrepancies mentioned in H1 of MDT and to the basic satisfaction ratings. An off-scale category was available in every case to allow people to opt out by checking 'No opinion'.

Basic satisfaction ratings were taken on my revised delightful–terrible scale. For example, the global item asked "How do you feel about your life as a whole right now?" and the response categories ran from "terrible" (= 1 point), through "mixed dissatisfying and satisfying" (= 4) to "delightful" (= 7).

Assessments of the discrepancies between what one has and wants were obtained in the next battery of questions. For example, the global item asked "Consider your life as a whole. How does it measure up to your general aspirations or what you want?" and the response categories ran from "not at all" (= 1), through "half as well as what you want" (= 4) to "matches or is better than what you want" (= 7).

Assessments of the discrepancies between what one has and relevant others have were obtained next. The global item asked "Consider your life as a whole. How does it measure up to the average for most people your own age in this area?" and the response categories ran from "far below average" (= 1), through "average" (= 4) to "far above average" (= 7).

Assessments of the discrepancies between what one has and deserves were next. The global item asked "Consider your life as a whole. How does it measure up to the life you think you deserve?" and the responses ran from "far below what is deserved" (= 1), through "matches exactly what is deserved" (= 4) to "far above what is deserved" (= 7).

Assessments of the discrepancies between what one has and needs were next. The global item asked "Consider your life as a whole. How does it measure up to what you think you need?" and the responses ran from "far below what is needed" (= 1), through "matches exactly what is needed" (= 4) to "far above what is needed" (= 7).

Assessments of the discrepancies between what one has and expected to have 3 years ago at this point in life were next. The basic question was briefly

"Compared to what you expected to have, does your life offer extremely less (= 1), about what you expected (= 4) or extremely more (= 7)?"

Assessments of the discrepancies between what one has and expects to have 5 years in the future were next. Unfortunately, the question was worded ambiguously.[1] Preceding the list of 12 domains, it was asked "... consider how you would rate your own life, as it is at present, in comparison to what you expect it will be five years from now. Do you expect it [later] to offer extremely less, much more, etc.?" The reference point of this question is life 5 years from now. However, the global item asked "Now, using the same scale, consider your life as a whole. How does it [now] measure up to what you expect five years from now?" The reference point of this question is life as it is now. If respondents noticed the difference, then their responses to the global item should have been roughly opposite to their domain item responses. In fact, the mean of the mean responses to the 12 domain items was 4.5 and the mean response to the global item was 4.4 (Exhibit 4), indicating that respondents apparently asnwered the thirteenth item on the page from the same point of view that they answered the other 12. Thus, although these 13 questions were consistently answered from the same reference point, this distant point differed from the current reference point used in all the other discrepancy items.

Assessments of the discrepancies between what one has and the best one has ever had in the past were next. The global item asked "Consider your life as a whole. How does it measure up to the best in your previous experience?" and the responses ran from "far below the previous best" (= 1), through "matches the previous best" (= 4) to "far above the previous best" (= 7).

Assessments of happiness with life as a whole were based on the question "Considering your life as a whole, would you describe it as very unhappy (= 1), unhappy (= 2 or 3), mixed (= 4), happy (= 5 or 6), or very happy (= 7)?"

The conditioners measured directly included age, sex and education. Self-esteem was measured indirectly using the domain satisfaction score, and social support was also measured indirectly using the mean of the satisfaction scores for family relations and friendships. I assumed that perceived self-esteem and perceived satisfaction with self-esteem would be highly correlated, and that if one had relatively satisfying relations with friends and family, then one had relatively good social support. Both of these assumptions are being tested with field studies now in progress, although they already have some support in the literature; e.g., see Turner, Frankel and Levin (1983) and Wills (1983). Instead of collecting data on incomes, which I suspected would be similar for most students or misleading as a result of scholarships, grants or bursaries, average length of weekly employment time was measured. In Canada, if not everywhere else, it is not likely that full-time students take on part-time paid employment unless they have financial problems. So the time invested in such employment might be a reasonable indirect measure of economic status. Ethnicity was not measured in this survey.

GENERAL RESULTS

Exhibit 4 summarizes the results from the 8 batteries of substantive questions. The third row from the bottom gives the means of the domain mean scores for the 8 sets of scores. The ratings on the delightful-terrible scale had the highest mean, 4.9. Life as a whole had a mean score of 5 on this scale,

EXHIBIT 4
Mean scores

	A Self now	B Self wants	C Self others	D Self de- served	E Self needs	F Self pro- gress	G Self future	H Self best	Mean B–H
Health	5.3	5.3	4.7	4.1	3.8	3.9	4.3	3.5	4.2
Financial security	4.2	3.8	4.1	3.7	3.2	3.7	4.6	3.4	3.8
Family rela- tions	5.2	5.3	4.9	4.2	3.9	4.2	4.3	4.1	4.4
Paid employ- ment	3.7	2.9	3.3	3.1	2.7	3.2	4.7	2.8	3.2
Friendships	5.2	5.2	4.7	4.1	3.8	4.2	4.4	4.0	4.3
Housing	5.1	4.7	4.5	4.0	3.9	4.1	4.5	3.7	4.2
Area lived in	5.1	4.9	4.6	4.1	4.0	4.1	4.5	3.7	4.3
Recreation	4.9	4.8	4.4	3.8	3.6	3.9	4.4	3.6	4.1
Religion	4.8	4.9	4.5	4.1	3.7	4.1	4.3	3.8	4.2
Self-esteem	5.1	5.1	4.7	3.9	3.7	4.2	4.6	4.2	4.3
Transporta- tion	4.7	4.5	4.2	3.8	3.6	3.9	4.5	3.6	4.0
Education	5.1	5.1	5.0	4.1	3.8	4.5	4.8	4.8	4.6
Mean	4.9	4.7	4.7	3.9	3.6	4.0	4.5	3.8	4.2/ 4.1
Whole life	5.0	4.9	4.8	4.0	3.7	4.2	4.4	4.1	4.3
Happiness	5.0								

which was exactly the same as the score for happiness with life as a whole. The Pearson correlation of these two global items was $r = 0.67$ ($P \leqslant 0.001$). The gap between what one has and needs was generally perceived as the greatest of the 7. It had a mean of 3.6 for the 12 domains and 3.7 for life as a whole. The discrepancies between what one has and wants, and what one has and relevant others have yielded the same means, 4.7. These were the highest means for the 7. On average, there was a difference of 0.15 between the mean of the mean domain scores and its corresponding global mean.

For the 12 domains, satisfaction with health had the highest mean, 5.3, and satisfaction with paid employment had the lowest mean, 3.7. For university undergraduates, these are quite reasonable results. Considering the means of mean domain discrepancy scores (in the extreme righthand column), it is

EXHIBIT 5

Multiple regression of global scores on domain scores

	Self wants	Self others	Self deserved	Self needs	Self progress	Self future	Self best
Percent of variance explained[a]	53	53	58	58	50	55	54
	$N=315$	$N=326$	$N=294$	$N=315$	$N=327$	$N=380$	$N=329$
Predictors	*Beta*	*Beta*	*Beta*	*Beta*	*Beta*	*Beta*	*Beta*
Health	0.105[d]	0.130[b]	e	e	0.099[d]	e	0.150[a]
Financial security	0.212[a]	0.186[a]	0.170[a]	0.233[a]	0.196[a]	0.173[b]	0.097[d]
Family relations	e	e	0.128[b]	e	e	0.111[c]	0.083[d]
Paid employment	e	e	0.100[d]	e	e	e	e
Friendships	0.189[a]	0.144[a]	0.112[c]	0.156[a]	0.176[a]	e	0.189[a]
Housing	0.195[a]	0.143[a]	e	e	e	e	e
Area lived in	e	e	0.205[a]	0.208[a]	0.094[d]	e	0.154[a]
Recreation	0.108[d]	e	0.142[a]	0.130[b]	0.138[b]	0.123[c]	e
Religion	e	0.082[d]	0.093[d]	e	e	0.095[d]	e
Self-Esteem	0.191[a]	0.266[a]	0.209[a]	0.243[a]	0.193[a]	0.167[a]	0.323[a]
Transportation	e	0.123[b]	e	e	e	0.126[d]	0.085[d]
Education	0.208[a]	0.260[a]	0.159[a]	0.249[a]	0.261[a]	0.186[a]	0.241[a]

[a] $P < 0.001$
[b] $P < 0.005$
[c] $P < 0.01$
[d] $P < 0.05$
[e] Significance level too low to enter equation.

clear that on average respondents' current university education tended to provide the smallest discrepancies. The mean of means for the 7 scales was 4.6. Again, on average it was paid employment that yielded the greatest discrepancy, 3.2.

Exhibits 5, 6, and 7 show the relative impact of domain scores on global scores for the 7 sorts of discrepancies. Exhibit 5 shows that for 3 types of discrepancies (self-others, self-deserved and self-best), the domain of self-esteem has the greatest impact on its corresponding global discrepancy score, and for 3 others (self-needs, self-progress and self-future) the domain of education has the greatest impact. For the self-wants discrepancy, the domain of financial security has the greatest impact on the global score. Only 3 of 12 domains have a significant impact on all of the 7 global discrepancy

EXHIBIT 6

Multiple regression of global scores on domain scores: Males

	Self wants	Self others	Self deserved	Self needs	Self progress	Self future	Self best
Percent of variance explained[a]	52	54	59	53	58	48	57
	$N=140$	$N=146$	$N=133$	$N=140$	$N=146$	$N=165$	$N=145$
Predictors	*Beta*	*Beta*	*Beta*	*Beta*	*Beta*	*Beta*	*Beta*
Health	0.211[b]	0.122[d]	0.131[d]	e	0.164[c]	e	0.228[a]
Financial security	0.210[b]	0.246[a]	0.289[a]	0.243[a]	0.239[a]	e	0.188[a]
Family relations	e	e	e	e	e	e	e
Paid employment	e	e	e	e	e	e	e
Friendships	0.188[c]	0.132[d]	0.142[d]	0.175[c]	0.211[a]	e	e
Housing	0.218[a]	0.183[c]	e	e	e	0.261[a]	e
Area lived in	e	e	0.262[a]	0.242[a]	e	e	0.150[c]
Recreation	e	e	0.131[d]	e	e	e	e
Religion	e	e	e	e	e	0.128[d]	e
Self-Esteem	0.158[d]	0.246[a]	0.239[a]	0.255[a]	0.258[a]	0.273[a]	0.468[a]
Transportation	e	e	e	e	e	e	e
Education	0.228[a]	0.296[a]	e	0.268[a]	0.306[a]	0.216[b]	0.265[a]

[a] $P < 0.001$
[b] $P < 0.005$
[c] $P < 0.01$
[d] $P < 0.05$
[e] Significance level too low to enter equation.

EXHIBIT 7

Multiple regression of global scores on domain scores: Females

	Self wants	Self others	Self deserved	Self needs	Self progress	Self future	Self best
Percent of variance explained[a]	55 $N=170$	49 $N=175$	56 $N=152$	62 $N=170$	47 $N=176$	60 $N=176$	54 $N=179$
Predictors	*Beta* e	*Beta* e	*Beta* e	*Beta*	*Beta* e	*Beta* e	*Beta* e
Health	e	e	e	0.119[d]	e	e	e
Financial security	0.221[a]	0.205[a]	e	0.146[b]	0.154[c]	0.192[c]	e
Family relations	e	e	0.206[a]	e	0.124[d]	0.139[c]	0.113[d]
Paid employment	e	e	0.159[b]	0.136[d]	e	e	e
Friendships	0.177[b]	0.156[c]	0.140[d]	0.165[b]	0.130[d]	e	0.237[a]
Housing	0.161[c]	e	e	e	e	e	e
Area lived in	e	0.156[c]	0.187[b]	0.172[a]	0.126[d]	e	0.182[a]
Recreation	0.149[d]	0.169[c]	0.124[d]	0.121[d]	0.165[c]	0.196[a]	e
Religion	0.128[d]	e	0.163[b]	e	0.186[b]	e	0.180[b]
Self-Esteem	0.197[b]	0.277[a]	0.178[b]	0.208[a]	0.125[d]	0.163[c]	0.256[a]
Transportation	e	e	e	e	e	0.155[d]	0.123[d]
Education	0.188[b]	0.237[a]	0.266[a]	0.228[a]	0.234[a]	0.145[b]	0.205[a]

[a] $P < 0.001$
[b] $P < 0.005$
[c] $P < 0.01$
[d] $P < 0.05$
[e] Significance level too low to enter equation.

scores, financial security, self-esteem and education.

Exhibits 6 and 7 show that males and females had slightly different profiles of domain impacts on global discrepancies. For both groups, only the domain of self-esteem had an impact on all of the 7 global discrepancy scores. However, males had on average 5.3 domains with significant impacts on their global discrepancy scores, while females averaged 7.1. That seems to indicate that female global discrepancy scores have a broader base than their male counterparts. In total figures, 37 (44%) of 84 possible domain gaps had significant impacts on corresponding global gaps for makes while 50 (60%) had significant impacts for females.

Exhibit 8 gives the results of regressing global satisfaction on 12 domains and 6 demographic variables. The most striking feature of the three regressions (for the whole group, males and females) is the relative insignificance of the demographic variables. As indicated earlier, most studies have found such variables to have relatively little impact on global satisfaction. Our program (*SPSS*) would not allow variables to enter regression equations unless they yielded values with a statistical significance level of 0.05, and that criterion was rigorous enough to keep out all the demographic variables. Presumably, the relatively homogeneous demographics of this sample of university under-

EXHIBIT 8

Multiple regression of satisfaction with life as a whole on satisfaction with 12 domains and 6 demographic variables

	Whole group	Males	Females
Percent of variance explained[a]	53 (N=296)	46 (N=140)	54 (N=149)
Predictors *Satisfaction with:*	*Beta*	*Beta*	*Beta*
Health	0.117[c]	e	e
Financial security	0.112[c]	0.179[b]	0.154[c]
Family relations	0.133[b]	e	0.142[d]
Paid employment	0.092[d]	e	e
Friendships	0.172[a]	0.235[a]	0.204[b]
Housing	0.121[b]	e	e
Area lived in	e	e	e
Recreation	0.122[c]	0.163[d]	0.143[d]
Religion	e	e	0.160[c]
Self-Esteem	0.308[a]	0.344[a]	0.290[a]
Transportation	e	e	e
Education	0.160[a]	0.208[b]	0.173[b]
Demographic variables			
Sex	e	—	—
Age	e	e	e
Marital status	e	e	e
Work status	e	e	e
Education level	e	e	e
Course of study	e	e	e

[a] $P < 0.001$
[b] $P < 0.005$
[c] $P < 0.01$
[d] $P < 0.05$
[e] Significance level too low to enter equation.

graduates was largely responsible for these variables having no distinctive explanatory power. Satisfaction in 2 domains had no impact on global satisfaction, namely, the area lived in and transportation. Satisfaction with self-esteem had the greatest relative impact on global satisfaction for all three groups, and satisfaction with friendships was second. Satisfaction with religion and family relations had no impact on global satisfaction for males, but some impact for females. Fifty-three percent of the variance in global satisfaction was explained by satisfaction in 9 domains for the whole group. For males,

EXHIBIT 9

Multiple regression of happiness with life as a whole on satisfaction with 12 domains and 6 demographic variables

	Whole group	Males	Females
Percent of variance explained[a]	39	33	43
	($N=296$)	($N=140$)	($N=149$)
Predictors *Satisfaction with:*	*Beta*	*Beta*	*Beta*
Health	0.168^a	0.173^d	0.189^b
Financial security	e	e	e
Family relations	0.141^b	e	0.174^c
Paid employment	0.180^a	0.231^a	0.137^d
Friendships	0.212^a	0.242^a	0.230^a
Housing	e	e	e
Area lived in	e	e	e
Recreation	e	e	e
Religion	e	e	e
Self-Esteem	0.255^a	0.290^a	0.249^a
Transportation	e	e	e
Education	0.123^c	e	0.142^d
Demographic variables			
Sex	e	–	–
Age	e	e	e
Marital status	e	e	e
Work status	e	e	e
Education level	e	e	e
Course of study	e	e	e

[a] $P \leqslant 0.001$
[b] $P \leqslant 0.005$
[c] $P \leqslant 0.01$
[d] $P \leqslant 0.05$
[e] Significance level too low to enter equation.

46% was explained by satisfaction in 5 domains and for females, 54% was explained by satisfaction in 7 domains. Again, therefore, the global satisfaction of females was influenced by more domains than that of males.

Exhibit 9 gives the results of regressing global happiness on 12 domains and 6 demographic variables. Again, the latter had no significant impact on happiness. Satisfaction in 6 domains had no impact on happiness, namely, the area lived in, transportation, religion, recreation, housing and financial security. Again, satisfaction with self-esteem had the greatest relative impact on happiness, and satisfaction with friendships was second. Satisfaction with

EXHIBIT 10

Comparison of satisfaction regressions for University Clerical Staff, Rural Seniors, Northern Community and Guelph Students

	1979 Clerical Staff	1981 Rural Seniors	1982 Northern Community	1984 Guelph University Undergraduates
Percent of variance explained in satisfaction with life as a whole[a]	57 (N=312)	49 (N=273)	53 (N=328)	53 (N=296)
Predictors Satisfaction with:	*Beta*	*Beta*	*Beta*	*Beta*
Health	0.107	0.180(2)	0.169(3)	0.117
Financial security	0.152(3)[d]	−0.011	0.242(1)	0.112
Family relations	0.348(1)	0.102	0.101	0.133
Paid employment	0.100	c	b	0.092
Friendships	0.195(2)	0.080	0.068	0.172(2)
Housing	−0.049	0.207(1)	0.095	0.121
Area lived in	b	0.010	0.133	b
Recreation	0.083	0.077	0.052	0.122
Religion	c	0.134	0.065	b
Self-Esteem	0.131	0.174(3)	0.192(2)	0.308(1)
Transportation	0.088	0.046	0.059	b
Government services	c	0.134	0.042	c
Spouse	c	0.057	c	c
Education	−0.026	c	c	0.160(3)

[a] $P < 0.001$
[b] Significance level too low to enter equation.
[c] Not in equation.
[d] Numbers in parentheses indicate the variable's rank of influence.

family relations and education had no impact on happiness for males, but some impact for females. Thirty-nine percent of the variance in happiness was explained by satisfaction in 6 domains for the whole group. For males, 33% was explained by satisfaction in 4 domains and for females, 43% was explained by satisfaction in 6 domains. Again, therefore, female happiness was influenced by more domains than that of males.

Exhibits 10 and 11 provide comparisons between this sample of university students and three previous samples described in Michalos 1980a, 1982a, and

EXHIBIT 11

Comparison of hapiness regressions for University Clerical Staff, Rural Seniors, Northern Community and Guelph Students

	1979 Clerical Staff	1981 Rural Seniors	1982 Northern Community	1984 Guelph University Under-graduates
Percent of variance explained in happiness with life as a whole[a]	45 (N=312)	32 (N=273)	36 (N=328)	39 (N=296)
Predictors Satisfaction with:	Beta	Beta	Beta	Beta
Health	0.121(3)	0.116(3)	0.181(2)	0.168
Financial security	0.092	0.057	0.211(1)	b
Family relations	0.384(1)	−0.028	0.090	0.141
Paid employment	0.033	c	0.092	0.180(3)
Friendships	0.225(2)	0.228(2)	0.011	0.212(2)
Housing	0.005	−0.010	0.095	b
Area lived in	b	0.014	0.048	b
Recreation	0.027	0.035	0.049	b
Religion	c	0.012	0.026	b
Self-Esteem	0.070	0.086	0.144(3)	0.255(1)
Transportation	0.050	0.046	b	b
Government services	c	0.080	0.033	c
Spouse	c	0.298(1)	c	c
Education	−0.033	c	c	c
Secure from crime	−0.048	c	c	0.123

[a] $P < 0.001$
[b] Significance level too low to enter equation.
[c] Not in equation.
[d] Numbers in parentheses indicate the variable's rank order of influence.

1983a. The first involved members of the University of Guelph's office and clerical staff, the second involved rural senior citizens in Huron County, Ontario, and the third involved all residents 18 years and older in the Northern Ontario community of Cochrane. Both exhibits show that the predictive power of domain satisfaction scores for global satisfaction and happiness is fairly stable across the 4 samples. Typically domain satisfaction scores can account for a bit over half the variance in global satisfaction scores, and a bit over a third of the variance in happiness scores. Exhibit 10 shows that satisfaction with self-esteem is the only variable to appear in the top 3 predictors of global satisfaction for 3 of the 4 samples. Exhibit 11 shows that satisfaction with friendships and health appear in the top 3 predictors of happiness for 3 of the 4 samples.

RESULTS FOR MDT

Exhibits 12 and 13 provide overviews of the success of MDT in its application to the undergraduate data-set. In these exhibits a successful prediction is understood as a predicted path coefficient with a (beta) value *and* a significance level of at least 0.05. This dual standard is a conservative combination of fairly common practice (Reis, 1982) and a proposal by Land (1969). A successful prediction ratio (ratio of successful to total predictions) may be used as one measure of a theory's adequacy, although it is certainly not the only or, perhaps, even the most important measure.

There were 771 successful out of a total of 2184 predictions, for a success rate of 35% (Exhibit 12). Only 528 of all these predictions involved the direct or indirect effects of perceived discrepancies, and these yielded 289 successes for a 55% rate of success. By "direct effects of perceived discrepancies" I mean predictions of satisfaction or happiness from perceived discrepancies, and by "indirect effects" I mean predictions of the gap between what one has and wants from the other six discrepancies. Sixty-two percent of the predicted indirect effects were successful, compared to 49% of the direct effects. The highest success rates were obtained for the two global variables, happiness (54%) and satisfaction with life as a whole (49%). The average domain satisfaction success rate was 34%, including a maximum of 37% for self-esteem and a minimum of 29% for education.

Successful prediction ratios provide a minimum measure of a theory's adequacy. A more substantial measure is provided by a theory's explanatory

EXHIBIT 12
Summary of prediction success rates, by dependent variables

	Whole group	Males	Females	Total
All effects				
N successes	305	225	241	771
N predictions	798	693	693	2184
Success rate (%)	38	33	35	35
All gap effects				
N successes	105	91	93	289
N predictions	176	176	176	528
Success rate (%)	60	52	53	55
Direct gap effects				
N successes	49	47	47	143
N predictions	98	98	98	294
Success rate (%)	50	48	48	49
Indirect gap effects				
N successes	56	44	46	146
N predictions	78	78	78	234
Success rate (%)	72	56	59	62
All effects by domains				
Happiness				
N successes	7	6	7	20
N predictions	13	12	12	37
Success rate (%)	54	50	58	54
% Var. exp.	49	45	53	
Global satisfaction				
N successes	32	25	24	81
N predictions	61	53	53	167
Success rate (%)	53	47	45	49
% Var. exp.	53	50	56	
Health satisfaction				
N successes	22	18	17	57
N predictions	61	53	53	167
Success rate (%)	36	34	32	34
% Var. exp.	50	46	53	
Financial security sat.				
N successes	21	19	20	60
N predictions	61	53	53	167
Success rate (%)	34	36	38	36
% Var. exp.	58	59	59	
Family relations sat.				
N successes	24	17	18	59
N predictions	61	53	53	167
Success rate (%)	39	32	34	35
% Var. exp.	79	77	81	

Exhibit 12 (continued)

	Whole group	Males	Females	Total
Paid employment sat.				
N successes	25	12	23	60
N predictions	61	53	53	167
Success rate (%)	41	23	43	36
% Var. exp.	59	55	68	
Friendships sat.				
N successes	21	17	19	57
N predictions	61	53	53	167
Success rate (%)	34	32	36	34
% Var. exp.	75	76	74	
Housing sat.				
N successes	24	18	16	58
N predictions	61	53	53	167
Success rate (%)	39	34	30	35
% Var. exp.	44	46	44	
Area sat.				
N successes	23	17	14	54
N predictions	61	53	53	167
Success rate (%)	38	32	26	32
% Var. exp.	48	49	46	
Recreation sat.				
N successes	21	14	19	54
N predictions	61	53	53	167
Success rate (%)	34	26	36	32
% Var. exp.	56	53	58	
Religion sat.				
N successes	21	13	17	51
N predictions	61	53	53	167
Success rate (%)	34	25	32	31
% Var. exp.	62	70	58	
Self-esteem sat.				
N successes	20	15	18	53
N predictions	53	45	45	143
Success rate (%)	38	33	40	37
% Var. exp.	58	54	61	
Transportation sat.				
N successes	24	20	15	59
N predictions	61	53	53	167
Success rate (%)	39	38	28	35
% Var. exp.	55	52	57	
Education sat.				
N successes	20	14	14	48
N predictions	61	53	53	167
Success rate (%)	33	26	26	29
% Var. exp.	35	34	37	

EXHIBIT 13

Prediction success rates, by predictors

Predictors	Whole group	Males	Females	Total	Direct	Indirect
Self-Wants						
N successes	14	14	14	42	42	0
N predictions	14	14	14	42	42	0
Rate (%)	100	100	100	100	100	0
Self-Others						
N successes	27	27	26	80	41	39
N predictions	27	27	27	81	42	39
Rate (%)	100	100	96	99	98	100
Self-Deserved						
N successes	16	9	13	38	17	21
N predictions	27	27	27	81	42	39
Rate (%)	59	33	48	47	40	54
Self-Needs						
N successes	17	15	18	50	13	37
N predictions	27	27	27	81	42	39
Rate (%)	63	56	67	62	31	95
Self-Progress						
N successes	9	8	9	26	10	16
N predictions	27	27	27	81	42	39
Rate (%)	33	30	33	32	24	41
Self-Future						
N successes	3	6	3	12	5	7
N predictions	27	27	27	81	42	39
Rate (%)	11	22	11	15	12	18
Self-Best						
N successes	19	12	12	43	16	27
N predictions	27	27	27	81	42	39
Rate (%)	70	44	44	53	38	69
Sex						
N successes	20	–	–	20	1	19
N predictions	105	–	–	105	14	91
Rate (%)	19			19	7	21
Age						
N successes	36	26	29	91	5	86
N predictions	105	105	105	315	42	273
Rate (%)	34	25	28	29	12	32
Work status						
N successes	27	25	17	69	6	63
N predictions	105	105	105	315	42	273
Rate (%)	26	24	16	22	14	23

Exhibit 13 (continued)

	Whole group	Males	Females	Total	Direct	Indirect
Education level						
N successes	6	3	11	21	2	19
N predictions	105	105	105	315	42	273
Rate (%)	6	3	11	7	5	7
Self-esteem						
N successes	40	28	29	97	20	77
N predictions	97	97	97	291	39	252
Rate (%)	41	29	30	33	51	31
Social support						
N successes	71	52	61	184	35	149
N predictions	105	105	105	315	42	273
Rate (%)	68	50	58	58	83	55

power. The percent of variance explained in one's dependent (criterion) variables by one's independent (explanatory, predictor) variables provides a good measure of a theory's explanatory power. Exhibit 12 lists the percent of variance explained in each of our basic 14 dependent variables beginning with happiness (49%) and global satisfaction (53%). On average 57% of the variance in domain satisfaction scores is explained by MDT, with a high of 79% for family relations and a low of 35% for education. To some extent the high percent of variance explained in satisfaction with family relations and friendships is the result of social support being defined by the mean of the mean scores for the former two variables. As it happened, the mean of each of the former two variables was 5.2, while the variance of the family relations variable was 1.51 and that of friendships was 1.44. Ignoring these possible anomalies, MDT was still able to explain 50% or more of the variance in 7 of the remaining 10 domain satisfaction scores. It was most successful in accounting for satisfaction with financial security (58%), paid employment (59%), recreation activity (56%), religion (62%) and self-esteem (58%).

Exhibit 13 summarizes the success rates of each of our predictor variables. The 7 discrepancy variables had an average success rate of 58%, ranging from 100% for the self-want discrepancy to 15% for the self-future discrepancy. That is, every time we predicted that the self-want discrepancy variable would have a significant effect, it did; but only 15% of the predicted effects of the self-future variable were confirmed. In fact, the self-others discrepancy variable was also practically infallible, with a success rate of 99%. The third most successful discrepancy predictor was self-needs (62%). Since I had never used this variable before, it was very encouraging to find it so successful. It surpassed the self-best (53%) predictor, which was the third basic variable in my earlier studies and the self-deserved (47%) predictor, which was another new one. The self-progress (32%) variable was also new and fairly successful.

The last two columns of Exhibit 13 list the numbers and percents of direct and indirect effects of our predictors. Since the self-wants discrepancy variable was only used in direct predictions of satisfaction and happiness, its 42 successes yielded a 100% prediction success rate. All other discrepancy variables were used to make direct and indirect predictions as indicated earlier. Thus, for example, the self-others discrepancy variable had 80 successful predictions, of which 41 were direct and 39 were indirect. Since 42 of the predictions made from this variable were direct, its success rate for direct predictions was $41/42 = 98\%$. Its success rate for indirect predictions was 100%. Hence, both the *total* and the *distribution* of predicted effects of this variable were almost exactly as MDT predicted. The self-needs discrepancy variable had the third best total (62%), indirect (95%) and average (63%) prediction success rates. In fact, the indirect prediction success rates were higher than the direct rates for each of the 6 variables that had both kinds of predictions, indicating a clear need for H3 in MDT.

The two satisfaction variables, self-esteem and social support, had total success rates of 33% and 58%, respectively (Exhibit 13). Unlike the discrepancy variables, the direct prediction success rates were higher than the indirect rates for these variables. For social support the direct rate was a very solid 83%, compared to a 55% indirect rate.

As indicated earlier, these variables were used as surrogate measures pending further tests with alternatives. Presumably the surrogate satisfaction measures would have some method effects resulting from the similarity of items (Diener, 1984). Still, whatever method effects there are, they seem to be at best erratic. For example, Exhibits 8 and 9 show that often there is no significant relation between global satisfaction, happiness and one or another domain satisfaction score in spite of the similarities in the format of the items. Furthermore, as I have just mentioned, the two surrogate variables in particular are not uniformly successful as predictors.

The four demographic predictors had an average total prediction success rate of 19% with a high of 29% for age and a low of 7% for educational level (Exhibit 13). In every case there were higher indirect than direct rates. Given the results presented earlier, one would have expected these variables to have low individual success rates, but there was no reason to expect that their indirect rates would be higher than their direct rates. This seems to demand some rethinking of H5 of MDT.

Exhibits 14 to 27 show the detailed results of applying MDT to happiness, global and twelve domains of satisfaction. Exhibit 14 graphically illustrates the application of MDT to satisfaction with life as a whole for 635 respondents. Fifty-three percent of the variance was explained. The solid lines leading to net satisfaction represent the results of regressing this variable on the other thirteen in the diagram. The dashed lines leading to self-wants represent the results of regressing this variable on the six discrepancy and six conditioning variables. Thirty-nine percent of the variance in self-wants was explained by those twelve predictors. The dotted lines leading to the column of six discrepancy variables from the six conditioners represent the results of regressing each of the former on the latter set. The number in each of the six discrepancy boxes indicates the percent of variance explained by the 6 conditioning variables. For example, the latter variables explained 19% of the variance in self-others scores, 10% in self-deserved scores, etc.

The three columns of numbers attached to the solid, dashed and dotted lines are standardized regression coefficients (Betas) or path coefficients. For example, the number 0.246[a] above the arrow from self-wants to net satisfaction is a path coefficient indicating that for every unit of change in self-wants there will be a change of 25% of a unit in net satisfaction (when both variables are standardized to have means of zero and standard deviations of one). Figuratively speaking, for every full step in self-wants, there will be a quarter of a step in net satisfaction. In order to interpret the dotted lines, follow each line first as far to the left and then as far down the page as it will go. For example, the number 0.303[a] at the head of the column on the left is on a line that goes all the way down to self-esteem. Following that, 0.174[a] goes all the way down to social support, and so on. The superscripts on these Betas indicate statistical significance levels. From Exhibit 14 on into Appendix A, I adopt the convention that a means $p \leqslant 0.001$, b: $p \leqslant 0.005$, c: $p \leqslant 0.01$ and d: $p \leqslant 0.05$.

Because Exhibit 14 is relatively difficult to read compared to the tables in Exhibits 15–27, I have not drawn any more diagrams. All other summaries

EXHIBIT 14

Satisfaction with life as a whole

Percent of variance explained: 53^a, $N = 635$

$^aP < 0.001$
$^bP < 0.005$
$^cP < 0.001$
$^dP < 00.05$

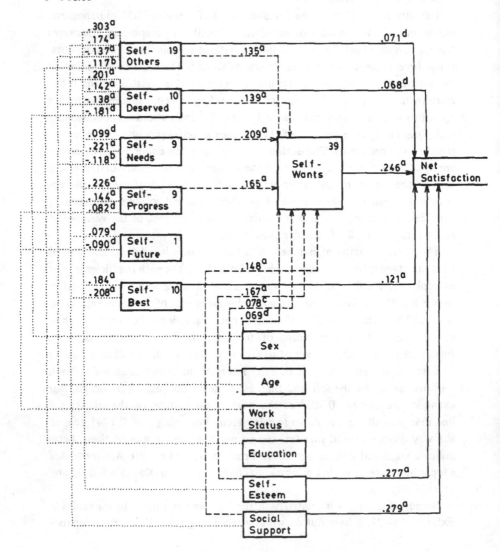

EXHIBIT 15

Happiness with life as a whole

Self-Others	Self-Deserved	Self-Needs	Self-Wants	Happiness
A = −0.137 [a]	A = −0.138 [a]	A = −0.118 [b]	SO = 0.135 [a]	SO = 0.129 [a]
S = 0	S = −0.081 [d]	S = 0	SD = 0.139 [a]	SD = 0.103 [b]
WS = 0	WS = 0	WS = 0	SN = 0.209 [a]	SN = 0
E = 0.117 [b]	E = 0	E = 0	SP = 0.165 [a]	SP = 0
SE = 0.303 [a]	SE = 0.142 [a]	SE = 0.099 [d]	SH = 0	SH = 0
SS = 0.174 [a]	SS = 0.201 [a]	SS = 0.221 [a]	SB = 0	SB = 0.214 [a]
R^2 = 0.19 [a]	R^2 = 0.10 [a]	R^2 = 0.09 [a]	A = 0.078 [c]	A = 0
			S = 0.069 [d]	S = 0
Self-Progress	**Self-Future**	**Self-Best**	WS = 0	WS = 0.086 [a]
			E = 0	E = 0
A = 0	A = 0	A = 0	SE = 0.167 [a]	SE = 0.183 [a]
S = 0	S = −0.090 [d]	S = 0	SS = 0.148 [a]	SS = 0.235 [a]
WS = −0.082 [d]	WS = 0	WS = 0	R^2 = 0.39 [a]	SW = 0.172 [a]
E = 0	E = 0	E = 0		R^2 = 0.49 [a]
SE = 0.226 [a]	SE = 0	SE = 0.184 [a]		N = 635
SS = 0.144 [a]	SS = 0.079 [d]	SS = 0.208 [a]		
R^2 = 0.09 [a]	R^2 = 0.01 [d]	R^2 = 0.10 [a]		

[a] $P \leqslant 0.001$
[b] $P \leqslant 0.005$
[c] $P \leqslant 0.01$
[d] $P \leqslant 0.05$
0 Significance level too low to enter equation.

of results of applying MDT are presented as in Exhibit 15, for happiness with life as a whole. In this exhibit, each set of figures represents a separate regression, with the word at the top of the set indicating the dependent variable. For example, the extreme right column indicates the results of regressing happiness on the thirteen predictors listed below it. The abbreviations are as follows for all these exhibits.

SO: Self-Other   A: Age
SD: Self-Deserved   S: Sex
SN: Self-Needs   WS: Work Status
SP: Self-Progress   E: Education
SH: Self-Future   SE: Self-Esteem
SB: Self-Best   SS: Social Support
SW: Self-Wants

Betas and their significance levels are listed, followed by the squared multiple

EXHIBIT 16

Satisfaction with health

Self-Others	Self-Deserved	Self-Needs	Self-Wants	Satisfaction
A = 0	A = 0	A = 0	SO = 0.390[a]	SO = 0.173[a]
S = 0	S = −0.102[b]	S = 0	SD = 0.079[d]	SD = 0.069[d]
WS = 0	WS = 0	WS = 0	SN = 0.134[a]	SN = 0
E = 0	E = 0	E = 0	SP = 0.104[b]	SP = 0
SE = 0.188[a]	SE = 0.127[a]	SE = 0.144[a]	SH = −0.101[a]	SH = 0
SS = 0	SS = 0	SS = 0	SB = 0.149[a]	SB = 0
R^2 = 0.03[a]	R^2 = 0.03[a]	R^2 = 0.02[a]	A = 0	A = −0.058[a]
			S = 0.108[a]	S = 0

Self-Progress	Self-Future	Self-Best		
			WS = 0	WS = 0
			E = 0	E = 0
A = 0	A = 0	A = 0	SE = 0.175[a]	SE = 0.088[b]
S = 0	S = 0	S = −0.106[c]	SS = 0	SS = 0.098[a]
WS = 0	WS = 0	WS = 0	R^2 = 0.49[a]	SW = 0.498[a]
E = 0	E = 0	E = 0		R^2 = 0.50[a]
SE = 0.213[a]	SE = 0	SE = 0.173[a]		N = 647
SS = 0	SS = 0.127[a]	SS = 0		
R^2 = 0.04[a]	R^2 = 0.02[a]	R^2 = 0.04[a]		

[a] $P \leqslant 0.001$
[b] $P \leqslant 0.005$
[c] $P \leqslant 0.01$
[d] $P \leqslant 0.05$
0 Significance level too low to enter equation.

correlation coefficient (R^2) and its significance level, and finally the number (N) of cases involved. The latter number is only given for the primary regression. For example, then, this column of numbers indicates that 49% of the variance in happiness with life as a whole was explained by MDT (cf. 39% in Exhibit 9), the most influential variable was social support (Beta = 0.235[a]) and the most influential discrepancy variable was self-wants (0.172[a]). The second column from the right indicates that 39% of the variance in self-wants scores was explained by the 12 predictors listed in that column, and the self-needs discrepancy variable was the most influential predictor (0.209[a]). The column headed "self-needs" indicates that 9% of the variance in this discrepancy variable was explained by the 6 variables listed below it, led by social support (0.221[a]).

It would obviously take more space than one can allow in an article to review each of the detailed Exhibits. However, it is possible to call your attention to a few notable features. Hereafter, it will be convenient to distin-

EXHIBIT 17

Satisfaction with financial security

Self-Others	Self-Deserved	Self-Needs	Self-Wants	Satisfaction
A $= -0.256^a$	A $= -0.170^a$	A $= -0.149^a$	SO $= 0.211^a$	SO $= 0.254^a$
S $= 0$	S $= 0$	S $= 0$	SD $= 0.155^a$	SD $= 0$
WS $= 0.156^a$	WS $= 0$	WS $= 0$	SN $= 0.319^a$	SN $= 0.178^a$
E $= 0$	E $= 0$	E $= 0$	SP $= 0$	SP $= 0$
SE $= 0$	SE $= 0$	SE $= 0$	SH $= 0$	SH $= 0$
SS $= 0.096^c$	SS $= 0.091^d$	SS $= 0.084^c$	SB $= 0.166^a$	SB $= 0.118^a$
$R^2 = 0.08^a$	$R^2 = 0.04^a$	$R^2 = 0.03^a$	A $= 0.119^a$	A $= 0$
			S $= 0$	S $= 0$
Self-Progress	Self-Future	Self-Best	WS $= 0$	WS $= 0$
			E $= 0$	E $= 0$
A $= -0.188^a$	A $= 0$	A $= 0.046^a$	SE $= 0$	SE $= 0$
S $= 0$	S $= 0$	S $= 0$	SS $= 0$	SS $= 0.076^b$
WS $= 0$	WS $= 0$	WS $= 0$	$R^2 = 0.46^a$	SW $= 0.356^a$
E $= 0$	E $= 0$	E $= 0$		$R^2 = 0.58^a$
SE $= 0$	SE $= 0$	SE $= 0$		N $= 646$
SS $= 0.127^a$	SS $= 0.119^b$	SS $= 0$		
$R^2 = 0.05^a$	$R^2 = 0.01^b$	$R^2 = 0.05^a$		

[a] $P < 0.01$
[b] $P < 0.05$
[c] $P < 0.01$
[d] $P < 0.05$
0 Significance level too low to enter equation.

guish two kinds of indirect effects, namely, effects on the self-wants discrepancy variable and effects on any of the other six discrepancy variables. I will refer to the former as "second-level" and to the latter as "third-level" effects.

Exhibits 14 and 15 show that social support has the greatest direct effect on happiness and global satisfaction, but not the greatest second-level effect. The perceived discrepancy between what one has and needs has the greatest second-level effect on these two global variables.

Given the enormous literature regarding the impact of social support on self-perceived health, one would have expected it to have had a similar significant impact on perceived satisfaction with health. Exhibit 16 shows that this is not the case for this data-set. On the other hand, self-esteem has significant second and third-level effects.

Satisfaction with financial security and paid employment tend to be dominated by the perceived self-wants discrepancy (Exhibits 17 and 19),

EXHIBIT 18

Satisfaction with family relations

Self-Others	Self-Deserved	Self-Needs	Self-Wants	Satisfaction
A $=-0.086^c$	A $= 0$	A $=-0.114^a$	SO $= 0.321^a$	SO $= 0.189^a$
S $= 0$	S $= 0$	S $= 0$	SD $= 0.114^a$	SD $= 0$
WS $= 0$	WS $=-0.097$	WS $= 0$	SN $= 0.199^a$	SN $= 0.113^a$
E $= 0$	E $= 0$	E $= 0$	SP $= 0$	SP $= 0$
SE $= 0$	SE $= 0$	SE $= 0$	SH $=-0.061^d$	SH $= 0$
SS $= 0.573^a$	SS $= 0.448^a$	SS $= 0.489^a$	SB $= 0.099^a$	SB $= 0$
$R^2 = 0.34^a$	$R^2 = 0.20^a$	$R^2 = 0.26^a$	A $= 0$	A $= 0$
			S $= 0$	S $=-0.042^d$
Self-Progress	Self-Future	Self-Best	WS $= 0$	WS $= 0$
			E $= 0$	E $= 0$
A $= 0$	A $= 0$	A $=-0.073^d$	SE $= 0$	SE $=-0.063^d$
S $= 0$	S $= 0$	S $= 0$	SS $= 0.251^a$	SS $= 0.537^a$
WS $=-0.073^d$	WS $=-0.144^a$	WS $= 0$	$R^2 = 0.60^a$	SW $= 0.222^a$
E $= 0$	E $= 0$	E $= 0$		$R^2 = 0.79^a$
SE $= 0$	SE $= 0$	SE $= 0$		$N = 641$
SS $= 0.404^a$	SS $= 0.176^a$	SS $= 0.411^a$		
$R^2 = 0.16^a$	$R^2 = 0.05^a$	$R^2 = 0.18^a$		

^{a} $P < 0.001$
^{b} $P < 0.005$
^{c} $P < 0.01$
^{d} $P < 0.05$
0 Significance level too low to enter equation.

while self-esteem has no effect at all on the former variable and almost no effect on the latter.

Curiously, self-esteem has relatively little impact on satisfaction with family relations and friendships (Exhibits 18 and 20). However, the social comparison variable (self-others) has strong second-level effects in both cases.

Satisfaction with housing in largely determined by the self-wants and self-others discrepancies, with the latter (self-others) mainly influenced positively by social support and work status, and negatively by age (Exhibit 21).

Satisfaction with housing is largely determined by the self-wants and self-tion are all strongly dominated by the self-wants and self-others discrepancies (Exhibits 23—26). Social support has significant first and third-level effects, but no second-level effects on satisfaction with recreation activity (Exhibit 23). Social comparison has a surprisingly high impact on satisfaction with religion, especially since the latter is defined simply as "your spiritual fulfilment" (Exhibit 25).

Given the variety of discrepancy hypotheses available in the literature, the

EXHIBIT 19

Satisfaction with paid employment

Self-Others	Self-Deserved	Self-Needs	Self-Wants	Satisfaction
A = −0.205[a]	A = 0	A = −0.126[c]	SO = 0.269[a]	SO = 0.244[a]
S = 0	S = 0	S = −0.112[d]	SD = 0.160[a]	SD = 0
WS = 0.520[a]	WS = 0.159[a]	WS = 0.290[a]	SN = 0.222[a]	SN = 0
E = 0	E = 0	E = 0	SP = 0	SP = 0.091[d]
SE = 0	SE = 0	SE = 0	SH = 0	SH = 0
SS = 0.088[d]	SS = 0.110[d]	SS = 0	SB = 0.094[d]	SB = 0
R^2 = 0.27[a]	R^2 = 0.03[a]	R^2 = 0.09[a]	A = 0	A = 0
			S = 0	S = 0

Self-Progress	Self-Future	Self-Best	WS = 0.182[a]	WS = 0.222[a]
			E = 0	E = 0
A = −0.152[a]	A = 0	A = −0.239[a]	SE = 0	SE = 0
S = 0	S = 0	S = 0	SS = 0	SS = .115[a]
WS = 0.202[a]	WS = −0.094[d]	WS = 0.493[a]	R^2 = 0.49[a]	SW = 0.390[a]
E = 0	E = 0	E = 0		R^2 = 0.59[a]
SE = 0	SE = 0.107[c]	SE = 0		N = 371
SS = 0.093[d]	SS = 0	SS = 0		
R^2 = 0.06[a]	R^2 = 0.02[c]	R^2 = 0.24[a]		

[a] $P \leqslant 0.001$
[b] $P \leqslant 0.005$
[c] $P \leqslant 0.01$
[d] $P \leqslant 0.05$
0 Significance level too low to enter equation.

question has been raised about the relative importance of each type, e.g., by Goodman (1974) and Diener (1984). The investigations reported in Michalos (1980a, 1982a, 1983a) indicated a fairly clear and consistent rank ordering of impact of perceived discrepancies on net satisfaction. In a total of 68 regressions, using three gap variables as predictors and some (domain or global) satisfaction or happiness variable as criteria, 65 times the gap between what one has and wants had the greatest impact (highest Beta value). The gap between what one has and relevant others have came in second 46 times, and the gap between what one has and the best one has ever had in the past came in third 50 times. There were only 6 times in which a variable involving the gap between what one has now and expects to have in five years was used, and in every case this variable ranked fourth behind the others and accounted for a negligible percent of the explained variance in the dependent variables.

Exhibit 28 summarizes the relative impacts of discrepancy types on satisfaction and happiness for this data-set. For example, the self-wants variable has the greatest impact 38 times, second-greatest 4 times and fourth-greatest

EXHIBIT 20

Satisfaction with friendships

Self-Others	Self-Deserved	Self-Needs	Self-Wants	Satisfaction
$A = 0$	$A = 0$	$A = 0$	$SO = 0.341^a$	$SO = 0.142^a$
$S = 0$	$S = 0$	$S = 0$	$SD = 0.081^c$	$SD = 0$
$WS = 0$	$WS = 0$	$WS = 0$	$SN = 0.096^c$	$SN = 0$
$E = 0$	$E = 0$	$E = 0$	$SP = 0$	$SP = 0$
$SE = 0.143^a$	$SE = 0$	$SE = 0.093^b$	$SH = 0$	$SH = 0$
$SS = 0.521^a$	$SS = 0.387^a$	$SS = 0.410^a$	$SB = 0.094^b$	$SB = 0.095^a$
$R^2 = 0.34^a$	$R^2 = 0.15^a$	$R^2 = 0.20^a$	$A = 0.082^b$	$A = 0$
			$S = 0$	$S = 0$
Self-Progress	**Self-Future**	**Self-Best**	$WS = 0$	$WS = 0$
			$E = 0$	$E = 0$
$A = 0$	$A = -0.109^a$	$A = 0$	$SE = 0.113^a$	$SE = 0$
$S = 0$	$S = 0$	$S = 0$	$SS = 0.262^a$	$SS = 0.540^a$
$WS = 0$	$WS = 0$	$WS = 0$	$R^2 = 0.56^a$	$SW = 0.243^a$
$E = 0$	$E = 0$	$E = 0$		$R^2 = 0.75^a$
$SE = 0.085^d$	$SE = 0$	$SE = 0$		$N = 650$
$SS = 0.336^a$	$SS = 0.089^d$	$SS = 0.426^a$		
$R^2 = 0.14^a$	$R^2 = 0.02^a$	$R^2 = 0.18^a$		

[a] $P < 0.001$
[b] $P < 0.005$
[c] $P < 0.01$
[d] $P < 0.05$
0 Significance level too low to enter equation.

once. Thus, the self-wants variable is typically the most influential of all seven discrepancy variables. The self-others variable is typically second. In order to aggregate all the rankings in Exhibit 28 to obtain a general view, I assigned each variable a weight. Six points were given to a variable for each time it was first, five points for each second, and so on to one for sixth place. Then the products were summed to get a total weight for each variable. Using this scheme, it is clear that the three discrepancy variables that I have worked with most are the three most influential, namely, self-wants, self-others and self-best.

In terms of the familiar theories reviewed earlier, one might say that Exhibit 28 shows that aspiration theory (self-wants) is superior to social comparison theory (self-others), that equity theory (self-deserved) is slightly superior to person-environment fit theory (self-needs), and that cognitive dissonance theory (insofar as it involves future expectations (self-future)) is the least powerful of the lot. Given the artificiality of the weighting scheme, the limitations of the data-set and the severe reduction of the familiar theories

EXHIBIT 21

Satisfaction with housing

Self-Others	Self-Deserved	Self-Needs	Self-Wants	Satisfaction
A $=-0.166^a$	A $=-0.098^d$	A $=-0.118^b$	SO $= 0.306^a$	SO $= 0.248^a$
S $= 0.080^d$	S $= 0$	S $= 0$	SD $= 0.084^d$	SD $= 0.114^b$
WS $= 0.128^a$	WS $= 0$	WS $= 0$	SN $= 0.113^c$	SN $= 0$
E $= 0$	E $= 0$	E $= 0.097^d$	SP $= 0.110^c$	SP $= 0.080^d$
SE $= 0$	SE $= 0$	SE $= 0$	SH $= 0$	SH $= 0$
SS $= 0.131^a$	SS $= 0$	SS $= 0.108^c$	SB $= 0.166^a$	SB $= 0$
$R^2 = 0.06^a$	$R^2 = 0.01^d$	$R^2 = 0.03^c$	A $= 0$	A $= 0$
			S $= 0$	S $= 0$
Self-Progress	Self-Future	Self-Best	WS $= 0$	WS $= 0$
			E $= 0$	E $= 0$
A $=-0.222^a$	A $= 0$	A $= 0$	SE $= 0$	SE $= 0.66^d$
S $= 0$	S $= 0$	S $= 0$	SS $= 0$	SS $= 0.147^a$
WS $= 0.84^d$	WS $= 0$	WS $= 0$	$R^2 = 0.37^a$	SW $= 0.325^a$
E $= 0.097^d$	E $= 0$	E $= 0.79^d$		$R^2 = 0.44^a$
SE $= 0$	SE $= 0$	SE $= 0$		$N = 644$
SS $= 0$	SS $= 0$	SS $= 0.089^d$		
$R^2 = 0.04^a$	$R^2 = 0$	$R^2 = 0.01^d$		

[a] $P < 0.001$
[b] $P < 0.005$
[c] $P < 0.01$
[d] $P < 0.05$
0 Signifiance level too low to enter equation.

to the few representative items in my questionnaire, one should not press the significance of this rank ordering very far. Still, I believe it is the first time anyone has ever tried to systematically assess the relative superiority of these theories.

Exhibit 29 is like the one before it, with the addition of self-esteem and social support. After self-wants and self-others, social support has the greatest relative impact out of the nine variables.

Appendix Exhibits A.1 to A.14 give detailed results of applying MDT to the happiness, global and domain satisfaction of males and females. The overviews given in Exhibits 12, 13, 28 and 29 cover this material too. On average MDT explained 48% of the variance in the global variables for males and 55% for females. For males, on average 56% of the variance in domain satisfaction was explained, compared to 58% for females. For both groups, the highest R^2's went to satisfaction with family relations and the lowest to satisfaction with education.

Again, only a few of the interesting results in these exhibits can be empha-

EXHIBIT 22

Satisfaction with area lived in

Self-Others	Self-Deserved	Self-Needs	Self-Wants	Satisfaction
A = 0	A = −0.088[d]	A = −0.083[d]	SO = 0.210[a]	SO = 0.234[a]
S = 0.086[d]	S = 0	S = 0	SD = 0	SD = 0.073[d]
WS = 0	WS = 0	WS = 0.104[c]	SN = 0.206[a]	SN = 0
E = 0	E = 0	E = 0	SP = 0.137[a]	SP = 0.076[d]
SE = 0	SE = 0	SE = 0	SH = −0.114[a]	SH = 0
SS = 0.097[c]	SS = 0.086[d]	SS = 0.082[d]	SB = 0.209[a]	SB = 0
R^2 = 0.02[d]	R^2 = 0.01[d]	R^2 = 0.02[d]	A = 0	A = 0
			S = 0	S = 0

Self-Progress	Self-Future	Self-Best		
			WS = 0.066[d]	WS = 0
			E = 0	E = 0
A = −0.186[a]	A = 0	A = 0	SE = 0	SE = 0
S = 0	S = 0	S = 0.077[d]	SS = 0	SS = 0.197[a]
WS = 0	WS = −0.116[b]	WS = 0	R^2 = 0.37[a]	SW = 0.408[a]
E = 0.089[d]	E = 0	E = 0		R^2 = 0.48[a]
SE = 0	SE = 0	SE = 0		N = 644
SS = 0	SS = 0	SS = 0.089[d]		
R^2 = 0.03[b]	R^2 = 0.01[b]	R^2 = 0.01[d]		

[a] $P < 0.001$
[b] $P < 0.005$
[c] $P < 0.01$
[d] $P < 0.05$
0 Significance level too low to enter equation.

sized. Notice, for example, that age has six negative third-level effects on female satisfaction with paid employment, but only one such effect for males (Exhibit A.6). Social support has only two effects on male satisfaction with recreation activity, but seven effects on female satisfaction (Exhibit A.10). Educational level has a single direct effect on male and female satisfaction with religion, but it is positive for males and negative for females (Exhibit A.11). Self-esteem has only one direct effect on male satisfaction with transportation, but it has one direct and three indirect effects on female satisfaction (Exhibit A.13). Work status has all six third-level effects on male satisfaction with transportation, but only one such effect for females.

DISCUSSION

Having completed our analysis of the Guelph undergraduate data-set with MDT, there are a few loose ends that should be nailed down. In the first place, it may have been noticed that all but one of the variables used here

EXHIBIT 23

Satisfaction with recreation activity

Self-Others	Self-Deserved	Self-Needs	Self-Wants	Satisfaction
A = 0	A = 0	A = 0	SO = 0.393^a	SO = 0.282^a
S = −0.094^c	S = 0	S = 0	SD = 0	SD = 0
WS = 0	WS = 0	WS = 0	SN = 0.129^a	SN = 0
E = 0	E = 0	E = 0	SP = 0.154^a	SP = 0
SE = 0.175^a	SE = 0.118^b	SE = 0.120^b	SH = 0	SH = 0
SS = 0.214^a	SS = 0.139^a	SS = 0.171^a	SB = 0.143^a	SB = 0.094^b
R^2 = 0.11^a	R^2 = 0.04^a	R^2 = 0.05^a	A = 0	A = 0
			S = 0	S = 0

Self-Progress	Self-Future	Self-Best	Self-Wants	Satisfaction
			WS = 0	WS = 0
			E = 0	E = 0
A = 0	A = −0.078^d	A = 0	SE = 0.091^b	SE = 0.057^d
S = 0	S = 0	S = 0	SS = 0	SS = 0.125^a
WS = 0	WS = 0	WS = 0	R^2 = 0.48^a	SW = 0.415^a
E = 0	E = 0	E = 0		R^2 = 0.56^a
SE = 0.157^a	SE = 0	SE = 0		N = 646
SS = 0.112^c	SS = 0	SS = 0.162^a		
R^2 = 0.05^a	R^2 = 0.01^d	R^2 = 0.03^a		

^{a} $P < 0.001$
^{b} $P < 0.005$
^{c} $P < 0.01$
^{d} $P < 0.05$
0 Significance level too low to enter equation.

(*viz.*, social support) are based on single item measures, in spite of the fact that generally speaking if all other things are equal, multi-item measures (indexes, scales) tend to have higher levels of reliability (Zeller and Carmines (1980); Anderson, Basilevsky and Hum (1983)). The main reason for using single item measures with some face validity here is that I am primarily interested in tracing the boundaries or scope of MDT in terms of its domains of applicability. I want to have a rough idea fairly early about where this sort of theory is likely to work. Besides this basic consideration, there is also the problem of increasing the length of the questionnaire with the use of multi-item measures. Moreover, as Schuessler (1982) had admirably shown, there is no guarantee that the more items a measure has, the more reliable it will be. For all these reasons, then, it seems wise to stay with single item measures for now.

The construct validity of the D-T scale of Andrews and Withey (1976) was thoroughly examined by these authors, and my delightful-terrible scale is simply a linguistically purer version of their scale. The original scale had

EXHIBIT 24

Satisfaction with religion

Self-Others	Self-Deserved	Self-Needs	Self-Wants	Satisfaction
A $=0$	A $=0$	A $=0$	SO $=0.340^a$	SO $=0.384^a$
S $=0$	S $=0$	S $=0$	SD $=0$	SD $=0$
WS $=0$	WS $=0$	WS $=0$	SN $=0.247^a$	SN $=-0.091^d$
E $=0$	E $=0$	E $=0$	SP $=0$	SP $=0$
SE $=0.182^a$	SE $=0.137^b$	SE $=0.157^b$	SH $=0$	SH $=0$
SS $=0.140^b$	SS $=0$	SS $=0.136^c$	SB $=0.154^a$	SB $=0.142^a$
$R^2=0.07^a$	$R^2=0.02^b$	$R^2=0.05^b$	A $=0$	A $=0$
			S $=0$	S $=0$
Self-Progress	Self-Future	Self-Best	WS $=0$	WS $=0$
			E $=0$	E $=0$
A $=0$	A $=0$	A $=0$	SE $=0.098^d$	SE $=0.104^b$
S $=0$	S $=0.107^d$	S $=0$	SS $=0.113^c$	SS $=0.073^d$
WS $=0$	WS $=0$	WS $=0$	$R^2=0.45^a$	SW $=0.400^a$
E $=0$	E $=0$	E $=0$		$R^2=0.62^a$
SE $=0.115^d$	SE $=0$	SE $=0.106^d$		$N = 396$
SS $=0.143^b$	SS $=0$	SS $=0.155^b$		
$R^2=0.04^b$	$R^2=0.01^d$	$R^2=0.04^b$		

a $P \leqslant 0.001$
b $P \leqslant 0.005$
c $P \leqslant 0.01$
d $P \leqslant 0.05$
0 Significance level too low to enter equation.

"approximately 65% valid variance" and "roughly eight percent of the total variance can be attributed to method effects" (Andrews and Withey, 1976, p. 189). I suppose that my delightful-terrible scale has fairly similar characteristics.

All of the perceived discrepancy measures are designed on the working assumption that people have distinct and identifiable levels of wants, needs, expectations and so on. But it is more likely that any levels of experienced wants, etc. are vaguely bounded by intervals which obscurely blend into perceivable chunks (Michalos, 1967). Following a suggestion from Samuel Stouffer, Rodman (1963) used the idea of an interval, "wider range of values" or "value-stretch" to account for the apparently contradictory findings in delinquency studies showing that society is based upon both a "common value system" and a "class-differentiated value system". Although I suspect it is misleading to describe perceptual limitations as some kind of an expanded range of values, I think we would all agree on the fuzziness of perceived discrepancies.

EXHIBIT 25
Satisfaction with self-esteem

Self-Others	Self-Deserved	Self-Needs	Self-Wants	Satisfaction
A = 0	A = 0	A = 0	SO = 0.458ᵃ	SO = 0.276ᵃ
S = −0.124ᵃ	S = −0.139ᵃ	S = −0.148ᵃ	SD = 0	SD = 0.068ᵈ
WS = 0	WS = 0	WS = 0	SN = 0.187ᵃ	SN = 0
E = 0	E = 0	E = 0	SP = 0	SP = 0
SS = 0.254ᵃ	SS = 0.160ᵃ	SS = 0.235ᵃ	SH = 0	SH = 0
R^2 = 0.08ᵃ	R^2 = 0.04ᵃ	R^2 = 0.07ᵃ	SB = 0.155ᵃ	SB = 0
			A = 0	A = 0
			S = 0	S = 0
Self-Progress	Self-Future	Self-Best	WS = 0	WS = 0
			E = 0	E = 0
A = 0	A = 0	A = 0.121ᵇ	SS = 0.080ᶜ	SS = 0.127ᵃ
S = −0.105ᶜ	S = 0	S = 0	R^2 = 0.50ᵃ	SW = 0.463ᵃ
WS = 0	WS = −0.108ᵇ	WS = 0		R^2 = 0.58ᵃ
E = 0	E = 0	E = 0		N = 644
SS = 0.222ᵃ	SS = 0.113ᵇ	SS = 0.236ᵃ		
R^2 = 0.06ᵃ	R^2 = 0.02ᵇ	R^2 = 0.06ᵃ		

ᵃ $P < 0.001$
ᵇ $P < 0.005$
ᶜ $P < 0.01$
ᵈ $P < 0.05$
0 Significance level too low to enter equation.

It may also have been noticed that, while all of the discrepancy measures are designed to run from the relatively unattractive (= 1) to the attractive (= 7), sometimes a score of 4 indicates a point of congruence and sometimes not. For example, for the self-wants measure 4 indicates "half as well as what you want" and for the self-deserved measure 4 indicates "matches exactly what is deserved". At this point, I don't know if these differences are important or not. However, at least for the self-deserved measure, it is important to have the congruence point at 4 in order to see what happens when people get more than they think they deserve. Examining cross-tabulations and a variety of measures of association between satisfaction and self-deserved discrepancy scores, I found no evidence of a U-shaped relationship. In particular, there was no evidence that satisfaction decreased as one perceived that one was getting more than one deserved. This is contrary to some results cited by Walster, Berscheid and Walster (1976).

Just as no evidence of a U-shaped relationship appeared, there was no evidence that what I call "conditioning variables" function as moderating

EXHIBIT 26
Satisfaction with transportation

Self-Others	Self-Deserved	Self-Needs	Self-Wants	Satisfaction
$A = -0.112^c$	$A = 0$	$A = 0.123^b$	$SO = 0.244^a$	$SO = 0.268^a$
$S = 0$	$S = 0$	$S = -0.077^d$	$SD = 0.109^d$	$SD = 0$
$WS = 0.103^c$	$WS = 0.103^c$	$WS = 0$	$SN = 0.254^a$	$SN = 0.151^a$
$E = 0$	$E = 0$	$E = 0$	$SP = 0.079^d$	$SP = 0$
$SE = 0$	$SE = 0$	$SE = 0$	$SH = 0$	$SH = 0$
$SS = 0$	$SS = 0$	$SS = 0.080^d$	$SB = 0.179^a$	$SB = 0$
$R^2 = 0.01^c$	$R^2 = 0.01^c$	$R^2 = 0.02^d$	$A = 0.128^a$	$A = 0.082^b$
			$S = 0$	$S = 0$

Self-Progress	Self-Future	Self-Best		
			$WS = 0$	$WS = 0$
			$E = 0$	$E = 0$
$A = -0.140^a$	$A = 0$	$A = -0.144^a$	$SE = 0$	$SE = 0.146^a$
$S = 0$	$S = 0$	$S = 0.081^d$	$SS = 0$	$SS = 0$
$WS = 0.113^b$	$WS = -0.083^d$	$WS = 0.172^a$	$R^2 = 0.51^a$	$SW = 0.408^a$
$E = 0$	$E = 0$	$E = 0$		$R^2 = 0.55^a$
$SE = 0$	$SE = 0.091^d$	$SE = 0$		$N = 631$
$SS = 0$	$SS = 0$	$SS = 0$		
$R^2 = 0.02^a$	$R^2 = 0.01^d$	$R^2 = 0.04^a$		

[a] $P \leqslant 0.001$
[b] $P \leqslant 0.005$
[c] $P \leqslant 0.01$
[d] $P \leqslant 0.05$
0 Significance level too low to enter equation.

variables as the latter is understood in LaRocco, House and French (1980) and Zedeck (1971). Examination of over 1700 pairs of equations including one with and one without a conditioning variable in the form of a product term revealed no significant changes in the predictive power of the equations. For example, the predictive strength of self-others discrepancy scores and age was the same as that of self-others scores, age and the product of self-others scores and age.

In correspondence concerning earlier work, Aubrey McKennell suggested that satisfaction and self-want discrepancy variables might merely be two measures of the same thing. Using the strategy recommended by Zeller and Carmines (1980) to distinguish method artifacts from substantive dimensions when factor analysis produces two factors from a data-set, it is possible to test this suggestion. The crux of Zeller and Carmines' argument is the simple observation that if two variables are measuring the same thing, then they ought to have similar relations to other "theoretically relevant external variables ... in terms of direction, strength, and consistency" (Zeller and

EXHIBIT 27
Satisfaction with education

Self-Others	Self-Deserved	Self-Needs	Self-Wants	Satisfaction
A $=0$	A $= 0$	A $=0$	SO $= 0.164^a$	SO $= 0.180^a$
S $=0$	S $=-0.082^d$	S $=0$	SD $= 0.133^a$	SD $= 0.087^d$
WS $=0$	WS $= 0$	WS $=0$	SN $= 0.283^a$	SN $= 0$
E $= 0.187^a$	E $= 0$	E $=0$	SP $= 0$	SP $= 0$
SE $= 0.202^a$	SE $= 0$	SE $=0$	SH $= 0$	SH $= 0$
SS $=0$	SS $= 0.116^b$	SS $= 0.132^a$	SB $= 0.101^c$	SB $= 0.198^a$
$R^2 = 0.08^a$	$R^2 = 0.02^b$	$R^2 = 0.02^a$	A $= 0$	A $= 0$
			S $= 0$	S $= 0$

Self-Progress	Self-Future	Self-Best	Self-Wants	Satisfaction
			WS $= 0$	WS $= 0$
			E $= 0$	E $= 0$
A $= 0$	A $= 0$	A $= 0.079^d$	SE $= 0.120^a$	SE $= 0$
S $=-0.088^d$	S $= 0$	S $= 0$	SS $= 0$	SS $= 0.179^a$
WS $= 0$	WS $=-0.134^a$	WS $= 0$	$R^2 = 0.28^a$	SW $= 0.285^a$
E $= 0$	E $= 0$	E $= 0$		$R^2 = 0.35^a$
SE $= 0$	SE $= 0$	SE $= 0.115^b$		$N = 645$
SS $= 0.126^a$	SS $= 0$	SS $= 0$		
$R^2 = 0.02^b$	$R^2 = 0.02^a$	$R^2 = 0.02^d$		

[a] $P < 0.001$
[b] $P < 0.005$
[c] $P < 0.01$
[d] $P < 0.05$
0 Significance level too low to enter equation.

Carmines, 1980, p. 97). Since this data-set includes 952 cases in which a satisfaction and a self-want discrepancy variable are related to a common third "theoretically relevant external variable", there are plenty of opportunities to apply the Zeller and Carmines test. I looked at every one of these triples, counting the relations as similar if the satisfaction and self-want variables both had significant associations to the third variable in the set (whether the associations were positive or negative), and counting the relations as different only if one of the former variables had a significant relation to the third. Clearly, my criterion of similarity of relations is easier to satisfy than that proposed by Zeller and Carmines. Nevertheless, similar relations were found in only 304 (32%) of the 952 sets of triples. I conclude, therefore, that the satisfaction and self-want discrepancy variables are not merely two measures of the same thing.

As indicated earlier, the predictive success and explanatory power of theories constitute reasonable and minimal measures of adequacy. Unfortunately, they do not constitute unambiguous measures. For example, one

EXHIBIT 28

Comparison of relative impacts of discrepancy types on satisfaction and happiness

	Firsts	Seconds	Thirds	Fourths	Fifths	Sixths	Sevenths	Total weight
Self wants	38	4	0	1	0	0	0	251
Self others	3	31	6	0	0	0	0	197
Self deserved	0	0	11	4	1	0	0	58
Self needs	0	1	9	3	0	0	0	50
Self progress	0	1	5	2	0	0	0	35
Self future	0	0	1	3	0	1	0	14
Self best	2	6	6	2	0	0	0	97

EXHIBIT 29

Comparison of relative impacts of discrepancy types, self-esteem and social support on satisfaction and happiness

	Firsts	Seconds	Thirds	Fourths	Fifths	Sixths	Sevenths	Total weight
Self wants	31	4	5	1	0	1	0	230
Self others	1	29	3	4	3	1	0	182
Self deserved	0	0	3	5	6	2	0	41
Self needs	0	0	7	4	2	0	0	44
Self progress	0	0	3	4	3	0	0	30
Self future	0	0	0	1	2	2	0	14
Self best	1	2	4	9	0	0	0	59
Self esteem	1	2	5	6	5	1	0	65
Social support	9	4	12	5	2	2	0	143

might be more interested in the comparative than in the absolute predictive success ratio of a theory. Does the theory have a success ratio better than chance, better than alternative available theories, or better than any logically possible alternatives? If one says success ratios should be better than chance, does that mean each prediction should have at most a 5% probability of success merely as a result of chance (i.e., the standard assumption about minimal statistical significance when testing particular hypotheses), that each prediction should have at least a 50% probability of success or, perhaps, that the total batting average of the theory, considering all the predictions derived from it, should be at least 50%? Exactly how should the infamous Principle of Indifference be applied here, if at all? I and others have shed enough ink on such questions in other places to allow me to neglect lengthy comment now. However, because I adopted the relatively naive adequacy measure of

Reichenbach (1949) and there is so much more to be said about such things, at least this one paragraph seems warranted. (Interested readers can find my most relevant views on these issues in Michalos 1969, 1971, 1976, 1980b, 1980c, 1983b.)

In an extremely provocative article, Zajonc (1980, p. 151) claimed that,

> Affect is considered by most contemporary theories to be postcognitive, that is, to occur only after considerable cognitive operations have been accomplished. Yet ... [he concludes] that affect and cognition are under the control of separate and partially independent systems that can influence each other in a variety of ways, and that both constitute independent sources of effects in information processing.

Although I have scrupulously tried to avoid any direct reference to affect and its relations to cognition, a few words are in order. (I will have a detailed discussion of these issues in my book on *A Pragmatic Theory of Value*.)

Basically, I believe that *affect* is an *effect* of cognitive and, more precisely, conative operations, as well as a *cause* of a variety of actions broadly construed (i.e., including cognition). This is suggested by Exhibits 1 and 2, but it is not made explicit. The perceptual core of MDT that is illustrated in Exhibit 2 shows net satisfaction as the effect of several antecedents, while the full theory illustrated in Exhibit 1 shows net satisfaction as the cause of action. My unstated assumption is that the causal antecedents specified in the basic hypotheses of MDT, H1–H6, are sufficient to produce any effects that are logically entailed by the concepts of satisfaction and happiness. Because any plausible conceptual analysis of net satisfaction and happiness would have to entail some reference to positive and negative affect, it follows that the working assumption of MDT is that any affective experiences connected to satisfaction and happiness are also caused by the antecedents specified in the theory.

Strictly speaking, then, the formulation of MDT that has guided this research is an oversimplification of my views about the relations between cognition, conation and affect. At this point my views are not entirely clear and it is, therefore, impossible for me to make MDT more precise. On the one hand, affect is a *signal* of previous cognition and conation; it is the felt aspect of thinking, wanting, needing and so on. On the other hand, affect is a *motivating force*; it is the felt aspect of attention, interest, purposiveness and so on. Research like that of Schwarz and Clore (1983) and Wills (1981) focuses on the motivating or causal nature of affect, while most of my research, including the present paper, has focused on the causal antecedents of affect insofar as affect is implied by satisfaction and happiness.

In his *magnum opus* of 1890, *The Principles of Psychology*, William James clearly recognized that cognitions are virtually always found fused with feelings and interests. So, theories that boldly (or naively) try to assign some priority to one or the other are almost certainly engaged in some sort of scientific oversimplification. James, of course, would have been the first to allow such speculation, for his view of theories was that "none is absolutely a transcript of reality, but any of them may be useful. Their great use is to summarize old facts and to lead to new ones." (From James' *Pragmatism* (1907) according to Barzun, 1983, p. 86). It is in this spirit that MDT has been proposed, with its relatively primitive view of the relation between cognition and affect.

Finally, some mention should be made of the voluntarism which is at the heart of MDT and my own brand of pragmatic philosophy. It is a familiar fact of everyone's experience and a well-documented fact of psychological research that people can be persuaded or can persuade themselves to be more or less satisfied or happy with a wide variety of features of their lives (Diener (1984), Schwarz and Clore (1983), Fordyce (1983), Michalos (1985)). At a minimum that implies that in some circumstances, some kind of cognitive activity has some kind of priority over some kind of affect. The particular kinds of cognitive activities and the resulting affective states posited by MDT have already been explained. What must be emphasized now is the immense practical significance of the proposed causal sequence. Insofar as MDT is a reliable and valid representation of reality, the idea of *managing* satisfaction and happiness is plausible. This, of course, has a bright as well as a dark side.

On the bright side, MDT provides a moderately confirmed theoretical justification for education and rational persuasion. After all, if peoples' satisfaction and happiness are functions of how they perceive and think about their own and others wants, needs, deserts, status, etc., then there is a fundamental role to be played by all (informal and formal) education institutions. People's satisfaction and happiness can be more or less cognitively well-founded, and reasonable people will want to be sure that they are essentially well-founded.

On the darker side, however, MDT provides the same moderately confirmed theoretical justification for those who are inclined, wittingly or not, to pernicious manipulation. Enough has been written about misleading advertising (Michalos, 1980d) and the role of freedom of information in democracies

(Galnoor, 1977), to allow us to add nothing here. For our purposes, the important point is that the very same psychological processes that make it possible to rightly persuade people of things that are true, good and beautiful, also make it possible to wrongly persuade people of their opposites, falsehoods, evil and ugliness. Wills (1981) reviews a depressingly long list of studies showing that people's satisfaction can be increased by making "downward comparisons" with less fortunate others. It would be sad if this sort of satisfaction and happiness management caught on, and instead of trying to improve the world, most people merely tried to make themselves feel good by either actively inflicting or acquiescing while others inflicted hardship on relatively defenseless people. Wills' research suggests that this scenario is far from fantastic. Clearly, then, besides having a socio-psychological theory that assures us that people's satisfaction and happiness can be managed, we must have a theory of value and a moral theory to help us identify *good management* in the broadest sense of these terms. These latter theories I hope to provide in my treatise on value. The present version of MDT is a first installment.

SUMMARY

In this article I have introduced a fairly thorough account of multiple discrepancies theory (MDT), briefly reviewed its historical antecedents and submitted it to some empirical testing . The tests were made on a sample of 700 undergraduate students from the University of Guelph's 1984 summer term . The main results were as follows:

(a) Of 2184 predictions made from MDT, 771 (35%) were successful;

(b) Of a subset of 528 predictions involving only effects of perceived discrepancies, 289 (55%) were successful;

(c) MDT explained 49% of the variance in reported happiness scores for the whole group, 53% in global satisfaction and 50% or more in seven out of twelve domain satisfaction scores;

(d) MDT was most successful in accounting for the variance in satisfaction with financial security (58%), paid employment (59%), recreation activity (56%), religion (62%) and self-esteem (58%);

(e) Prediction success rates from six discrepancy variables to the self-wants variable were higher than the rates from the same six variables to satisfaction and happiness, indicating that the impact of the six variables on our main dependent variables is most often indirect rather than direct;

(f) On average, the global satisfaction and happiness of females was influenced by satisfaction in more domains than that of males;

(g) In five out of six cases, MDT explained more of the variance in happiness and global satisfaction than an analytic model positing global well-being as a linear function of domain satisfactions;

(h) Some evidence was produced suggesting that in terms of relative explanatory power, a rank ordering may be formed with aspiration theory at the top, followed by the theories of social comparison, equity, person-environment fit and finally cognitive dissonance;

(i) The voluntaristic, pragmatic philosophy underlying MDT was emphasized, including its immense practical significance for good or evil.

APPENDIX A

EXHIBIT A.1
Satisfaction with life as a whole

Males

Self-Others	Self-Deserved	Self-Needs	Self-Wants	Satisfaction
A = 0	A = −0.165[b]	A = −0.125[d]	SO = 0.173[b]	SO = 0.110[d]
WS = 0	WS = 0	WS = 0	SD = 0	SD = 0
E = 0	E = 0	E = 0	SN = 0.261[a]	SN = 0
SE = 0.260[a]	SE = 0.176[b]	SE = 0.149[c]	SP = 0.186[a]	SP = 0
SS = 0.237[a]	SS = 0.138[d]	SS = 0.187[b]	SH = 0	SH = −0.093[d]
R^2 = 0.16[a]	R^2 = 0.09[a]	R^2 = 0.09²	SB = 0	SB = 0.129[c]
			A = 0	A = 0
Self-Progress	**Self-Future**	**Self-Best**	WS = 0	WS = 0
			E = 0	E = 0
A = 0	A = 0	A = 0	SE = 0.176[a]	SE = 0.252[a]
WS = −0.132[d]	WS = −0.119[d]	WS = 0	SS = 0.122[d]	SS = 0.262[a]
E = 0	E = 0	E = 0	R^2 = 0.38[a]	SW = 0.266[a]
SE = 0.218[a]	SE = 0	SE = 0.209[a]		R^2 = 0.50[a]
SS = 0.145[c]	SS = 0	SS = 0.186[b]		N = 283
R^2 = 0.09[a]	R^2 = 0.01[d]	R^2 = 0.10[a]		

Females

Self-Others	Self-Deserved	Self-Needs	Self-Wants	Satisfaction
A = −0.137[c]	A = 0	A = −0.121[d]	SO = 0.111[d]	SO = 0
WS = 0	WS = 0	WS = 0	SD = 0.167[b]	SD = 0.104[c]
E = 0.158[b]	E = 0	E = 0	SN = 0.185[a]	SN = 0
SE = 0.337[a]	SE = 0	SE = 0	SP = 0.167[a]	SP = 0
SS = 0.142[c]	SS = 0.305[a]	SS = 0.268[a]	SH = 0	SH = 0
R^2 = 0.20[a]	R^2 = 0.09[a]	R^2 = 0.08[a]	SB = 0	SB = 0.130[b]
			A = 0	A = 0
Self-Progress	**Self-Future**	**Self-Best**	WS = 0	WS = 0
			E = 0	E = 0
A = 0	A = −0.141[c]	A = 0	SE = 0.166[a]	SE = 0.305[a]
WS = 0	WS = 0	WS = 0	SS = 0.165[a]	SS = 0.278[a]
E = 0	E = 0	E = 0	R^2 = 0.40[a]	SW = 0.256[a]
SE = 0.235[a]	SE = 0	SE = 0.160[b]		R^2 = 0.56[a]
SS = 0.140[c]	SS = 0.150[b]	SS = 0.228[a]		N = 340
R^2 = 0.09[a]	R^2 = 0.04[a]	R^2 = 0.10[a]		

EXHIBIT A.2
Happiness with life as a whole

Males

Self-Others	Self-Deserved	Self-Needs	Self-Wants	Happiness
A = 0	A = -0.165^b	A = -0.125^d	SO = 0.173^b	SO = 0.152^b
WS = 0	WS = 0	WS = 0	SD = 0	SD = 0.109^b
E = 0	E = 0	E = 0	SN = 0.261^a	SN = 0
SE = 0.260^a	SE = 0.176^b	SE = 0.149^c	SP = 0.186^a	SP = 0
SS = 0.237^a	SS = 0.138^d	SS = 0.187^b	SH = 0	SH = 0
R^2 = 0.16^a	R^2 = 0.09^a	R^2 = 0.09^a	SB = 0	SB = 0.270^a
			A = 0	A = 0
			WS = 0	WS = 0
			E = 0	E = 0
Self-Progress	Self-Future	Self-Best	SE = 0.176^a	SE = 0.175^a
			SS = 0.122^d	SS = 0.205^a
A = 0	A = 0	A = 0	R^2 = 0.38^a	SW = 0.108^d
WS = -0.132^d	WS = -0.119^d	WS = 0		R^2 = 0.45^a
E = 0	E = 0	E = 0		N = 283
SE = 0.218^a	SE = 0	SE = 0.209^a		
SS = 0.145^c	SS = 0	SS = 0.186^b		
R^2 = 0.09^a	R^2 = 0.01^d	R^2 = 0.10^a		

Females

Self-Others	Self-Deserved	Self-Needs	Self-Wants	Happiness
A = -0.137^c	A = 0	A = -0.121^d	SO = 0.111^d	SO = 0.113^c
WS = 0	WS = 0	WS = 0	SD = 0.167^b	SD = 0
E = 0.158^b	E = 0	E = 0	SN = 0.185^a	SN = 0.125^b
SE = 0.337^a	SE = 0	SE = 0	SP = 0.167^a	SP = 0
SS = 0.142^c	SS = 0.305^a	SS = 0.268^a	SH = 0	SH = 0
R^2 = 0.20^a	R^2 = 0.09^a	R^2 = 0.08^a	SB = 0	SB = 0.164^a
			A = 0	A = 0
Self-Progress	Self-Future	Self-Best	WS = 0	WS = 0.095^c
			E = 0	E = 0
A = 0	A = -0.141^c	A = 0	SE = 0.166^a	SE = 0.219^a
WS = 0	WS = 0	WS = 0	SS = 0.165^a	SS = 0.246^a
E = 0	E = 0	E = 0	R^2 = 0.40^a	SW = 0.207^a
SE = 0.235^a	SE = 0	SE = 0.160^b		R^2 = 0.53^a
SS = 0.140^c	SS = 0.150^b	SS = 0.228^a		N = 340
R^2 = 0.09^a	R^2 = 0.04^a	R^2 = 0.10^a		

EXHIBIT A.3
Satisfaction with health

Males

Self-Others	Self-Deserved	Self-Needs	Self-Wants	Satisfaction
A $=0$	A $=0$	A $=0$	SO $=$ 0.427[a]	SO $=$ 0.189[a]
WS $=0$	WS $=0$	WS $=0$	SD $=$ 0	SD $=$ 0
E $=0$	E $=0$	E $=0$	SN $=$ 0.128[c]	SN $=$ 0
SE $=0.180$[b]	SE $=0.155$[b]	SE $=0.117$[d]	SP $=$ 0.139[c]	SP $=$ 0
SS $=0$	SS $=0$	SS $=0$	SH $=-0.129$[b]	SH $=-0.088$[d]
$R^2=0.03$[b]	$R^2=0.02$[b]	$R^2=0.01$[d]	SB $=$ 0.105[d]	SB $=$ 0
			A $=$ 0	A $=$ 0
Self-Progress	Self-Future	Self-Best	WS $=$ 0	WS $=$ 0
			E $=$ 0	E $=$ 0
A $=0$	A $=0$	A $=$ 0	SE $=$ 0.160[a]	SE $=$ 0
WS $=0$	WS $=0$	WS $=-0.137$[d]	SS $=$ 0.106[d]	SS $=$ 0.167[a]
E $=0$	E $=0$	E $=$ 0	$R^2=$ 0.48[a]	SW $=$ 0.491[a]
SE $=0.150$[c]	SE $=0$	SE $=$ 0.115[d]		$R^2=$ 0.46[a]
SS $=0$	SS $=0.115$[d]	SS $=$ 0		$N =$ 296
$R^2=0.02$[c]	$R^2=0.01$[d]	$R^2=$ 0.02[c]		

Females

Self-Others	Self-Deserved	Self-Needs	Self-Wants	Satisfaction
A $=0$	A $=0$	A $=$ 0	SO $=$ 0.364[a]	SO $=0.168$[a]
WS $=0$	WS $=0$	WS $=-0.129$[c]	SD $=$ 0	SD $=0.129$[b]
E $=0.178$[a]	E $=0$	E $=$ 0.112[d]	SN $=$ 0.178[a]	SN $=0$
SE $=0$	SE $=0$	SE $=$ 0	SP $=$ 0.126[c]	SP $=0$
SS $=0$	SS $=0$	SS $=$ 0.163[b]	SH $=-0.081$[d]	SH $=0$
$R^2=0.03$[a]	$R^2=0$	$R^2=$ 0.04[a]	SB $=$ 0.190[a]	SB $=0$
			A $=$ 0	A $=0$
Self-Progress	Self-Future	Self-Best	WS $=$ 0	WS $=0$
			E $=$ 0	E $=0$
A $=0$	A $=0$	A $=0$	SE $=$ 0.151[a]	SE $=0.160$[a]
WS $=0$	WS $=0$	WS $=0$	SS $=$ 0	SS $=0$
E $=0$	E $=0$	E $=0$	$R^2=$ 0.49[a]	SW $=0.493$[a]
SE $=0.257$[a]	SE $=0$	SE $=0.206$[a]		$R^2=0.53$[a]
SS $=0$	SS $=0.149$[b]	SS $=0$		$N =341$
$R^2=0.06$[a]	$R^2=0.02$[b]	$R^2=0.04$[a]		

EXHIBIT A.4
Satisfaction with financial security

Males

Self-Others	Self-Deserved	Self-Needs	Self-Wants	Satisfaction
A = −0.296[a]	A = −0.157[c]	A = −0.188[a]	SO = 0.245[a]	SO = 0.284[a]
WS = 0.179[b]	WS = 0	WS = 0	SD = 0.250[a]	SD = 0
E = 0	E = 0	E = 0	SN = 0.246[a]	SN = 0.172[a]
SE = 0	SE = 0	SE = 0	SP = 0	SP = −0.100[d]
SS = 0.122[d]	SS = 0	SS = 0	SH = 0	SH = −0.077[d]
R^2 = 0.11[a]	R^2 = 0.02[c]	R^2 = 0.03[a]	SB = 0.113[d]	SB = 0.153[b]
			A = 0.125[c]	A = 0
Self-Progress	Self-Future	Self-Best	WS = 0	WS = 0
			E = 0	E = 0
A = −0.234[a]	A = 0	A = −0.282[a]	SE = 0	SE = 0
WS = 0	WS = 0	WS = 0.171[b]	SS = 0	SS = 0
E = 0	E = 0	E = 0	R^2 = 0.42[a]	SW = 0.401[a]
SE = 0	SE = 0	SE = 0		R^2 = 0.59[a]
SS = 0	SS = 0	SS = 0		N = 293
R^2 = 0.05[a]	R^2 = 0	R^2 = 0.08[a]		

Females

Self-Others	Self-Deserved	Self-Needs	Self-Wants	Satisfaction
A = −0.176[a]	A = −0.182[a]	A = −0.109[d]	SO = 0.180[a]	SO = 0.200[a]
WS = 0.132[d]	WS = 0	WS = 0	SD = 0	SD = 0.120[c]
E = 0	E = 0	E = 0	SN = 0.415[a]	SN = 0.155[b]
SE = 0	SE = 0	SE = 0	SP = 0	SP = 0.128[b]
SS = 0	SS = 0	SS = 0	SH = 0	SH = 0
R^2 = 0.03[b]	R^2 = 0.03[a]	R^2 = 0.01[d]	SB = 0.225[a]	SB = 0
			A = 0.091[d]	A = 0
Self-Progress	Self-Future	Self-Best	WS = 0	WS = 0
			E = 0	E = 0
A = −0.136[c]	A = 0	A = −0.116[d]	SE = 0	SE = 0
WS = 0	WS = 0	WS = 0.182[a]	SS = 0.079[d]	SS = 0.112[b]
E = 0	E = 0	E = 0	R^2 = 0.51[a]	SW = 0.324[a]
SE = 0	SE = 0	SE = 0		R^2 = 0.59[a]
SS = 0.211[a]	SS = 0.182[a]	SS = 0		N = 341
R^2 = 0.06[a]	R^2 = 0.03[a]	R^2 = 0.03[b]		

EXHIBIT A.5
Satisfaction with family relations

Males

Self-Others	Self-Deserved	Self-Needs	Self-Wants	Satisfaction
A = -0.127^c	A = 0	A = -0.123^c	SO = 0.378^a	SO = 0.160^a
WS = 0	WS = 0	WS = 0	SD = 0	SD = 0
E = 0	E = 0	E = 0	SN = 0.281^a	SN = 0.173^a
SE = 0	SE = 0	SE = 0	SP = 0	SP = 0
SS = 0.532^a	SS = 0.443^a	SS = 0.535^a	SH = 0	SH = 0
R^2 = 0.31^a	R^2 = 0.19^a	R^2 = 0.32^a	SB = 0.104^d	SB = 0
			A = 0	A = 0
Self-Progress	Self-Future	Self-Best	WS = 0	WS = 0
			E = 0	E = 0
A = 0	A = 0	A = 0	SE = 0	SE = 0
WS = 0	WS = 0	WS = 0	SS = 0.156^b	SS = 0.485^a
E = 0	E = 0	E = 0	R^2 = 0.57^a	SW = 0.222^a
SE = -0.122^d	SE = 0	SE = 0		R^2 = 0.77^a
SS = 0.413^a	SS = 0.160^c	SS = 0.358^a		N = 290
R^2 = 0.15^a	R^2 = 0.02^c	R^2 = 0.13^a		

Females

Self-Others	Self-Deserved	Self-Needs	Self-Wants	Satisfaction
A = 0	A = 0	A = -0.116^c	SO = 0.300^a	SO = 0.219^a
WS = 0	WS = -0.148^b	WS = 0	SD = 0.154^a	SD = 0
E = 0	E = 0	E = 0	SN = 0.165^a	SN = 0.085^c
SE = 0	SE = 0	SE = 0	SP = 0	SP = 0
SS = 0.607^a	SS = 0.468^a	SS = 0.468^a	SH = 0	SH = 0
R^2 = 0.37^a	R^2 = 0.23^a	R^2 = 0.23^a	SB = 0	SB = 0
			A = 0	A = 0
Self-Progress	Self-Future	Self-Best	WS = 0	WS = 0
			E = 0	E = 0
A = 0	A = 0	A = 0	SE = 0	SE = -0.069^c
WS = 0	WS = -0.198^a	WS = 0	SS = 0.340^a	SS = 0.544^a
E = 0	E = 0	E = 0	R^2 = 0.62^a	SW = 0.215^a
SE = 0	SE = 0	SE = 0		R^2 = 0.81^a
SS = 0.430^a	SS = 0.189^a	SS = 0.473^a		N = 341
R^2 = 0.18^a	R^2 = 0.07^a	R^2 = 0.22^a		

EXHIBIT A.6
Satisfaction with paid employment

Males

Self-Others	Self-Deserved	Self-Needs	Self-Wants	Satisfaction
A =0	A =0	A =0	SO = 0.377[a]	SO = 0.324[a]
WS = 0.478[a]	WS = 0	WS = 0.228[a]	SD = 0.168[c]	SD = 0
E =0	E =0	E =0	SN = 0.171[d]	SN = 0
SE =0	SE =0	SE =0	SP = 0	SP = 0
SS =0.172[b]	SS =0	SS =0	SH = 0	SH = 0
R^2 = 0.26[a]	R^2 = 0	R^2 = 0.05[a]	SB = 0	SB = 0
			A = 0	A = 0
Self-Progress	**Self-Future**	**Self-Best**	WS = 0.196[a]	WS = 0.240[a]
			E = 0	E = 0
A =0	A =0	A = −0.196[b]	SE = 0	SE = 0
WS = 0	WS = 0	WS = 0.387[a]	SS = 0	SS = 0
E =0	E =0	E = 0	R^2 = 0.49[a]	SW = 0.334[a]
SE =0	SE =0	SE = 0		R^2 = 0.55[a]
SS =0	SS =0	SS = 0		N = 173
R^2 =0	R^2 =0	R^2 = 0.14[a]		

Females

Self-Others	Self-Deserved	Self-Needs	Self-Wants	Satisfaction
A = −0.270[a]	A = −0.182[c]	A = −0.176[c]	SO = 0.228[a]	SO = 0.195[a]
WS = 0.529[a]	WS = 0.224[a]	WS = 0.319[a]	SD = 0.167[c]	SD = 0.188[a]
E = 0	E = 0	E = 0	SN = 0.326[a]	SN = 0
SE = 0	SE = 0	SE = 0	SP = 0	SP = 0
SS = 0	SS = 0	SS = 0	SH = 0	SH = 0.133[b]
R^2 = 0.27[a]	R^2 = 0.05[a]	R^2 = 0.10[a]	SB = 0	SB = 0
			A = 0	A = 0
Self-Progress	**Self-Future**	**Self-Best**	WS = 0.203[a]	WS = 0.231[a]
			E = 0	E = 0
A = −0.152[d]	A = −0.126[d]	A = −0.270[a]	SE = 0	SE = 0
WS = 0.266[a]	WS = 0	WS = 0.595[a]	SS = 0	SS = 0.169[a]
E = 0	E = 0	E = 0	R^2 = 0.49[a]	SW = 0.369[a]
SE = 0	SE = 0	SE = 0		R^2 = 0.68[a]
SS = 0.121[d]	SS = 0.163[b]	SS = 0		N = 192
R^2 = 0.08[a]	R^2 = 0.04[a]	R^2 = 0.34[a]		

EXHIBIT A.7

Satisfaction with friendships

Males

Self-Others	Self-Deserved	Self-Needs	Self-Wants	Satisfaction
A = 0	A = 0	A = 0	SO = 0.387[a]	SO = 0.201[a]
WS = 0	WS = 0	WS = 0	SD = 0	SD = 0
E = 0	E = 0	E = 0	SN = 0.087[d]	SN = 0
SE = 0.170[a]	SE = 0	SE = 0.190[a]	SP = 0.100[d]	SP = 0
SS = 0.547[a]	SS = 0.361[a]	SS = 0.413[a]	SH = 0	SH = 0
R^2 = 0.38[a]	R^2 = 0.13[a]	R^2 = 0.25[a]	SB = 0	SB = 0.101[b]
			A = 0.093[c]	A = 0
Self-Progress	Self-Future	Self-Best	WS = 0	WS = 0
			E = 0	E = 0
A = 0	A = 0	A = 0	SE = 0.122[b]	SE = 0
WS = 0	WS = 0	WS = 0	SS = 0.304[a]	SS = 0.528[a]
E = 0	E = 0	E = 0	R^2 = 0.60[a]	SW = 0.191[a]
SE = 0	SE = 0	SE = 0		R^2 = 0.76[a]
SS = 0.348[a]	SS = 0	SS = 0.433[a]		N = 294
R^2 = 0.12[a]	R^2 = 0	R^2 = 0.19[a]		

Females

Self-Others	Self-Deserved	Self-Needs	Self-Wants	Satisfaction
A = 0	A = 0	A = 0	SO = 0.331[a]	SO = 0.082[d]
WS = 0	WS = 0	WS = 0	SD = 0	SD = 0
E = 0	E = 0	E = 0	SN = 0.147[b]	SN = 0
SE = 0.117[c]	SE = 0	SE = 0	SP = 0	SP = 0.104[b]
SS = 0.502[a]	SS = 0.417[a]	SS = 0.407[a]	SH = 0	SH = 0
R^2 = 0.30[a]	R^2 = 0.17[a]	R^2 = 0.16[a]	SB = 0.132[b]	SB = 0
			A = 0.081[d]	A = 0
Self-Progress	Self-Future	Self-Best	WS = 0	WS = 0
			E = 0	E = 0
A = 0	A = −0.204[a]	A = 0	SE = 0.104[c]	SE = 0
WS = 0	WS = 0	WS = 0.138[b]	SS = 0.237[a]	SS = 0.556[a]
E = 0	E = 0	E = 0	R^2 = 0.52[a]	SW = 0.284[a]
SE = 0.129[c]	SE = 0	SE = 0		R^2 = 0.74[a]
SS = 0.329[a]	SS = 0	SS = 0.408[a]		N = 345
R^2 = 0.15[a]	R^2 = 0.04[a]	R^2 = 0.19[a]		

EXHIBIT A.8
Satisfaction with housing

Males

Self-Others	Self-Deserved	Self-Needs	Self-Wants	Satisfaction
$A = -0.231^a$	$A = 0$	$A = 0$	$SO = 0.369^a$	$SO = 0.244^a$
$WS = 0.186^a$	$WS = 0$	$WS = 0$	$SD = 0.219^a$	$SD = 0.175^a$
$E = 0$	$E = 0$	$E = 0$	$SN = 0$	$SN = 0$
$SE = 0$	$SE = 0$	$SE = 0$	$SP = 0.184^a$	$SP = 0$
$SS = 0.180^a$	$SS = 0$	$SS = 0.154^c$	$SH = 0$	$SH = 0$
$R^2 = 0.10^a$	$R^2 = 0$	$R^2 = 0.02^c$	$SB = 0$	$SB = 0$
			$A = 0$	$A = 0.098^d$
Self-Progress	Self-Future	Self-Best	$WS = 0$	$WS = 0$
			$E = 0$	$E = 0$
$A = -0.218^a$	$A = 0$	$A = -0.169^c$	$SE = 0$	$SE = 0$
$WS = 0.179^b$	$WS = 0$	$WS = 0.120^d$	$SS = 0$	$SS = 0.187^a$
$E = 0$	$E = 0$	$E = 0.172^c$	$R^2 = 0.38^a$	$SW = 0.353^a$
$SE = -0.138^c$	$SE = 0$	$SE = 0$		$R^2 = 0.46^a$
$SS = 0$	$SS = 0$	$SS = 0$		$N = 290$
$R^2 = 0.06^a$	$R^2 = 0$	$R^2 = 0.04^b$		

Females

Self-Others	Self-Deserved	Self-Needs	Self-Wants	Satisfaction
$A = 0$	$A = 0$	$A = -0.121^d$	$SO = 0.295^a$	$SO = 0.275^a$
$WS = 0$	$WS = 0$	$WS = 0$	$SD = 0$	$SD = 0$
$E = 0$	$E = 0$	$E = 0.167^b$	$SN = 0.218^a$	$SN = 0$
$SE = 0$	$SE = 0$	$SE = 0$	$SP = 0$	$SP = 0.183^a$
$SS = 0.116^d$	$SS = 0$	$SS = 0$	$SH = 0$	$SH = 0$
$R^2 = 0.01^d$	$R^2 = 0$	$R^2 = 0.02^c$	$SB = 0.236^a$	$SB = 0$
			$A = 0.102^d$	$A = 0$
Self-Progress	Self-Future	Self-Best	$WS = 0$	$WS = 0$
			$E = 0$	$E = 0$
$A = -0.214^a$	$A = -0.106^d$	$A = 0$	$SE = 0$	$SE = 0.111^c$
$WS = 0$	$WS = 0$	$WS = 0$	$SS = 0$	$SS = 0.117^c$
$E = 0.152^c$	$E = 0$	$E = 0$	$R^2 = 0.36^a$	$SW = 0.301^a$
$SE = 0$	$SE = 0$	$SE = 0$		$R^2 = 0.44^a$
$SS = 0$	$SS = 0.127^d$	$SS = 0$		$N = 341$
$R^2 = 0.04^a$	$R^2 = 0.02^c$	$R^2 = 0$		

EXHIBIT A.9

Satisfaction with area lived in

Males

Self-Others	Self-Deserved	Self-Needs	Self-Wants	Satisfaction
A $=-0.118^d$	A $=-0.200^a$	A $=-0.188^b$	SO $=$ 0.257^a	SO $=0.228^a$
WS $=$ 0	WS $=$ 0.120^d	WS $=$ 0.141^d	SD $=$ 0	SD $=0.125^c$
E $=$ 0	E $=$ 0	E $=$ 0	SN $=$ 0.215^a	SN $=0$
SE $=$ 0	SE $=$ 0	SE $=$ 0	SP $=$ 0.275^a	SP $=0$
SS $=$ 0.121^d	SS $=$ 0	SS $=$ 0	SH $=-0.095^d$	SH $=0$
$R^2 =$ 0.03^c	$R^2 =$ 0.04^b	$R^2 =$ 0.04^b	SB $=$ 0	SB $=0$
			A $=$ 0	A $=0$
Self-Progress	Self-Future	Self-Best	WS $=$ 0	WS $=0$
			E $=$ 0	E $=0$
A $=-0.176^b$	A $=$ 0	A $=0$	SE $=$ 0	SE $=0$
WS $=$ 0	WS $=-0.120^d$	WS $=0$	SS $=$ 0	SS $=0.225^a$
E $=$ 0	E $=$ 0	E $=0$	$R^2 =$ 0.35^a	SW $=0.420^a$
SE $=$ 0	SE $=$ 0	SE $=0$		$R^2 =0.49^a$
SS $=$ 0	SS $=$ 0	SS $=0.125^d$		N $=291$
$R^2 =$ 0.03^b	$R^2 =$ 0.01^d	$R^2 =0.01^d$		

Females

Self-Others	Self-Deserved	Self-Needs	Self-Wants	Satisfaction
A $=0$	A $=0$	A $=0$	SO $=$ 0.208^a	SO $=0.235^a$
WS $=0$	WS $=0$	WS $=0$	SD $=$ 0	SD $=0$
E $=0.125^d$	E $=0$	E $=0$	SN $=$ 0.217^a	SN $=0$
SE $=0.125^d$	SE $=0$	SE $=0$	SP $=$ 0	SP $=0.136^b$
SS $=0$	SS $=0$	SS $=0$	SH $=-0.171^a$	SH $=0$
$R^2 =0.03^b$	$R^2 =0$	$R^2 =0$	SB $=$ 0.352^a	SB $=0$
			A $=$ 0	A $=0$
Self-Progress	Self-Future	Self-Best	WS $=$ 0	WS $=0$
			E $=$ 0	E $=0$
A $=-0.178^b$	A $=-0.145^c$	A $=0$	SE $=$ 0	SE $=0$
WS $=$ 0	WS $=$ 0	WS $=0$	SS $=$ 0	SS $=0.176^a$
E $=$ 0.138^d	E $=$ 0	E $=0$	$R^2 =$ 0.41^a	SW $=0.417^a$
SE $=$ 0	SE $=$ 0	SE $=0$		$R^2 =0.46^a$
SS $=$ 0	SS $=$ 0.114^d	SS $=0$		N $=343$
$R^2 =$ 0.03^b	$R^2 =$ 0.03^b	$R^2 =0$		

EXHIBIT A.10

Satisfaction with recreation activity

Males

Self-Others	Self-Deserved	Self-Needs	Self-Wants	Satisfaction
A $= 0$	A $= 0$	A $= 0$	SO $= 0.386^a$	SO $= 0.355^a$
WS $= 0$	WS $= 0$	WS $= 0$	SD $= 0.190^a$	SD $= 0$
E $= 0$	E $= 0$	E $= 0$	SN $= 0$	SN $= 0$
SE $= 0.200^a$	SE $= 0.215^a$	SE $= 0.171^b$	SP $= 0.154^c$	SP $= 0$
SS $= 0.171^b$	SS $= 0$	SS $= 0$	SH $= 0$	SH $= 0$
$R^2 = 0.09^a$	$R^2 = 0.04^a$	$R^2 = 0.03^b$	SB $= 0.111^d$	SB $= 0$
			A $= 0$	A $= 0$
Self-Progress	Self-Future	Self-Best	WS $= 0$	WS $= 0$
			E $= 0$	E $= 0$
A $= 0$	A $= 0$	A $= 0$	SE $= 0$	SE $= 0.113^c$
WS $= -0.120^d$	WS $= 0$	WS $= 0$	SS $= 0$	SS $= 0.111^c$
E $= 0$	E $= 0$	E $= 0$	$R^2 = 0.47^a$	SW $= 0.377^a$
SE $= 0.155^c$	SE $= 0$	SE $= 0$		$R^2 = 0.53^a$
SS $= 0$	SS $= 0$	SS $= 0$		$N = 295$
$R^2 = 0.03^b$	$R^2 = 0$	$R^2 = 0$		

Females

Self-Others	Self-Deserved	Self-Needs	Self-Wants	Satisfaction
A $= 0$	A $= 0$	A $= 0$	SO $= 0.394^a$	SO $= 0.200^a$
WS $= 0$	WS $= 0$	WS $= 0$	SD $= 0$	SD $= 0$
E $= 0.151^b$	E $= 0$	E $= 0$	SN $= 0.124^c$	SN $= 0.136^b$
SE $= 0.161^b$	SE $= 0$	SE $= 0$	SP $= 0.121^d$	SP $= 0$
SS $= 0.231^a$	SS $= 0.228^a$	SS $= 0.241^a$	SH $= 0$	SH $= 0$
$R^2 = 0.13^a$	$R^2 = 0.05^a$	$R^2 = 0.06^a$	SB $= 0.180^a$	SB $= 0$
			A $= 0$	A $= 0$
Self-Progress	Self-Future	Self-Best	WS $= 0$	WS $= 0$
			E $= 0$	E $= 0$
A $= 0$	A $= -0.111^d$	A $= 0$	SE $= 0.170^a$	SE $= 0$
WS $= 0$	WS $= 0$	WS $= 0$	SS $= 0$	SS $= 0.136^a$
E $= 0$	E $= 0$	E $= 0$	$R^2 = 0.52^a$	SW $= 0.478^a$
SE $= 0.176^b$	SE $= 0$	SE $= 0$		$R^2 = 0.58^a$
SS $= 0.164^b$	SS $= 0.109^d$	SS $= 0.234^a$		$N = 341$
$R^2 = 0.07^a$	$R^2 = 0.02^c$	$R^2 = 0.05^a$		

EXHIBIT A.11

Satisfaction with religion

Males

Self-Others	Self-Deserved	Self-Needs	Self-Wants	Satisfaction
A $= 0$	A $= 0$	A $= 0$	SO $= 0.433^a$	SO $= 0.327^a$
WS $= 0$	WS $= 0$	WS $= 0$	SD $= 0$	SD $= 0$
E $= 0$	E $= 0$	E $= 0$	SN $= 0.332^a$	SN $= -0.152^c$
SE $= 0$	SE $= 0$	SE $= 0.260^a$	SP $= 0$	SP $= 0$
SS $= 0.212^b$	SS $= 0$	SS $= 0$	SH $= 0$	SH $= 0$
$R^2 = 0.04^b$	$R^2 = 0$	$R^2 = 0.06^a$	SB $= 0$	SB $= 0.189^a$
			A $= 0$	A $= 0$
Self-Progress	Self-Future	Self-Best	WS $= 0$	WS $= 0$
			E $= 0$	E $= 0.105^c$
A $= 0$	A $= 0$	A $= 0$	SE $= 0$	SE $= 0.108^c$
WS $= 0$	WS $= 0$	WS $= 0$	SS $= 0.135^d$	SS $= 0$
E $= 0$	E $= 0$	E $= 0$	$R^2 = 0.45^a$	SW $= 0.531^a$
SE $= 0$	SE $= 0$	SE $= 0$		$R^2 = 0.70^a$
SS $= 0.149^d$	SS $= 0$	SS $= 0.207^b$		$N = 173$
$R^2 = 0.02^d$	$R^2 = 0$	$R^2 = 0.04^b$		

Females

Self-Others	Self-Deserved	Self-Needs	Self-Wants	Satisfaction
A $= 0$	A $= 0$	A $= 0$	SO $= 0.259^a$	SO $= 0.400^a$
WS $= 0$	WS $= 0$	WS $= 0$	SD $= 0$	SD $= 0$
E $= 0$	E $= 0$	E $= 0$	SN $= 0.241^a$	SN $= 0$
SE $= 0.275^a$	SE $= 0$	SE $= 0$	SP $= 0$	SP $= 0.165^b$
SS $= 0$	SS $= 0.184^b$	SS $= 0.167^c$	SH $= 0$	SH $= 0$
$R^2 = 0.07^a$	$R^2 = 0.03^b$	$R^2 = 0.02^c$	SB $= 0.239^a$	SB $= 0$
			A $= 0$	A $= 0$
Self-Progress	Self-Future	Self-Best	WS $= 0$	WS $= 0$
			E $= 0$	E $= -0.111^c$
A $= 0$	A $= -0.142^d$	A $= 0$	SE $= 0.184^a$	SE $= 0.127^c$
WS $= 0$	WS $= 0$	WS $= 0$	SS $= 0$	SS $= 0.103^d$
E $= 0$	E $= 0$	E $= 0$	$R^2 = 0.45^a$	SW $= 0.248^a$
SE $= 0.157^d$	SE $= 0$	SE $= 0$		$R^2 = 0.58^a$
SS $= 0.165^c$	SS $= 0$	SS $= 0.179^b$		$N = 219$
$R^2 = 0.06^a$	$R^2 = 0.02^d$	$R^2 = 0.03^b$		

EXHIBIT A.12

Satisfaction with self-esteem

Males

Self-Others	Self-Deserved	Self-Needs	Self-Wants	Satisfaction
$A = 0$	$A = 0$	$A = 0$	$SO = 0.438^a$	$SO = 0.228^a$
$WS = 0$	$WS = 0$	$WS = 0$	$SD = 0.131^d$	$SD = 0.170^a$
$E = 0$	$E = 0$	$E = 0$	$SN = 0.151^d$	$SN = 0$
$SS = 0.227^a$	$SS = 0.134^d$	$SS = 0.223^a$	$SP = 0$	$SP = 0$
$R^2 = 0.05^a$	$R^2 = 0.02^d$	$R^2 = 0.05^a$	$SH = 0$	$SH = -0.096^d$
			$SB = 0$	$SB = 0$
Self-Progress	Self-Future	Self-Best	$A = 0$	$A = 0$
			$WS = 0$	$WS = 0$
$A = 0$	$A = 0$	$A = 0$	$E = 0$	$E = 0$
$WS = 0$	$WS = -0.134^d$	$WS = 0$	$SS = 0.094^d$	$SS = 0.160^a$
$E = 0$	$E = 0$	$E = 0$	$R^2 = 0.42^a$	$SW = 0.400^a$
$SS = 0.156^c$	$SS = 0$	$SS = 0.174^b$		$R^2 = 0.54^a$
$R^2 = 0.02^c$	$R^2 = 0.02^d$	$R^2 = 0.03^b$		$N = 293$

Females

Self-Others	Self-Deserved	Self-Needs	Self-Wants	Satisfaction
$A = 0$	$A = 0$	$A = 0$	$SO = 0.247^a$	$SO = 0.305^a$
$WS = 0$	$WS = 0$	$WS = -0.123^d$	$SD = 0.143^d$	$SD = 0$
$E = 0$	$E = 0$	$E = 0$	$SN = 0.314^a$	$SN = 0$
$SS = 0.294^a$	$SS = 0.198^a$	$SS = 0.276^a$	$SP = 0$	$SP = 0$
$R^2 = 0.08^a$	$R^2 = 0.04^a$	$R^2 = 0.08^a$	$SH = 0$	$SH = 0$
			$SB = 0.154^a$	$SB = 0$
Self-Progress	Self-Future	Self-Best	$A = 0.146^a$	$A = 0$
			$WS = 0$	$WS = 0$
$A = 0$	$A = 0$	$A = 0.129^c$	$E = 0$	$E = 0$
$WS = 0$	$WS = 0$	$WS = 0$	$SS = 0.089^d$	$SS = 0.115^b$
$E = 0$	$E = -0.134^c$	$E = 0$	$R^2 = 0.54^a$	$SW = 0.491^a$
$SS = 0.291^a$	$SS = 0.140^c$	$SS = 0.285^a$		$R^2 = 0.61^a$
$R^2 = 0.08^a$	$R^2 = 0.03^b$	$R^2 = 0.09^a$		$N = 340$

EXHIBIT A.13

Satisfaction with transportation

Males

Self-Others	Self-Deserved	Self-Needs	Self-Wants	Satisfaction
A $= -0.213^a$	A $= 0$	A $= -0.193^a$	SO $= 0.258^a$	SO $= 0.282^a$
WS $= 0.188^b$	WS $= 0.160^c$	WS $= 0.222^a$	SD $= 0$	SD $= 0$
E $= 0$	E $= 0$	E $= 0$	SN $= 0.230^a$	SN $= 0.176^b$
SE $= 0$	SE $= 0$	SE $= 0$	SP $= 0.168^b$	SP $= 0$
SS $= 0$	SS $= 0$	SS $= 0$	SH $= 0$	SH $= 0$
$R^2 = 0.05^a$	$R^2 = 0.02^c$	$R^2 = 0.06^a$	SB $= 0.205^a$	SB $= 0$
			A $= 0.103^d$	A $= 0.083^d$
Self-Progress	Self-Future	Self-Best	WS $= 0$	WS $= 0$
			E $= 0$	E $= 0$
A $= -0.244^a$	A $= 0$	A $= -0.276^a$	SE $= 0$	SE $= 0.117^b$
WS $= 0.119^d$	WS $= -0.133^d$	WS $= 0.213^a$	SS $= 0$	SS $= 0$
E $= 0$	E $= 0$	E $= 0$	$R^2 = 0.48^a$	SW $= 0.377^a$
SE $= 0$	SE $= 0$	SE $= 0$		$R^2 = 0.52^a$
SS $= 0$	SS $= 0$	SS $= 0$		$N = 285$
$R^2 = 0.05^a$	$R^2 = 0.01^d$	$R^2 = 0.08^a$		

Females

Self-Others	Self-Deserved	Self-Needs	Self-Wants	Satisfaction
A $= 0$	A $= 0$	A $= 0$	SO $= 0.247^a$	SO $= 0.243^a$
WS $= 0$	WS $= 0$	WS $= 0$	SD $= 0.143^d$	SD $= 0.177^a$
E $= 0$	E $= 0$	E $= 0$	SN $= 0.314^a$	SN $= 0$
SE $= 0$	SE $= -0.119^d$	SE $= -0.157^b$	SP $= 0$	SP $= 0$
SS $= 0$	SS $= 0$	SS $= 0$	SH $= 0$	SH $= 0$
$R^2 = 0$	$R^2 = 0.01^d$	$R^2 = 0.02^b$	SB $= 0.154^a$	SB $= 0$
			A $= 0.146^a$	A $= 0.092^c$
Self-Progress	Self-Future	Self-Best	WS $= 0$	WS $= 0$
			E $= 0$	E $= 0$
A $= 0$	A $= 0$	A $= 0$	SE $= 0.089^d$	SE $= 0.169^a$
WS $= 0$	WS $= 0$	WS $= 0.130^c$	SS $= 0$	SS $= 0$
E $= 0$	E $= 0$	E $= 0$	$R^2 = 0.54^a$	SW $= 0.415^a$
SE $= 0$	SE $= 0$	SE $= 0$		$R^2 = 0.57^a$
SS $= 0$	SS $= 0.174^a$	SS $= 0$		$N = 336$
$R^2 = 0$	$R^2 = 0.03^a$	$R^2 = 0.01^c$		

EXHIBIT A.14

Satisfaction with education

Males

Self-Others	Self-Deserved	Self-Needs	Self-Wants	Satisfaction
A $=0$	A $=0$	A $=0$	SO $= 0.218^a$	SO $= 0.158^b$
WS $= 0$	WS $= 0$	WS $= 0$	SD $= 0$	SD $= 0$
E $= 0.172^b$	E $= 0$	E $= 0$	SN $= 0.291^a$	SN $= 0$
SE $= 0.178^b$	SE $= 0$	SE $= 0$	SP $= 0$	SP $= 0$
SS $= 0$	SS $= 0.155^c$	SS $= 0.149^c$	SH $= 0$	SH $= 0$
$R^2 = 0.06^a$	$R^2 = 0.02^c$	$R^2 = 0.02^c$	SB $= 0.191^a$	SB $= 0.205^a$
			A $= 0$	A $= 0$
Self-Progress	Self-Future	Self-Best	WS $= 0$	WS $= 0$
			E $= 0$	E $= 0$
A $= 0$	A $= 0$	A $= 0$	SE $= 0$	SE $= 0$
WS $= 0$	WS $= -0.239^a$	WS $= 0$	SS $= 0$	SS $= 0.251^a$
E $= 0$	E $= 0$	E $= 0$	$R^2 = 0.26^a$	SW $= 0.286^a$
SE $= 0$	SE $= 0$	SE $= 0$		$R^2 = 0.34^a$
SS $= 0.130^d$	SS $= 0$	SS $= 0.130^d$		N $= 295$
$R^2 = 0.01^d$	$R^2 = 0.05^a$	$R^2 = 0.01^d$		

Females

Self-Others	Self-Deserved	Self-Needs	Self-Wants	Satisfaction
A $= 0$	A $= 0$	A $= 0$	SO $= 0.151^b$	SO $= 0.209^a$
WS $= 0$	WS $= 0$	WS $= 0$	SD $= 0.183^b$	SD $= 0$
E $= 0.191^a$	E $= 0$	E $= 0$	SN $= 0.310^a$	SN $= 0.130^c$
SE $= 0.232^a$	SE $= 0$	SE $= 0$	SP $= 0$	SP $= 0.111^d$
SS $= 0$	SS $= 0$	SS $= 0.112^d$	SH $= 0$	SH $= 0$
$R^2 = 0.09^a$	$R^2 = 0$	$R^2 = 0.01^d$	SB $= 0$	SB $= 0.153^b$
			A $= 0$	A $= 0$
Self-Progress	Self-Future	Self-Best	WS $= 0$	WS $= 0.095^c$
			E $= 0$	E $= 0$
A $= 0$	A $= 0$	A $= 0$	SE $= 0.149^b$	SE $= 0$
WS $= 0$	WS $= 0$	WS $= 0$	SS $= 0$	SS $= 0.092^d$
E $= 0$	E $= 0$	E $= 0$	$R^2 = 0.28^a$	SW $= 0.258^a$
SE $= 0$	SE $= 0$	SE $= 0$		$R^2 = 0.37^a$
SS $= 0$	SS $= 0$	SS $= 0$		N $= 341$
$R^2 = 0$	$R^2 = 0$	$R^2 = 0$		

[a] $P \leqslant 0.001$
[b] $P \leqslant 0.005$
[c] $P \leqslant 0.01$
[d] $P \leqslant 0.05$
0 Significance level too low to enter equation.

APPENDIX B

Definitions

Health	The present state of your general, overall health (relatively free of common and chronic illnesses).
Financial security	How well your income (including investments, property, etc.) takes care of your daily needs and provides funds for unexpected or unplanned expenses.
Family relations	Kind of contact and frequency of contact you have with your family members. This includes personal contact, phone calls, and letters.
Paid employment	Any work for wages, salaries or fees.
Friendship	Kind of contact and frequency of contact you have with your friends. This includes personal contact, phone calls, and letters.
Housing	The present type, atmosphere and state of the home you live in at the time. Suitability of the home (e.g., apartment, house, farm, room, etc.).
Area you live in	The general place in which you live, including climate, location and lifestyle.
Recreation activity	Personal recreation activities you engage in for pure pleasure when you are not doing normal daily chores or some type of work. This includes relaxing, reading, T.V., regular get togethers, church activities, arts and crafts, exercises, trips, etc.
Religion	Your spiritual fulfillment.
Self-Esteem	How good you feel about yourself; your sense of self-respect.
Transportation	In general, how well public and private transportation meets your needs (e.g., convenience, expense).
Education	Your formal education as provided in the university you are presently attending.
No opinion	This is a catch-all box covering not applicable, can't remember, no comment, etc.

ACKNOWLEDGMENT

* I would like to thank the following people for their help with various aspects of the research presented in this paper: all the instructors who let me use their class time to administer my questionnaire, F. M. Andrews, A. Dyer, H. Esser, W. Glatzer, H. J. Krupp. D. C. Poff, U. E. Simonis, and W. Zapf. Earlier versions were presented at the University of Mannheim, J. W. Goethe-University of Frankfurt and the International Institute for Environment and Society at the Wissenschaftszentrum Berlin. In all these places, I received helpful comments from people attending the seminars, for which I am very grateful.

NOTE

[1] My colleague, Dr. Linda Wood, pointed this out after most of the data for this study were collected.

BIBLIOGRAPHY

Abbey, A. and F. M. Andrews: 1985, 'Modeling the psychological determinants of life quality', Social Indicators Research 16, pp. 1–34.

Abelson, R. P. et al. (eds.): 1968, Theories of Cognitive Consistency: A Sourcebook (Rand McNally and Co., Chicago).

Adams, J. S.: 1965, 'Inequity in social exchange', in Advances in Experimental Social Psychology, ed. by L. Berkowitz (Academic Press, New York), pp. 267–300.

Adams, J. S. and S. Freedman: 1976, 'Equity theory revisited: comments and annotated bibliography', in Advances in Experimental Social Psychology, ed. by L. Berkowitz and E. Walster (Academic Press, New York), pp. 43–90.

Anderson, A. B., A. Basilevski, and D. P. J. Hum: 1983, 'Measurement: Theory and techniques', in Handbook of Survey Research, ed. by P. H. Rossi, J. D. Wright and A. B. Anderson (Academic Press, New York), pp. 231–287.

Andrews, F. M. and R. F. Inglehart: 1979, 'The structure of subjective well-being in nine western societies', Social Indicators Research 6, pp. 75–90.

Andrews, F. M. and S. B. Withey: 1976, Social Indicators of Well-Being (Plenum Press, New York).

Appelgryn, A. E. and C. Plug: 1981, 'Application of the theory of relative deprivation to occupational discrimination against women', South African Journal of Psychology 11, pp. 143–147.

Barnett, L. R. and M. T. Nietzel: 1979, 'Relationship of instrumental and affectional behaviors and self-esteem to marital satisfaction in distressed and nondistressed couples', Journal of Consulting and Clinical Psychology 47, pp. 946–957.

Barzun, J.: 1983, A Stroll with William James (University of Chicago Press, Chicago).

Berkowitz, L.: 1968, 'The study of urban violence: some implications of laboratory studies of frustration and aggression', American Behavioral Scientist 11, pp. 14–17.

Bledsoe, J. C., D. J, Mullen, and G. J. Hobbs: 1980, 'Validity of the Mullen diagnostic survey for leadership improvement', Perceptual and Motor Skills 59, pp. 838–846.

Booth, R. F., M. S. McNally, and N. H. Berry: 1979, 'Hospital corpsmen perceptions of working in a fleet Marine force environment', Military Medicine 144, pp. 31–34.

Campbell, A. P., P. E. Converse, and W. L. Rodgers: 1976, The Quality of American Life (Russell Sage Foundation, New York).

Canter, D. and K. Rees: 1982, 'A multivariate model of housing satisfaction', International Review of Applied Psychology 31, pp. 185–208.

Caplan, R. D.: 1979, 'Social support, person-environment fit, and coping', in Mental Health and the Economy, ed. by L. A. Ferman and J. P. Gordus (Upjohn Institute, Kalamazoo, Michigan), pp. 89–137.

Caplan, R. D.: 1983, 'Person-environment fit: Past, present, and future', in Stress Research, ed. by C. L. Cooper (John Wiley and Sons, New York), pp. 35–77.

Cherrington, D. J. and J. L. England: 1980, 'The desire for an enriched job as a moderator of the enrichment-satisfaction relationship', Organizational Behavior and Human Performance 25, pp. 139–159.

Cook, K. S.: 1975, 'Expectations, evaluations, and equity', American Sociological Review 40, pp. 372–388.

Crosby, F.: 1976, 'A model of egoistical relative deprivation', Psychological Review 83, pp. 85–113.

Crosby, F. J.: 1982, Relative Deprivation and Working Women (Oxford University Press, New York).

Davis, J. A.: 1959, 'A formal interpretation of the theory of relative deprivation', Sociometry 22, pp. 280–296.

Diener, E.: 1984, 'Subjective well-being', Psychological Bulletin 95, pp. 542–575.

Duncan, O. D.: 1975, 'Does money buy satisfaction?', Social Indicators Research 2, pp. 267–274.

Durbin, P. T.: 1980, A Guide to the Culture of Science, Technology and Medicine (The Free Press, New York).

Edwards, W. and A. Tversky: 1967, Decision Making (Penguin Books, Middlesex).

Festinger, L.: 1957, A Theory of Cognitive Dissonance (Stanford University Press: Stanford, California).

Fisher, J. D., A. Nadler, and S. Whitcher-Alagna: 1982, 'Recipient reactions to aid', Psychological Bulletin 91, pp. 27–54.

Fordyce, M. W.: 1983, 'A program to increase happiness: Further studies', Journal of Counseling Psychology 30, pp. 483–498.

Galnoor, I.: 1977, ed., Government Secrecy in Democracies (Harper & Row, Pub., New York).

Glenn, N. D.: 1981, 'The well-being of persons remarried after divorce', Journal of Family Issues 2, pp. 61–75.

Goodman, P. S.: 1966, A Study of Time Perspective: Measurement and Correlates (Doctoral Disseration, Cornell University).

Goodman, P. S.: 1974, 'An examination of referents used in the evaluation of pay', Organizational Behavior and Human Performance 12, pp. 170–195.

Goodman, P. S. and A. Friedman: 1971, 'An examination of Adams' theory of inequity', Administrative Science Quarterly 16, pp. 271–288.

Gottlieb, B. H.: 1984, 'Social support and the study of personal relationships', paper presented at the Second International Conference on Personal Relationships, July 22–27, 1984, in Madison, Wisconsin.

Gurr, T. R.: 1970, Why Men Rebel (Princeton University Press: Princeton, N.J.).

Harrison, R. V.: 1978, 'Person-environment fit and job stress', Stress at Work, ed. by C. L. Cooper and R. Payne (John Wiley, New York), pp. 175–205.

Harrison, R. V.: 1983, 'The person-environment fit model and the study of job stress', Human Stress and Cognition in Organizations: An Integrated Perspective, ed. by T. A. Beehr and R. S. Bhagat (John Wiley, New York).

Hatfield, E., D. Greenberger, J. Traupmann, and P. Lambert: 1982, 'Equity and sexual satisfaction in recently married couples', Journal of Sex Research 18, pp. 18–32.

Hatfield, J. D. and R. C. Huseman: 1982, 'Perceptual congruence about communication as related to satisfaction: Moderating effects of individual characteristics', Academy of Management Journal 25, pp. 349–358.

Harsanyi, J. C.: 1982, 'Morality and the theory of rational behaviour', Utilitarianism and

Beyond, ed. by A. Sen and B. Williams (Cambridge University Press, Cambridge), pp. 39–62.

James, W.: 1890, The Principles of Psychology (reprinted 1950 by Dover Pub., New York).

Kauder, E.: 1965, A History of Marginal Utility Theory (Princeton Press, Princeton, N.J.).

Kuhn, A.: 1974, The Logic of Social Systems (Jossey-Bass, San Francisco).

Kurella, S.: 1979, 'The social needs of patients and their satisfaction with medical care: a survey of medical inpatients in the community hospitals of the German Democratic Republic', Academy Postgraduate Medical Education 13A, pp. 737–742.

Land, K. C.: 1969, 'Principles of path analysis', in Sociological Methodology, ed. by E. F. Borgatta and G. W. Bohrnstedt (Jossey-Bass, San Francisco), pp. 3–37.

LaRocco, J. M., J. S. House, and J. R. P. French: 1980, 'Social support, occupational stress, and health', Journal of Health and Social Behaviour 21, pp. 202–218.

Lewin, K. et al.: 1944, 'Level of aspiration', Personality and Behaviour Disorders, ed. by J. McV. Hunt (Ronald Press Co., New York), pp. 333–378.

Luce, R. D., and H. Raiffa: 1957, Games and Decisions (John Wiley and Sons, New York).

Merton, R. K. and A. S. Kitt: 1950, 'Contributions to the theory of reference group behavior', in Continuities in Social Research, ed. by R. K. Merton and P. F. Lazarsfeld, pp. 40–105.

Michalos, A. C.: 1967, 'Postulates of rational preference', Philosophy of Science 34, pp. 18–22.

Michalos, A. C.: 1969, Principles of Logic (Prentice-Hall, Englewood Cliffs).

Michalos, A. C.: 1971, The Popper-Carnap Controversy (Martinus Nijhoff, Hague).

Michalos, A. C.: 1976, 'The morality of cognitive decision-making', in Action Theory, ed. by M. Brand and D. Walton (D. Reidel, Dordrecht), pp. 325–340.

Michalos, A. C.: 1978, Foundations of Decision-Making (Canadian Library of Philosophy, Ottawa).

Michalos, A. C.: 1979, 'Life changes, illness and personal life satisfaction in a rural population', Social Science and Medicine 13A, pp. 175–181.

Michalos, A. C.: 1980a, 'Satisfaction and happiness', Social Indicators Research 8, pp. 385–422.

Michalos, A. C.: 1980b, 'Philosophy of science: historical, social and value aspects', in A Guide to the Culture of Science, Technology and Medicine, ed. by P. T. Durbin (The Free Press, New York), pp. 197–281.

Michalos, A. C.: 1980c, 'A reconsideration of the idea of a science court', Research in Philosophy and Technology 3, pp. 10–28.

Michalos, A. C.: 1980d, 'Advertising: Its logic, ethics and economics', in Informal Logic, ed. by J. A. Blair and R. H. Johnson (Edgepress, Inverness, California), pp. 93–111.

Michalos, A. C.: 1982a, 'The satisfaction and happiness of some senior citizens in rural Ontario', Social Indicators Research 11, pp. 1–30.

Michalos, A. C.: 1982b, North American Social Report. Vol. V: Economics, Religion, and Morality (D. Reidel, Dordrecht).

Michalos, A. C.: 1983a, 'Satisfaction and happiness in a rural northern resource community', Social Indicators Research 13, pp. 224–252.

Michalos, A. C.: 1983b, 'Technology assessment, facts and values', in Philosophy and Technology, ed. by P. T. Durbin and F. Rapp (D. Reidel Pub. Co., Dordrecht), pp. 59–81.

Michalos, A. C.: 1985, 'Job satisfaction, marital satisfaction and the quality of life: A review and a preview', in Research on The Quality of Life, ed. by F. M. Andrews (University of Michigan Press, Ann Arbor).

Oldham, G. R. et al.: 1982, 'The selection and consequences of job comparisons', Organizational Behavior and Human Performance 29, pp. 84–111.

Oldham, G. R. and H. E. Miller: 1979, 'The effect of significant other's job complexity on employee reactions to work', Human Relations 32, pp. 247–260.

Oliver, R. L.: 1980, 'A cognitive model of the antecedants and consequences of satisfaction decisions', Journal of Marketing Research 17, pp. 460–469.

Patchen, M.: 1961, The Choice of Wage Comparisons (Prentice-Hall, Englewood Cliffs, N.J.).

Reichenbach, H.: 1949, Theory of Probability, 2nd ed. (University of California Press, Berkeley).

Reis, H. T.: 1982, 'An introduction to the use of structural equations: Prospects and problems', Review of Personality and Social Psychology 3, pp. 255–287.

Rhyne, D.: 1981, 'Bases of marital satisfaction among men and women', Journal of Marriage and the Family 43, pp. 941–955.

Rodman, H.: 1963, 'The lower-class value stretch', Social Forces 42, pp. 205–215.

Ross, C. E., J. Mirowsky, and R. S. Duff: 1982, 'Physician status characteristics and client satisfaction in two types of medical practice', Journal of Health and Social Behavior 23, pp. 317–329.

Runciman, W. G.: 1966, Relative Deprivation and Social Justice (University of California Press, Berkeley).

Schuessler, K. F.: 1982, Measuring Social Life Feelings (Jossey-Bass Pub., San Francisco).

Schwarz, N. and G. L. Clore: 1983, 'Mood, misattribution, and judgments of well-being: Informative and directive functions of affective states', Journal of Personality and Social Psychology 45, pp. 513–523.

Shaftesbury, Lord: 1711, An Inquiry Concerning Virtue and Merit (London).

Suls, J. and G. S. Sanders: 1982, 'Self-evaluations through social comparison: A developmental analysis', Review of Personality and Social Psychology 3, pp. 171–197.

Turner, R. J., B. G. Frankel, and D. M. Levin: 1983, 'Social support: Conceptualization, measurements, and implications for mental health', Research in Community and Mental Health 3, pp. 67–111.

Veenhoven, R.: 1984, Conditions of Happiness (D. Reidel Pub. Co., Dordrecht).

Walster, E., E. Berscheid, and G. W. Walster: 1976, 'New directions in equity research', in Advances in Experimental Social Psychology, ed. by L. Berkowitz and E. Walster (Academic Press, New York), pp. 1–42.

Weaver, C. N.: 1980, 'Job satisfaction in the United States in the 1970s', Journal of Applied Psychology 65, pp. 364–367.

Weintraub, Z.: 1981, 'The relationship between job satisfaction and work performance', Revista de Psihologia 27, pp. 59–67.

Williams, R. M. Jr.: 1975, 'Relative deprivation', in The Idea of Social Structure: Papers in Honor of Robert K. Merton, ed. by L. A. Coser (Harcourt Brace Jovanovich, New York), pp. 355–378.

Wills, T. A.: 1981, 'Downward comparison principles in social psychology', Psychological Bulletin 90, pp. 245–271.

Wills, T. A.: 1983, 'Social comparison in coping and help-seeking', in New Directions in Helping, Volume 2: Help-Seeking, ed. by B. M. DePaulo, A. Nadler and J. D. Fisher (Academic Press, New York), pp. 109–141.

Zajonc, R. B.: 1980, 'Feeling and thinking: Preferences need no inferences', American Psychologist 35, pp. 151–175.

Zedeck, S.: 1971, 'Problems with the use of 'moderator' variables', Psychological Bulletin 76, pp. 295–310.

Zeller, R. A. and E. G. Carmines: 1980, Measurement in the Social Sciences: The Link Between Theory and Data (Cambridge University Press, Cambridge).

University of Guelph, Ontario
and
Institute of Public Affairs,
Dalhousie University,
Halifax, Nova Scotia B3H 3J5,
Canada.

MICHAEL W. FORDYCE

14. A REVIEW OF RESEARCH ON
THE HAPPINESS MEASURES: A SIXTY SECOND
INDEX OF HAPPINESS AND MENTAL HEALTH

(Received 12 April, 1987)

ABSTRACT. Eighteen years of research using the Happiness Measures (HM) is reviewed in relation to the general progress of well-being measurement efforts. The accumulated findings on this remarkably quick instrument, show good reliability, exceptional stability, and a record of convergent, construct, and discriminative validity unparalleled in the field. Because of this, the HM is offered as a potential touchstone of measurement consistency in a field which generally lacks it.

Personal happiness is generally held to be the most important goal in life. Throughout history, it has been seen as the ultimate end of temporal existence. Aristotle's ancient view that "happiness is so important, it transcends all other worldly considerations" differs little form William James' more modern, psychological observation that "happiness is for most men, at all times, the secret motive of all they do . . ."

Despite the obvious importance of this basic human concern, the social sciences have only in the last decades turned any real, research attention to the topic (for reasons that Fordyce, 1981a, and Kammann et al., 1979, discuss elsewhere). Although late getting started, research on happiness has mushroomed exponentially in recent years (cf. Diener and Griffin, 1982; Michalos, 1985a) and the results of this growing effort are currently most impressive. It is now widely accepted that happiness and related topics of subjective well-being can be measured and studied with reliability and validity (cf. Campbell, 1976; Diener, 1984; Fordyce, 1974b, 1986; Kammann et al., 1979; Veenhoven, 1984) and the emerging research understanding of happiness is quite substantial. Much is now known regarding the nature of happiness, the factors which contribute to it, and the attributes of happy individuals (cf. Diener, 1984; Fordyce, 1974b, 1978, 1981a, 1981b, 1986; Veenhoven, 1984). Theoretical models are coming to the fore (Diener,

373

Alex C. Michalos (ed.), Citation Classics from Social Indicators Research, 373–399.
© 2005 Springer. Printed in the Netherlands.

1984; Fordyce, 1978, 1981b; Kammann and Flett, 1983; Michalos, 1980, 1985b; and Veenhoven, 1984). And even more exciting, a number of recent studies report interventions based on this accumulated research knowledge, to significantly increase the happiness-levels of normal adults (Fordyce, 1977, 1983; Fraser et al., 1985; Lichter et al., 1980).

Notwithstanding the tremendous progress in the field, there is one, somewhat nagging problem: the consistency of happiness and well-being measurement. To be more specific, the field of well-being research is plagued with a rather unique over-abundance of instrumentality. Perhaps more than in any other field in psychology, happiness researchers face a bewildering multitude of measurement possibilities.

There are the straightforward, "How happy are you?" items (with three responses: "very happy", "pretty happy", and "not too happy") used in the classic, national surveys of Gurin et al. (1960), Bradburn and Caplovitz (1965), Converse and Robinson (1966), and the many studies by Campbell and his fellows at the Institute for Social Research.

There have been a multitude of single-item scales developed over the years; the most recent and oft cited being those by Andrews and Withey (1976), Cantril (1965), Wessman and Ricks (1966), and the seven-point scales used by Kammann and Flett (1983a), and Michalos (1985b), as dependent variables in their research.

A plethora of multi-item scales and questionnaires also exist: e.g., Bradburn's Affect Balance Scale (1969), Campbell, Converse, and Rodger's Index of General Affect (1976), Fordyce's Psychap Inventory (1983, 1986), the Satisfaction with Life Survey (Diener et al., in press), Kammann and Flett's Affectometer-2 (1983b), Nagpal and Sell's Subjective Well-Being Inventory (1985), Tellegen's DPQ Well-Being Scale (1979), and Underwood and Froming's Mood Survey (1980), yet these represent only a small fraction of such measures, some of which date as far back as Watson (1930), and others just in the design-stage.

Beyond these, one must consider scores of assessment devices that tap such happiness-allied fields as life-satisfaction, positive affect, geriatric morale, and satisfaction with specific life-domains (such as one's job or marriage).

There are also a host of widely recognized, clinical instruments designed to identify depressed (i.e., "unhappy") individuals (e.g., Beck's

Depression Inventory, 1978; Lubin's Depression Adjective Checklists, 1967; Krug and Laughlin's IPAT Depression Scale, 1970). And to compound it all, many of the most respected clinical and personality inventories (such as the MMPI), contain some form of emotional morale subscale in their protocol.

To the newcomer in this field, it would appear the alternatives are endless — and the perception is largely true. Over the years, no measure of happiness has emerged as a standard reference-point for ongoing study. In fact, just the opposite seems to be the case. Historically, every new researcher investigating happiness has tended to develop a new test to measure it, with little or no reference to past measurement efforts. Only in recent years has this trend been broken (with the comparative studies on measurement by Fordyce, 1986; Diener, 1984; Kammann et al., 1981; and Larson et al., 1985), and it now appears that measurement efforts in the field are beginning to mature and trying to coalesce.

Given this background, the present article focuses on one, very simple happiness measure which has been around for a long time: the Happiness Measures (HM). Considered by some to be the "grand-daddy" of them all, the Happiness Measures — an especially quick and simple measure — has been the most researched and extensively validated, index of happiness proffered the field. This paper provides a review of its current status.

DESCRIPTION OF THE HAPPINESS MEASURES

The *Happiness Measures* consist of two, self-reporting items measuring emotional well-being: (1) an 11-point, happiness/unhappiness scale, and (2) a question asking for the time spent in "happy", "unhappy", and "neutral" moods (see Appendix I).

The scale used in the HM is based on the pioneering work of Wessman and Ricks (1966). Their well-validated scale was expanded and refined by Fordyce (1972, 1973b) to its present form. The present HM scale is unique in two respects: (1) it provides the widest range-of-response and variance of any established scale, and (2) it contains anchoring descriptions at each point on the scale (to insure a better cross-comparability of subject response).

The percentage question (which asks the subject to estimate the amount of time spent in happy, unhappy, and neutral moods), was added to provide a quantitative measure to compliment the qualitative scale. It also adds an index of unhappy mood, which (according to the work of Bradburn, 1969; Bryant and Veroff, 1982; Diener and Emmons, 1984; and Zevon and Tellegen, 1982), plays a somewhat independent role in the overall assessment of subjective well-being. The neutral percentage was included to allow the happy and unhappy mood estimates to vary independently. Originally, it was thought that the neutral estimate would yield close-to-zero correlations with happiness factors, but instead a long history of use shows that neutral mood is more unhappy than happy, and correlations show a consistently negative pattern of association with happiness factors.

Together, the *scale* and *percentage estimates* provide what Diener, in his timely review (1984), considered as the most important qualities of a well-being instrument: measures of *frequency* and *intensity* of affect. The HM *scale* is a measure of intensity (or quality) of happiness; the *percentage estimates*, a measure of its frequency (or quantity).

ADMINISTRATION AND SCORING

The HM is remarkably easy to administer and score. Directions for the examinee are provided on the sheet and most individuals can complete it without further instruction. Few examinees take more than a minute to finish, and the instrument is virtually scored as it's answered.

The *scale score* and the three *percentage estimates* — as they are marked — are used directly as raw scores. The *combination score* (combining the *scale* and *happy* % in equal weights) requires only minimal calculation (i.e., *combination* = [*scale score* × 10 + *happy* %]/2).

Generally, because of its stronger reliability and validity data (see sections below), the *combination score* is used as the primary criterion for happiness in research. However, in most studies all five HM scores have been examined, for each has its own interesting (and often independent) associations with other studied factors. Indeed, given the four basic scores the HM provides as it is completed, other combinations of the raw data are possible. Kammann, Farry, and Herbison (1981) used the HM to produce a "net-time happiness score" (subtracting the *unhappy % estimate* from the *happy % estimate*), and others (like Larson *et al.*, 1985), have treated the subscales quite independently in their analyses.

It is also important to point out, that although the HM has been primarily used to measure happiness in a more general, "on the average" way, it can also be used to measure happiness over more specific time-periods (e.g., "this year", "last month", "today", etc.) as was done in Fordyce's study of daily mood-change (1972) and in more recent studies which successfully attempted to increase the happiness-level of normal adults (Fordyce, 1977, 1983).

RELIABILITY

The reliability data on the HM has always been good. Fordyce (1987) reports test-retest coefficients (for the *combination score*) of 0.98 ($n = 111$) for a two day period; 0.86 ($n = 105$) to 0.88 ($n = 58$) for two weeks; 0.81 ($n = 57$) for one month; and 0.62 ($n = 71$) and 0.67 ($n = 27$) for four months ($p < 0.001$ in each case) — (reliabilities of the other HM scores have been comparable). Larson *et al.*, found similar results in their comparative analysis of current well-being measures (1985). Their reliability data showed HM *scale score* coefficients of 0.59 ($n = 34$) for one month and 0.59 ($n = 76$) for two months; and 0.81 ($n = 34$) for one month and 0.60 ($n = 76$) for two months on the *happy percentage estimate* — the strongest of the reliabilities shown for the popular, single-item measures they analyzed.

In other related studies, the HM was given in a repeated series of four, over-time testings (one-and-a-half weeks apart) — the average reliability being 0.85 (Fordyce, 1983); and in another study (Fordyce, 1983a), three weeks of daily HM ratings correlated 0.70 to an "in-general" taking of the instrument given at the end of the daily ratings, and 0.60 when given 15 weeks later.

Despite the strong reliability data reported over the years for the HM, there is always a legitimate question as to how enduring happiness actually is or ought to be. Most investigators see happiness as a reasonably enduring phenomenon (cf. Diener, 1984; Veenhoven, 1984), and the collected data using the HM seems to support this contention. Still, unlike many, more stable personality traits, one's happiness can change quite dramatically over time, especially if life-situations change. The Happiness Measures have demonstrated an ability to measure such changes in several studies. Fordyce, for example, found the HM sensitive to short-term change in his experiments to increase the personal happiness of normal adults (1977, 1983) and, likewise, servicable in a study of day-to-day happiness change (1972, 1973a).

STABILITY

Perhaps more important in measuring an inevitably changing phenomenon like happiness than its reliability, is an instrument's stability-of-measurement over time and samples. And in this regard, the data is quite clear: over several dozen testings — involving a great variety of ages, occupations, and socio-economic backgrounds — the internal-consistency coefficients, score means, score variances, and intercorrelational patterns with concurrent variables (see Validity sections below) have shown an extremely high degree of similarity over the years (Fordyce, 1987). Such stable, (and remarkably consistent) statistics suggest that the HM tends to measure the same properties, to the same degree, over various samples, and over time.

VALIDITY STUDIES

The validity of the Happiness Measures as a measure of emotional well-being and global mental health has been extensively investigated. Over the years, studies have examined its convergence with other happiness instruments, its construct validity, its ability to discriminate between known happy and unhappy groups, and its association with widely-accepted characteristics of mental health.

Convergent Validity

The HM has demonstrated a strong and consistent convergence with a wide array of recognized happiness, well-being, and emotion instruments (see Table I).

In Fordyce's ongoing assessment of the HM (1972, 1973a, b, 1977, 1983, 1986, 1987), validity studies have repeatedly compared the HM

TABLE I

A summary of converent validity correlations from three studies comparing the
Happiness Measures to other indices of subjective well-being[a]

Test subscales & study reference	HM scores				
	Combina- tion	Scale	Happy %	Unhappy %	Net Happy*
Affectometer-2 happiness score (Kammann & Flett)					
Fordyce, 1987	0.71	0.69	0.65	−0.61	—
Kammann et al., 1981	—	—	—	—	0.68
Affectometer-2 7-point happiness scale (Kammann & Flett)					
Fordyce, 1987	0.76	0.77	0.64	−0.66	—
Kammann et al., 1981	—	—	—	—	0.66
Andrews & Withey's D-T scale					
Larson et al., 1985	—	0.58	0.56	—	—
Kammann et al., 1981	—	—	—	—	0.70
Andrews & Withey's 'circles'					
Kammann et al., 1981	—	—	—	—	0.73
Andrews & Withey's 'Faces'					
Kammann et al., 1981	—	—	—	—	0.66
Beck Depression Inventory depression index					
Fordyce, 1987	−0.54	−0.51	−0.49	−0.52	—
Bradbrun's affect balance score (ABS)					
Larson et al., 1985	—	0.52	0.41	—	—
Larson et al., 1985	—	0.52	0.41	—	—
Kammann et al., 1981	—	—	—	—	0.61
Bradburn's positive affect score					
Larson et al., 1985	—	0.53	0.56	—	—
Bradburn's negative affect score					
Larson et al., 1985	—	−0.33	−0.35	—	—
Campbell et al., index of affect					
Larson et al., 1985	—	0.65	0.62	—	—
Kammann et al., 1981	—	—	—	—	0.66
Cantril's self anchoring ladder					
Larson et al., 1985	—	0.58	0.51	—	—
Clinical Analysis Questionnaire suicidal depression scale					
Fordyce, 1987	−0.54	−0.57	−0.46	0.58	—

(Table I continued)

Test subscales & study reference	HM scores				
	Combination	Scale	Happy %	Unhappy %	Net Happy*
Clinical Analysis Questionnaire low energy depression scale					
Fordyce, 1987	−0.65	−0.52	−0.66	0.61	—
Depression Adjective Checklist (Form A)					
Fordyce, 1987	−0.79	−0.80	−0.69	0.51	—
Depression Adjective Checklist (Form B)					
Fordyce, 1987	−0.66	−0.72	−0.57	0.63	—
Depression Adjective Checklist (Form C)					
Fordyce, 1987	−0.55	−0.51	−0.53	0.40	—
Depression Adjective Checklist (Form D)					
Fordyce, 1987	−0.55	−0.62	−0.44	0.46	—
Diener *et al.*, satisfaction with life scale (SWLS)					
Larson *et al.*, 1985	—	0.64	0.60	—	—
Gurin *et al.*, 3-choice question					
Larson *et al.*, 1985	—	0.55	0.53	—	—
Kammann *et al.*, 1981	—	—	—	—	0.46
IPAT Depression Scale					
Fordyce, 1987	−0.48	−0.40	−0.45	0.30	—
Minnesota Counselling Inventory positive mood scale					
Fordyce, 1987	0.47	0.42	0.37	−0.27	—
Minnesota Multiphasic Personality Inventory depression scale					
Fordyce, 1987	−0.38	−0.27	−0.38	0.27	—
Multiple Affect Adjective Checklist depression scale					
Fordyce, 1987	−0.73	−0.73	−0.68	0.66	—
Profile of Mood States depression scale					
Fordyce, 1987	−0.66	−0.68	−0.56	0.73	—
Psychap Inventory achieved happiness scale (Form A)					
Fordyce, 1987	0.67	0.66	0.58	−0.66	—
Psychap Inventory achieved happiness scale (Form B)					
Fordyce, 1987	0.69	0.68	0.60	−0.66	—
Psychap Inventory achieved happiness scale (Form C)					
Fordyce, 1987	0.63	0.60	0.55	−0.56	—

(Table I continued)

Test subscales & study reference	HM scores				
	Combina-tion	Scale	Happy %	Unhappy %	Net Happy*
Psychap Inventory achieved happiness scale (Form D)					
Fordyce, 1987	0.67	0.64	0.58	−0.61	—
Michalos' 7-point happiness scale					
Fordyce, 1987	0.72	0.69	0.64	−0.62	—
Tellegen's DPQ well-being scale					
Larson *et al.*, 1985	—	0.71	0.60	—	—
Underwood & Fromming's Mood Survey					
Larson *et al.*, 1985	—	0.74	0.70	—	—

[a] This table presents a summary of statistics gathered by three independent research teams. The data from Kammann *et al.*, represents a single sample (*n* = 118); statistics from Larson *et al.*, are the median correlations from three separate testings (*n* = 34—176); data from Fordyce are median correlations from numerous replications (*n* ranging from 46 to 123); dashes indicate comparisons that were not made. All correlations are significant (*p* < 0.01).

* Kammann *et al.*, used a 'net-time happy score' (i.e., subtracting the unhappy % score from the happy % score) in their analysis.

to numerous well-being indices. The collected data (Fordyce, 1987), show strongly significant, positive correlations between the HM and such happiness indices as the Affectometer-2 (Kammann and Flett, 1986), the *achieved happiness scale* of the Psychap Inventory (PHI; Fordyce, 1986) the Subjective Well-Being Inventory (Nagpal and Sell, 1985), the Wessman and Ricks Scale (1966), and a number of simple happiness scales (e.g., those used by Kammann and Flett, 1983a, and Michalos, 1985b). Marked, negative relationships have also been shown between the HM and indices of unhappiness like the Beck Depression Inventory (BDI; Beck, 1978), the Depression Adjective Check Lists (DACL; Lubin, 1967), the IPAT Depression Scale (IPAT-D; Krug and Laughlin, 1970), and the depression subscales of the Clinical Analysis Questionnaire (CAQ; Cattell *et al.*, 1970), Minnesota Counseling Inventory (MCI; Berdie and Layton, 1957), Minnesota Multiphasic Personality Inventory (MMPI; Hathaway and McKinley, 1951), Multiple Affect Adjective Checklist (MAACL; Zuckerman and Lubin,

1965), and Profile of Mood States (POMS; McNair et al., 1971). Most of these comparisons have been replicated several times, using different samples, and some of the comparisons have been independently confirmed by others (e.g., Corwin and Teigue, 1984; Cejka, 1986).

More recently, two groups of researchers have conducted comparative assessments of well-being measures in which the HM was included.

Kammann, Farry, and Herbison (1981) compared twelve, current indices of happiness, including the widely cited measures of Andrews and Withey (1976), Bradburn and Caplovitz (1969), Campbell et al. (1976), Wessman and Ricks (1966), as well as their own Affectometer. Results indicated the HM to be among the top five in convergence with these other indices.

Diener, along with his associates Larson and Emmons, also conducted comparative studies of well-being measures. Included were the HM, along with measures by Andrews and Withey (1967), Bradburn and Caplovitz (1965), Campbell et al. (1976), Cantril (1965), Gurin et al., (1960), Tellegen (1979), and scales of their own design. In their 1985 report (Larson et al., 1985), the HM was found to be among the strongest in convergent validity of all measures, and the very strongest of the single-item measures they compared. And, in a later report (Diener, 1984), where twenty well-being indices were assessed, it was concluded that "the 11-point Fordyce scale showed the strongest correlations with daily affect and with life-satisfaction of any measure we assessed ..." and that the HM's "... positive and negative frequency estimates provide convergent, construct, and criteria validities that are equal to or superior to those found for the Bradburn scale ..." (i.e., the Braburn Affect Balance Scale [Bradburn, 1969] — widely cited as a model of frequency measurement).

Construct Validity

A measure of happiness should relate in a reliable and predictable way to the numerous personality, attitudinal, and life-style characteristics that have long been established about happy persons in the literature. In this regard, the Happiness Measures have accumulated more validational data than any other well-being measure.

Fordyce, for example, has compared the Happiness Measures to a broad array of recognized tests and inventories (1972, 1973a, b, 1977, 1983, 1985, 1987). In this continuious effort, HM scores have been correlated to concurrently derived scores on the California Personality Inventory (CPS; Gough, 1957), Caring Relationship Inventory (CRI; Shostrom, 1970), Clinical Analysis Questionnaire (CAQ; Cattell *et al.*, 1970), Comrey Personality Scales (CPS; Comrey, 1970), Edwards Personal Preference Schedule (EPPS; Edwards, 1959), Eysenck Personality Questionnaire (EPQ; Eysenck and Eysenck, 1975), Greer Fear Survey (Greer, 1965), Health Problems Checklist (HPC; Schinka, 1984a), IPAT Anxiety Scale (IPAT-A; Cattell and Scheier, 1963), Laswell Values Ranking (Laswell, 1953), Marital Evaluation Checklist (Navran, 1984), Minnesota Counseling Inventory (MCI; Berdie and Layton, 1957), Minnesota Multiphasic Personality Inventory (MMPI; Hathaway and McKinley, 1951), Motivational Analysis Test (MAT; Cattell *et al.*, 1959), Morris Ways To Live Survey (Morris, 1956), Myers-Briggs Type Indicator (MBTI; Myers, 1962), Multiple Affect Adjective Checklist (MAACL; Zuckerman and Lubin, 1965), Pair Attracion Inventory (PAI; Shostrom, 1970), Personal Orientation Inventory (POI; Shostrom, 1963), Personal Problems Checklist (PPC; Schinka, 1984b), Personality Research Form (PRF; Jackson, 1967), Profile of Mood States (POMS; McNair *et al.*, 1971), Psychap Inventory (PHI; Fordyce, 1986), Rokeach Value Scales (Rokeach, 1968), Satisfaction and Happiness Survey (Michalos, 1985b), Schedule of Recent Experiences (SRE; Holmes, 1984), Sixteen Personality Factor Questionnaire (16PFQ; Cattell and Eber, 1957), Subjective Well-Being Inventory (SWBI; Nugpal and Sell, 1985), and Survey of Values (Allport *et al.*, 1953). Table II provides a sumarized review of the data Fordyce has collected, as well as data from the correlational investigations of others (Cejka, 1986; Corwin and Teigue, 1984; Dillman, 1979; Teique and Brandon, 1984). The table is taken from a complete presentation given in the *Research and Tabular Supplement for the Happiness Measures* (Fordyce, 1987).

The data in Table II shows strong relationships between the HM and concurrent measures of the personality characteristics established for happiness in past research. Reviewing the data as a whole, a number of trends appear: persons scoring happily on the HM have a personality profile on these other tests which suggest a low level of fear, hostility,

TABLE II

A summary of correlations between the Happiness Measures and other personality tests and inventories across studies

Test names and subscales	HM scores				
	Combination	Scale	Happy %	Unhappy %	Neutral %
Affectometer-2 (n = 46)*					
Happiness score	0.71	0.69	0.65	−0.61	−0.18ns
7-Point scale	0.76	0.77	0.64	−0.66	−0.13ns
Beck Depression Inventory (BDI) (n = 46)*					
Depression score	−0.54	−0.51	−0.49	0.52	0.31
Clinical Analysis Questionnaire (CAQ) (n = 65)*					
Hypochondriasis	−0.46	−0.43	−0.44	0.55	0.19ns
Suicidal depression	−0.54	−0.57	−0.46	0.58	0.20ns
Anxious depression	−0.25	−0.19ns	−0.26	0.29	0.14ns
Low-energy depression	−0.65	−0.52	−0.66	0.61	0.42
Guilt/resentment	−0.57	−0.48	−0.57	0.55	0.35
Bored/withdrawn	−0.58	−0.55	−0.53	0.50	0.33
Paranoia	−0.30	−0.26	−0.30	0.42	0.10ns
Psychopathic deviate	0.39	0.34	0.38	−0.21ns	−0.33
Schizophrenia	−0.50	−0.47	−0.47	0.57	0.22ns
Psychasthenia	−0.37	−0.31	−0.37	0.30	0.27
Inadaquacy	−0.61	−0.62	−0.54	0.56	0.31
Comrey Personality Personality Scales (CPS) (n = 84)*					
Activity	0.30	0.37	0.23	−0.10ns	−0.11ns
Emotional stability	0.52	0.61	0.43	−0.41	−0.05ns
Extroversion	0.42	0.45	0.40	−0.20ns	−0.22
Depression Adjective Checklists (DACL)					
Form A (n = 58)*	−0.79	−0.80	−0.69	0.51	0.36
Form B (n = 46)*	−0.66	−0.72	−0.57	0.63	0.26
Form C (n = 46)*	−0.55	−0.51	−0.53	0.40	0.25
Form D (n = 46)*	−0.55	−0.62	−0.44	0.46	0.27
Edwards Personal Preference Survey (EPPS) (n = 65)*					
Autonomy	0.37	0.45	0.25	−0.32	−0.13ns
Affiliation	0.38	0.37	0.40	−0.28	−0.23ns
Aggression	−0.39	−0.33	−0.31	0.27	0.05ns
Eysenck Personality Questionnaire (EPQ) (n = 47)*					
Extroversion	0.56	0.57	0.53	−0.43	−0.30
Neutroticism	−0.41	−0.42	−0.38	0.51	−0.02ns
Greer Fear Survey Schedule (n = 87)					
Fear score	−0.23	−0.19ns	−0.27	0.24	n/c

(Table II continued)

Test names and subscales	HM scores				
	Combina-tion	Scale	Happy %	Unhappy %	Neutral %
Health Problems Checklist (HPC) (*n* = 58)					
General health	−0.43	−0.33	−0.44	0.29	0.42
Total health problems	−0.35	−0.26	−0.36	0.32	0.41
IPAT Anxiety Scale (IPAT-A) (*n* = 65)					
Covert anxiety	−0.74	−0.66	−0.70	0.54	0.50
Overt anxiety	−0.59	−0.51	−0.56	0.48	0.38
Total anxiety	−0.65	−0.58	−0.61	0.54	0.40
IPAT Depression Scale (IPAT-D) (*n* = 108)					
Depression score	−0.48	−0.40	−0.45	0.30	0.39
Marital Evaluation Checklist (MEC) (*n* = 34)					
Relationship problems	−0.54	−0.45	−0.64	0.42	0.63
Minnesota Counselling Inventory (MCI) (*n* = 146)					
Family relations	0.31	0.21	0.31	−0.25	−0.19
Social relations	0.41	0.38	0.32	−0.23	−0.16ns
Emotional stability	0.43	0.44	0.36	−0.41	−0.15ns
Conformity	0.25	0.27	0.17ns	−0.29	−0.02ns
Reality adjustment	0.49	0.49	0.41	−0.43	−0.18
Mood	0.47	0.42	0.37	−0.27	−0.20ns
Leadership	0.41	0.38	0.33	−0.27	−0.19
Minnesota Multiphasic Personality Inventory (MMPI) (*n* = 58)					
Depression (D)	−0.38	−0.27	−0.38	0.27	0.37
Psychopathy (Pd)	−0.42	−0.28	−0.44	0.32	0.39
Psychasthenia (Pt)	−0.34	−0.30	0.31	0.31	0.25
Schizophrenia (Sc)	−0.35	−0.29	−0.33	0.30	0.29
Introversion (Si)	−0.39	−0.37	−0.33	0.26	0.34
Anxiety (A)	−0.35	−0.33	−0.31	0.26	0.29
Motivational Analysis Test (MAT) (*n* = 98)					
Fear	−0.23	−0.23	−0.23	0.16ns	0.17ns
Super ego	0.25	0.27	0.20ns	−0.30	−0.02ns
Pugnacity/sadism	−0.34	−0.30	−0.30	0.25	0.19ns
Swetheart/spouse	0.26	0.14ns	0.32	−0.28	−0.19ns
Multiple Affect Adjective Checklist (MAACL) (*n* = 71)*					
Anxiety	−0.67	−0.67	−0.63	0.68	0.35
Depression	−0.73	−0.73	−0.68	0.66	0.44
Hostility	−0.64	−0.58	−0.65	0.62	0.38

(*Table II continued*)

Test names and subscales	HM scores				
	Combina-tion	Scale	Happy %	Unhappy %	Neutral %
Myers-Briggs Type Indicator (MBTI) (*n* = 98)*					
Extroversion	0.61	0.64	0.53	−0.53	−0.25
Pair Attraction Inventory (PAI) (*n* = 56)					
Actualized relationship	0.63	0.59	0.66	−0.48	−0.33
Hawks (tense relations)	−0.33	−0.38	−0.29	0.37	0.32
Personal Orientation Inventory (POI) (*n* = 58)*					
Time-competence	0.46	0.43	0.41	−0.47	−0.07ns
Inner-directedness	0.55	0.50	0.54	−0.56	−0.17ns
Self-actualized value	0.50	0.46	0.53	−0.41	−0.32
Feeling reactivity	0.31	0.34	0.29	−0.33	−0.06ns
Spontaniety	0.36	0.36	0.30	−0.29	−0.11ns
Self-regard	0.60	0.57	0.58	−0.61	−0.17ns
Nature of humankind	0.29ns	0.33	0.19ns	−0.29ns	−0.04ns
Synergy	0.41	0.35	0.40	−0.28ns	−0.28ns
Acceptance of aggression	0.32	0.32	0.34	−0.26ns	−0.20ns
Intimate relationships	0.45	0.45	0.44	−0.46	−0.13ns
Personal Problems Checklist (PPC) (*n* = 108)					
Social problems	−0.37	−0.28	−0.38	0.21	0.35
Financial problems	−0.26	−0.24	−0.22	0.28	0.10ns
Emotional problems	−0.33	−0.27	−0.32	0.17ns	0.25
Attitude problems	−0.32	−0.20	−0.34	0.37	0.16ns
Total personal problems	−0.29	−0.22	−0.28	0.23	0.21
Personality Research Form (PRF) (*n* = 58)					
Affiliation	0.35	0.34	0.29	−0.20	−0.30
Change	0.34	0.36	0.27	−0.22ns	−0.25
Exhibition	0.35	0.31	0.32	−0.30	−0.27
Profile of Mood States (POMS) (*n* = 98)*					
Tension	−0.51	−0.47	−0.47	0.58	0.15ns
Depression	−0.66	−0.68	−0.56	0.73	0.14ns
Anger	−0.40	−0.46	−0.42	0.47	0.17ns
Vigor	0.63	0.61	0.55	−0.54	−0.28
Fatigue	−0.55	−0.52	−0.48	0.51	0.21
Confusion	−0.52	−0.49	−0.48	0.56	0.17ns

(Table II continued)

Test names and subscales	HM scores				
	Combina-tion	Scale	Happy %	Unhappy %	Neutral %

Psychap Inventory (PHI) (n = 123)*

Form A:
Achieved Happiness	0.67	0.66	0.58	−0.66	−0.23
Happy Personality	0.53	0.48	0.49	−0.50	−0.28
Happy Attitudes & Values	0.56	0.57	0.47	−0.58	−0.18
Happy Life Style	0.55	0.52	0.49	−0.50	−0.29
Total Score	0.69	0.66	0.61	−0.67	−0.29

Form B:
Achieved Happiness	0.69	0.68	0.60	−0.66	−0.27
Happy Personality	0.64	0.58	0.59	−0.56	−0.33
Happy Attitudes & Values	0.57	0.57	0.49	−0.53	−0.26
Happy Life Style	0.52	0.47	0.48	−0.41	−0.34
Total Score	0.69	0.66	0.61	−0.62	−0.33

Form C:
Achieved Happiness	0.63	0.60	0.55	−0.56	−0.28
Happy Personality	0.57	0.48	0.56	−0.49	−0.37
Happy Attitudes & Values	0.55	0.52	0.50	−0.52	−0.26
Happy Life Style	0.55	0.51	0.50	−0.42	−0.34
Total Score	0.69	0.63	0.64	−0.60	−0.38

Form D:
Achieved Happiness	0.67	0.64	0.58	−0.61	−0.29
Happy Personality	0.60	0.53	0.57	−0.54	−0.33
Happy Attitudes & Values	0.56	0.55	0.47	−0.53	−0.22
Happy Life Style	0.55	0.47	0.52	−0.42	−0.36
Total Score	0.68	0.63	0.62	−0.61	−0.35

Satisfaction & Happiness Survey (SHS) (n = 107)*
Current	0.60	0.58	0.55	−0.53	−0.24
Want	0.39	0.37	0.33	−0.35	−0.14
Peers	0.50	0.42	0.50	−0.45	−0.26
Deserve	0.47	0.44	0.43	−0.32	−0.30
Need	0.42	0.44	0.37	−0.49	−0.02ns
Expected	0.46	0.38	0.44	−0.45	−0.21
Future	0.33	0.33	0.26	−0.25	−0.15
Past best	0.54	0.54	0.44	−0.47	−0.20
Self-esteem	0.54	0.48	0.50	−0.42	−0.28
Social support	0.45	0.41	0.41	−0.37	−0.21
7-point scale	0.72	0.69	0.64	−0.62	−0.30

(*Table II continued*)

Test names and subscales	HM scores				
	Combina-tion	Scale	Happy %	Unhappy %	Neutral %
Schedule of Recent Experiences (SRE) (*n* = 65)					
Stress events (6 mos. to 1 year previous)	−0.30	−0.16ns	−0.36	0.26	0.27
Sixteen Personality Factor Questionnaire (16PFQ) (*n* = 65)*					
Outgoing	0.31	0.32	0.27	−0.23ns	−0.19ns
Emotionally stable	0.43	0.42	0.42	−0.62	−0.08ns
Happy-go-lucky	0.30	0.27	0.34	−0.14ns	−0.34
Conscientious	0.29	0.30	0.26	−0.08ns	−0.26
Venturesome	0.29	0.32	0.26	−0.15ns	−0.10ns
Guilt-prone	−0.47	−0.39	−0.46	0.50	0.28
High self-concept	0.40	0.44	0.33	−0.45	−0.21ns
Tense	−0.37	−0.40	−0.35	0.50	0.13ns

* This table presents a summarization of the collected data on the HM. In cases where the comparison has been replicated more than once, an asterisk is given next to the sample size. In such cases the correlations represent the MEDIAN of the replications. Unmarked samples are from single, non-replicated, comparisons. For brevity, the table excludes the listing of test subscales which have not shown consistently significant relationships with the HM.

All correlations are significant ($p < 0.05$) unless designated with ns (non-significant).

tension, anxiety, guilt, confusion, anger, and other negative emotion; a high degree of energy, vitality, and activity; a high level of self-esteem and a generally self-actualized, healthy, and emotionally stable personality; a strong social-orientation coupled with outgoing, spontaneous, extroverted characteristics; a marked absence of health concerns, personal problems, and psychopathology; healthy, satisfying, and warm love and social relationships; a life-style typified as involved, active, social, and meaningfully productive; and an attitudinal approach to life that is optimistic, worry-free, present-oriented, internally-locused, and well-directed. This description is quite in line with, indeed perhaps exemplifies, our current understanding of the "happy personality." But beyond this, this description also closely approximates what the literature in psychology views as the major criteria of optimal mental health.

Discriminative Validity

Ideally, a measure of happiness should statistically discriminate between known happy and unhappy groups, and the Happiness Measures has shown such discriminative validity in a number of studies. Fordyce (1987) has sampled numerous, socially-stratified groups over the years in his studies. Cullington and Plummer (1984) and Salazar *et al.*, (1984) have done similar work. The results of such inter-socioeconomic testings have been in accord with the predictions that would be made from past research: i.e., groups of higher social, economic, or occupational standing score higher (usually, significantly so) on the HM (cf. Fordyce, 1987). In addition, data from Hall (1984), Hodges (1985), Linden (1984), and Salazar *et al.*, (1984) has consistently indicated significant differences between HM scores obtained from from various "troubled" populations (e.g., hospitalized depressives, crisis intake-clients, individuals or couples seeking counseling, etc.) and those of more normal samples.

PSYCHOMETRIC CHARACTERISTICS

Beyond studies dealing with the reliability and validity of the Happiness Measures, a number of investigations have delt with more specific psychometric concerns.

Response Bias

The HM has been compared to a variety of response-bias measures over the years (Fordyce, 1987). These include such response-bias indices as the Crowne-Marlowe Social Desirability Scale (Crowne and Marlowe, 1960) and a number of response bias scales contained on other, more extensive inventories (i.e., the CPS, EPQ, MCI, MMPI, and PRE — as referenced above). Over a dozen such response-bias comparisons have been analyzed, and most have proven non-significant. Still, a few significant results have emerged which indicate the HM may be susceptible to bias from some examinees tending to portray themselves in a favorable light. Collectively, the findings indicate some caution should be exercised in the intrepretation of individual profiles, but for general research use, it appears that the HM can be considered relatively free of bias.

Repeated Use and Sensitization Effects

In most work using the HM as a happiness-criterion, a single, "in general" testing has been used. However, the HM appears to have equal utility in repeated-measures and pretest-posttest designs (e.g., Fordyce, 1972, 1973a, b, 1977, 1983). In a series of studies (Fordyce 1973b, 1977) it was concluded, using Solomon designs, that previous takings of the HM do not appear to bias subsequent takings in any systematic way. In addition, there appears to be close correspondence between the average of a series of daily HM takings and a single, "in general" taking evaluating the same time-period (Fordyce, 1973a). However, in comparing the two methods (averaged daily-ratings *vs.* a one-shot, "general" rating) the one-shot administration proved more valid and less susceptible to response bias than the averaging method — supporting the way the HM and other well-being measures have been typically employed in research.

Sex, Age, and Racial Differences

There appears to be little discrimination in response to the HM due to sex, age, or race.

Sex differences have been most extensively examined (Fordyce, 1987), and in scores of testings over many years, sex differences have been generally nonsignificant. Additionally, other testing characteristics (i.e., interscore correlational patterns, correlations with outside criteria, etc.) show little sex difference. The data on age and race has, likewise, proven nonsignificant — although these factors have not received a great deal of study with the HM. Overall, work with the HM coincides with the literature which finds no particular sex differences in happiness, and only slight relationships regarding age and race factors (Diener, 1984; Fordyce, 1974b; Veenhoven, 1984).

Norms

For preliminary research use, Table III provides normative data on a

TABLE III

Normative means and standard deviations for preliminary uses
$(n = 3050)$[a]

Score	Mean	S.D.
Combination score	61.66	17.84
Scale score	6.92	1.75
Happy % estimate	54.13	21.52
Unhappy % estimate	20.44	14.69
Neutral % estimate	25.43	16.52

[a] Sample characteristics: mean age 26.3; age range 16—73; 1237 males; 1813 females; adult community college students with varied educational, socio-economic, regional, ethnic, and occupational backgrounds.

sample of 3050 community college students. As typical of community colleges, the sample varies widely in age (mean = 26.3; range = 16—73), occupation, academic ability, socio-economic background, and mental health status. The normative sample should be considered more widely representative of young-adult Americans than might be obtained in other college samples.

For more specific research, means and other data from a number of occupational, special socio-economic, and clinical groups are also available (Fordyce, 1987).

DISCUSSION

As we examine the 15 years of study on the Happiness Measures, a number of conclusions come to the fore. The first and most obvious, is the extensive nature of the collected data. It would be safe to classify the HM as the most thoroughly analyzed well-being measure developed in the field. This is not to say it is the best of the instruments (although there is some evidence to support the contention) — it is only to say that the Happiness Measures have been tested and retested with respect to reliability, validity, and other important characteristics to an extent that far exceeds the efforts reported for other instruments. And from the collected data, it would appear that the Happiness Measures demonstrate strong reliability; remarkable stability; relative freedom from response, sex, age, and race bias; and an exceptionally wide background of evidence supporting it's convergent, construct, concurrent, and discriminative validity.

The second general conclusion regarding the Happiness Measures is how deceptively simple an instrument it is. Happiness instruments have often been very simple (e.g., scales or one-item questions), yet what has has always been fascinating is how such simple questions elicit such an enormous amount of relevant information about an individual's life. The Happiness Measures are like this. The HM is amazingly simple: it's quick to administer (taking less than a minute to complete) — and it's actually scored as it's answered. Yet what it shows about a person's life, their basic emotional well-being, and their global mental health is most remarkable. The collected evidence suggests that a simple, one-minute testing using the HM can provide a general assessment of emotional, social, and mental health functioning that closely rivals hours of testing using the most respected clinical instruments in the field. Indeed, it could be paraphrased from Winston Churchill: "never has so much, about so many, been obtained by so little . . ."

The third conclusion regards the ultimate value of measurement investigation itself. Inevitably, our efforts to examine the measurement of happiness and subjective well-being offers new insights into the the nature of the phenomenon we are attempting to study. It is, as Kammann and Flett discuss (1983b), a process of ". . . double discovery . . . finding out simultaneously what it is that we are measuring and what factors are linked to it . . ." (p. 31). In this regard, the present paper provides the first published summary of an extensive reservior of data on personal happiness, which, in general, provides a strong, independent confirmation of the basic findings reported in the literature, and, in specific, adds even more, new findings to our understanding of happiness (cf. Fordyce, 1987).

The final conclusion regards the maturing of our field of research. It is currently quite clear that research on happiness and subjective well-being has grown to substantial proportions in recent years and that our present understanding of happiness in the literature is quite extensive. Much is now known about the nature of happiness, its objective and situational correlates, and the personality characteristics of happy individuals. What is also intriguing, is how consistent and stable the happiness findings have been across cultures, between varied samples, and over time. Indeed, "the findings on happy people have proven to be so consistent that the nature of happiness is far more stable, understandable, and basically universal than most have ever expected" (Fordyce, 1981a, p. 8). Yet what is most remarkable of all, is the fact that these consistent findings have occurred despite any real consistency of measurment. Indeed, since practically every research group has chosen a new well-being instrument of its own design, what we have, essentially, is a situation of consistent results borne of inconsistent methods!

In a previous paper, the author considered this situation to be most fortuitous, ". . . since if great inconsistency in resultant findings occurred in the field, happiness studies would be in a thoroughly confused and confounded state" (Fordyce, 1886, p. 27). Apparently (and most fortunately, for those in the field), "no matter how you decide to ask people how happy they are, the results are the same" (Fordyce, 1986, p. 27).

We have been quite lucky so far — probably because the phenomenon we seek to measure is so basic and global to human personality (cf. Fordyce, 1986; Kammann and Flett, 1983b). But for our field to mature scientifically, measurement efforts must begin to coalesce rather than disperse. The beginings of such an effort toward convergence has recently begun in the literature (Fordyce, 1986; Diener, 1984; Kammann et al., 1981; Larson et al., 1985), and the conclusions of this paper represent a further step in this same direction.

More than anything else, the value of the Happiness Measures lies in its extensive validity data. The HM appears to be exceptional in this regard, and should be considered as an appropriate touchstone for the future research in the the field.

APPENDIX I

a. The Happiness Measures
b. Profile sheet for the Happiness Measures

DATE _____

NAME _____

AGE _____ SEX _____

EMOTIONS QUESTIONNAIRE

PART I DIRECTIONS: Use the list below to answer the following question: IN GENERAL, HOW HAPPY OR UNHAPPY DO YOU USUALLY FEEL? Check the *one* statement below that best describes *your average happiness.*

Check just one of these boxes!

☐ 10. Extremely happy (feeling ecstatic, joyous, fantastic!)

☐ 9. Very happy (feeling really good, elated!)

☐ 8. Pretty happy (spirits high, feeling good.)

☐ 7. Mildly happy (feeling fairly good and somewhat cheerful.)

☐ 6. Slightly happy (just a bit above neutral.)

☐ 5. Neutral (not particularly happy or unhappy.)

☐ 4. Slightly unhappy (just a bit below neutral.)

☐ 3. Mildly unhappy (just a little low.)

☐ 2. Pretty unhappy (somewhat "blue", spirits down.)

☐ 1. Very unhappy (depressed, spirits very low.)

☐ 0. Extremely unhappy (utterly depressed, completely down.)

PART II DIRECTIONS: Consider your emotions a moment further. *On the average,* what percent of the time do you feel happy? What percent of the time do you feel unhappy? What percent of the time do you feel neutral (neither happy nor unhappy)? Write down your best estimates, as well as you can, in the spaces below. Make sure the three figures add-up to equal 100%.

ON THE AVERAGE:

The percent of time I feel happy _____ %

The percent of time I feel unhappy _____ %

The percent of time I feel neutral _____ %

TOTAL: ___100___ %

PROFILE SHEET FOR HAPPINESS MEASURES

NAME _____ DATE TESTED _____

OCCUPATION _____ AGE _____ SEX _____

	INTENSITY (I) SCALE SCORE	FREQUENCY (F)			(I + F) COMBINATION SCORE	
		% HAPPY	% UNHAPPY	% NEUTRAL		
						80
DESCRIPTION of SCORES:		100 ___ 95 ___			100 ___	
						70
Extremely happy	10 ___	90 ___ 85 ___			95 ___ 90 ___	
Very happy	9 ___	80 ___ 75 ___	0 ___ 5 ___	0 ___	85 ___ 80 ___	
		70 ___			75 ___	60
Pretty happy	8 ___	65 ___	10 ___	10 ___	70 ___	
		60 ___	15 ___	20 ___	65 ___	
Mildly happy	7 ___	55 ___	20 ___			
		50 ___		30 ___	60 ___	50
Slightly happy	6 ___	45 ___	25 ___		55 ___	
		40 ___	30 ___	40 ___	50 ___	
		35 ___			45 ___	
Neutral	5 ___	30 ___	35 ___	50 ___	40 ___	40
		25 ___	40 ___			
		20 ___		60 ___	35 ___	
Slightly unhappy	4 ___	15 ___	45 ___		30 ___	
Mildly unhappy	3 ___	10 ___	50 ___	70 ___	25 ___	30
		5 ___	55 ___		20 ___	
Pretty unhappy	2 ___	0 ___	60 ___	80 ___	15 ___ 10 ___	
			65 ___	90 ___	5 ___	20
Very unhappy	1 ___		70 ___			
Extremely unhappy	0 ___		75 ___	100 ___	0 ___	
						10

Raw Scores _____ _____ _____ _____ _____

© Copyright. Dr. Michael W. Fordyce

NOTE

The Happiness Measures and other research materials cited in this article are available upon request from Michael Fordyce, Edison Community College, Fort Myers, FL 33907, U.S.A — telephone (813) 489—9000.

REFERENCES

Allport, G., Vernon, P., and Lindsey, G.: 1953, Study of Values (Houghton Mifflin, New York).
Andrews, F. and Withey, S. R.: 1976, Social Indicators of Well-Being (Plenum Press, New York).
Beck, A.: 1978, Beck Depression Inventory (Center for Cognitive Therapy, Philadelphia).
Berdie, R. and Layton, W.: 1957, Minnesota Counseling Inventory (Psychological Corporation, New York).
Bradburn, N.: 1969, The Structure of Psychological Well-Being (Aldine, Chicago).
Bradburn, N. and Caplovitz, D.: 1965, Reports on Happiness (Aldine, Chicago).
Bryant, F. and Veroff, J.: 1982, 'The structure of psychological well-being', Journal of Personality and Social Psychology 43, pp. 653—673.
Campbell, A.: 1976, 'Subjective measures of well-being', American Psychologist 31, 117—124.
Campbell, A., Converse, P., and Rogers, W. L.: 1976, The Quality of American Life (Russell Sage Foundation, New York).
Cantril, H.: 1965, The Pattern of Human Concerns (Rutgers University Press, New Brunswick, New Jersey).
Cattell, R. B. and Eber, H. W.: 1957, Sixteen Personality Factor Questionnaire (Institute for Personality and Ability Testing, Champaign, Illinois).
Cattell, R., Horn, J., Sweney, A., and Radcliff, J.: 1959, Motivational Analysis Test (Institute for Personality and Ability Testing, Champaign, Illinois).
Cattell, R. and Scheier, I.: 1963, IPAT Anxiety Scale (Institute for Personality and Ability Testing, Champaign, Illinois).
Cattell, R.: 1970, Clinical Analysis Questionnaire (Institute for Personality and Ability Testing: Champaign, Illinois).
Cejka, E.: 1986, 'Intercorrelational data between the Happiness Measures, Psychap Inventory, and other mood tests' (Unpublished data, reported in in Fordyce, 1987).
Comrey, A. L.: 1970, Comrey Personality Scales (Educational and Industrial Testing Services, San Diego).
Corwin, R. and Teigue, I.: 1984, 'Comparative reliability and validity of three happiness tests: The Happiness Measures, Psychap Inventory, and Affectometer-2' (Unpublished data and analysis, presented in Fordyce, 1987).
Crowne, D. P. and Marlowe, D.: 1960, 'A new scale of social desirability independent of psychopathology', Journal of Consulting Psychology 24, 349—354.
Cullington, M., Plummer, K., Diggs, B., and Courter, D.: 1984 'A testing of 5th, 7th, 9th, and 11th grade students using the Psychap Inventory and the Happiness Measures' (Unpublished data and analysis, presented in Fordyce, 1987).
Diener, E. and Griffin, S.: 1982, Subjective Well-Being: Happiness, Life Satisfaction and Morale (Unpublished Bibliography, University of Illinois at Urbana-Champaign).

Diener, R.: 1984, 'Subjective well-being', Psychological Bulletin 95 (3), pp. 542—575.

Diener, E. and Emmons, R.: 1984, 'The independence of positive and negative affect', Journal of Personality and Social Psychology 47, pp. 871—883.

Diener, R., Emmons, R., Larson, R., and Grifin, S.: (in press), 'The Satisfaction with Life Scale: A measure of life satisfaction', Journal of Personality Assessment.

Dillman, B.: 1979, 'Marital status, relationship styles, and individual happiness' (Unpublished, analyzed data, reported in Fordyce, 1987).

Edwards, A. L.: 1959, Edwards Personal Preference Schedule (Psychological Corporation, New York).

Eysenck, H. J. and Eysench, S.: 1975, Eysenck Personality Questionnaire. (Educational and Industrial Testing Service, San Diego).

Fordyce, M. W.: 1972, 'Happiness, its daily variation and its relation to values', Dissertation Abstracts International 33, 1266B (University Microfilms No. 72—23, 491).

Fordyce, M.: 1973a, 'Measuring happiness' (Unpublished paper, Edison Community College, Fort Myers, Florida).

Fordyce, M.: 1983b, 'Further validation of the Happiness Measures' (Unpublished paper, Edison Community College, Fort Myers, Florida).

Fordyce, M.: 1974a, 'More psychometric data on human happiness' (Unpublished paper, Edison Community College, Fort Myers, Florida).

Fordyce, M.: 1974b, Human Happiness: The Findings of Psychological Research (Unpublished book, Edison Community College, Fort Myers, Florida)

Fordyce, M.: 1977, 'Development of a program to increase personal happiness', Journal of Counseling Psychology 24 (6), 511—521.

Fordyce, M.: 1978, The Psychology of Happiness: The Book Version of the Fourteen Fundamentals (Unpublished book, Edison Community College, Fort Myers, Florida).

Fordyce, M.: 1981a, The Psychology of Happiness: A Brief Version of the Fourteen Fundamentals (Cypress Lake Media, Fort Myers, Florida).

Fordyce, M.: 1981b, The Psychology of Happiness: The Audio-Cassette Course on the Fourteen Fundamentals (Cypress Lake Media, Fort Myers, Florida).

Fordyce, M.: 1983, 'A program to increase happiness: Further studies', Journal of Counseling Psychology 30 (4), 483—498.

Fordyce, M.: 1985, The Psychap Inventory: Software for Administration, Scoring, and Intrepretative Reporting (Microcomputer diskette, IBM compatible, Cypress Lake Media, Fort Myers, Florida).

Fordyce, M.: 1986, 'The Psychap Inventory; A multi-scale test to measure happiness and its concomitants', Social Indicators Research 18, pp. 1—33.

Fordyce, M.: 1987, Research and Tabular Supplement for the Happiness Measures (1987 edition), (Cypress Lake Media, Fort Myers, Florida).

Fraser, S., Cesa, I., Alba, A., Perera, S., Jorgenson, B., Schulte, L., and Titoian, L.: 1985 (April), 'Novel experiences, friendships, emotional fluctuations and happiness' (Paper presented at the Western Psychological Association annual convention, San Jose, California).

Gough, H.: 1957, California Personality Inventory (Consulting Psychologists Press: Palo Alto, California).

Gurin, G., Veroff, J., and Feld, S.: 1960, Americans View Their Mental Health (Basic Books, New York).

Hall, R.: 1984, 'Happiness Measures testing of depressed in-patients at a private psychiatric hospital' (Unpublished data, presented in Fordyce, 1987).

Hathaway, S. R. and McKinley, J. C.: 1951, Minnesota Multiphasic Personality Inventory (The Psychological Corporation, New York).

Headey, B., Holmstrom, E., and Wearing, A.: 1984, 'Well-being and ill-being: Different dimensions?', Social Indicators Research 14, pp. 115—139.

Hodges, R.: 1985, 'Happiness Measures testing of patients at a state psychiatric hospital' (Unpublished data, presented in Fordyce, 1987).

Holmes, T.: 1984, Schedule of Recent Experiences (Professional Assessment Resources, Odessa, Florida).

Jackson, D.: 1967, Personality Research Form (Research Psychologists Press, Port Huron, Michigan).

Kammann, R., Christie, D., Irwin, R., and Dixon, G.: 1979, 'Properties of an inventory to measure happiness (and psychological health)', New Zealand Psychologist 8, pp. 1—9.

Kammann, R., Farry, M., and Herbison, P.: 1981, 'The measurement and content of the sense of well-being' (Unpublished paper, University of Otago, Dunedin, New Zealand).

Kammann, R. and Flett, R.: 1983a, 'Affectometer 2: A scale to measure current level of general happiness', Australian Journal of Psychology 35(2), 259—265.

Kammann, R. and Flett, R.: 1983b, Sourcebook for Measuring Well-Being with Affectometer-2 (Why not? Foundation, Dunedin, New Zealand).

Krug, S. and Laughlin, J.: 1970, IPAT Depression Checklist (Institute for Personality and Ability Testing, Champaign, Illinois).

Larson, R., Diener, E., and Emmons, R.: 1985, 'An evaluation of subjective well-being measures', Social Indicators Reserach 17, pp. 1—17.

Lichter, S., Kaye, K., and Kammann, R.: 1980, 'Increasing happiness through cognitive retraining', New Zealand Psychologist 9, pp. 57—64.

Linden, K.:1984, 'Testing of clients in a private practice setting with the Happiness Measures' (Unpublished data, presented in Fordyce, 1987).

Lubin, G.: 1967, Depression Adjective Check Lists (Educational and Industrial Testing Service, San Diego).

McNair, D., Lorr, M. and Droppleman, L.: 1971, Profile of Mood States (Educational and Industrial Testing Service, San Diego).

Michalos, A.: 1980, 'Satisfaction and happiness', Social Indicators Research 8, pp. 385—422.

Michalos, A.: 1985a, 'Job satisfaction, marital satisfaction and the quality of life: A review and a preview', in F. M. Andrews (ed), Research in Quality of Life (Institute for Social Research, Ann Arbor, Michigan).

Michalos, M.: 1985, 'Multiple discrepancies theory (MDT)', Social Indicators Research 16, pp. 347—413.

Morris, C.: 1956, Varieties of Human Values (Harper & Row, New York).

Myers, I.: 1962 Myers-Briggs Type Indicator (Educational Testing Service, Princeton, New Jersey).

Nagpal, R., and Sell, H.: 1985, Subjective Well-Being (World Health Organization, New Delhi.

Navran, L.: 1985, Marital Evaluation Checklist (Psychological Assessment Resources, Odessa, Florida.

Rokeach, M.: 1967, Beliefs, Attitudes, and Values (Bassey, New York).

Salazar, C., Plummer, K., Corwin, R., Gardner, J., Gran, S., Hall, R., Kralik, A., McElwee, M., Titterington, A., and Walker, A.: 1984, 'A comparison of happiness testings on ten unique groups using the Happiness Measures and Psychap Inventory' (Unpublished data and analysis, presented in Fordyce, 1987).

Schinka, J.: 1984b, Personal Problems Checklist (Psychological Assessment Resources, Odessa, Florida).

Schinka, J.: 1984a, Health Problems Checklist (Psychological Assessment Resources, Odessa, Florida).

Shostrom, E.: 1963, Personal Orientation Inventory (Educational and Industrial Testing Service, San Diego).

Shostrom, E.: 1966, Caring Relationship Inventory (Educational and Industrial Testing Service, San Diego).

Shostrom, E.: 1970, Pair-Attraction Inventory (Educational and Industrial Testing Service, San Diego).

Teigue, I. and Brandon, M.: 1984, 'Intercorrelations between the Happiness Measures, Psychap Inventory, the Myers-Briggs Type Indicator and the Edwards Personal Preference Survey' (Unpublished data presented in Fordyce 1987).

Tellegen, A.: 1979, Differential Personality Questionnaire (Unpublished materials, University of Minnesota).

Underwood, B. and Fromming, W.: 1980, 'The Mood Survey: A personality measure of happy and sad moods', Journal of Personality Assessment 44, 404—414.

Veenhoven, R.: 1984, Conditions of Happiness (D. Reidel, Dordrecht).

Watson, G.: 1930, 'Happiness among adult students of education', Journal of Educational Psychology 21, pp. 79—109.

Wessman, A. E. and Ricks, D. F.: 1966, Mood and Personality (Holt, Rinehart and Winston, New York).

Zevon, M. A. and Tellegen, A.: 1982, 'The structure of mood change: An idiographic/nomothetic analysis', Journal of Personality and Social Psychology 43, pp. 111—122.

Zuckerman, M. and Lubin, B.: 1965, Multiple Affect Adjective Check List (Educational and Industrial Testing Service, San Diego).

Edison Community College,
16000 College Parkway,
Ford Myers, FA 33907—5164,
U.S.A.

BRUCE HEADEY, RUUT VEENHOVEN, AND ALEX WEARI

15. TOP-DOWN VERSUS BOTTOM-UP THEORIES OF SUBJECTIVE WELL-BEING*

(Received 22 May, 1990)

ABSTRACT. This paper addresses issues of causal direction in research on subjective well-being (SWB). Previous researchers have generally assumed that such variables as domain satisfactions, social support, life events, and levels of expectation and aspiration are causes of SWB. Critics have pointed out that they could just as well be consequences (Costa and McCrae, 1980; Veenhoven, 1988). In some contexts this has been referred to as the top-down versus bottom-up controversy (Diener, 1984). The main purpose is to propose a general statistical model which holds promise of resolving this controversy. The model can be used when three or more waves of panel data are available. It is used here to assess causal direction between six domain satisfactions (marriage, work, leisure, standard of living, friendship and health) and SWB. Data are drawn from four waves of an Australian Quality of Life panel survey (1981—1987) with an initial sample size of 942.

One of the most fundamental problems in research on subjective well-being (SWB) is uncertainty about which variables cause SWB and which are consequences. Almost all previous research has been about the causes of SWB. However most of the variables described as causes have only been shown to be *correlates* of SWB, and might conceivably be consequences, or perhaps both causes and consequences. Diener (1984) has distinguished between bottom-up and top-down theories of SWB. Bottom-up causation is where particular variables cause SWB and top-down causation is where SWB produces certain outcomes.

Among the variables commonly treated as causes of SWB are domain satisfactions, social support, major life events and reference standards (expectations, aspirations, sense of equity etc.). Several reviewers have pointed out that all these variables could conceivably be consequences of SWB and have urged greater attention to issues of causal direction (Costa and McCrae, 1980; Diener, 1984; Veenhoven, 1984, 1987). Informally, however, there has been a tendency to dismiss these exhortations as requiring investigation of hopelessly confounded

Alex C. Michalos (ed.), Citation Classics from Social Indicators Research, 401–420.
© 2005 *Springer. Printed in the Netherlands.*

chicken-and-egg issues; 'there is no point in asking which came first the chicken or the egg'.

The main purpose of the present paper is to propose a statistical model which holds promise of resolving issues of causal direction. The model can be used if three or more waves of data are available from the same panel of respondents. The purpose of the model is to estimate the *net effects* of a variable of interest on SWB and of SWB on the variable. Estimated effects need to be net of spurious covariation due to possible joint dependence of both variables on other variables, whether these other variables are included in the model (which they are if measured) or omitted (if unmeasured). We shall refer to the net effect of a variable of interest on SWB as a bottom-up (BU) effect, and the net effect of SWB on the variable as a top-down (TD) effect.

This paper focusses on linkages between domain satisfactions and SWB. The six domains selected for analysis — marriage, work, material standard of living, leisure, friendship and health — have consistently been found to be strong correlates of SWB (Andrews and Withey, 1976; Argyle, 1987; Campbell, Converse and Rodgers, 1976; Headey, Holmstrom and Wearing, 1985). Most researchers have assumed that a bottom-up model is appropriate and, more precisely, that a linear additive combination of domain satisfactions accounts for SWB (Andrews and Withey, 1976; Argyle, 1987; Campbell *et al.*, 1976; Headey *et al.*, 1985). In other words, the whole is the sum of the parts; satisfaction with life is a result of marriage satisfaction, job satisfaction, leisure satisfaction etc. Contrary to this view, Diener (1984) notes that high inter-correlations among domain satisfactions could be taken as evidence for a top-down model. The correlations suggests that domain satisfactions could be just a spin-off from overall levels of life satisfaction. A third possibility, implied by Costa and McCrae (1980), is that apparent causal relationships between domain satisfactions and measures of SWB are spurious, with both sets of variables being dependent on stable personal traits, notably extraversion and neuroticism.

Matters become more complex when it is recognised that the three models outlined above are not mutually exclusive. To give an example, the correlation between marriage satisfaction and SWB may be partly due to the influence of marriage on life satisfaction, partly due to the influence of life on marriage, and partly spurious. Furthermore, contrary to what previous reviews have implied, there is no strong reason to expect that the same pattern of relationships holds for all domains. As will be seen, the evidence indicates that the relative strength of BU and TD effects varies from domain to domain.

This paper should be read as an exploratory analysis of two-way causation, using panel data. It is hoped that the statistical model proposed here has broad application in SWB research. However it should be emphasised that results are only as good as the statistical assumptions underlying them. It is desirable to vary assumptions to se if results are substantially affected (sensitivity analysis). Where possible, the effects of alternative assumptions have been tested in this paper and results appear not to change much. Nevertheless the model requires careful scrutiny and results need replicating before they can be accepted with confidence.

METHODS

Sample

Data to estimate the models come from four waves of the Australian Quality of Life Panel Study (1981, 1983, 1985, 1987). The panel study is conducted in Australia's most densely populated state, Victoria. A stratified probability sample of 942 persons was drawn in 1981. By 1987 649 respondents remained. House movers are usually traced (over 350 respondents moved between 1981 and 1987) but, inevitably, panel loss is fairly substantial. Checks have shown that the means and standard deviations of all variables (except age) have remained virtually unchanged over the four waves. It is hoped that the study will continue for a decade until 1991.

Measures

Life Satisfaction. It is generally agreed that at least three dimensions of SWB need to be distinguished: cognitive life satisfaction, positive affect and negative affect (Andrews and Withey, 1976; Argyle, 1987; Diener, 1984). In the present paper we focus on life satisfaction. This was measured by Andrews and Withey's (1976) Life-as-a-whole Index. The index requires twice asking respondents, 'How do you feel about your life-as-a-whole?' The two items were approximately twenty minutes apart on the interview schedule. The response scale was a 9-point Delighted-Terrible scale, expanded from Andrews and Withey's 7-point scale to reduce bunching at the top end (Headey *et al.*, 1984).

The Life-as-a-whole Index is considered one of the most reliable and valid measures of cognitive life satisfaction (Diener, 1984; Veenhoven, 1984). The two items were included as separate indicators in our LISREL measurement models (see below).

Domain satisfactions. Levels of satisfaction with the domains of marriage, work, standard of living, leisure, friendship and health were measured on a 9-point Delighted-Terrible scale. For all domains multiple items were used to enhance reliability. For inclusion in measurement models the items measuring each domain were combined into two equal sub-sets. This had the effect of producing two adequately reliable indicators, whereas inclusion of all items separately would have meant that some indicators had low reliability.

Personality. The Eysenck Personalty Invenory, Form B (Eysenck and Eysenck, 1964) measures extraversion and neuroticism. For inclusion in the measurement model the 24 indicators of extraversion were split into sub-sets of 12, as were the 24 indicators of neuroticism.

Socio-economic status. The three indicators were gross family income, the occupational status of the main breadwinner and the educational level of the respondent.

The other two measures included in models were sex (male = 1, female = 2) and age. Both were assumed to be 100% reliable in measurement models.

Data Analysis: Assessing Causal Direction

A concept of causation which statisticians often work with requires that in order to say that *A* causes *B* one has to show that:

1. *A* and *B* are correlated;

2. The correlation is not entirely spurious;

3. A precedes B in time (changes in A precede changes in B).

The biggest difficulty faced in SWB research, and survey research generally, relates to the third condition. Take the relationship between a domain satisfaction (DS) and life satisfaction (LS). In a panel survey several measures of both variables are obtained, and the scores of many respondents change. However no direct observation is possible of whether changes in DS precede or follow changes in LS. In order to get round this problem statisticians have persistently proposed methods based on the idea that if the relationship between DS_1 (domain satisfaction at time 1) and LS_2 (life satisfaction at time 2) is stronger than between LS_1 and DS_2, then the direction of causation is predominantly from DS to LS. On the other hand if $LS_1 \rightarrow DS_2 > DS_1 \rightarrow LS_2$, then causation runs mainly form LS to DS.

Kessler and Greenberg (1981) in their thorough review of alternative methods based on this reasoning conclude that, if three or more waves of panel data are available, the following model is particularly promising. It is promising (a) because no instrumental variables are required (and the search for appropriate instruments is often fruitless) and (b) because few restrictive assumptions are required.

The usual problem with models which include two-way causation is that some equations are not identified (i.e. there are too many unknowns and too few pieces of information). However, as Kessler and Greenberg (1981) demonstrate, their 3-wave model is identified if one includes the two equality constraints show in Figure 1.[1] $LS_1 \rightarrow LS_2$ is assumed equal to $LS_2 \rightarrow LS_3$ and $DS_1 \rightarrow LS_2$ is assumed equal to $DS_2 \rightarrow LS_3$. On both theoretical and empirical grounds these assumptions appear well justified in the Australian data. Note, in particular, that correlations among variables are much the same within each wave of data (see Appendix I).

The model includes both lagged and contemporaneous links between DS and LS. The cross-lagged links are in accordance with the usual understanding of causation in which causes must precede effects. The concept of contemporaneous or simultaneous causation is more problematic, because it defies the time sequence requirement. However statisticians, especially econometricians, often include simultaneous

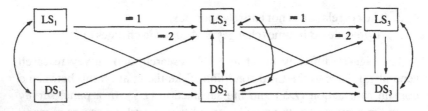

Key:

DS = Domain satisfaction
LS = Life satisfaction
1, 2, 3 = time points
= 1 an imposed equality
= 2 an imposed equality

Fig. 1. Kessler and Greenberg's three-wave model with two imposed equalities.

causation in their models in situations where time sequence cannot, in practice, be directly observed, but where causal lags can be assumed to be fairly short and, certainly, shorter than the interval between observations (e.g. between surveys).

Unfortunately there is another difficulty. Although the model is in principle identified, one is likely to find that, in actually estimating equations, problems of multicollinearity are encountered. In particular, estimates of the lagged and contemporaneous effects of a predictor variable (e.g. $DS_1 \rightarrow LS_2$ and $DS_2 \rightarrow LS_2$) are likely to be too highly correlated to be reliable.[2] So, in practice, in any given computer run, one is forced to drop from the model *either* the cross-lagged links between *DS* and *LS or* the contemporaneous, reciprocal links. All is not lost, however. Models with only lagged links and only contemporaneous links can be run consecutively. Provided that the *signs* of the lagged and contemporaneous estimates showing causation running from, for example, *DS* to *LS* are the same, then the two estimates may be regarded as consistent, although both will be conservative if the 'true' causal (time) lag falls between the two points of observation (cf. Greenberg and Kessler, 1982).[3]

In the present paper there are perhaps reasons for believing that contemporaneous links come closer to providing accurate estimates than lagged links. On *a priori* grounds one might expect that, if they had any effect at all, changes in domain satisfactions would have fairly rapid effects on life satisfaction. Similarly, changes in life satisfaction might be expected soon to affect domain satisfactions. At a more practical level it should be noted that interviews in the Australian panel study are conducted at two year intervals. It seems most unlikely that the causal effects analysed here take anything like two years to be felt. Supporting this view is the fact that contemporaneous correlations in the data are somewhat higher than lagged correlations (Appendix I). In practice we shall rely primarily on contemporaneous estimates of reciprocal causation. We will find, however, that the lagged estimates not only have the same signs as contemporaneous estimates but are not a great deal lower.

The general model used to obtain results given in this paper embodies several modifications of Kessler and Greenberg's model. Five separate sets of equalities were imposed. They reflect a theory that the 'true' relationships in the structural (causal) model should be the same in all four waves of data. Technically the effect of the equalities was to assist with identification problems and to provide extra degrees of freedom in arriving at maximum likelihood estimates (see below).

Two features of the model were included to test hypotheses about the possible spuriousness of links between domain satisfactions and LS (i.e. their joint dependence on other variables). Five stable personal characteristics — sex, age, socio-economic status, extraversion and neuroticism — were included as exogenous variables. The first three may be regarded as standard background variables which need to be routinely 'controlled', while extraversion and neuroticism were included because Costa and McCrae (1980) hypothesize that apparent causal relationships between DS and LS are spurious due to these personality traits which they, among others, have shown to be very stable over a lifetime. Exogenous variables are of course assumed to be causes not consequences of DS and LS, and in so far as relationships between DS and LS are due to joint dependence on exogenous variables, the model allows these effects to be partialled out, providing a more accurate estimate of the BU and TD effects of chief interest. It should be noted that only time 1 (1981) measures of these stable exogenous variables have been included.[4] They are assumed to be related directly to DS and LS only at time 1. (However if direct links to later measures of DS and

LS are inserted, then bottom-up and top-down results of main interest are virtually unaffected).

Spuriousness could also be due to variables omitted from the model. The effects of such variables are obtained by estimating correlations between error terms of equations for *DS* and *LS* (Kessler and Greenberg, 1981). (The correlated errors are labelled ➡ 5 in Fig. 2).

It needs to be recognised that, in estimating a model of this kind, we are assuming that relationships among variables are in equilibrium. If the equilibrium assumption were not met, it would be inappropriate to use structural equation methods (Kenny, 1979; Rogosa *et al.*, 1982; Rogosa and Willett, 1985). In regard to the present model, the reader is asked to inspect the correlations, means and standard deviations in Appendix 1 to confirm that relationships across waves appear to be very close to equilibrium. (Appendix I covers only one application of the model. Relevant statistics for other applications are available from the authors).

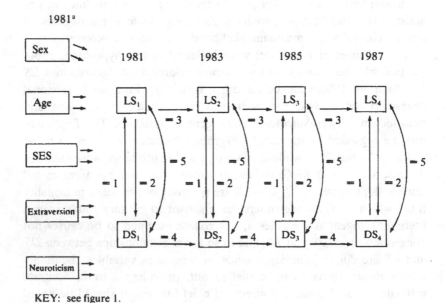

KEY: see figure 1.
   a. These variables are directly linked to *DS* and *LS* only at time 1 (1981)

Fig. 2. General model with 4 waves of data.

To summarize: the chief purpose of the model is to estimate the effects of variables of interest on SWB and vice-versa. For reasons given, we treat contemporaneous reciprocal estimates as the best available, calculating lagged estimates primarily to check that the signs of the coefficients are the same. Spurious effects due to both included and omitted exogenous variables are also estimated in order to get more accurate estimates of the net effects of variables of interest on SWB and vice-versa.[5] Problems of identification have been dealt with primarily by imposing equalities which seem justified on grounds of theory.

The Measurement Model

The previous section dealt with possible relationships in a structural equation or causal model. It is also necessary to provide a measurement model; a model specifying linkages between underlying concepts and the survey items used to measure concepts. Whenever the same variables are measured at successive time points, there is a risk of misestimating relationships due to measurement errors made on the first occasion being repeated on later occasions. However, provided that there are at least two indicators for each concept, autocorrelated error can be estimated if three or more waves of data are available (Kessler and Greenberg, 1981). In the measurement model which accompanied the structural model, autocorrelated error terms were estimated whenever the same indicator (survey question) was repeatedly used to measure the same concept. We thus allowed for the possibility of first, second and third order autocorrelated error. Furthermore, error terms relating to the same indicator were constrained to be equal, because it is reasonable to assume that the degree of error would be the same on each occasion (i.e. we assumed first, second and third order methods effects; see Andrews and Withey, 1976). Details are given in Appendix II.

LISREL

The ideal software for present purposes is LISREL IV (Joreskog and Sorbom, 1978).[6] LISREL first estimates a measurement model in order to calculate disattenuated (estimated 'true') correlations among the concepts in the structural model. It then uses these correlations to calculate the coefficients in the causal model (maximum likelihood estimates).

LISREL has the flexibility to perform the tasks needed to estimate our models. It can accept equality constraints, it can estimate correlations among error terms in the structural model, and it can estimate autocorrelated error in the measurement model.

The LISREL runs for this paper were based on correlation matrices and, in presenting results, *standardized* (not metric) maximum likelihood estimates are given. The use of standardized estimates is often considered appropriate when, as is the case here, all variables of interest have arbitrary metrics. The use of standardized estimates makes it easy to assess the relative magnitude of *BU* and *TD* effects, since estimates are constrained to fall between −1 and +1. It should be noted, however, that all models were re-run using variance-covariance matrices as inputs into LISREL in order to obtain metric (unstandardized) estimates. In all cases the metric results told essentially the same story as the standardized results given below.

RESULTS

As noted above, most previous researchers have assumed but not demonstrated that a bottom-up model adequately summarizes relationships between domain satisfactions and life satisfaction. A more complicated picture emerges from the following pages. Of the six major life domains analyzed, there is one case of reciprocal causation, three of (mainly) top-down causation and two of spuriousness.

We first give results relating to marriage satisfaction and life satisfaction.

The model indicates two-way causation. Being happily married increases one's life satisfaction (*BU* = 0.18), but it is also true that happy people are more likely to maintain happy marriages ... while miserable people tend to have miserable marriages (*TD* = 0.12). No statistically significant differences were found between results for men and women.

It should be remembered that these statistically significant *BU* and

TD coefficients are net of the effects of the stable personal characteristics included in the model, and of the effects of omitted exogenous variables (estimated at 0.10). Costa and McCrae's (1980) hypothesis that stable personal characteristics account for apparent causal relationships between domain satisfactions and life satisfaction appears incorrect in regard to the marriage domain.

It is essential to check that the lagged *BU* and *TD* estimates have the same signs as the contemporaneous estimates. For this model the lagged *BU* estimate was 0.08 and the lagged *TD* estimate was 0.07 (both coefficients are just significant at the 0.05 level). For reasons given above, it seems likely that the contemporaneous estimates are closer to being accurate.[7]

Since this is the first set of results presented, a number of technical points need to be made; points which also apply to subsequent models. A initial comment is that the model fits the data very satisfactorily. LISREL models can be evaluated by several measures of fit. For this model *Chi*-square divided by degrees of freedom was 1.60 (Carmines and McIver, 1981), Hoelter's (1983) Critical Number (*CN*) was 258.62, and the mean absolute residual was 0.04. It should also be noted that the standard errors and LISREL diagnostics relating to correlations among parameter estimates indicated no symptoms of multicollinearity.

A number of *sensitivity analyses* indicate that reasonable variations in model specification do not affect the basic result that marriage satisfaction influences life satisfaction and vice-versa. If the correlated error terms are dropped (the terms marked $=$ 5 in Fig. 2), the betas change to *BU* $=$ 0.25 and *TD* $=$ 0.20. A valuable check, available with four waves of panel data (Kessler and Greenberg, 1981), is to remove one pair of equality constraints between *MS* and *LS* and to see if the estimates for the free parameters are approximately the same as for the constrained parameters. In fact they are (*BU* $=$ 0.14, *TD* $=$ 0.15). A further possibility is to allow the exogenous variables to affect marriage and life satisfaction at all later time point as well as at time 1. Again, the reciprocal causation results of chief interest are scarcely affected. (It may be noted that, because of the large number of imposed equality constraints, the model is still identified.)

Next, how is life satisfaction linked to job satisfaction and material

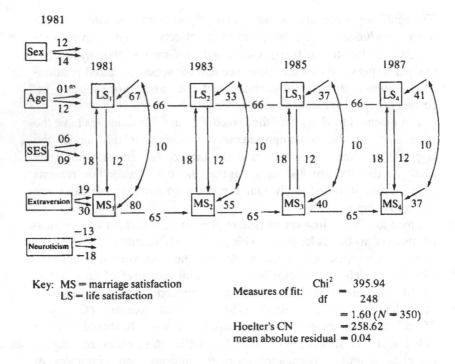

Key: MS = marriage satisfaction
      LS = life satisfaction

Measures of fit: $\dfrac{Chi^2}{df}$ = $\dfrac{395.94}{248}$

= 1.60 (N = 350)

Hoelter's CN   = 258.62
mean absolute residual = 0.04

Fig. 3. Does marriage satisfaction cause life satisfaction, or vice-versa, or both?

standard of living? A well established but puzzling finding is that most people, even those in low status and routine jobs, report fairly high levels of job satisfaction and satisfaction with their standard of living. Our panel data show that satisfaction with work and standard of living are just a spin-of (consequences) of life satisfaction and have no causal effect at all. The contemporaneous estimates (lagged estimates in parentheses) were:

Job satisfaction $BU = -0.07^{ns} (-0.03^{ns})$
$TD = 0.24 (0.19)$
Standard of living satisfaction $BU = -0.04^{ns} (-0.02^{ns})$
$TD = 0.18 (0.12)$

It is well known from much previous research that low status people in Western countries are not much less satisfied with their lives-as-a-whole than high status people (Veenhoven, 1984). In view of the results just given, it seems that this is the main reason for them not being much less satisfied than others with their work and living standards.

Now leisure satisfaction. A surprising finding in previous research is that leisure satisfaction correlates as highly if not more highly with life satisfaction than any other domain (Andrews and Withey, 1976; Campbell et al., 1976; Headey et al., 1985). In a bottom-up framework this result is puzzling because one would not, on a priori grounds, be inclined to accept that leisure mattered most to life satisfaction. Application of the reciprocal causation model helps to resolve the puzzle because it transpires that the bottom-up link is insignificant ($BU = 0.06^{ns}$), whereas the top-down link is moderately strong ($TD = 0.17$). The effect of omitted exogenous variables, given by the correlated error term (marked as $= 5$ in Fig. 2) is also strong (0.24). The equivalent lagged estimates confirm this pattern of results: $BU = -0.05^{ns}$, $TD = 0.12$. In short, the high correlations between leisure and life satisfaction, reported in previous studies, appear to have led to inappropriate causal inferences. Leisure satisfaction is partly just a spin-off of SWB, and the relationship is partly spurious.

Several studies have concluded that satisfaction with friendships and social support are a major determinant of SWB (Argyle, 1987). But results from our model, giving contemporaneous links, show that neither bottom-up nor top-down links between friendship satisfaction and life satisfaction are statistically significant at the 0.05 level ($BU = -0.01^{ns}$, $TD = 0.06^{ns}$). The equivalent lagged estimates were $BU = -0.01^{ns}$, and $TD = 0.04^{ns}$. In other words the correlation between friendship satisfaction and life satisfaction ($r = 0.49$) appears to be spurious. The main explanation for this result is that the model includes extraversion as an exogenous variable antecedent to both friendship and life satisfaction. This causal ordering, while hopefully justified, means that, in effect, extraversion is permitted to account for as much variance as possible before the reciprocal effects of friendship and life satisfaction on each other are assessed. Extraversion is highly related to friendship satisfaction ($Beta = 0.52$) and fairly highly to life satisfaction

(*Beta* = 0.36), so the consequences of assumptions about causal ordering are non-trivial. The friendship domain is one in which Costa and McCrae's spuriousness hypothesis is partly confirmed.

Finally, health. The panel survey includes measures of self-reported health and health satisfaction but provides no independent medical checks. Application of the standard model indicates no significant links from health satisfaction to life satisfaction or vice-versa. The association between the variables (r = 0.36) is spurious, with extraversion and neuroticism being related to both, neuroticism particularly to health (dis)satisfaction. Health, then, is a second domain in which Costa and McCrae's spuriousness hypothesis is confirmed.

Table I summarizes contemporaneous and lagged estimates between life satisfaction and the six domain satisfactions considered in this paper.

It can be seen that all pairs of contemporaneous and lagged estimates have the same signs and, indeed, that the magnitudes of most

TABLE I

Contemporaneous and lagged reciprocal relationships between domain satisfactions and life satisfaction

| Domain | Type of Effect[b] | Relationship with Life Satisfaction | |
		Contemporaneous Effects	Lagged Effects
Marriage	*BU*	0.18	0.08
	TD	0.12	0.07
Job	*BU*	-0.07^{ns}	-0.03^{ns}
	TD	0.24	0.19
Standard of	*BU*	-0.04^{ns}	-0.02^{ns}
Living	*TD*	0.18	0.12
Leisure	*BU*	-0.06^{ns}	-0.05^{ns}
	TD	0.17	0.12
Friendship	*BU*	-0.01^{ns}	-0.01^{ns}
	TD	0.06^{ns}	0.04^{ns}
Health	*BU*	0.02^{ns}	0.00^{ns}
	TD	0.05^{ns}	0.05^{ns}

[a] Standardized maximum likelihood estimates (betas).
[b] *BU* — bottom-up effects; *TD* — top-down effects.
[ns] Not significant at the 0.05 level.

pairs are similar. Substantively, this means that reasonable confidence can be placed in our interpretation of the relative importance of *BU* and *TD* effects.

DISCUSSION

The main purpose of this paper has been to present a general statistical model which may help to clarify issues of causal direction in SWB research. Because the model embodies numerous non-obvious assumptions, it is important to vary assumptions and check if results are substantially affected. It is also important to see if results replicate in other data sets. However if the results in this paper are confirmed, they stand a good deal of conventional wisdom on its head. Most researchers have held a bottom-up view of links between domain satisfactions and life satisfaction. Even those who have recognised the possibility of top-down causation have tended to pose the issue in either-or terms; either all relationships must be top-down or all bottom-up. The results given above paint a more complicated picture. The marriage domain is characterized by two-way causation. The work, leisure and standard of living domains show top-down causation, and the observed correlations between life satisfaction and both friendship and health satisfaction appear to be spurious. These results hold under a variety of assumptions, although not in most cases if we (misguidedly?) drop the assumption that relationships could be wholly or partly spurious (i.e. dropping the correlated error terms in Fig. 2 does make a difference).

The implications of the unexpected degree of support for top-down theory need to be carefully considered. Some might infer that the results lend support to the view that life satisfaction (or, more generally, *SWB*) is a fairly stable trait rather than a fluctuating state (Diener, 1984). While not directly dissenting from this interpretation, our view is that the state-trait controversy applied to SWB research offers few insights. We have estimated the stability of *SWB* measures at around 0.55—0.60 for two, four and six year intervals (Headey and Wearing, 1989). This may be regarded as a fairly high degree of stability, but it is also true that about a quarter of the population shift by over a standard deviation in these time periods.

In future work the intention is to apply the same approach to analyzing causal relationships between SWB and other variables besides domain satisfactions. As noted above, it is open to question whether variables like social support, levels of expectation and aspiration, perceptions of role performance and reports of life events are causes or consequences of *SWB* ... or whether, indeed, apparent relationships are spurious. It will also be desirable to extend the analysis to other dimensions of *SWB* besides cognitive life satisfaction. Top-down and bottom-up theories of SWB are likely to remain in contention for the foreseeable future. In this paper we have proposed a statistical model which, it is hoped, offers promise of disentangling the causal network.

APPENDIX

APPENDIX I
Means, SDs and correlations for variables in Fig. 3

Matrix to be analyzed

	1	2	3	4	5	6	7	8	9	10
1	1.000									
2	0.821	1.000								
3	0.467	0.502	1.000							
4	0.418	0.484	0.682	1.000						
5	0.520	0.463	0.299	0.311	1.000					
6	0.493	0.528	0.311	0.324	0.875	1.000				
7	0.325	0.412	0.515	0.538	0.491	0.541	1.000			
8	0.356	0.414	0.512	0.578	0.465	0.530	0.696	1.000		
9	0.498	0.427	0.257	0.330	0.605	0.618	0.359	0.371	1.000	
10	0.428	0.450	0.286	0.363	0.571	0.671	0.423	0.463	0.838	1.000
11	0.245	0.274	0.367	0.373	0.317	0.357	0.499	0.481	0.414	0.483
12	0.314	0.379	0.407	0.518	0.353	0.429	0.516	0.592	0.485	0.564
13	0.462	0.436	0.247	0.329	0.527	0.549	0.323	0.361	0.730	0.700
14	0.430	0.481	0.277	0.365	0.519	0.609	0.338	0.385	0.670	0.732
15	0.269	0.345	0.362	0.422	0.333	0.384	0.461	0.473	0.407	0.466
16	0.286	0.390	0.351	0.461	0.283	0.337	0.402	0.480	0.422	0.498
17	0.062	0.097	0.089	0.109	0.006	0.073	0.080	0.053	0.092	0.130
18	0.005	−0.025	0.111	0.022	−0.003	0.043	0.059	−0.039	0.037	0.063
19	0.151	0.115	0.161	0.082	0.138	0.083	0.145	0.108	0.072	0.026
20	0.060	0.049	0.124	0.104	0.089	0.057	0.111	0.033	0.121	0.094
21	0.092	0.057	−0.002	−0.004	0.061	−0.011	−0.050	−0.009	0.033	−0.007
22	0.054	0.125	0.105	0.164	0.065	0.030	0.116	0.115	0.059	0.073
23	0.203	0.186	0.235	0.202	0.108	0.053	0.174	0.154	0.40	0.085
24	−0.180	−0.145	−0.223	−0.201	−0.243	−0.202	−0.197	−0.156	−0.196	−0.166
25	−0.190	−0.184	−0.238	−0.212	−0.201	−0.184	−0.175	−0.162	−0.200	−0.182

Appendix I (Continued)

Matrix to be analyzed

	11	12	13	14	15	16	17	18	19	20
11	1.000									
12	0.685	1.000								
13	0.298	0.406	1.000							
14	0.386	0.485	0.877	1.000						
15	0.503	0.586	0.405	0.446	1.000					
16	0.478	0.623	0.479	0.530	0.720	1.000				
17	0.108	0.127	0.096	0.135	0.056	0.064	1.000			
18	0.019	0.025	0.75	0.85	0.034	0.012	0.079	1.000		
19	0.065	0.015	0.046	−0.006	0.063	0.047	−0.170	−0.031	1.000	
20	0.110	0.066	0.114	0.043	0.055	0.052	−0.025	0.083	0.482	1.000
21	0.022	−0.008	0.029	−0.033	−0.013	−0.054	−0.104	−0.099	0.298	0.318
22	0.116	0.140	0.053	0.078	0.084	0.140	0.028	−0.274	0.039	0.032
23	0.083	0.155	0.010	0.042	0.147	0.106	0.004	−0.051	0.056	0.097
24	−0.179	−0.137	−0.179	−0.159	−0.206	−0.147	0.201	−0.050	−0.208	−0.231
25	−0.145	−0.119	−0.190	−0.152	−0.175	−0.129	0.126	−0.154	−0.198	−0.236

Matrix to be analyzed

	21	22	23	24	25
21	1.000				
22	−0.061	1.000			
23	0.038	0.419	1.000		
24	−0.231	−0.105	−0.223	1.000	
25	−0.205	−0.035	−0.204	0.750	1.000

Key to variables			$\bar{X}$	(SD)				$\bar{X}$	(SD)
(1)	Marriage		7.1	(1.6)	(15)	Life		7.0	(1.3)
(2)	Satisfaction	81	7.5	(1.2)	(16)	Satisfaction	87	7.0	(1.1)
(3)	Life		7.1	(1.3)	(17)	Sex	81	1.5	(0.5)
(4)	Satisfaction	81	7.1	(1.2)	(18)	Age	81	37.1	(12.8)
(5)	Marriage		7.1	(1.4)	(19)			4.6	(1.6)
(6)	Satisfaction	83	7.5	(1.2)	(20)	SES	81	3.8	(1.3)
(7)	Life		7.1	(1.2)	(21)			3.7	(1.5)
(8)	Satisfaction	83	7.0	(1.5)	(22)			7.2	(2.1)
(9)	Marriage		7.2	(1.3)	(23)	Extraversion	81	7.2	(1.9)
(10)	Satisfaction	85	7.2	(1.2)	(24)			5.5	(2.7)
(11)	Life		7.1	(1.1)	(25)	Neuroticism	81	5.3	(2.6)
(12)	Satisfaction	85	7.1	(1.1)					
(13)	Marriage		7.0	(1.4)					
(14)	Satisfaction	87							

APPENDIX II
Measurement model for figure 3

Loadings for indicators of endogenous concepts	Error term of endogenous indicators	Auto-correlated error
MS_{81} (1) 0.82	0.25	First
(2) 0.93	0.09	indicator
		of $MS = 0.08$
LS_{81} (1) 0.80	0.33	
(2) 0.81	0.30	Second
		indicator
MS_{83} (1) 0.95	0.25	of $MS = -0.01$
(2) 1.0	0.00	
		First
LS_{83} (1) 0.78	0.32	indicator
(2) 0.83	0.30	of $LS = 0.02$
MS_{85} (1) 0.93	0.21	Second
(2) 0.98	0.09	indicator
		of $LS = 0.05$
LS_{85} (1) 0.81	0.39	
(2) 0.88	0.23	
MS_{87} (1) 0.90	0.18	
(2) 0.97	0.07	
LS_{87} (1) 0.85	0.33	
(2) 0.87	0.25	

Loadings for indicators of exogenous concepts	Error terms of exogenous indicators
Sex 1.0*	0.01
Age 1.0*	0.00
SES (1) 0.69	0.52
(2) 0.68	0.53
(3) 0.46	0.79
Extraversion (1) 0.66	0.56
(2) 0.88	0.61
Neuroticism (1) 0.88	0.23
(2) 0.85	0.27

Structural Equation Model

One matrix in the structural equation model could not conveniently be printed in Fig. 3. This is the matrix of correlations among exogenous concepts.

Correlations among exogenous concepts

	(1)	(2)	(3)	(4)	(5)
Sex (1)	1.00				
Age (2)	0.08	1.00			
SES (3)	−0.16	0.00	1.00		
Extraversion (4)	0.03	−0.26	0.09	1.00	
Neuroticism (5)	0.19	−0.11	−0.39	−0.25	1.00

NOTES

* We particularly thank Ronald C. Kessler of the University of Michigan for his advice on statistical issues. We are also very grateful for comments from Frank M. Andrews of the University of Michigan and Mariah Evans and Jonathan Kelley of Australian National University. Constructive comments from an anonymous SIR reader also led to significant revisions.

[1] If more equality constraints are imposed, then over-identified equations result. This is highly desirable for estimation purposes.

[2] This occurs whenever the model is nearly in equilibrium (i.e. when correlations among variables in successive waves of data are approximately the same). The effect is the same as under-identification; successive waves are not supplying new information.

[3] Greenberg and Kessler (1982) state that the correct estimate must be *between* the lagged and contemporaneous estimates. We are grateful to Frank M. Andrews of the University of Michigan for the observation made in the text.

[4] It appears odd to refer to age as a stable variable. However the *relative* ages of Australian panel members have of course remained entirely stable and this is what matters for the structural equation modelling which follows. Of the other exogenous variables, sex and SES are clearly stable over a 6-year period. The personality traits, extraversion and neuroticism, have been shown to be highly stable in much previous work (e.g. Costa and McCrae, 1984). In the present study both traits have been almost 100% stable.

[5] In other words the covariance between a variable of interest and SWB is treated as having four components: (1) the effect of the variable on *SWB* (2) the effect of *SWB* on the variable (3) joint dependence on exogenous variables included in the model and (4) joint dependence on omitted exogenous variables.

[6] LISREL IV is preferable to later versions of LISREL. Kessler and Greenberg's (1981) demonstration that their 3-wave model is identified refers to the *reduced form* of the structural equations (not to the structural equations as such) and these are employed in LISREL IV. Later versions of LISREL directly estimate the structural equations.

[7] It may also be noted that LISREL diagnoses less satisfactory fits between model and data when lagged estimates are used. For discussion of the measures of fit employed see p. 91.

REFERENCES

Andrews, F. M. and Withey, S. B.: 1976, Social Indicators of Well-Being (Plenum, New York).

Argyle, M.: 1987, The Psychology of Happiness (Methuen, London).

Bradburn, N. M.: 1969, The Structure of Psychological Well-Being (Aldine, Chicago).

Campbell, A., Converse, P. E., and Rodgers, W. R.: 1976, The Quality of American Life (Sage, New York).

Carmines, E. G. and McIver, J. P.: 1981, 'Analysing models with unobserved variables', in G. W. Bohrnstedt and E. F. Borgatta (eds.), Social Measurement: Current Issues (Beverley Hills, Sage).

Costa, P. T. and McCrae, R. R.: 1980, 'Influence of extraversion and neuroticism on subjective well-being', Journal of Personality and Social Psychology 38, 668—78.

Costa, P. T. and McCrae, R. R.: 1984, 'Personality as a lifelong determinant of well-being', in C. Malatesta and C. Izard (eds.), Affective Processes in Adult Development and Agiing (Beverley Hills, Sage).

Diener, E.: 1984, 'Subjective well-being', Psychological Bulletin 95, 542—75.

Eysenck, H. J. and Eysenck, S. B. G.: 1964, Manual of the Eysenck Personality Inventory (Hodder and Stoughton, London).

Greenberg, D. F. and Kessler, R. C.: 1982, 'Equilibrium and identification in linear panel models', Sociological Methods and Research 10, 435—51.

Headey, B. W., Holmstrom, E. L. and Wearing, A. J.: 1985, 'Models of well-being and ill-being', Social Indicators Research 17, 211—34.

Headey, B. W. and Wearing, A. J.: 1988, 'The sense of relative superiority: central to well-being', Social Indicators Research 20, pp. 497—516.

Headey, B. W. and Wearing, A. J.: 1990, What Makes for Happiness? A Theory of Subjective Well-Being (forthcoming).

Hoelter, J. W.: 1983, 'The analysis of covariance structure', Sociological Methods and Research 11, 325—44.

Joreskog, K. G. and Sorbom, D.: 1978, LISREL IV (International Educational Services, Chicago).

Kenny, D. A.: 1979, Correlation and Causality (Wiley, New York).

Kessler, R. C. and Greenberg, D. F.: 1981, Linear Panel Analysis (Academic Press, New York).

Kohn, M. L. and Schooler, C.: 1983, Work and Personality (Ablex, Norwood, N.J.).

Rogosa, D. R., Brandt, D., and Zimowski, M.: 1982, 'A growth curve approach to the measurement of change', Psychological Bulletin 90, 726—48.

Rogosa, D. R. and Willet, J. B.: 1985, 'Understanding correlates of change by modeling individual differences in growth', Psychometrika 50, 203—28.

Veenhoven, R.: 1984, Conditions of Happiness (Reidel, Dordrecht).

Veenhoven, R.: 1988, 'The utility of happiness', Social Indicators Research 20, 333—54.

Pol. Science Dept.,
University of Melbourne,
Parkville,
Victoria 3052, Australia.

ED DIENER

16. ASSESSING SUBJECTIVE WELL-BEING:
PROGRESS AND OPPORTUNITIES

(Accepted 30 July, 1993)

ABSTRACT. Subjective well-being (SWB) comprises people's longer-term levels of pleasant affect, lack of unpleasant affect, and life satisfaction. It displays moderately high levels of cross-situational consistency and temporal stability. Self-report measures of SWB show adequate validity, reliability, factor invariance, and sensitivity to change. Despite the success of the measures to date, more sophisticated approaches to defining and measuring SWB are now possible. Affect includes facial, physiological, motivational, behavioral, and cognitive components. Self-reports assess primarily the cognitive component of affect, and thus are unlikely to yield a complete picture of respondents' emotional lives. For example, denial may influence self-reports of SWB more than other components. Additionally, emotions are responses which vary on a number of dimensions such as intensity, suggesting that mean levels of affect as captured by existing measures do not give a complete account of SWB. Advances in cognitive psychology indicate that differences in memory retrieval, mood as information, and scaling processes can influence self-reports of SWB. Finally, theories of communication alert us to the types of information that are likely to be given in self-reports of SWB. These advances from psychology suggest that a multimethod approach to assessing SWB will create a more comprehensive depiction of the phenomenon. Not only will a multifaceted test battery yield more credible data, but inconsistencies between various measurement methods and between the various components of well-being will both help us better understand SWB indictors and group differences in well-being. Knowledge of cognition, personality, and emotion will also aid in the development of sophisticated theoretical definitions of subjective well-being. For example, life satisfaction is theorized to be a judgment that respondents construct based on currently salient information. Finally, it is concluded that measuring negative reactions such as depression or anxiety give an incomplete picture of people's well-being, and that it is imperative to measure life satisfaction and positive emotions as well.

ASSESSING SUBJECTIVE WELL-BEING:
PROGRESS AND OPPORTUNITIES

Since the Golden Age of Greek philosophy, western thinkers have been concerned with understanding "happiness." Aristotle laid down this agenda when he defined happiness as the summum bonum, the supreme good. He maintained that happiness is the only value which is final and sufficient: final in that all else is merely a means to this end, and sufficient in that once happiness is attained, nothing else is desired. It is little wonder, then, that scholars have been seeking this holy grail ever

421

Alex C. Michalos (ed.), Citation Classics from Social Indicators Research, 421–475.
© 2005 *Springer. Printed in the Netherlands.*

since. It is also unsurprising, given the difficulties that thinkers have in defining this concept, that folk wisdom maintains that happiness is highly desirable, but elusive. Nonetheless, researchers have created a number of self-report scales to measure "happiness." In recent decades behavioral scientists focused a spotlight on happiness, although relabeling the concept under new rubrics such as subjective well-being (SWB), morale, positive affect, and life satisfaction.

The overwhelming majority of work on subjective well-being has been based on self-report assessment. One widespread SWB measure is Bradburn's (1969) Affect Balance Scale which separately measures "positive" and "negative" affect. The respondent is asked whether, in the past few weeks, he or she experienced a series of 10 feelings such as "Depressed or very unhappy" and "On top of the world." Larsen *et al.* (1985) report that this scale performs more poorly than several others, perhaps there are too few questions, in light of the narrowness of most items (e.g., "Upset because someone criticized you"). Nonetheless, the scale was the first to separately assess long-term levels of negative and positive affect.

A short, one-item scale to measure global well-being was developed by Andrews and Withey (1976) and has been used extensively in large-scale survey work. The question asks respondents "How do you feel about your life as a whole?" and instructs them to frame their answer in terms of what has happened in the last year and what they expect in the near future. The seven response options vary from "delighted" to "terrible" and the scale is therefore often called the D-T Scale. In the work of Andrews and Withey, this item is averaged across two administrations given about 20 minutes apart during the interview. The scale was designed to reflect both affective and cognitive components of well-being, and in a cluster analysis falls near the center of well-being items. A LISREL analysis showed the scale to have a surprisingly high validity coefficient (0.77) for two administrations of a single item (Andrews and Robinson, 1991). A similar scale was created by Fordyce (1988). His major question specifically mentions "happiness," and the response options list emotions varying from "elation" to "utter despair." Additional questions ask about the percent of time the respondent feels happy and unhappy. Thus, this scale is likely to reflect emotional well-being to a great extent and a life satisfaction judgment to a lesser extent than the D-T scale. Fordyce (1988) advertises the scale as one which shows "good reliability, exceptional stability, and a record of convergent, construct, and discriminative validity unparalleled in the field" (p. 355).

In contrast to the above scales, the Affectometer 2 (Kammann and Flett, 1983) and the Satisfaction with Life Scale (Diener *et al.*, 1985; Pavot and Diener, 1993b) are multi-item scales which are purposefully designed to more narrowly measure affective well-being and life satisfaction, respectively. The Affectometer 2 measures the balance of pleasant and unpleasant feelings in recent experience with items such as "I smile and laugh a lot" and "Nothing seems very much fun anymore." The Satisfaction with Life Scale (SWLS) was explicitly designed to measure cognitive judgments of life satisfaction rather than affect per se. Sample items, answered on a scale varying from "Strongly agree" to "Strongly disagree," are "If I could live my life over, I would change almost nothing," and, "My life is close to my ideal."

A number of reviews of well-being measurement are available and these focus primarily on the psychometric evaluation of existing scales (Andrews and Robinson, 1991; Diener, 1984; George and Bearon, 1980; Larsen *et al.*, 1985; McKennell, 1974; Nydegger, 1977; Veenhoven, 1984). There are also a number of reviews of the historical definitions of happiness (Jones, 1953; Tatarkiewicz, 1976; Veenhoven, 1984). Finally, there are existing reviews of the correlates of subjective well-being (Andrews and Withey, 1976; Diener, 1984; Diener and Larsen, 1993; Veenhoven, 1984).

In the current review, I examine evidence showing that long-term well-being is a meaningful construct. There are cross-situational consistencies and temporal stabilities in subjective well-being. Further, I briefly review the evidence which demonstrates that self-report measures of SWB display adequate levels of validity and reliability. Despite the past success of SWB measures, information is accumulating in psychology which suggests that current measures and definitions of subjective well-being can be advanced. A major purpose of the present paper is to review advances in psychology as they relate to the assessment of well-being. Progress in basic areas of psychology now make possible more sophisticated understanding and measurement of subjective well-being. In the final section, recommendations are made for improving the definition and measurement of SWB.

PROGRESS TO DATE:
THE CURRENT STATUS OF SWB MEASUREMENT

Defining Subjective Well-Being

Definitions of subjective well-being are often not made explicit in the literature, but are only implied by the measures which are used. Nonetheless, a current composite definition of SWB can be gleaned from the major works in the field. Diener (1984) suggests that there are three hallmarks to the area of SWB: First, it is subjective — it resides within the experience of the individual. Second, it is not just the absence of negative factors, but also includes positive measures. Third, it includes a global assessment rather than only a narrow assessment of one life domain. Although these hallmarks serve to delimit the area of study, they are not complete definitions of subjective well-being.

Veenhoven (1984) defines subjective well-being as the degree to which an individual judges the overall quality of her or his life as a whole in a favorable way. In other words, subjective well-being is how well the person likes the life he or she leads (p. 22). Andrews and Withey (1976) define subjective well-being as "both a cognitive evaluation and some degree of positive or negative feelings, i.e., affect" (p. 18). Veenhoven (1984) follows their lead in asserting that individuals use two components in evaluating their lives: their affects and their thoughts (p. 25). The affective component is hedonic level, the pleasantness experienced in feelings, emotions, and moods. Campbell, Converse, and Rodgers (1976) define satisfaction, the cognitive component, as "the perceived discrepancy between aspiration and achievement, ranging from the perception of fulfillment to that of deprivation. Satisfaction implies a judgmental or cognitive experience while happiness suggests an experience of feeling or affect" (p. 8).

Of course the most useful definition of subjective well-being will be based on a compelling theory. The implicit theory of SWB in the above definitions is the following. Humans are not only capable of appraising events, life circumstances, and themselves, but they make such appraisals continually. Appraisals of things in terms of goodness-badness is a human universal. Following the theory of Lazarus (1991), such appraisals are seen as leading to emotional reactions, which can be either pleasant or unpleasant. Other things being equal, pleasant experiences are perceived as desirable and valuable. Thus, a person who has pleasant emotional experiences is more likely to perceive his or her life as being desirable and positive.

People with high subjective well-being are those who make a preponderance of positive appraisals of their life events and circumstances. People who are "unhappy" are those who appraise a majority of factors in their life as harmful or as blocking their goals. Life satisfaction is a global judgment that people make when they consider their life as a whole, whereas the hedonic component of subjective well-being is the presence of ongoing pleasant affect (due to positive appraisals of ongoing events) much of the time and infrequent unpleasant affect (resulting from few on-line negative appraisals).

Life satisfaction and hedonic level are likely to correlate because both are influenced by appraisals of one's life events, activities, and circumstances. At the same time, life satisfaction and hedonic level are likely to diverge to some degree because life satisfaction is a global summary of one's life as a whole, whereas hedonic level consists of ongoing reactions to events (and may also be influenced by unconscious goals and biological factors which may influence mood). In support of this reasoning, Campbell, Converse, and Rodgers et al. (1976) found that there is a strong general SWB factor, but that there are also components of SWB which may behave differently under some circumstances. Research shows that affect and cognitive satisfaction judgments can diverge (Andrews and Withey, 1976; Horley and Little, 1985; Judge, 1990; Lawton, 1983; Liang, 1985; Stock et al., 1986), although many measures include both components (Chamberlain, 1988). Affective well-being and satisfaction sometimes move in different directions over time and have different correlates (Beiser, 1974; Campbell et al., 1976; DeHaes et al., 1987; Kushman and Lane, 1980). However, life satisfaction and affective well-being tend to fall together on a common well-being factor when a second order factor analysis is performed (Liang, 1985; McNeil et al., 1986), although this second order structure may not be longitudinally invariant (McCulloch, 1991). Thus, SWB is composed of partially separable affective and cognitive components, which nevertheless correlates at levels sufficient to say that they are parts of a higher order construct.

In the literature, the term "happiness" is sometimes used synonymously with subjective well-being. Most authors, however, avoid the use of the term "happiness" because of its varied popular meanings. For example, happiness may refer to the global experience of well-being, to the current feeling of joy, or to the experience of much positive affect over time. In contrast, the terms used in this field now possess more specific meanings. Subjective well-being refers to the global experience of positive reactions to one's life, and includes all of the lower-order components such as life satisfaction and hedonic level. Life satisfaction refers to a conscious global judgment of one's life. Hedonic level or balance refers to the pleasantness minus unpleasantness of one's emotional life.

Subjective well-being is likely to have both stable and changeable components. One's appraisals of ongoing life events can change, and therefore one's hedonic level can change. But at the same time, one's emotions are likely to return to an average baseline which is set by one's temperament and one's general life circumstances. Thus, although immediate emotions may change constantly, one's long-term subjective well-being is likely to have considerable stability. Similarly, one's life satisfaction might change if one's life circumstances change dramatically. There are likely to be many life circumstances, however, which are consistent over time and this leads to a degree of stability in life satisfaction.

One can decompose subjective well-being into finer and finer units. For example, life satisfaction can be broken down into satisfaction with various domains: work, love, and so forth. These domains in turn can be broken down more finely. Similarly, emotion can be divided into finer and finer categories. Unpleasant affect can be broken into discrete emotions such as anger, which can in turn be decomposed into anger over various types of events. The more global categories of hedonic level, life satisfaction, and subjective well-being serve a useful scientific role, however, because people show coherencies between their well-being in different domains (e.g., Campbell et al., 1976) and because specific positive or negative emotions tend to covary to some extent (e.g., McConville and Cooper, 1992). In other words, the reasons to study more molar as well as more molecular categories is that the smaller categories cohere in larger units. Thus, broader categories of well-being are useful scientifically because they point to more global psychological phenomena. At the same time, there are many circumstances in which narrow aspects of subjective well-being are scientifically useful.

Although useful as a starting point, the above definitions and theory must be refined as advances occur in the field. One message of this paper is that advances in other areas of psychology, including cognition and emotion, now allow us to proceed beyond the theory above. If we examine contributions in other areas of psychology, we can offer more refined definitions of subjective well-being and prescribe more sophisticated measurement approaches.

Existence of Long-Term Well-Being

Although well-being researchers recognize the influence of momentary factors in influencing life satisfaction and affective well-being, they are most interested in longer-term subjective well-being. Rather than study emotions which fluctuate from moment-to-moment, SWB researchers are primarily interested in factors which lead to specific levels of well-being over periods of weeks, months, or years. Thus, it is imperative to first demonstrate that there is some stability in moods and life satisfaction which transcends the moment-to-moment fluctuations which exist. Although verbal definitions of SWB have been advanced as described above, these definitions will be important only insofar as the phenomena they describe actually possess long term coherence at the empirical level.

SWB shows some temporal stability. For example, Headey and Wearing (1989) found stabilities in the 0.5 to 0.6 range over a six year period and Chamberlain and Zika (1992) found that the average six-month reliability across well-being measure was 0.69. Wessman and Ricks (1966) report a two-year stability of 0.67 for hedonic level. Others also report strong temporal reliabilities (e.g., Bradburn, 1969; Campbell et al., 1976; Kammann and Flett, 1983). Costa and McCrae

(1988) report an impressive 0.57 correlation between spouse-ratings and self-ratings of positive affect separated by six years and a correlation of 0.49 for negative affect. Given these stabilities, one cannot conceive of well-being as simply a momentary phenomenon without enduring aspects. Because several of the studies relied on both self reports and informant reports, a methodological explanation of the temporal stabilities of SWB in terms of self-report artifacts seems untenable. Thus, long-term levels of life satisfaction and hedonic level do exist.

Further, SWB has cross-situational consistency. Diener and Larsen (1984) found that average pleasant and unpleasant affect correlated 0.58 and 0.70, respectively, across social versus alone situations, and 0.70 and 0.74 across work versus recreation situations. They found that life satisfaction judgments on single occasions correlated 0.44 between social and alone situations, but 0.92 when they aggregated life satisfaction reports over time. Furthermore, Pavot *et al.* (1991) found life satisfaction rating for a target person completed by family members correlated 0.54 with friends' assessments of the target's life satisfaction. This is impressive because the parents and friends observed the subjects in quite different situations. Further, the use of informants again rules out an explanation based on common self-report method variance. Thus, studying long-term levels of well-being is defensible because temporally stable and cross-situationally consistent levels of longer-term SWB clearly exist.

Psychometric Qualities of Self-Report Measures

Research on SWB has relied almost exclusively on self-report assessment. Empirical analyses of these measures reveal that they are somewhat valid and reliable. In the first place, the scales tend to converge with each other. For example, Pavot *et al.* (1991) report that the Satisfaction with Life Scale (Diener *et al.*, 1985) converges with the Life Satisfaction Index-A at r = 0.81, and Sandvik *et al.* (1993) found that the single-item scales of Andrews and Withey and Fordyce correlated at 0.62. Encouragingly, Rodgers *et al.* (1988) estimate that half of the variance in happiness measures is due to the underlying well-being construct, and only about one tenth of the variance is normally due to method.

It is possible to measure subjective well-being with methods other than traditional self-report. For example, a person's well-being might be estimated by friends and measured with informant reports, or it might be measured with the coding of vocal tone and facial expressions during an interview. Several nonself-report measures of SWB will be described later in the paper. Self-report measures of subjective well-being display moderate convergence with nonself-report measures of well-being (e.g., Costa and McCrae, 1988; Jasper, 1930; Lawton, 1972; Lawton *et al.*, 1984; Neugarten *et al.*, 1961; Stones and Kozma, 1980; Washburne, 1941; Wood *et al.*, 1969). For example, Sandvik *et al.* (1993) found that Andrews and Withey's D-T scale correlated 0.58 with informant reports of well-being. They report that daily reports of mood over a six week period correlated 0.66 with the D-T scale given at a prior time. They also found that the Affectometer correlated 0.80 with a factor score comprised of nontraditional measures of SWB, and the single item Fordyce scale correlated 0.68 with this factor. Furthermore, they found that the nonself-report measures converged with each other. For example, they report that an event memory measure (the number of good minus bad events recalled) correlated 0.34 with informant reports of well-being. Pavot *et al.* (1991) reported that peer estimated and self-reported life satisfaction correlated 0.54 and 0.64 in two studies, and that peer-related and self-related affect balance correlated 0.51 and 0.57 in the two studies. Despite this moderate convergence of self-report and nonself-report measures of SWB, it will be argued that the size of these correlations provides insufficient justification for using only self-report assessment in the future. The convergence of self-report and nonself-report measures is ample to suggest that these measures contain substantial amounts of common variance, which points to a coherent phenomenon, but are modest enough to indicate that the various types of measures also capture nonoverlapping aspects of SWB which need to be separately measured. In other words, self-reports of SWB are often likely to yield interesting theoretical results because they do partly reflect common aspects of global well-being. These self-report measures, however, are unlikely to fully capture SWB phenomena because they converge only moderately with measures which tap well-being via other methodologies.

As suggested earlier, SWB measures have moderate temporal reliabilities. In addition, the measures possess Cronbach alphas (Larsen *et al.*, 1985) which indicate a good degree of internal consistency in the scales. For example, the alpha of the Satisfaction with Life Scale (Pavot and Diener, 1993b) is about 0.84. A related issue is the degree of factorial invariance of the scales. If the factor structure of the scales remains similar across very different groups of respondents, it suggests that the measures are assessing a psychological universal with general properties. Fortunately the scales have tended to show factorial invariance across groups (Lawrence and Liang, 1988; MacKinnon and Keating, 1989; Wilson *et al.*, 1985). For instance, a cross-cultural comparison of the Philadelphia Geriatric Center Morale Scale in Japan and the U.S. revealed that the factor structure of the scale was similar in the two countries (Liang *et al.*, 1987). Similarly, Andrews (1991) reports evidence showing that the structure of well-being measures has remained stable in the U.S. from 1972 to 1988. Watson *et al.* (1984) and Balatsky and Diener (1993) both found that affect formed two clear global factors in different cultures. Nevertheless, Shao (1992) and Balatsky and Diener (1992) found that the alphas for the Satisfaction with Life Scale were much lower in China and Russia, respectively, than in the U.S. This suggests that the items do not cohere together in a unified whole as well in those cultures. The factorial invariance of SWB measures across cultures deserves greater research attention. Similarly the second order factor structure of subjective well-being measures over time (e.g. McCulloch, 1991) also deserves further study.

Despite adequate reliabilities of SWB scales, they appear to be sensitive to change (Horley and Lavery, 1991). For instance, Headey and Wearing (1989) found in a longitudinal study that favorable and adverse life events influenced SWB beyond the predictive effects of personality. Atkinson (1982) reported test-retest correlations of about 0.50 for respondents who reported no major life changes, but smaller stabilities for subjects reporting changes. Chamberlain and Zika (1992) found that current hassles predicted well-being in addition to past well-being. Pavot and Diener (1993) review evidence suggesting that SWB measures improve for clients in therapy. Thus, despite the moderate temporal reliabilities of the scales, they do move in response to changed circumstances. These findings are important for two reasons. First, they indicate that subjective well-being measures are sensitive to change. Second, they indicate that subjective well-being is not identical to personality — it can be influenced by life events, especially recent ones.

A concern with all self-report instruments is whether the language used influences responding. Research among those with different languages within the same countries is encouraging in that few differences in reported well-being are found. For example, Flemish and French speaking Belgians, Swiss of different languages (Inglehart, 1977), and French and English speaking Canadians (Blishen and Atkinson, 1980) report similar levels of well-being when the same measure is translated into different languages. This is encouraging because it suggests that the specific words used do not have a substantial influence on the overall score. Nevertheless, the scales have been used in very similar cultures, so language comparability has not been strongly tested. What is needed is a demonstration that items cluster together in a similar manner across very different cultures. The issue is not only whether words can be adequately translated, but whether the concepts themselves are comparable across cultures.

Individual differences in social desirability in responding is a potential artifact (Carstensen and Cone, 1983) in interpreting SWB scores because the SWB measures correlate at moderate levels with desirability scales (e.g., Campbell et al., 1976; Kammann and Flett, 1983). Social desirability, however, is now seen as a substantive individual difference (Furnham, 1986; Hogan and Nicholson, 1988; Weinberger, 1990) and not necessarily as an artifact (Diener et al., 1993; McCrae and Costa, 1983). For example, "social desirability" scores may correlate with conformity and avoidance of thinking about unpleasant affect, both of which correlate with well-being. Thus, controlling individual differences in "social desirability" may not enhance the validity of SWB scales. This has been shown to be true in reference to well-being measures in several studies (e.g. McCrae, 1986). For example, Diener, Sandvik, Pavot, and Gallagher (1991) found that a measure which controlled for "social desirability" correlated more poorly with nonself-report measures of well-being. In addition, Diener et al. (1991)

discovered that controlling for Crowne-Marlowe social desirability in the relationship between self-report and non-self report measures of well-being reduced the size of the correlations. Similarly, Kozma and Stones (1988) found that controlling social desirability in the correlation between SWB measures and an external criterion did not improve the zero-order correlations. Thus, individual differences in "social desirability" are related to personality content that is related to subjective well-being, and scoring high on "social desirability" does not indicate a threat to the validity of SWB scores. This does not mean that impression management does not decrease the validity of the SWB scales. What it does mean is that current social desirability scales do not correct for such impression management because they tap personality content which is actually related to SWB. Thus, controlling for social desirability scores may simultaneously reduce the effects of impression management and also substantive personality influences on well-being, with no net increase in validity.

An alternative method of assessing the effects of social desirability is to collect half of the data in face-to-face interviews and the other half of the data in anonymous or quasi-anonymous group settings. In the former setting, impression management should be magnified, whereas in the latter it should be reduced. Thus, the effects of impression management on responding can be assessed. It can be determined not only whether mean scores differ in the two conditions, but also standard deviations and validity coefficients can be examined. Fujita, Smith, and Diener (1993), using this strategy with American college students, found no differences in the validity of SWB measures when they were obtained in interviews versus in quasi-anonymous questionnaires. This method represents a powerful way of examining self-presentational difference between groups.

Conclusion

Self-report measures of well-being appear to possess adequate psychometric properties. The reader is referred to Andrews and Robinson (1991), Andrews and Withey (1976), and Sandvik, Diener, and Seidlitz (1993) for further material on the psychometrics of SWB scales. Although the data are encouraging, several issues demand further study. For example, sophisticated multimeasure factor analytic studies are needed to separate true change in the latent constructs from unreliability due to error of measurement. Additional work is needed on factorial invariance across very different cultures. Finally, research on social desirability is needed which differentiates self-deception versus other-deception (e.g., Paulhus, 1988).

CORRELATES OF SWB

Many demographic variables have been correlated with SWB, with the typical finding being that advantaged groups such as the wealthy are slightly happier than others (e.g., Diener et al., 1985; Diener et al., 1993). For example, Campbell, Converse, and Rodgers reported that the unemployed were the unhappiest group they studied. Nevertheless, some advantaged groups such as men and the highly educated do not always report higher levels of well-being (e.g., Campbell et al., 1976; Diener, 1984). In general, resources such as health, income, and physical attractiveness have shown surprisingly small correlations with SWB, whereas personality variables have been much stronger predictors (Costa et al., 1987; Diener and Larsen, 1993). Diener and Diener (1993) reported that self-esteem correlated about 0.53 with life satisfaction in eight western countries and an average of 0.47 across the 31 diverse countries they examined. Some correlates of subjective well-being such as being married (Glenn and Weaver, 1978) may be due to pre-existing personality differences rather than solely to the situation of marriage per se (Scott et al., 1992). A number of psychological characteristics such as maturity (Alker and Gawin, 1978) have proven to be strong correlates of SWB. Emmons (1986) found that past goal success predicted positive affect, ambivalence over one's strivings predicted negative affect, and that the importance of one's strivings predicted life satisfaction. Global subjective well-being usually correlates at moderate to high levels with satisfaction with particular aspects of one's life (Diener, 1984). For example, Campbell (1981) reported that life satisfaction correlated 0.55 with satisfaction with the self and 0.37 with work satisfaction. There are cross-cultural differences in happiness and life satisfaction (e.g., Balatsky and Diener, 1992; Diener and Diener, 1993; Diener, Diener and Diener, 1993; Shao, 1992) which are not completely explained by income differences (Diener, Suh, Smith, and Shao, 1994). Finally, differences in SWB covary with the discrepancies one perceives between what one has, what others have, and what one had in the past (Michalos, 1991). Thus, SWB scales show interesting theoretical patterns of relations to other variables.

More sophisticated analyses are desirable in examining the correlates of subjective well-being in order to determine the causal interconnections of variables. For example, certain life events such as divorce may be a hardship for some people and a blessing for others. Additional measures of the meaning of life events for each individual should provide more powerful insights into the genesis of subjective well-being. Longitudinal research can help disentangle whether subjective well-being is the cause or effect of predictor variables. For example, Scott, Diener, and Fujita (1992) hypothesized that marriage might be an effect of high subjective well-being rather than simply a cause of it. Headey *et al.* (1991) used a longitudinal panel survey to examine the direction of influence between variables. Even experimental designs are sometimes possible (e.g. Kozma *et al.*, 1990; Pavot and Diener, 1993a). For instance, Fujita (1993) found in an experimental assignment of college roommates that social comparison did not influence satisfaction judgments. Thus, there are more powerful designs to determine the causes of subjective well-being than simple cross-sectional correlations, and these designs should be used more frequently.

DIVERGENT VALIDITY

The divergent validity of subjective well-being measures has been extensively explored at the single-measure level. For example, a meta-analysis by Okun and Stock (1987) showed that subjective well-being measures were moderately associated with adjustment (0.38), with neuroticism (0.33) with work satisfaction (0.33), and with family satisfaction (0.29), but were more substantially related to each other (0.52). Although SWB is highly related, as would be expected, with constructs such as optimism (Carver and Gaines, 1987) and self-esteem (Diener and Emmons, 1985; Fordyce, 1988), these correlations do not approach unity. For example, Marshall *et al.* (1992) found an average correlation between optimism and positive affect of 0.35 and an average correlation between pessimism and negative affect of 0.27.

Another finding which points to the divergent validity of SWB scales is the fact that additional variables can predict subjective well-being beyond the predictive power of variables to which SWB might be seen as identical (Diener and Diener, 1993). For example, extraversion and neuroticism are both predictors of SWB and might be viewed as the temperament underpinnings to a predilection towards positive and negative affect, respectively. Agreeableness and conscientiousness, however, predict SWB incrementally over the influence of E and N (McCrae and Costa, 1991). Furthermore, Costa and McCrae (1980) found that the average correlation between positive affect and extraversion was 0.20, while between negative affect and neuroticism it was 0.38. These findings suggest that extraversion and neuroticism, although correlates of SWB, cannot be seen as synonymous with SWB. The fact that subjective well-being reacts to life changes and life events (e.g., Atkinson, 1982; Ormel and Schaufeli, 1991; Tran et al., 1991) also indicates that it is not isomorphic with personality traits.

More sophisticated approaches to the divergent validity of SWB scales using multi-method matrices or confirmatory factor analyses are rare. Larsen and Diener (1985), using MTMM, found that hedonic level was independent of emotional intensity. Andrews and Withey (1976) found in several studies that global evaluations of one's life formed a core cluster which was separable from satisfaction with various life domains. Smith et al. (1989) found, however, that the LOT measure of optimism correlated as strongly with negative affect as with an alternative measure of optimism. Fujita (1991) employed LISREL and found that extraversion and long-term positive affect were highly related constructs and found that long-term negative affect and neuroticism were not distinguishable. Similarly, Watson and Clark (1984) have argued that negative affectivity and neuroticism are the same thing. Positive and negative affect, however, each appear to make independent contributions to life satisfaction (Pavot and Diener, 1993b).

Clearly, a more systematic mapping of the interrelation of subjective well-being and related constructs is needed. Such a mapping must be based on the use of multiple measures for each construct so that the effects of error can be assessed and the relation of both manifest variables and latent traits can be estimated. In addition, it would be valuable to explore the relation of personality measures such as extraversion, optimism, and neuroticism to both shorter- and longer-term measures of positive and negative affect because short-term measures of SWB may be more strongly affected by events, whereas longer-term measures may be more strongly tied to temperament.

ADVANCING SUBJECTIVE WELL-BEING MEASUREMENT: DEVELOPMENTS IN OTHER AREAS OF PSYCHOLOGY

The evidence reviewed above indicates that coherent levels of long-term well-being exist, and that the typical self-report measurement of SWB produces psychometric indices that are as good or better than those in many areas. Nevertheless, recent advances in a number of subdisciplines of psychology indicate that the exclusive reliance on self-report measures of SWB has limitations. and that theoretical and empirical advances are probable if additional types of measures are employed.

The study of subjective well-being has its roots in survey research. One of the early scales simply asked respondents "how things are these days," and gave them three response choices: "very happy," "pretty happy," and "not too happy" (Gurin et al., 1960). Although recent scales such as the Satisfaction with Life Scale (Diener et al., 1985) tend to use more items, and offer more finely graded response options, they still rely on straightforward self-reports. Yet, in recent years progress in various areas such as emotion theory and cognitive psychology have important implications for the way SWB is conceived and for the self-report measurement of well-being. I review several of the relevant advances below, and explicate their implications for the measurement of well-being. Next, the ramifications of these findings for definitions and theory are discussed, and additional measurement methods are described.

The Multiple Components of Emotion

The reader is referred to Frijda (1986), Lazarus (1991), and Oatley and Jenkins (1992) for more complete discussions of emotion. Emotion is defined here following Lazarus (1991), as organized psychophysiological reactions which occur because of self-relevant information in the environment (p. 38). It is now widely agreed that emotion is composed of behavioral, nonverbal, motivational, physiological, experimental, and cognitive components (Scherer, 1984). For example, Plutchik (1984) defines emotions as a response to a stimulus which involves experienced feeling, neural and autonomic arousal, goal directed behavior, expressive reactions, and appraisal.

Many emotions evidence typical facial expressions (Ekman *et al.*, 1972; Izard, 1971). Smiling for joy is a cultural universal (e.g., Ekman, 1984). Cacioppo *et al.* (1986) discovered that even when facial muscle movements are not visible, EMG activity occurs in the face in reaction to emotional stimuli. Emotions include nonobservable events such as subjective experience, as well as appraisal and coping processes (Lazarus, 1991). Emotions are also accompanied by action readiness (e.g., Frijda, 1986), a motor component (Zajonc, 1984a). For instance, angry persons show physical preparation for attack and fearful persons evidence a readiness to flee. The physiological component of emotion includes activation of the autonomic system, and emotional feelings are often accompanied by physiological reactions (Ekman *et al.*, 1983). Thus, emotion appears to be a complex process, with experience being only one component. Furthermore, there is now mounting evidence that although the various components of emotion do covary, they show some degree of independence (e.g., Frijda, 1986; Leventhal, 1984; Schwartz, 1982; Tyrer, 1976; Zajonc, 1984b). Therefore a measure of one component is not a sure indicator of other components of the emotion system. The self-reports of affective well-being which form the basis of the vast majority of SWB research rely almost totally on cognitive labelling of emotions, and thus largely ignore the remaining parts of the emotion system. Because the labelling of emotions reflected in self-report is imperfectly related to the other emotional channels, self-reports do not give a complete view of the affective life of an individual.

Compounding the limitations of self-report, if respondents are asked to report their emotional well-being, the researcher depends on subjects labelling their emotions in the same way that the experimenter and other subjects do. This is not always a safe assumption (Kagan, 1984). For example, my mother claims never to have been unhappy in her life, although she will admit to being sad or fearful. Apparently she uses the word "unhappy" in a way that makes her self-reports not comparable to the reports of many other people. The issue is not whether she is right or wrong, but rather that individuals, cohorts, or other groups may not give the exact same meaning to words. Because it is likely that individuals, groups, and cultures use emotion labels differently (Russell, 1991) a total reliance on self-reports of emotion is risky.

Thus, if we are to validly assess the affective portion of SWB, we must examine more than the cognitive labels respondents give their emotions. In addition to the imprecision and variability of emotion words, the fact that emotion has a number of components which are only moderately correlated makes it imperative that we assess other emotion channels if we want to obtain a complete picture of people's affective well-being.

It might be argued that self-report is the only way to assess the experiential component of emotion, and that subjective well-being is most related to subjective experience. It is not self-evident, however, that self-reports are either direct measures of experience or the only measures of experience. For example, behavioral preferences and depth of processing memory measures might be just as valid measures of experience. Self-reports do not have privileged status as the only measures of experience, and researchers should creatively engineer additional ways to assess subjective experience. As Izard (1992) wrote, "feeling states must be studied by multiple methods that yield convergent data" (p. 563).

Denial

Related to the emotional labelling problem described above is the fact that individuals may deny or ignore their emotional reactions. A modular view of the brain (Gazzaniga, 1985) suggests that the subcortical centers from which emotions emanate show some degree of independence from the verbal center of the brain (MacLean, 1975;

Panksepp, 1982). For example, Haggard and Isaacs (1966) found that patients showed momentary facial expressions of which they were not aware when discussing emotionally conflictual topics. The language centers in the left cerebral hemisphere may be partly dissociated from the emotion centers in the right cerebral hemisphere (Borod, 1992; Galin, 1974), thus making verbal reports of emotions imperfect indicants of other types of emotional reactions.

There are individual differences in the degree to which the components of emotion are dissociated. Recent work shows that some individuals strongly deny or avoid their emotional reactions (e.g., Bonanno and Singer, 1990; Gudjonsson, 1981; Schwartz, 1983; Weinberger, 1990). These individuals either do not label unpleasant emotions, do not attend to their emotional reactions, or isolate emotional information from their left cerebral hemisphere (Davidson, 1983). Yet these same people show evidence that they are experiencing emotional reactions in nonverbal channels. For example, although avoiders deny negative emotions, they show greater speech disfluencies under stress (Weinberger et al., 1979), evidence greater physiological reactivity (e.g., King et al., 1986; Levenson and Mades, 1980), and are rated as having greater facial anxiety (Asendorpf and Scherer, 1983).

Although repression is usually not conceptualized in Freudian terms by modern emotion theorists, most would agree that individuals differ in the degree to which they attend to their emotional reactions. An edited volume by Singer (1990) presents an excellent overview of the effects of denial and repressive coping on the memory for unpleasant affective experiences. For example, Davis reviews evidence showing that individuals identified as repressors have a more difficult time retrieving emotional experiences from memory. She found that "repressors" were able to remember many fewer emotional memories in a free recall task, but were almost equal to nonrepressors in a cued recall task. Davis concluded that "repressors may be individuals with a propensity to engage in less elaborative processing of their own emotional experiences, with a consequent reduction in the richness of associative pathways among affect-related experiences stored in memory" (p. 402). This line of research suggests that personality may influence subjective well-being, not simply in terms of temperament propensities to experience specific types of affect, but also in terms of certain individuals avoiding emotional reactions. Multi-channel emotional assessment thus becomes imperative because the researcher otherwise cannot fully understand the cause of self-reported levels of negative affect.

Assessing denial. There are a number of scales to assess individual differences in denial of distress or the avoidance of emotional feelings (e.g., Weinberger, 1990). Other measures have also been used to assess denial or avoidance of emotion: The Crowne-Marlowe Scale of Social Desirability (usually in combination with an anxiety scale), Byrne's Repression-Sensitization Scale, and a dichotic listening task (Bonanno and Singer, 1990). When used in conjunction with self-report SWB measures, these scales may help the researcher interpret the SWB responses. For example, subjective well-being may be interpreted in a different light for emotional avoiders versus nonavoiders. The subjective well-being of emotional avoiders may be accompanied by stress in other channels, for example in physiological reactions. In contrast, if an emotional nonavoider reports a high level of SWB, it is more likely that she will show a dearth of negative emotional reactions in other channels as well. Differences between self-report and reports by knowledgeable informants or behavioral information can also be employed to help infer the denial of negative emotions. Physiological recordings have also been used; if a person reacts in the physiological channel, but says he is not feeling emotional, denial might be inferred. Finally, emotionally avoidance may be present if a person denies feeling unpleasant emotions, but the presence of negative affect is evident in mood sensitive tasks. Discrepancies will sometimes be noted between self-reports and measures which depend more heavily on nonself-report channels. When self-reports yield less negative affect, the investigator might suspect emotional avoidance or denial. The inclusion of other scales such as those measuring avoidance or self-presentation (Paulhus, 1988) will also aid in diagnosing avoidance. Further, an anonymity-identifiability manipulation can also help separate self-presentation from emotional avoidance effects. If an anonymity manipulation has no influence on responses, emotional avoidance would be suspected in the case in which self-reports reveal less unpleasant affect than nonself-report items.

In order to fully understand the nature of a group's SWB, we need to understand the role that denial or avoidance coping plays in their emotional life. For example, Allman (1990) found that the SWB report of wheelchair-bound respondents correlated very highly with their Crowne-Marlowe scores, and this might indicate that repression of negative affect was integral to the happiness of the disabled subjects. At this time there appear to be two major approaches to assessing the denial of negative affect: direct measures of denial such as Weinberger's scales, and searching for a discrepancy between self-reports and other types of measures.

Conclusion. It is evident that scientists cannot gain a complete measure of people's emotional reactions only from self-report. Self-reported affect and reactions in other emotional channels show only moderate convergence. Certain people do not admit to emotional reactions, but may show motoric, physiological, and facial evidence of affective responses. Some individuals have a more difficult time retrieving emotional material from memory. Thus, researchers must employ additional measures besides self-reports to tap the nonverbal channels of emotion and to veridically assess emotional reactions across individuals.

Emotion Is Multifaceted

In addition to the various response components of emotion described earlier, affect also varies in other ways besides simple hedonic level or valence. For example, there are a number of separate unpleasant emotions such as sadness, fear and anger (Izard, 1972; Plutchik, 1980; Tomkins and McCarter, 1964), and describing the emotions only as "negative affect" may lose substantial information. Furthermore, in addition to mean hedonic level, we can also describe emotions in terms of peak amplitude and variability. For instance, two individuals who possess the same average hedonic level may differ greatly in emotional intensity (Larsen and Diener, 1987) or emotional variability (Diener and Larsen, 1986). Current measures of SWB fail to capture the full richness of emotional life. The following examination of the relation of the duration versus peak amplitude of emotion to SWB demonstrates that a more intricate conception of emotional life would be beneficial. Although aspects of emotion such as duration and intensity are not fully understood, ignoring these distinctions or lumping them together will hardly produce better understanding.

Time and intensity of emotions. Diener *et al.* (1990) argue that the total amount of time a person experiences pleasant emotions versus unpleasant emotions (regardless of the peak intensity of emotions experienced) forms the basis of affective well-being. Diener *et al.* (1990) found that the relative frequency of pleasant affect was necessary and sufficient to produce high scores on both self-report and nonself-report well-being measures. In support of this conclusion, Andrews and Withey (1976) found that a question assessing the frequency of pleasant versus unpleasant emotions over time loaded most highly of 50 global well-being measures on the central component of subjective well-being.

In terms of evidence showing that peak intensity contributes little to global SWB as currently measured, Larsen and Diener (1985) discovered that emotional intensity was distinct from SWB in a multitrait-multimethod examination of long-term affect measures, and Larsen *et al.* (1985) found that emotional intensity and well-being measures loaded on two separate factors. Diener *et al.* (1990) offer a number of reasons why intense positive emotions are not as strongly related to well-being as are frequent positive experiences. Chief among these reasons is that intense positive emotions are very rare (thus contributing little to long-term well-being), and that intense positive emotions often have countervailing costs (Diener *et al.*, 1991). Intense emotions are rare — extremely intense joy was virtually never reported by college age students (Diener *et al.*, 1990). In contrast, some level of pleasant affect was reported by college students over 70% of the time. Thus, the amount of time one experiences pleasant affect can have a greater influence than the rare intense moments. In terms of countervailing costs, intense positive emotions often follow unpleasant emotional periods and often depend on psychological conditions which would have resulted in intense negative emotions had circumstances not turned out favorably. Thus, the long-run effect of intense pleasant emotions may not be that positive because their net effect may be slight when countervailing unpleasant emotions are also considered (see Diener *et al.*, 1991, for a more thorough exposition).

Thus, a tenable hypothesis is that global emotional SWB can be defined as the proportion of time one experiences pleasant emotions. I note, however, that even if peak intensity does not strongly influence the level of SWB reported by a respondent, it is likely to influence the quality of the person's emotional life. Two people could be equally "happy," but might experience their happiness in different ways if one has low intensity emotions and the other has large mood swings. The evidence that SWB depends more directly on the time/duration of pleasant emotions than on their intensity is tentative. If, however, SWB researchers systematically assess various aspects of emotion such as duration, intensity, and variability, a more definitive conclusion can be reached regarding how various parameters of emotion influence SWB.

Positive and negative affect. In recent years it has become debatable whether one should combine pleasant and unpleasant emotions into a single valence score. An unexpected finding in mood research is that positive and negative emotions often form independent dimensions (Bradburn, 1969; Diener and Emmons, 1985; Zevon and Tellegen, 1982). In addition, a number of investigators have discovered different correlates for pleasant and unpleasant affect (Beiser, 1974; Costa and McCrae, 1980; Emmons and Diener, 1985; Headey *et al.*, 1985; Lawton, 1983). Baker *et al.* (1992) trace different environmental and genetic influences for positive and negative affect. Despite these findings, the independence of pleasant and unpleasant emotions is still a contentious issue (e.g., Diener *et al.*, 1985; Watson, 1988) and the empirical work is mixed. For example, several researchers have found a strong inverse correlation between positive and negative affect (e.g., Kammann *et al.*, 1979; Zautra *et al.*, 1988), whereas others have found tiny correlations between the two (e.g., Zevon and Tellegen, 1982).

How can we reconcile the discrepant findings on the relation of pleasant and unpleasant affect? Investigators have found that the relation between the two depends on the time frame sampled (Diener and Emmons, 1985; Staats *et al.*, 1989), on the intensity of the emotions sampled (Diener and Emmons, 1985; Diener and Iran-Nejad, 1986; Watson, 1988), on the type of response scale used (Brenner, 1975; Warr *et al.*, 1983), on the particular pleasant and unpleasant emotions sampled (Watson, 1988), on whether verbal or nonverbal measures are employed (Ketelaar, 1989), and on whether acquiescence response set is controlled (Lorr *et al.*, 1989). Therefore, a simple answer as to whether positive and negative affect are independent is not possible. Strict independence of positive and negative affect are found when a restricted set of mood adjectives is factor analyzed, and a varimax rotation is applied (which guarantees independence).

Diener and Iran-Nejad (1986) found that the relationship between positive and negative emotions is not homoscedastic. The relation between pleasant and unpleasant affect formed an L pattern rather than the "cigar" ellipse of homoscedastic correlations. The L pattern emerged because at a low level of intensity of one type of emotion, people could feel virtually any level of the other type of emotion, from very low to very high. Although low levels of the two types of emotion frequently occurred together, intense levels never occurred together. This pattern thus suggests that simple correlations and factor analysis might not fully capture the complex relation between the two types of emotion at varying levels of intensity.

Another problem is that factor analysis may be an inappropriate analytical tool because the trace line between mood adjective words and the underlying emotional feeling is not monotonic. For many mood words of intermediate intensity, a person may report feeling just as much of them when expressing a feeling a distance below that mood word as when he or she is the same distance above that mood word. For such data, Coomb's (1964) unfolding analysis might be a more appropriate statistical technique than is factor analysis.

Green *et al.* (1993) showed that measures of positive and negative affect varied inversely, but only at modest levels. When measurement error was controlled through a latent factor analysis based on multiple measures, however, the two correlated inversely at an extremely strong level. Diener, Fujita, and Smith (1993) followed up this lead by examining both discrete emotions and positive and negative affect using a LISREL analysis of multiple measures of each construct. They found that positive and negative affect were statistically separable into two factors even though they were strongly inversely correlated when measurement error was controlled. That is, positive and negative affect were clearly separable, although not orthogonal, thus suggesting that they should be measured separately. Furthermore, there were relations between specific discrete emotions which could not be accounted for by the general structure, indicating that for some purposes it will also be useful to separately assess specific emotions. They found, however, strong convergence between the positive emotions and between the negative emotions. This indicates that global positive affect and negative affect are useful categories and account for much of the variance in discrete emotions.

Conclusion. A simple self-report of mean hedonic level is unlikely to capture the full complexity of emotional well-being. Although positive and negative affect may not be entirely independent, it nevertheless seems desirable to separately assess each because they show some degree of autonomous variation, at least under certain measurement conditions. Furthermore, in many SWB studies, scientists can also assess specific emotions such as anger, fear, joy, and sadness because global pleasant and unpleasant emotion categories may not fully capture important differences between people in emotional experience. In addition, measurement methods which allow the assessment of dimensions such as peak intensity, emotional episode duration, and total time experiencing specific emotions will yield a much more unabridged picture of people's emotional lives. For this reason, experience sampling methods in which people's emotions are sampled over time will be described in future sections. Many previous measures of SWB give a single summary score of respondents' emotional lives. Clearly, such a single score is unlikely to capture the richness of a person's emotional well-being. At the same time, individuals in single session self-reports are unlikely to be able to accurately separate out and report complex facets of their emotional experiences. Thus, measures which validly capture additional emotions and dimensions seem desirable.

Cognitive Processing of Self-Report Items

The conventional view of SWB measures assumes that people simply access their state of morale from memory and then report it. But people must search for information in memory and perform computations on that information in order to give a report in acceptable form. Torangeau and Rasinski (1988), in discussing a model of attitudes which is applicable to well-being measurement, suggest that respondents must interpret attitude questions, search working and long-term memory for relevant information, and seek standards of comparison in order to present appropriate output. People must construct an answer to self-report measures based on information stored in memory. Because individuals rely on search, computational, and constructivist processes in order to arrive at the answer to self-report SWB items, scores are often influenced by situational factors which affect these processes.

Memory. In order to answer well-being questions, subjects must consult working and/or long-term memory and construct their report based on the material in consciousness. It is well known that people will often use heuristic shortcuts (Kahneman *et al.*, 1982) rather than thoroughly search their memory for answers to questions. Because the amount of information available on which well-being judgments can be made is enormous, the respondent is usually forced to take short-cuts. Whereas some information required is not easily available in memory or is stored in incomplete fashion, other information is readily available because it was recalled more recently (Wyer and Srull, 1989). For example, Skelton and Strohmetz (1990) demonstrated that priming can influence the reporting of physical symptoms. Larsen (1992) has shown that neuroticism influences the selective recall of physical symptoms compared to symptoms reported on a daily basis. A number of studies have shown that prior questions can influence responses to the subsequent well-being items (Schwarz and Strack, 1990; Sinclair *et al.*, 1989; Wellens *et al.*, 1989), possibly because these questions make specific information more salient to the respondents.

Memory biases also depend on the dimensions of mood which are retrieved. Thomas and Diener (1990) found that subjects tend to overestimate their emotional intensity, but underestimate the frequency of their positive affect. They found that subjects were somewhat accurate at estimating the relevant frequency of their emotions, but very poor at estimating the intensity of their unpleasant emotions. Furthermore, negative intensity estimates were biased by the frequency of the emotions. Diener *et al.* (1984) found that happy individuals overestimated their average positive affect and that unhappy individuals overestimated their average negative affect.

Another type of memory bias revolves around subject's current mood. Because of state-dependent and mood-congruent effects (Blaney, 1986), people may recall more positive experiences when in a good mood, and may therefore overestimate their degree of long-term happiness if in that state. Similarly, people may be able to recall more negative experiences when in a bad mood, and therefore give a lower SWB estimate when in that state.

To further complicate matters, memory seems to be a constructive process rather than a retrieval of discrete information (Mandler, 1985). What this means is that the respondent will not simply recall an accurate picture of his past emotional life. The memories are constructed or reconstructed by subjects depending of their beliefs, and other material in consciousness at the time. Thus, single-occasion reports of long-term mood obviously do not perfectly reflect an individual's on-line affective reactions.

Controlling memory effects. One way to obtain memories which accurately represent the person's life is to lead respondents through a life review before presenting the well-being questions. Such a life review can decrease the chances that one salient memory will exert a disproportionate influence on the SWB report. Another alternative is to use experience sampling (e.g., Csikszentmihalyi and Larson, 1987), including audio tape or portable computer aided recording, to gain a relatively accurate picture of on-line mood. In experience sampling, the researcher relies on memory because she asks respondents how they feel at the moment. Similarly, we can obtain satisfaction ratings on a daily basis over a period of time to reduce recall biases (e.g., Pavot et al., 1991). Procedures which shorten the time period on which respondents report and which reinforce the subjects for systematically searching memory should enhance accuracy and thereby increase the validity of measures. If daily or moment reports are obtained over a long enough time period, an estimation of the subjects' long-term SWB can be made. Nevertheless, self-reports of emotion over time are still subject to some of the other artifacts mentioned above. Further, the reactive effects of experience sampling or daily recording (Hammen and Glass, 1975; Harmon et al., 1980) have not yet been studied in depth.

Mood as information. Because a thorough memory search is so difficult and time-consuming, participants may simply consult their mood at the moment in order to determine their subjective well-being (Schwarz and Clore, 1983). Schwarz and Strack (1990) showed that both life satisfaction and happiness judgments can be affected by current moods (see also Kozma *et al.*, 1990). Even seemingly trivial factors such as sunny weather or finding a dime in a phone booth can induce people to report higher life satisfaction scores! People can discount the effect of their current mood if attention is called to it, but otherwise use this easily available mood information to give a quick answer to well-being questions.

Diener *et al.* (1991) reasoned that in real testing situations current mood often is not a problem because it correlates moderately with enduring mood. They suggested that the correlation between long-term mood and current mood implies that the constant variance added by current mood is usually nonspurious, whereas the error variance would tend to be random because of the multiplicity of other factors influencing current mood. They examined the effects of current mood on SWB measures after controlling for the effects of long-term mood as measured by nonself-report measures such as peer reports. Diener *et al.* (1991) found that on one measurement occasion out of three, current mood added significantly to the prediction of happiness measures taken at that time, although the effect was modest. They concluded that the influence of current mood on happiness scales is often slight, but is certainly worth controlling and measuring.

Moods generated by the interview situation are of particular concern. For example, Schwarz and Strack (1990) report that individuals who were asked about a recent hospitalization thereafter reported less well-being. Similarly, Lehman *et al.* (1987) found that people who lost a spouse or child in an auto accident many years earlier still reported being less happy. It could be, however, that the reminder of the loss by the interviewer created a negative mood which then influenced their well-being report. A related complication is that influences such as current mood could also affect the reporting of other variables such as life events (Cohen *et al.*, 1988). Thus, correlations might result from the influence of current mood on both well-being reports and on the independent variables.

Controlling current mood effects. We can infer the influence of current mood on global SWB reports by measuring both current mood and longer-term subjective well-being. If groups differ to a greater degree in standardized terms on current mood than they do on long-term well-being estimates, there is a chance that a current mood artifact could be operating. We can control the influence of current mood by assessing well-being on several occasions and by insuring that testing is conducted so that a population's current mood at the time of testing is likely to be similar to its long-term average. For example, if a researcher wanted to assess long-term mood, she would not want to study a group entirely on sunny spring days after a dreary winter, or after the local team won a championship. Finally, researchers must be alert to factors within the interview (e.g., prior questions) which could influence the mood of participants.

Scaling. A number of situational and individual difference variables can influence how subjects use response scales. Schwarz and Strack (1990) and Branscombe and Diener (1987) showed that moods and events can serve as contrast or assimilation anchors when well-being judgments are made. For example, people reporting a hospitalization in the distant past reported greater happiness because this unhappy event served as a contrast anchor (Schwarz and Strack, 1990). Similarly, when subjects heard another person tell of an unfortunate medical condition, they rated their own life satisfaction as higher. Finally, when a handicapped person was in their visual field, subjects also reported more happiness (Strack *et al.*, 1990). In contrast, reports of one's own *recent* hospitalization lowered well-being responses because of the information these reports contained on one's current life. In a similar vein, Dermer *et al.* (1979) found that people rated their lives as worse or better depending on whether they had previously read descriptions which painted a favorable or unfavorable picture of past living conditions.

In addition to the contrast and assimilation effects noted above, there is the problem that individuals may use scale responses differently. For example, how can we be sure that one respondent's "4" is higher than another subject's "3," much less know the size of the interval between the two responses? Diener *et al.* (1990) contend that scales which measure the time people experience various types of affect are in principle of ratio quality. A person who experiences pleasant affect 80% of the time is twice as happy in a meaningful sense compared to a person who feels it 40% of the time. Therefore, if we can accurately assess frequency of pleasant and unpleasant affect (e.g., with the experience sampling method), strong scale properties might exist even across individuals. In contrast, scales which assess the intensity of affect might not even be ordinal. For instance, one person's "very intense" emotion may be less intense than another's "moderately intense" emotion.

Controlling scaling effects. Several procedures in psychometrics are utilized to reduce the scaling problems noted above. One is to provide subjects with concrete anchors for each choice so that responses are more likely to mean the same thing from time to time and across subjects. Another precaution is to use constant conditions in testing so that transitory effects are reduced. Although we can control situational influences on scaling in part by standardized testing conditions, we can also assess them by using repeated measurements under systematically varying conditions. Nevertheless, as long as we rely entirely on self-reports to assess SWB, we cannot be sure to what degree an adjustment of the response scale (Tversky and Griffin, 1991) has influenced the subject's responses.

Conclusion. Experimental work on memory and scaling clearly demonstrates that one-time self-reports of well-being are not simple readouts of people's underlying state of SWB. Situational factors can influence what participants recall and how they scale their responses, and thus can influence self-reports of SWB. These facts point to the desirability of more sophisticated measurement of well-being.

Communication Effects

The need to communicate the answer to well-being questions to the experimenter can influence the responses subjects furnish. For example, when respondents were interviewed by an attractive experimenter, life satisfaction judgments were higher than when made anonymously. But when interviewed by a disabled experimenter, subjects reported less happiness, apparently because they did not want to appear too happy (Strack *et al.*, 1990).

Hogan (1983) suggests that reports to questionnaires are self-presentations which follow certain strategies and norms. As such, it would be naive to interpret them in a way that does not recognize their dramaturgical quality. It is well known that respondents may adjust their output to create a desired impression. What is less well known is that there are additional communication effects involved in subjects' interpretations of the questions posed by the researcher.

Interpretation of questions. The context for subjects' interpretation of questions is provided both by the interview situation and by other preceding questions (Strack *et al.*, 1991). For instance, an experimenter might ask a subject how satisfied she is with her work, and then with her family. In another study, the order of questions might be about satisfaction with the marriage, and then satisfaction with the family. In the first study, the subject's satisfaction with the family is likely to include information about the marriage because the family includes the spouse. But in the second study, the subject may interpret the family question to mean the family other than the spouse because information on marriage satisfaction was already requested. Schwarz and Strack (1990) interpret SWB responses within a "Gricean" communication framework (Grice, 1975) which asserts that one of the norms of communication is that it should not be redundant. Thus, differences between the two hypothetical studies above could result from the contextual meaning of the question, *even if an identical question were used.* If the marriage is viewed quite positively, the second study might find lower family satisfaction, even if the actual satisfaction were identical for the groups, because subjects are likely to omit a positive component from their family satisfaction response.

Social desirability. Different groups may possess varying norms for how desirable it is to be happy or how undesirable it is to be unhappy (Sommers, 1984). Furthermore, groups and cultures may differ in how normative it is to express or admit these emotions. Taylor (1977, p. 33) wrote, "Some cultures place considerable value on portraying life as a pain in the neck. Six to 8% of the inhabitants of most modern countries admit to unhappiness but about half of Frenchmen do so." The implication is that the French appear more happy because of a norm which approves the expression of dissatisfaction with life. Such norms, however, might actually lead to experiencing more unpleasant emotions. Thus, we should investigate normative differences in terms of their producing both actual and artifactual differences in well-being. We can measure norms for happiness — the degree to which individuals believe that experiencing pleasant or unpleasant affect or specific emotions is appropriate and desirable. We can also assess the degree to which subjects believe that *expressing* certain emotions is desirable. Differences between groups in reported well-being can then be interpreted in light of group norms for experiencing or expressing positive and negative emotions. Ouweneel and Veenhoven (1991) and Diener, Suh, Smith, and Shao (1994) concluded that differences in desirability had little influence on reports of subjective well-being.

The effects of situational social desirability in terms of varying anonymity of responses is another potential problem. Because being happy is often considered normatively desirable (Sommers, 1984), people may report higher levels of happiness when queried in a face-to-face interview than on an anonymous questionnaire (King and Buchwald, 1982; Smith, 1979; Sudman, 1967), although studies on this issue are mixed (Fujita *et al.*, 1993).

Conclusion. A variety of communication effects may influence self-reports of SWB and make them less reliable indicators of people's long-term emotional states. First, impression management effects are problematical in some testing situations. Furthermore, social desirability may differ from group to group and testing situation to testing situation. Finally, communication effects are not simply self-presentational; the interview situation can also influence the way subjects interpret questions.

Systematically varying anonymity can be used profitably to assess the degree to which group averages reflect a propensity on the part of respondents to appear happy to others. For example, King and Buchwald (1982) found that men and women both increased their happiness responses when interviewed nonanonymously, but that this difference was approximately equivalent for both sexes. This finding suggested that a desire to seem happy to others does not differentially influence the reports of men and women. Other ways of inferring self-presentational effects are through social desirability scales (e.g., Paulhus, 1988) and through the comparison of scores from traditional SWB scales with scores from scales which control social desirability (e.g., Sandvik, Diener, and Seidlitz's Forced Choice Measure, 1993). Finally, we can assess people's norms for being happy, and for communicating this to others. If people differ in their beliefs about the desirability of being happy or acting happy, their SWB responses can be interpreted in this light.

ADVANCING THE THEORETICAL DEFINITION OF SUBJECTIVE WELL-BEING

In light of the findings from other fields, we can now move forward in terms of defining and measuring subjective well-being. Recall that SWB was defined earlier as people's evaluations of their lives. These evaluations might be assessed both in terms of cognitive appraisals (satisfaction) and in term of affect (the pleasantness of one's moods and emotions resulting from the appraisals of ongoing events in the person's life). It is now possible to define SWB in more sophisticated and complex ways.

Cognition and Life Satisfaction

Compelling findings in cognitive psychology, especially from the laboratories of Fritz Strack and Norbert Schwarz, indicate that it may be incorrect to think that people usually simply recall a stored life satisfaction judgment and report it. Instead, people seem to form a life satisfaction judgment in response to the interview situation. Because they form the judgment at the moment, it can be influenced by the memories and life domains which are salient at the time, as well as by what comparison standards are particularly prominent. This reasoning suggests that life satisfaction for most people is not likely to be a Platonic form, stored in a discrete and simple way. Rather, it is a complex judgment which can be altered and updated. As such, it can be subject to the influence of current mood and of situational influences which make certain memories of life domains salient. At the same time, life satisfaction judgments are likely to show some stability because many people have made and stored judgments about specific aspects of their lives, and because the life circumstances on which life judgments rest tend to be stable.

The implications of conceptualizing life satisfaction as an ongoing judgment which is updated in terms of the immediate situation are manifold. First, it will not be possible to measure the exact level of life satisfaction because it is not an entity which is invariant. It is a judgment which will depend on how the respondent makes the valuation and under what circumstances. This means that many factors must be similar in order to compare life satisfaction judgments made in different studies. Further, it means that it will be desirable to measure life satisfaction on a number of occasions if the researcher is interested in obtaining a long-term stable average. On the other hand, differences in life satisfaction in various circumstances become the object of legitimate inquiry when life satisfaction is thought of in this way. Variations in life satisfaction judgments will not necessarily be conceived as arising entirely from measurement error, but may come about because of the situations in which the judgments are made.

Differences in comparison standards are one reason that life satisfaction judgments may vary. Such differences, however, need not be thought of narrowly in terms of the problem of inducing individuals to all use the same standards. People may actually compare their lives to different standards in different circumstances. They may use an absolute standard in terms of their goals, but people may also compare to other persons, to their ideals, to their past, and so forth. The differences in life satisfaction resulting from comparison to different standards need not be thought of as measurement error. Rather, these differences can be thought of as theoretically interesting variations in the way life judgments are made.

The need to communicate life satisfaction judgments to others may change the actual judgment made. It is not simply that respondent may retrieve a judgment, but alter it at output because he wants to regulate the impression made on the researcher. It may be that the respondent actually considers different information and constructs a different life satisfaction judgment depending on the specific interview situation.

Once again, situational influences on satisfaction judgments are important to study.

What this line of reasoning suggests is the importance of examining the processes by which people make life satisfaction judgments. Rather than being seen as error, differences in life satisfaction judgments become the object of exciting scientific work. Of course, the baby must not be thrown out with the bath water. There are some long-term coherencies to life satisfaction judgments, and the source of these coherencies is a legitimate question for researchers. Although transient factors can influence life satisfaction judgments, it is also interesting to explore why there are stabilities in life satisfaction across many years and across situations.

Emotion and Hedonic Level

Subjective well-being theorists can also learn much from recent work on emotion. For example, it is now widely agreed that there are important discrete emotions such as fear, anger, sadness, and joy. It is still not agreed whether these discrete emotions have separate biological bases, or whether they rest on prototypical appraisals which are likely to be universal in all cultures. Nevertheless, both theoretical (e.g., Izard, 1971) and empirical (Shaver et al., 1987) work has arrived at the conclusion that there are a finite number of important emotions which are separable. This suggests that SWB researchers often should, when time permits, assess a number of specific emotions rather than global hedonic level. Individuals may arrive at the same hedonic level through different emotional paths. Thus, understanding the correlates of hedonic level will be aided by knowledge of the specific pleasant and unpleasant emotions which individuals experience. Furthermore, subjective well-being can now be defined more specifically as comprising certain emotions which are unpleasant (e.g., sadness, jealousy, and fear) and certain ones which are pleasant (e.g., affection and joy).

Similarly, defining and appraising subjective well-being can be improved by considering long-term emotion to have more facets than simple hedonic level, which is the average pleasantness level of a person's affect over time. Parameters such as a person's emotional intensity (Larsen and Diener, 1987), emotional range (Larsen and

Cutler, 1992), and mood variability (Diener and Larsen, 1986) are also necessary to fully describe a person's affective life and subjective well-being. Two persons might have the same average hedonic level, but one may experience many varied and intense positive and negative emotions, whereas the other might experience a few mild emotions. Although their subjective well-being would be equivalent in terms of the average pleasantness of their affect, their quality of experience would be quite different. Furthermore, the antecedents and consequences of their emotions would likely be different. Thus, research on emotions suggests that a more complex assessment of long-term affect would benefit our understanding of subjective well-being.

A final way that advances in the field of emotion can contribute to our understanding of subjective well-being is by indicating which are the key components of emotion: action readiness, conscious experience, physiological reactions, nonverbal reactions such as vocal and facial parameters, and cognitive appraisals and labelling of emotions. The one-time measures of subjective well-being are like to heavily tap cognitive labelling aspects of emotion, and to some degree emotional experience. Other facets of emotion are less likely to be directly reflected in SWB self-report measures. Under most circumstances there will be incomplete agreement between measures of various emotional channels. For example, some individuals may deny negative emotions and not label them, even though they show signs of emotion in terms of action readiness or nonverbal behavior. Self-reports may be the best single measure of emotional experience, but they are limited in terms of the channels of emotion they are likely to accurately capture. Therefore, assessing additional emotional channels will help SWB researchers to determine the genesis of self-reports of affect, and yield a broader understanding of the emotional differences between individuals.

Time Frame and SWB Reports

Measures of subjective well-being can be phrased so that they reflect different time frames. For example, the SWLS item, "If I could live my life over, I would change almost nothing," is likely to elicit responses referring to a large segment of the person's life. In contrast, the SWLS item, "I am satisfied with my life," might draw responses which refer to the respondent's entire life or only to the person's present life. The causes and consequences of SWB measured in terms of different time frames are likely to differ. For example, temperament is likely to have a bigger influence on measures that have a longer-frame, and recent daily hassles will have a greater influence on measures which reflect a shorter time-frame. Although SWB researchers are interested in reactions which are not merely momentary mood, there is not a time frame which is "correct." Instead, different time frames all fall within the boundaries of subjective well-being and can produce interesting findings. But researchers should be aware that the time frame of their measures is likely to influence the correlations of SWB they uncover.

An additional issue about time is the fact that measures will differ in terms of accurately reflecting on-line experience. More reconstructive and judgmental processes will be involved for questions tapping long periods of time, whereas measures which rely on the experience sampling method will more accurately reflect on-line experience. Either variable might be of interest to the researcher, but she should understand the limitations of the measures used in terms of each phenomenon. Global measures given at a single session are unlikely to accurately reflect on-line emotional experiences, and are likely to be biased by memory heuristics as well as by the respondent's beliefs about his or her emotions. If the researcher desires to assess the respondent's construction of his or her emotions, the global measure is likely to be valuable. On the other hand, if the researcher uses an experience sampling or daily recording method, more fidelity is likely in the measure in reference to on-line emotional experience. But the measure is less likely to capture respondents' meta-moods — their conceptualization of their emotions.

The Satisfaction and Hedonic Level Relation

Finally, advances in the field of cognition, emotion, and personality suggest ways of conceptualizing the relation between life satisfaction and long-term affect. Just as life satisfaction arises from a judgment by the person of his or her life, affect also arises from cognitive appraisals. In the case of emotion, however, the appraisals are ongoing reactions to events. Thus, the emotion system produces hedonic level which is much more reactive to short-term life events. In contrast, life satisfaction judgments may take a more Olympian perspective and are more likely to involve a big picture of the person's life. Hassles or uplifts during the past week may have less impact on a life satisfaction judgment, whereas they may impact hedonic level substantially. In contrast, the fact that a person won the Nobel prize many years ago may substantially increase her life satisfaction, but may have little impact on her hedonic level over the last week. The relation between life satisfaction and hedonic level is likely to be substantial, but is unlikely to have one set value. The size of the relation will depend on the time frame of the affect and satisfaction questions, on the degree to which the person's conscious and unconscious motives differ, and on numerous other factors. Life satisfaction is dependent on global appraisals of life, appraisals which are guided to some extent by the immediate situation and current mood. Hedonic level, in contrast, is dependent on the on-line, often unconscious, appraisals the person makes of ongoing events. Such a conceptualization should aid SWB researchers in exploring the covariation between the two in a more theoretical way.

Contributions in other areas of psychology lead us to conceive of subjective well-being in a more differentiated, less monolithic way. The goal will then be, not to discover *the* cause of SWB, but rather to understand the antecedents of various types of SWB parameters. Subjective well-being cannot be considered to be a brute, incontrovertible fact, but will, like all scientific phenomena, depend on the types of measures used to assess it.

DEVELOPING NEW MEASURES

The evidence indicates that self-report measures of SWB are psychometrically adequate. At the same time, there are reasons to believe that the typical one-time self-reports of well-being, including my Satisfaction with Life Scale, have a host of potential shortcomings (e.g., see Diener and Fujita, 1994). We can greatly reduce the spurious influences on self-reports of SWB described earlier by using latent variables which depend on maximally different measures of the construct. It is also likely that multiple sources of nonself-report data such as those recommended below will better integrate the study of subjective well-being with basic psychological knowledge about emotion and cognition. Finally, the inclusion of additional types of measures in SWB batteries will yield a more complete picture of the various components of emotion. Thus, although self-report is usually the measure of choice if only one method of assessment can be used, additional types of measurement can help investigators triangulate and better understand the phenomenon. Below I describe a variety of new, nontraditional methods of SWB assessment:

a. Recording of nonverbal behaviors, either in natural settings or in reaction to stimuli sampled from the subjects' lives, can supplement self-reports. Paravocal, gestural, postural, and facial assessment can all give valuable information about subjects' emotions. For example, subjects could be videotaped while they are interviewed about their lives. Their micromomentary facial expressions and vocal tone could then be scored for emotional reactions, in addition to the verbal content of their answers. Some of the nonverbal channels such as vocal tone are less controllable than self-report (Babad et al., 1989; DePaulo and Rosenthal, 1979) and these are less likely to be contaminated by impression management. Further, these recordings will reflect emotional components which are not directly mediated by language.

b. Reports by significant others have potential as sources of information about well-being, although they have several inherent limitations. For example, because informants are not directly privy to their acquaintance's feelings, they must infer these from outward behaviors. Thus, their reports are more likely to be based on nonverbal behaviors and what the acquaintance says about his or her experiences. Furthermore, informants may skew their reports so as to be positive about their friend. Finally, informants often see their acquaintance in only one setting, and thus may not know their friend's full range of emotions. Despite these limitations, informant reports are valuable because they provide another source of data without compounding the errors of self-report, and because they are likely to reflect a different mix of emotional components than self-report measures. Although these reports tend to primarily assess external manifestations of well-being, they are not subject to some of the same sources of error as self-report and are therefore complementary to it. Sandvik et al. (1993) found that when a number of informant reports were aggregated, they converged substantially with other measures of SWB.

c. Although still in its infancy, the measurement of hormones and other physiological indices has promise. For example, electromyographic facial recording while a subject watches slides of her life and her close associates is a potential source of information. Similarly, cortisol, norepinephrine, and so forth could provide alternative sources of information about a subject's emotional well-being. Vitaliano *et al.* (1993) offer an excellent example of how life satisfaction may be related to heart rate reactivity and recovery. Physiological measures are not without flaws, but they have strengths which are complementary to those of self-report. For example, many physiological measures are unlikely to be altered by self-presentation effects.

d. Cognitive measures such as depth of processing have thus far received little attention in assessing well-being. We find that memory production measures of happy and unhappy events can provide valuable information about subjects' happiness (Sandvik *et al.*, 1993; Seidlitz and Diener, 1993) while being much less subject to some sources of error (e.g., self-presentational style) which are problematical for self-report. People high and low in subjective well-being are likely to differ in their chronically accessible constructs. Therefore, memory, priming, and attentional paradigms borrowed from experimental cognitive psychology offer promise as alternative measures of SWB.

e. Behavioral information (e.g., crying, sleep disturbances, alcohol consumption, activity level, and lack of appetite) offers another form of information about well-being.

f. Moods can be assessed on-line in the behavioral sampling technique pioneered by Csikszentmihalyi (e.g., Csikszentmihalyi *et al.*, 1977). For a discussion of the validity and reliability of this technique, see Csikszentmihalyi and Larson (1987) and Hormuth (1986). Because people are "beeped" at random moments, and record their current moods immediately, there is much less chance for memory distortion than there is when one asks subjects to summarize information from long periods of time. An extension of this technique is to require respondents to write down their moods each evening for that particular day. Despite the obvious strengths of the experience sampling technique, problems such as reactivity have not been thoroughly explored. Nevertheless, the experience sampling method seems to be a more accurate way of assessing mood than requesting global self-reports.

g. The recording of cognitive content (e.g., thoughts about self-worth, goals, helplessness, and success) can provide additional information about SWB beyond emotion based self-reports. For example, people's thoughts can be sampled when they are beeped at random moments, and these cognitions can be coded for rumination, and so forth. Appraisals of important life situations by the respondent would also be a valuable method for gaining a more complete assessment of respondents' SWB.

h. In-depth interviews about people's lives can provide qualitative information (Thomas and Chambers, 1989; Wood and Johnson, 1989) on well-being which is not subject to number use artifacts. Another advantage of such data is that they can be customized to a specific respondent's life. In addition, qualitative material can then be rated by coders and such ratings may be more resistant to idiosyncratic differences in scaling between subjects.

i. Mood sensitive tasks are available (Clark, 1983; Friswell and McConkey, 1989; Goodwin and Williams, 1982; Hama and Tsuda, 1989; Ketelaar, 1989; Mayer et al., 1988) which could be used as indicants of a person's moods, especially when repeated over time. If mood sensitive tasks are used on several occasions and indicate that a person is depressed or elated, a measure of SWB is obtained which does not share many of the pitfalls of self-report. At this time, it is not yet clear what types of mood sensitive tasks perform robustly across age groups, and which tasks show mood effects which are not swamped by stable individual differences in reaction time and so forth.

j. Tversky and Griffin (1991) remind us that economists rely on choice behavior as their major dependent variable, as a reflection of quality of life. SWB researchers also could use choice as a reflection of life satisfaction. For example, rather than simply obtain self-reports of satisfaction, a researcher could ask subjects which aspect of their lives they would choose to change and not change if they could do so. These descriptions could then be coded by raters for the degree of change the person would like in her life.

Clinical psychologists have long been wary of an uncritical acceptance of self-reports, and therefore have often sought additional information about their clients in behavioral measures, in nonverbal signs of emotion, and in the reports of significant others. It is time that SWB researchers adopt such a catholic approach to assessment. Where the measures converge, greater confidence can be placed in the results. If the measures diverge, the researcher can gain greater insights into how and why groups and individuals differ in SWB. Although additional measures can be expensive and time-consuming, their use seems imperative if we are to truly understand the SWB differences between groups.

Applied Research: The Survey Practitioner

What recommendations can be given to the survey researcher who has limited time with each respondent and who cannot use intrusive methods (e.g., physiological recording)? Survey field workers can systematically introduce a number of factors into the assessment session to increase the validity of their measures. Interviewers can allow adequate time for subjects to consider their responses, can reinforce careful responding, and can repeat wording and give very explicit instructions (Stimson, 1988). Naturally, it is desirable to keep these behaviors constant across interviews.

Survey researchers should consider measuring at least the three major components of well-being: satisfaction, positive affect, and negative affect, and measures of specific moods and emotions may be desirable as well. In addition, a measure of current momentary mood is very desirable in survey situations because it will allow the researcher to infer the influence of temporary mood states on the SWB measures.

Survey researchers also should carefully consider the context in which the well-being questions are asked. For example, the effects of question order must be considered. Instituting certain safeguards such as repeating the well-being questions at both the beginning and end of the interview will pay dividends in terms of more reliable measurement and as a check on contextual effects. When possible, researchers can administer well-being questions on two occasions in order to achieve a more stable judgment. Finally, survey researchers can sometimes include brief alternative measures of well-being: (a) ratings of subjects' affective facial expressions, (b) ratings of paravocal factors (for example, based on a tape recording), (c) memory production measures of good and bad events or factors in the subjects' lives, and (d) the questioning of informants.

FUTURE RESEARCH

The issues outlined in this paper present exciting opportunities for study and theory building. For instance, the new measures of well-being proposed above will require much development and testing. There are many questions for future research, for example:

a. Given the diversity of emotion theories, can we develop a common set of emotions which broadly reflect affective well-being across cultures? Will the pleasantness value of various emotions have to be assessed on an individual basis, or will it be possible to develop universal pleasantness or unpleasantness values for the basic emotions?

b. What is the relation of life satisfaction to emotional well-being? How do happiness and life satisfaction interrelate?

c. What factors influence emotional well-being as consciously labelled by the individual, and what factors influence emotional reactions which are not labelled?

d. To what degree does the pleasantness of an emotion covary with its degree of judged desirability or normativeness in a culture, and what factors influence this relation?

e. What is the influence of one's beliefs about happiness and of emotional self-presentation on happiness reports? To what degree is this influence spurious, and to what degree do these factors influence actual subjective well-being?

f. Can we develop an assessment battery which will reflect each of the components of affect and satisfaction, and optimally protect against likely self-report artifacts?

CONCLUSION

The study of subjective well-being is growing into a major area in the social sciences. It is imperative that we build this area on a solid measurement foundation. The major message is simply this: SWB measures are good, but they can be better. Measures of subjective well-being often simply ask respondents how happy or satisfied they are. These existing measures served surprisingly well during the initial stages of study in this field. But measurement should be an increasingly sophisticated enterprise in any scientific area. Therefore, increasing the quality of well-being measures and theoretical definitions of well-being offers an important vehicle for the field to progress.

The theory and measurement of subjective well-being were not well connected in the past with related areas of psychology such as emotion and cognition. The present paper begins constructing bridges to these areas by discussing well-being measurement in terms of the components of emotion, the concept of emotional avoidance, and the role of memory and judgment in making satisfaction judgments. Because measurement is so intertwined with theory, it is natural that conceptual bridges between SWB and other areas of psychology begin in this area. Several major conclusions can be drawn from the material reviewed in this paper.

1. Whenever possible, researchers should use multiple measures of SWB, both to reduce and assess error of measurement, but also to assess the multiple components of SWB. Self-reports of subjective well-being are adequate in a traditional psychometric sense. If one could choose only one type of SWB measure, in most cases it would be a self-report instrument because such measures have shown acceptable levels of validity and reliability. Nevertheless, measurement of SWB can be improved considerably by the addition of other methods of measurement such as experience sampling. Self-report measures covary strongly enough with other

types of measures to indicate that they are tapping some common SWB variance, but moderately enough to indicate that other types of measures will yield additional information.

2. A single score is likely to over-simplify the phenomenon of SWB. Multiple scores which capture multiple aspects of SWB such as various discrete emotions, emotional intensity, and life satisfaction are likely to lead to more sophisticated theories and understanding. Although positive and negative affect are not strictly independent in many measurement situations, they show enough unique variation and differing patterns of correlations with other variables to recommend that they be assessed separately.

3. Memory, judgment, and attentional processes must be considered in order to understand how respondents create their responses to SWB measures. Variations in these processes under varying measurement conditions can produce error variance in the measures which hitherto has been overlooked by researchers. Furthermore, understanding these processes will lead to a better theoretical understanding of subjective well-being.

4. Subjective well-being should not be reified as a concrete thing. There are clearly aspects of SWB which are often stable and consistent, and these coherencies are of deep scientific interest. Yet, it must be remembered that SWB is composed of a number of types of ongoing reactions in the individual, and these reactions will best be understood as processes, not as entities. At the same time, there are long-term stabilities and cross-situational consistencies in these processes which make the study of long-term well-being a defensible endeavor.

5. Researchers have often exclusively emphasized the negative reactions of individuals. Positive reactions in terms of pleasant affect and life satisfaction are of equal theoretical importance and should be afforded equal scientific attention.

In every area of the psychological sciences, concepts are originally conceived in relatively simple terms. Over time more complex views of these phenomena emerge, and measurement methods are created which reflect the more complex theoretical approach. The area of subjective well-being has been served by a relatively rudimentary concept of well-being, and the resulting measures have been extremely simple. Enough knowledge has now been accumulated, however, to indicate the needed advances in the concept of subjective well-being, and in this paper I recommend new measurement methods which reflect a more refined theory of what constitutes subjective well-being.

REFERENCES

Alker, H. A. and F. Gawin: 1978, 'On the intrapsychic specificity of happiness', Journal of Personality 46, pp. 311—322.

Allman, A. L.: 1990, Subjective Well-Being of People with Disabilities: Measurement Issues (Unpublished masters thesis, University of Illinois).

Andrews, F. M.: 1991, 'Stability and change in levels and structure of subjective well-being: USA 1972 and 1988', Social Indicators Research 25, pp. 1—30.

Andrews, F. M. and J. P. Robinson: 1991, 'Measures of subjective well-being', in J. P. Robinson, P. Shaver, and L. Wrightsman (eds.), Measures of Personality and Social Psychological Attitudes (Academic Press, San Diego), pp. 61—114.

Andrews, F. M. and S. B. Withey: 1976, Social Indicators of Well-Being: America's Perception of Life Quality (Plenum, New York).

Asendorpf, J. B. and K. R. Scherer: 1983, 'The discrepant repressor: Differentiation between low anxiety, high anxiety, and repression of anxiety by autonomic-facial-verbal patterns of behavior', Journal of Personality and Social Psychology 45, pp. 1334—1346.

Atkinson, T.: 1982, 'The stability and validity of quality of life measures', Social Indicators Research 10, pp. 113—132.

Babad, E., F. Bernieri, and R. Rosenthal: 1989, 'Nonverbal communication and leakage in the behavior of biased and unbiased teachers', Journal of Personality and Social Psychology 56, pp. 89—94.

Baker, L. A. , I. L. Cesa, M. Garz, and C. Mellins: 1992, 'Genetic and environmental influences on positive and negative affect: Support for a two-factor theory', Psychology and Aging 7, pp. 158—163.

Balatsky, G. and E. Diener: 1993, 'Subjective well-being among Russian students', Social Indicators Research 28, pp. 225—243.

Beiser, M.: 1974, 'Components and correlates of mental well-being', Journal of Health and Social Behavior 15, pp. 320—327.

Blaney, P. H.: 1986, 'Affect and memory: A review', Psychological Bulletin 99, pp. 229—246.

Blishen, B. and T. Atkinson: 1980, 'Anglophone and francophone differences in perceptions of the quality of life in Canada', in A. Szalai and F. M. Andrews (eds.), The Quality of Life: Comparative Studies (Sage, London).

Bonanno, G. A. and J. L. Singer: 1990, 'Repressive personality style: Theoretical and methodological implications for health and pathology', in J. L. Singer (ed.), Repression and Dissociation: Implications for Personality Theory, Psychopathology, and Health (University of Chicago Press, Chicago), pp. 455—470.

Borod, J. C.: 1992, 'Interhemispheric and intrahemispheric control of emotion: A focus on unilateral brain damage', Journal of Consulting and Clinical Psychology 60, pp. 339—348.

Bradburn, N. M.: 1969, The Structure of Psychological Well-Being (Aldine, Chicago).

Branscombe, N. R. and E. Diener: 1987, Consequences of Priming of Emotions:

Contrast and Assimilation Effects (Paper presented at the 95th Annual Meeting of the American Psychological Association, New York).

Brenner, B.: 1975, 'Quality of affect and self-evaluated happiness', Social Indicators Research 2, pp. 315—331.

Cacioppo, J. T., R. E. Petty, M. E. Losch, and H. S. Kim: 1986, 'Electromyographic activity over facial muscle regions can differentiate the valence and intensity of affective reactions', Journal of Personality and Social Psychology 50, pp. 260—268.

Campbell, A.: 1981, The Sense of Well-Being in America (McGraw Hill, New York).

Campbell, A., P. E. Converse, and W. L. Rodgers: 1976, The Quality of American Life (Russell Sage Foundation, New York).

Carstensen, L. L. and J. D. Cone: 1983, 'Social desirability and the measurement of psychological well-being in elderly persons', Journal of Gerontology 38, pp. 713—715.

Carver, C. S. and J. G. Gaines: 1987, 'Optimism, pessimism, and post-partum depression', Cognitive Therapy and Research 11, pp. 449—462.

Chamberlain, K.: 1988, 'On the structure of well-being', Social Indicators Research 20, pp. 581—604.

Chamberlain, K. and S. Zika: 1992, 'Stability and change in subjective well-being over short time periods', Social Indicators Research 26, pp. 101—117.

Clark, D. M.: 1983, 'On the induction of depressed mood in the laboratory: Evaluation and comparison of the Velten and musical procedures', Advances in Behavioral Research and Therapy 5, pp. 27—49.

Cohen, L. H., L. C. Towbes, and R. Flocco: 1988, 'Effects of induced mood on self-reported life events and perceived and received social support', Journal of Personality and Social Psychology 55, pp. 669—674.

Coombs, C. H.: 1964, A Theory of Data (Wiley, New York).

Costa, P. T. and R. R. McCrae: 1980, 'Influence of extraversion and neuroticism on subjective well-being: Happy and unhappy people', Journal of Personality and Social Psychology 38, pp. 668—678.

Costa, P. T. and R. R. McCrae: 1988, 'Personality in adulthood: A six-year longitudinal study of self-reports and spouse ratings on the NEO personality inventory', Journal of Personality and Social Psychology 54, pp. 853—863.

Costa, P., R. McCrae and A. Zonderman: 1987, 'Environmental and dispositional influences on well-being: Longitudinal follow-up of an American national sample', British Journal of Psychology 78, pp. 299—306.

Csikszentmihalyi, M. and R. Larson: 1987, 'Validity and reliability of the experience-sampling method', Journal of Nervous and Mental Disorders 175, pp. 526—536.

Csikszentmihalyi, M., R. Larson, and S. Prescott: 1977, 'The ecology of adolescent activity and experience', Journal of Youth and Adolescence 6, pp. 281—294.

Davidson, R. J.: 1983, 'Affect, repression, and cerebral asymmetry', in L. Temoshok, C. VanDyke, and L. S. Zegans (eds.), Emotions in Health and Illness (Grune & Stratton, New York), pp. 123—135.

Davis, P. J.: 1990, 'Repression and the inaccessibility of emotional memories', in J. L. Singer (ed.), Repression and Dissociation: Implications for Personality Theory, Psychopathology and Health (University of Chicago Press, Chicago), pp. 387—404.

DeHaes, J. C., B. J. W. Pennink, and K. Welvaart: 1987, 'The distinction between affect and cognition', Social Indicators Research 19, pp. 367—378.

DePaulo, B. M. and R. Rosenthal: 1979, 'Ambivalence, discrepancy, and deception in nonverbal communication', in R. Rosenthal (ed.), Skill in Nonverbal Communication (Oelgeschlager, Gunn & Hain, Cambridge, MA), pp. 204—248.

Dermer, M., S. J. Cohen, E. Jacobsen, and E. A. Anderson: 1979, 'Evaluative judgments of aspects of life as a function of vicarious exposure to hedonic extremes', Journal of Personality and Social Psychology 37, pp. 247—260.

Diener, E.: 1984, 'Subjective well-being', Psychological Bulletin 95, pp. 542—575.
Diener, E., C. R. Colvin, W. Pavot, and A. Allman: 1991, 'The psychic costs of intense positive emotions', Journal of Personality and Social Psychology 61, pp. 492—503.
Diener, E. and M. Diener: 1993, Self-Esteem and Life Satisfaction Across 31 Countries (Sixth Meeting of the International Society for the Study of Individual Differences, Baltimore).
Diener, E., M. Diener, and C. Diener: 1993, 'Factors predicting the subjective well-being of nations', manuscript submitted for publication.
Diener, E. and R. Emmons: 1985, 'The independence of positive and negative affect', Journal of Personality and Social Psychology 47, pp. 1105—1117.
Diener, E., R. A. Emmons, R. J. Larsen, and S. Griffin: 1985, 'The satisfaction with life scale', Journal of Personality Assessment 49, pp. 71—75.
Diener, E. and F. Fujita: 1994, 'Methodological pitfalls and solutions in satisfaction research', in A. C. Samli and M. J. Sirgy (eds.), New Dimensions in Marketing/Quality-of-life Interface (Quorum Books, Westport, Connecticut).
Diener, E., F. Fujita, and H. Smith: 1993, The Death of Social Desirability: An Empirical Demonstration (Manuscript in Preparation, University of Illinois).
Diener, E., J. Horwitz, and R. A. Emmons: 1985, 'Happiness of the very wealthy', Social Indicators Research 16, pp. 263—274.
Diener, E. and A. Iran-Nejad: 1986, 'The relationship in experience between various types of affect', Journal of Personality and Social Psychology 50, pp. 1031—1038.
Diener, E. and R. J. Larsen: 1984, 'Temporal stability and cross-situational consistency of affective, behavioral, and cognitive responses', Journal of Personality and Social Psychology 47, pp. 871—883.
Diener, E. and R. J. Larsen: 1986, The Emotionally Reactive Individual: Intensity, Variability, and Stimulus Responsivity (Unpublished manuscript).
Diener, E. and R. J. Larsen: 1993, 'The experience of emotional well-being', in M. Lewis and J. M. Haviland (eds.), Handbook of Emotions (Guilford, New York), pp. 405—415.
Diener, E., R. J. Larsen and R. A. Emmons: 1984, 'Person X situation interactions: Choice of situations and congruence response models', Journal of Personality and Social Psychology 47, pp. 580—592.
Diener, E., R. J. Larsen, S. Levine, and R. A. Emmons: 1985, 'Intensity and frequency: Dimensions underlying positive and negative affect', Journal of Personality and Social Psychology 48, pp. 1253—1265.
Diener, E., E. Sandvik, and W. Pavot: 1990, 'Happiness is the frequency, not the intensity, of positive versus negative affect', in F. Strack, M. Argyle, and N. Schwarz (eds.), Subjective Well-Being: An Interdisciplinary Perspective (Pergamon, New York), pp. 119—136.
Diener, E., E. Sandvik, W. Pavot, and D. Gallagher: 1991, 'Response artifacts in the measurement of subjective well-being', Social Indicators Research 24, pp. 35—56.
Diener, E., E. Sandvik, L. Seidlitz, and M. Diener: 1992, 'The relationship between income and subjective well-being', Social Indicators Research 28, pp. 195—223.
Diener, E., H. Smith, and F. Fujita: 1993, The Structure of Long-Term Affect (Manuscript in preparation, University of Illinois).
Diener, E., M. Suh, H. Smith, and L. Shao: 1994, 'National and cultural differences in reported subjective well-being: Why do they occur?' Social Indicators Research (in press).
Ekman, P.: 1984, 'Expression and the nature of emotion', in K. R. Scherer and P. Ekman (eds.), Approaches to Emotion (Lawrence Erlbaum, Hillsdale, NJ), pp. 319—344.

Ekman, P., W. V. Friesen, and P. Ellsworth: 1972, Emotion in the Human Face: Guidelines for Research and an Integration of Findings (Pergamon Press, New York).

Ekman, P., R. W. Levenson, and W. V. Friesen: 1983, 'Autonomic nervous system activity distinguishes between emotions', Science 221, pp. 1208—1210.

Emmons, R. A.: 1986, 'Personal strivings: An approach to personality and subjective well-being', Journal of Personality and Social Psychology 51, pp. 1058—1068.

Emmons, R. A. and E. Diener: 1985, 'Personality correlates of subjective well-being', Journal of Personality and Social Psychology 11, pp. 89—97.

Fordyce, M. W.: 1988, 'A review of research on the happiness measures: A sixty second index of happiness and mental health', Social Indicators Research 20, pp. 355—381.

Frijda, N. H.: 1986, The Emotions (Cambridge University Press, Cambridge).

Friswell, R. and K. M. McConkey: 1989, 'Hypnotically induced mood', Cognition and Emotion 3, pp. 1—26.

Fujita, F.: 1991, An Investigation of the Relationship Between Extraversion, Neuroticism, Positive Affect and Negative Affect (Unpublished Masters Thesis, University of Illinois).

Fujita, F.: 1993, The Effects of Naturalistic Social Comparison on Satisfaction (Doctoral dissertation, University of Illinois).

Fujita, F., H. Smith, and E. Diener: 1993, Variations in Anonymity and the Validity of Well-Being Reports (Manuscript submitted for publication).

Furnham, A.: 1986, 'Response bias, social desirability, and dissimulation', Personality and Individual Differences 7, pp. 385—400.

Galin, D.: 1974, 'Implications for psychiatry of left and right cerebral specialization', Archives of General Psychiatry 31, pp. 572—583.

Gazzaniga, M. S.: 1985, The Social Brain: Discovering the Networks of the Mind (Basic Books, New York).

George, L. K. and L. B. Bearon: 1980, Quality of Life in Older Persons: Meaning and Measurement (Human Sciences Press, New York).

Glenn, N. D. and C. N. Weaver: 1978, 'A multivariate, multisurvey study of marital happiness', Journal of Marriage and the Family 40, pp. 269—281.

Goodwin, A. M. and M. G. Williams: 1982, 'Mood induction research — its implications for clinical depression', Behavior Research and Therapy 20, pp. 373—382.

Green, D. P., S. Goldman, and P. Salovey: 1993, 'Measurement error masks bipolarity in affect ratings', Journal of Personality and Social Psychology 64, pp. 1029—1041.

Grice, H. P.: 1975, 'Logic and conservation', in P. Cole and J. L. Morgan (eds.), Syntax and Semantics: Speech Acts (Academic Press, New York), pp. 41—58.

Gudjonsson, G. H.: 1981, 'Self-reported emotional disturbance and its relation to electrodermal reactivity, defensiveness and trait anxiety', Personality and Individual Differences 2, pp. 47—52.

Gurin, G., J. Veroff, and S. Feld: 1960, Americans View Their Mental Health (Basic Books, New York).

Haggard, E. A. and K. S. Isaacs: 1966 'Micromomentary facial expression as indicators of ego mechanisms in psychotherapy', in L. A. Gottschalk and A. H. Auerbach (eds.), Methods of Research in Psychotherapy (Appleton-Century-Crofts, New York).

Hama, H. and K. Tsuda: 1989, Analysis of Emotions Evoked by Schematic Faces and Measured with Clynes' Sentograph (Paper presented at the Fourth International Meeting of the International Society for Research on Emotions, Paris, France).

Hammen, C. and D. R. Glass: 1975, 'Activity, depression, and evaluation of reinforcement', Journal of Abnormal Psychology 84, pp. 718—721.

Harmon, T. M., R. O. Nelson, and S. C. Hayes: 1980, 'Self-monitoring of mood versus activity by depressed clients', Journal of Consulting and Clinical Psychology 48, pp. 30—38.

Headey, B., E. Holmstrom, and A. Wearing: 1985, 'Models of well-being and ill-being', Social Indicators Research 17, pp. 211—234.

Headey, B., R. Veenhoven, and A. Wearing: 1991, 'Top-down versus bottom-up theories of subjective well-being', Social Indicators Research 24, pp. 81—100.

Headey, B. and A. Wearing: 1989, 'Personality, life events, and subjective well-being: Toward a dynamic equilibrium model', Journal of Personality and Social Psychology 57, pp. 731—739.

Hogan, R.: 1983, 'A socioanalytic theory of personality', in M. M. Page (ed.), Person-ality — Current Theory and Research: 1982 Nebraska Symposium on Motivation (University of Nebraska Press, Lincoln, Nebraska), pp. 55—89.

Hogan, R. and R. A. Nicholson: 1988, 'The meaning of personality test scores', American Psychologist 43, pp. 621—626.

Horley, J. and J. J. Lavery: 1991, 'The stability and sensitivity of subjective well-being measures', Social Indicators Research 24, pp. 113—122.

Horley, J. and B. R. Little: 1985, 'Affective and cognitive components of global subjective well-being measures', Social Indicators Research 17, pp. 189—197.

Hormuth, S. E.: 1986, 'The sampling of experiences in situ', Journal of Personality 54, pp. 262—293.

Inglehart, R: 1977, The Silent Revolution: Changing Values and Political Styles Among Western Publics (Princeton University Press, Princeton, NJ).

Izard, C. E.: 1971, The Face of Emotion (Appleton-Century-Crofts, New York).

Izard, C. E.: 1972, Patterns of Emotions: A New Analysis of Anxiety and Depression (Academic Press, New York).

Izard, C. E.: 1992, 'Basic emotions, relations among emotions, and emotion-cognition relations', Psychological Review 99, pp. 561—565.

Jasper, H. H.: 1930, 'The measurement of depression-elation and its relation to a measure of extraversion-introversion', Journal of Abnormal and Social Psychology 25, pp. 307—318.

Jones, H. M.: 1953, The Pursuit of Happiness (Harvard University Press, Cambridge, MA).

Judge, T.: 1990, Job Satisfaction As a Reflection of Disposition: Investigating the Rela-tionship and Its Effects on Employee Adaptive Behaviors (Doctoral dissertation, University of Illinois).

Kagan, J.: 1984, 'The idea of emotion in human development', in C. E. Izard, J. Kagan, and R. B. Zajonc (eds.), Emotions, Cognition, and Behavior (Cambridge University Press, Cambridge).

Kahneman, D., P. Slovic, and A. Tversky (eds.): 1982, Judgment Under Uncertainty: Heuristics and Biases (Cambridge University Press, New York).

Kammann, R., D. Christie, R. Irwin, and G. Dixon: 1979, 'Properties of an inventory to measure happiness (and psychological health)', New Zealand Psychologist 8, pp. 1—9.

Kammann, R. and R. Flett (1983). Coursebook for Measuring Well-Being with the Affectometer 2 (Why Not? Foundation: Dunedin, New Zealand).

Ketelaar, T.: 1989, Examining the Dimensions of Affect in the Domain of Mood-Sensitive Tasks (Unpublished master's thesis, Purdue University, West Lafayette, IN).

King, A. C., C. L. Albright, C. B. Taylor, W. L. Haskell, and R. F. Debusk: 1986, The Repressive Coping Style: A Predictor of Cardiovascular Reactivity and Risk (Presented at the annual meeting of the Society of Behavioral Medicine, San Francisco).

King, D. A. and A. M. Buchwald: 1982, 'Sex differences in subclinical depression: Administration of the Beck Depression Inventory in public and private disclosure situations', Journal of Personality and Social Psychology 42, pp. 963—996.

Kozma, A., S. Stone, M. J. Stones, T. E. Hannah, and K. McNeil: 1990, 'Long- and short-term affective states in happiness: Model, paradigm, and experimental evidence', Social Indicators Research 22, pp. 119—138.

Kozma, A. and M. J. Stones: 1988, 'Social desirability in measures of subjective well-being: Age comparisons', Social Indicators Research 20, pp. 1—14.

Kushman, J. and S. Lane: 1980, 'A multivariate analysis of factors affecting perceived life satisfaction and psychological well-being among the elderly', Social Science Quarterly 61, pp. 264—277.

Larsen, R. J.: 1992, 'Neuroticism and selective encoding and recall of symptoms: Evidence from a combined concurrent-retrospective study', Journal of Personality and Social Psychology, pp. 480—488.

Larsen, R. J. and S. E. Cutler: 1992, 'The complexity of individual emotional lives: A process analysis of affect structure (Manuscript submitted for publication, University of Michigan).

Larsen, R. J. and E. Diener: 1985, 'A multitrait-multimethod examination of affect structure: Hedonic level and emotional intensity', Personality and Individual Differences 6, pp. 631—636.

Larsen, R. J. and E. Diener: 1987, 'Emotional response intensity as an individual difference characteristic', Journal of Research in Personality 21, pp. 1—39.

Larsen, R. J., E. Diener and R. A. Emmons: 1985, 'An evaluation of subjective well-being measures', Social Indicators Research 17, pp. 1—18.

Lawrence, R. H. and J. Liang: 1988, 'Structural integration of the Affect Balance Scale and the Life Satisfaction Index A: Race, sex, and age differences', Psychology and Aging 3, pp. 375—384.

Lawton, M. P.: 1972, 'The dimensions of morale', in D. P. Kent, R. Kastenbaum, and S. Sherwood (eds.), Research, Planning and Action for the Elderly (Behavioral Publications, New York).

Lawton, M. P.: 1983, 'The varieties of well-being', Experimental Aging Research 9, pp. 65—72.

Lawton, M. P., M. H. Kleban, and E. DiCarlo: 1984, 'Psychological well-being in the aged', Research on Aging 6, pp. 67—97.

Lazarus, R. S.: 1991, Emotion and Adaptation (Oxford University Press, New York).

Lehman, D. R., C. B. Wortman, and A. F. Williams: 1987, 'Long-term effects of losing a spouse or child in a motor vehicle crash', Journal of Personality and Social Psychology 52, pp. 218—231.

Levenson, R. W. and L. L. Mades: 1980, Physiological Response, Facial Expression, and Trait Anxiety: Two Methods for Improving Consistency (Paper presented at the Society for Psychophysiological Research, Vancouver, British Columbia).

Leventhal, H.: 1984, 'A perceptual motor theory of emotion', in K. R. Scherer and P. Ekman (eds.), Approaches to Emotion (Lawrence Erlbaum: Hillsdale, NJ), pp. 271—292.

Liang, J.: 1985, 'A structural integration of the Affect Balance Scale and the Life Satisfaction Index A', Journal of Gerontology 40, pp. 552—461.

Liang, J., H. Asano, K. A. Bollen, E. F. Kahana, and D. Maeda: 1987, 'Cross-cultural comparability of the Philadelphia Geriatric Center Morale Scale: An American-Japanese comparison', Journal of Gerontology 42, pp. 37—43.

Lorr, M., A. Qing Shi, and R. P. Youniss: 1989, 'A bipolar multifactor conception of mood states', Personality and Individual Differences 10, pp. 155—159.

MacKinnon, N. J. and L. J. Keating: 1989, 'The structure of emotions: Canada-United States comparisons', Social Psychology Quarterly 52, pp. 70—83.

MacLean, P. D.: 1975, 'Sensory and perceptive factors in emotional functions in the triune brain', in L. Levi (ed.), Emotions: Their Parameters and Measurement (Raven Press, New York).

Mandler, G.: 1985, Cognitive Psychology: An Essay in Cognitive Science (Erlbaum, Hillsdale, NJ).

Marshall, G. N., C. B. Wortman, J. W. Kusulas, K. L. Hervig, and R. R. Vickers: 1992, 'Distinguishing optimism from pessimism: Relations to fundamental dimensions of mood and personality', Journal of Personality and Social Psychology 62, pp. 1067—1074.

Mayer, J. D., M. H. Mamberg, and A. J. Volanth: 1988, 'Cognitive domains of the mood system', Journal of Personality 56, pp. 453—486.

McConville, C. and C. Cooper: 1992, 'The structure of moods', Personality and Individual Differences 8, pp. 909—919.

McCrae, R. R.: 1986, 'Well-being scales do not measure social desirability', Journal of Gerontology 41, pp. 390—392.

McCrae, R. R. and P. T. Costa: 1983, 'Social desirability scales: More substance than style', Journal of Consulting and Clinical Psychology 51, pp. 882—888.

McCrae, R. R. and P. R. Costa: 1991, 'Adding liebe and arbeit: The full five-factor model and well-being', Personality and Social Psychology Bulletin 17, pp. 227—232.

McCulloch, B. J.: 1991, 'A longitudinal investigation of the factor structure of subjective well-being: The case of the Philadelphia Geriatric Center Morale Scale', Journal of Gerontology 46, pp. 251—258.

McKennell, A.: 1974, 'Surveying subjective welfare: Strategies and methodological considerations', in B. Strumpel (ed.), Subjective Elements of Well-Being (Organization for Economic Development and Cooperation, Paris), pp. 45—72.

McNeil, J. K., M. J. Stones, and A. Kozma: 1986, 'Subjective well-being in later life: Issues concerning measurement and prediction', Social Indicators Research 18, pp. 35—70.

Michalos, A.: 1991, Global Report on Student Well-Being. Volume 1: Life Satisfaction and Happiness (Springer Verlag, New York).

Neugarten, B. L., R. J. Havighurst, and S. S. Tobin: 1961, 'The measurement of life satisfaction', Journal of Gerontology 16, pp. 134—143.

Nydegger, C. N. (ed.): 1977, Measuring Morale: A Guide to Effective Assessment (Gerontological Society, Washington, DC).

Oatley, K. and J. M. Jenkins: 1992, 'Human emotions: Function and dysfunction', Annual Review of Psychology 43, pp. 55—85.

Okun, M. A. and W. A. Stock: 1987, 'A construct validity study of subjective well-being measures: An assessment via quantitative research syntheses', Journal of Community Psychology 15, pp. 481—492.

Ormel, J. and W. B. Schaufeli: 1991, 'The stability and change in psychological distress and their relationship with self-esteem and locus of control: A dynamic equilibrium model', Journal of Personality and Social Psychology 60, pp. 288—299.

Ouweneel, P. and R. Veenhoven: 1991, 'Cross-national differences in happiness: Cultural bias or societal quality', in N. Bleichrodt and P. J. D. Drenth (eds.), Contemporary Issues in Cross-Cultural Psychology (Swets & Zeitlinger, Amsterdam), pp. 168—184.

Panksepp, J.: 1982, 'Toward a general psychobiological theory of emotions', The Behavioral and Brain Sciences 5, pp. 407—467.

Paulhus, D. L.: 1988, Assessing Self Deception and Impression Management in Self-Reports: The Balanced Inventory of Desirable Responding (Department of Psychology, University of British Columbia, Vancouver, B.C., Canada V6T 1Y7).

Pavot, W. and E. Diener: 1993a 'The affective and cognitive context of self-reported measures of subjective well-being', Social Indicators Research 28, pp. 1—20.

Pavot, W. and E. Diener: 1993b, 'A review of the satisfaction with life scale', Psychological Assessment 5, pp. 164—172.

Pavot, W., E. Diener, C. R. Colvin, and E. Sandvik: 1991, 'Response artifacts in the measurement of subjective well-being', Social Indicators Research 24, pp. 35—56.

Pavot, W., E. Diener and F. Fujita: 1990, 'Extraversion and happiness', Personality and Individual Differences 11, pp. 1299—1306.

Plutchik, R.: 1980, Emotion: A Psychoevolutionary Synthesis (Harper & Row, New York).

Plutchik, R.: 1984, 'Emotions: A general psychoevolutionary theory', in K. R. Scherer and P. Ekman (eds.), Approaches to Emotion (Erlbaum, Hillsdale, NJ), pp. 197—219.

Rodgers, W. L., A. R. Herzog and F. M. Andrews: 1988, 'Interviewing older adults: Validity of self-reports of satisfaction', Psychology and Aging 3, pp. 264—272.

Russell, J. A.: 1991, 'Culture and the categorization of emotions', Psychological Bulletin 110, pp. 426—450.

Sandvik, E., E. Diener, and L. Seidlitz: 1993, 'The assessment of well-being: A comparison of self-report and nonself-report strategies', Journal of Personality 61, pp. 317—342.

Scherer, K. R.: 1984, 'On the nature and function of emotion: A component process approach', in K. R. Scherer and P. Ekman (eds.), Approaches to Emotion (Lawrence Erlbaum: Hillsdale, NJ), pp. 293—318.

Schwartz, G. E.: 1982, 'Psychophysiological patterning of emotion revisited: A systems perspective', in C. E. Izard (ed.), Measuring Emotions in Infants and Children (Cambridge University Press, Cambridge), pp. 67—93.

Schwartz, G. E.: 1983, 'Disregulation theory and disease: Applications to the repression/ cerebral disconnection/cardiovascular disorder hypothesis', International Review of Applied Psychology 32, pp. 95—118.

Schwarz, N. and G. Clore: 1983, 'Mood, misattribution, and judgments of well-being: Informative and directive functions of affective states', Journal of Personality and Social Psychology 45, pp. 513—523.

Schwarz, N. and F. Strack: 1991, 'Evaluating one's life: A judgment model of subjective well-being', in F. Strack, M. Argyle and N. Schwarz (eds.), Subjective Well-Being: An Interdisciplinary Perspective (Pergamon, Oxford), pp. 27—48.

Scott, C., E. Diener, and F. Fujita: 1992, Personality Versus the Situational Effect in the Relation Between Marriage and Subjective Well-Being (Unpublished manuscript, University of Illinois).

Seidlitz, L. and E. Diener: 1993, 'Memory for positive versus negative life events: Theories for the differences between happy and unhappy persons', Journal of Personality and Social Psychology 64, pp. 654—664.

Shao, L.: 1992, Multilanguage Comparability of Life Satisfaction and Happiness Measures in Mainland Chinese and American Students (Unpublished Master Thesis, University of Illinois).

Shaver, P., J. Schwartz, D. Kirson, and C. O'Connor: 1987, 'Emotional knowledge: Further exploration of a prototype approach', Journal of Personality and Social Psychology 52, pp. 1061—1086.

Sinclair, R. C., M. M. Mark, and T. R. Wellens: 1989, Administration of the Beck Depression Inventory on Self-Report of Mood State: A Case in Contrast (Paper presented at the Midwest Psychological Association Meeting, Chicago).

Singer, J. L. (ed.): 1990, Repression and Dissociation: Implications for Personality Theory, Psychotherapy, and Health (University of Chicago Press, Chicago).

Skelton, J. A. and D. B. Strohmetz: 1990, 'Priming symptom reports with health related cognitive activity', Personality and Social Psychology Bulletin 16, pp. 449—464.

Smith, T. W.: 1979, 'Happiness: Time trends, seasonal variations, intersurvey differences, and other mysteries', Social Psychology Quarterly 42, pp. 18—30.

Smith, T. W., M. K. Pope, F. Rhodewalt, and J. L. Poulton: 1989, 'Optimism, neuroticism, coping and symptom reports: An alternative interpretation of the Life Orientation Test', Journal of Personality and Social Psychology 56, pp. 640—648.

Sommers, S.: 1984, 'Reported emotions and conventions of emotionality among college students', Journal of Personality and Social Psychology 46, pp. 207—215.

Staats, S., C. Partlo, and N. Adam: 1989, When Time Frame Makes a Difference (Paper presented at the 61st Annual Meeting of the Midwestern Psychological Association, Chicago).

Stimson, R. J.: 1988, Problems of Research on Spatial Behavior in Large Scale Urban Environments: Methodological Issues in Minimizing Error and Bias to Produce Valid and Reliable Data (Paper presented at the 24th International Congress of Psychology, Sydney, Australia).

Stock, W. A., M. A. Okun, and M. Benin: 1986, 'Structure of subjective well-being among the elderly', Psychology and Aging 1, pp. 91—102.

Stones, M. J. and A. Kozma: 1980, 'Issues relating to the usage and conceptualization of mental health constructs employed by gerontologists', International Journal of Aging and Human Development 11, pp. 269—281.

Strack, F., N. Schwarz, B. Chassein, D. Kern, and D. Wagner: 1990, 'Salience of comparison standards and the activation of social norms: Consequences for judgments of happiness and their communication', British Journal of Social Psychology 29, pp. 303—314.

Strack, F., N. Schwarz, and M. Wanke: 1991, 'Semantic and pragmatic aspects of context effects in social and psychological research', Social Cognition 9, pp. 111—125.

Sudman, S.: 1967, 'Reducing the Cost of Surveys. NORC Monographs in Social Research (Aldine, Chicago).

Tatarkiewicz, W.: 1976, Analysis of Happiness (Martinus Nijhoff, The Hague, Netherlands).

Taylor, C.: 1977, 'Why measure morale?', in C. Nydegger (ed.), Measuring Morale: A Guide to Effective Assessment (Gerontological Society, Washington, D.C.), pp. 30—33.

Thomas, D. and E. Diener: 1990, 'Memory accuracy in the recall of emotions', Journal of Personality and Social Psychology 59, pp. 291—297.

Thomas, L. E. and K. D. Chambers: 1989, 'Phenomenology of life satisfaction among elderly men: Quantitative and qualitative views', Psychology and Aging 4, pp. 284—289.

Tomkins, S. S. and R. McCarter: 1964, 'What and where are the primary affects? Some evidence for a theory', Perceptual and Motor Skills 18, pp. 119—158.

Torangeau, R. and K. A. Rasinski: 1988, 'Cognitive processes underlying context effects of attitude measurement', Psychological Bulletin 103, pp. 299—314.

Tran, T. V., R. Wright and L. Chatters: 1991, 'Health, stress, psychological resources, and subjective well-being among older blacks', Psychology and Aging 6, pp. 100—108.

Tversky, A. and D. Griffin: 1991, 'Endowment and contrast in judgments of well-being', in F. Strack, M. Argyle, and N. Schwarz (eds.), Subjective Well-Being: An Interdisciplinary Perspective (Pergamon, New York), pp. 101—118.

Tyrer, P.: 1976, The Role of Bodily Feelings in Anxiety (Oxford Press, New York).

Veenhoven, R.: 1984, Conditions of Happiness (D. Reidel, Dordrecht).

Vitaliano, P. P., V. M. Paulsen, J. Russo, and S. L. Bailey: 1993, Cardiovascular Recovery: Biopsyosocial Concomitants in Older Adults (Manuscript submitted for publication, University of Washington, Seattle).

Warr, P., J. Barter and G. Brownbridge: 1983, 'On the independence of negative and positive affect', Journal of Personality and Social Psychology 44, pp. 644–651.

Washburne, J. N.: 1941, 'Factors related to the social adjustment of college girls', Journal of Social Psychology 13, pp. 281–289.

Watson, D.: 1988, 'The vicissitudes of mood measurement: Effects of varying descriptors, time frames, and response formats on measures of positive and negative affect', Journal of Personality and Social Psychology 55, pp. 128–141.

Watson, D. and L. A. Clark: 1984, 'Negative affectivity: The disposition to experience aversive emotional states', Psychological Bulletin 96, pp. 465–490.

Watson, D., L. A. Clark, and A. Tellegen: 1984, 'Cross-cultural convergence in the structure of mood: A Japanese replication and comparison with U.S. findings', Journal of Personality and Social Psychology 47, pp. 127–144.

Weinberger, D. A.: 1990, 'The construct validity of the repressive coping style', in J. L. Singer (ed.), Repression and Dissociation: Implications for Personality Theory, Psychopathology, and Health (University of Chicago Press, Chicago), pp. 337–386.

Weinberger, D. A., G. E. Schwartz, and R. J. Davidson: 1979, 'Low-anxious, high-anxious, and repressive coping styles: Psychometric patterns and behavioral and physiological responses to stress', Journal of Abnormal Psychology 88, pp. 369–380.

Wellens, T. R., J. S. Tanaka, and A. T. Panter: 1989, 'The Role of Item Order in the Assessment of Dysphoric Affect (Paper presented at the Midwest Psychological Association Meeting, Chicago).

Wessman, A. E. and D. F. Ricks: 1966, Mood and Personality (Holt, New York).

Wilson, G. A., J. W. Elias, and L. J. Brownlee: 1985, 'Factor invariance and the life satisfaction index', Journal of Gerontology 40, pp. 344–346.

Wood, L. A. and J. Johnson: 1989, 'Life satisfaction among the rural elderly: What do the numbers mean?', Social Indicators Research 21, pp. 379–408.

Wood, V., M. L. Wylie, and B. Sheafor: 1969, 'An analysis of a short self-report measure of life satisfaction: Correlation with rater judgments', Journal of Gerontology 24, pp. 465–469.

Wyer, R. S. and T. K. Srull: 1989, Memory and Cognition in its Social Context (Erlbaum, Hillsdale, NJ).

Zajonc, R. B.: 1984a, 'The interaction of affect and cognition', in K. R. Scherer and P. Ekman (eds.), Approaches to Emotion (Lawrence Erlbaum, Hillsdale, NJ), pp. 239–246.

Zajonc, R. B.: 1984b, 'On the primacy of affect', in K. R. Scherer and P. Ekman (eds.), Approaches to Emotion (Lawrence Erlbaum, Hillsdale, NJ), pp. 259–270.

Zautra, A. J., C. A. Guarnaccia, and J. W. Reich: 1988, 'Factor structure of mental health measures for older adults', Journal of Consulting and Clinical Psychology 56, pp. 514–519.

Zevon, M. A. and A. Tellegen: 1982, 'The structure of mood change: An idiographic/nomothetic analysis', Journal of Personality and Social Psychology 43, pp. 111–122.

Psychology Department,
University of Illinois,
Champaign IL 61820,
U.S.A.

RUUT VEENHOVEN

17. IS HAPPINESS A TRAIT?

Tests of the Theory that a Better Society does not Make People any Happier[1,2,3]

(Accepted 16 May, 1993)

ABSTRACT. One of the ideological foundations of the modern welfare states is the belief that people can be made happier by providing them with better living conditions. This belief is challenged by the theory that happiness is a fixed 'trait', rather than a variable 'state'. This theory figures both at the individual level and at the societal level. The individual level variant depicts happiness as an aspect of personal character; rooted in inborn temperament or acquired disposition. The societal variant sees happiness as a matter of national character; embedded in shared values and beliefs. Both variants imply that a better society makes no happier people.

Happiness can be regarded as a trait if it meets three criteria: (1) temporal stability, (2) cross-situational consistency, and (3) inner causation. This paper checks whether that is, indeed, the case.

The theory that happiness is a personal-character-trait is tested in a (meta) analysis of longitudinal studies. The results are: (1) Happiness is quite stable on the short term, but not in the long run, neither relatively nor absoloutely. (2) Happiness is not insensitive to fortune or adversity. (3) Happiness is not entirely built-in: its genetic basis is at best modest and psychological factors explain only part of its variance.

The theory that happiness is a national-character-trait is tested in an analysis of differences in average happiness between nations. The results point in the same direction: (1) Though generally fairly stable over the last decades, nation-happiness has changed profoundly in some cases, both absolutely and relatively. (2) Average happiness in nations is clearly not independant of living conditions. The better the conditions in a country, the happier its citizens. (3) The differences cannot be explained by a collective outlook on life.

It is concluded that happiness is no immutable trait. There is thus still sense in striving for greater happiness for a greater number.

Alex C. Michalos (ed.), Citation Classics from Social Indicators Research, 477–536.
© 2005 *Springer. Printed in the Netherlands.*

1. INTRODUCTION

The Pursuit of Happiness

Happiness is a main goal in present day Western society. Individually, people try to shape their lives in such ways that they can enjoy them. Politically, there is massive support for policies that aim at greater happiness for everybody. It is widely believed that we can get happier than we are. There is also consensus that we should not acquiesce in current unhappiness.

The belief that we *can* get happier is rooted in the Humanistic view of man. Rather than a helpless being expelled from Paradise, man is seen as autonomous, and able to improve his condition by the use of reason. This view was at the core of the 19th century Utopian movement and is still at the ideological basis of the 20th century Welfare States. Planned social reform, guided by scientific research, is expected to result in a better society with happier citizens.

The conviction that we *should* try to improve happiness is rooted in Enlighted thought as well. The notion that happiness is to be preferred above unhappiness figured already in ancient Greek moral philosophy. In the 19th century it crystallized into the Utilitarian doctrine that the moral value of all action depends on the degree to which it contributes to the 'greatest happiness for the greatest number'. Though few accept happiness as the only and ultimate goal in life, it is generally agreed that happiness is worth pursuing. Happiness ranks high in public opinion surveys on value priorities. See a.o. Harding (1985: 231.)

This ideology is not unchallenged however. It is argued that happiness is not the most valuable goal and it is claimed that we cannot get happier even if we would want to.

The objection that happiness is not worth pursuing rests partly in religious doctrines that glorify suffering. Such doctrines figure in Calvinist moral philosophy and in some variants of Hinduism. Objections come also from advocates of other endvalues who are eager to depreciate the competitor. Many Marxists for instance reject happiness as something 'false', equality being the only 'true' value they accept. Such moral objections find support in theories about adverse effects of happiness. Happiness is said to make people politically uncritical, socially unresponsive and morally decadent. Mild unhappiness would be preferable in the long run. Elsewhere I have examined these claims empirically and found most of them untrue. See Veenhoven (1988, 1989.)

The objection that we cannot raise happiness, even if we wanted to, rests on two lines of thought. The first is that we are unable to change society according to plan; this is the theme of limits to social engineering. The second denunciation is that even successful improvement of society would help little. A better society would not make people any happier. This latter objection draws on two theories: One theory holds that happiness is 'relative'. Any improvement in living conditions would soon result in a rise in standards of comparison and would therefore leave us as (un)happy as before. The other theory is that happiness is a fixed 'trait' rather than a variable 'state'. Improvements of external living conditions would therefore not result in greater happiness, the evaluation of life being largely determined by an internal disposition to enjoy it. Elsewhere I have tested the theory that happiness is relative (Veenhoven, 1991). That theory was largely refuted. This paper considers the claim that happiness is a fixed trait. This latter theory will appear to lose considerable ground as well.

The Idea of Fixed Happiness

The notion that happiness is essentially unalterable figures in psychological thinking as well as in sociological thought.

Psychologists who adhere to this view think of happiness or unhappiness as a stable disposition towards life rather that as the variable outcome of an ongoing evaluation of it. Some even regard happiness as a 'personality' trait: that is a tendency to react (judge life) similarly across different situations. Chronic states, as manifested in some forms of pathological unhappiness (depression, ahedonia), are believed to be the rule.

Sociologists in this tradition see the happiness of individuals as a reflection of collective 'national character'. The outlook on life implied in common values and beliefs is seen to pervade individual perceptions and evaluations. As collective outlook is largely an invariant matter, individual judgements geared by it are seen to be rather static as well.

Personal Character
The idea of a 'happy personality' has several variations. One is that people are born as either happy or unhappy. In this view happiness is a *temperamental disposition*, possibly based in the neurophysiological structure of pleasure centers in the brain. Some people would be apt to feel cheerfull and hence be positive about their life, even in difficult conditions, whereas others are prone to depression and hence judge their lives negatively, even in favourable situations. See a.o. Tellegen (1988).

Another variation is that happiness is an *acquired disposition*. Some people would develop a positive attitude towards life, whereas others would become sour. In this vein Lieberman (1970: 74) wrote: "... at some point in life, before even the age of 18, an individual becomes geared to a certain stable level of satisfaction, which – within a rather broad range of environmental circumstances – he maintains throughout life".

Whatever the variant, the idea of happiness as a personality trait implies that people tend to remain as happy or unhappy as they are, and that improvement or detoriation in their living conditions does not make them more or less happy. An explicit account of this implication can be found with Costa *et al.* (1987: 305), who write: "... happiness is ultimately also independant of health, youth, power and other life circumstances ... ".

National Character
The idea that there are happy and unhappy nations is part of common sense knowledge. For example: the Italians are seen as easygoing and light-hearted, whereas the Swedes are attributed a gloomy outlook on life. Comparision of average scores on survey questions about happiness show striking differences between nations, though typically not the ones predicted (see table 3).

Sociologists who have considered these differences also refer to cultural variation in outlook. Inkeles (1990/91: 93) for instance attributes the difference in happiness between nations to "national creed". "Given the tendency to report oneself as happy or unhappy seems to be a relatively stable characteristic of given national populations, in short a statistically reliable measure of the feeling state of the nation,

would seem to justify describing it as truly a national character trait".
Likewise Inglehart (1990: 30) writes that cross-national differences in
happiness "reflect cognitive cultural norms, rather than individual grief
and joy". He sees these norms as rooted in "profound differences in
outlook" between nations.

Two issues tend to be confused in discussions on this matter: 'cultural
bias' in measurement of happiness and 'culturally induced difference'
in happiness itself. The attention has been focused very much on the
issue of measurement bias (Ostroot and Snyder, 1985, Veenhoven, 1986,
Ouweneel and Veenhoven, 1989). Yet most relevant in the discussion
at issue here is the presumed effect of cultures on the evaluation of life
as such.

Approach

The aim of this paper is to explore the tenability of these claims empirically. Is happiness really that unalterable a matter that it is not worth
trying to reach out for more? To answer this question I will take stock
of the available research findings and check whether happiness appears
to be static or not.

First I will check the claim that happiness is in itself a rather invariant
'personality trait'. I will consider the available longitudinal studies on
happiness to assess its stability over time, as well as its sensitivity to
fortune and adversity. I will also inspect whether the evaluation of life is
largely determined by 'inner' psychological characteristics rather than
by 'external' living conditions. That analysis will be at the individual
level.

Next I will consider the hypothesis that average happiness in nations
reflects a collective 'idea fixe' rather than the actual quality of life in
the country. For that purpurse I will consider the stability of average
happiness in nations: how stable is it over time, how dependant on
living conditions in the nations and how much rooted in shared values
and beliefs. That analysis will be at the societal level.

Concept of Happiness

The answer to these questions depends on the precise concept of happiness used. Some things called happiness are more static than others. 'Frustration-tolerance' is for instance likely to be more stable than 'elated mood'. The current confusion about variability of happiness is in fact largely due to sloppy conceptualisation of the matter.

The concept of happiness used here is in line with the Utilitarian conception of happiness as the 'sum of pleasures and pains'. The focus is on the 'subjective' appreciation of life and not on any 'objective' qualities of the individual himself or his living conditions. Happiness is defined *as the degree to which an individual evaluates the overall quality of his/her life-as-a-whole positively.* This definition is delineated in more detail in Veenhoven (1984: ch 2). Within this concept two components of happiness are distinguished. The first component is *hedonic level of affect*, which is the degree to which pleasant affective experiences outbalance unpleasant ones generally. The second component is called *contentment* and concerns the degree to which the individual perceives his wants to have been met. These components represent respectively 'affective' and 'cognitive' appraisals of life and are seen to figure as sub-totals in the overall evaluation of life, called *overall happiness*.

Measures of Happiness

Happiness as defined here can be measured by means of questioning. Various claims to the contrary have been disproven empirically. (Research reviewed in Veenhoven, 1984: ch 3). Though measurable in principle, not all the questions and scales that are used measure this kind of happiness validly. Elsewhere I have reviewed current indicators and distinguished between acceptable and unacceptable ones (Veenhoven, 1984: ch 4). This paper considers only data based on indicators that were deemed acceptable. As a consequence several well known studies on this matter are left out. The studies used here were located by means of the World Database of Happiness (Veenhoven, 1992).

Concept of Trait

The term 'trait' is used in contrast to 'state'. A trait is seen as a durable characteristic of a person or society, that is in some way 'built-in'. A trait is a 'chronic' phenomenon. On the other hand a state is thought of as something essentially variable, that is continually (re-)produced. Traits are typically seen as causes, states as results.

Several criteria have been suggested to mark the difference more sharply. See Chaplin et al. (1988). Three of these are relevant for the problem at hand here, (1) temporal stability, (2) cross-situational consistency, and (3) internal (rather than external) causation. These three criteria will be used in the following tests of the theory that happiness is a trait.

2. IS HAPPINESS A PERSONAL TRAIT?

The question whether happiness can be characterized as a stable personal 'trait' rather than a variable 'state' is not new: trait-state discussions have raged in many fields of psychology. In the field of subjective well-being the issue was already under debate in the thirties (Young, 1937). Recent contributions to this discussion have been made by Aron and Aron (1987), Costa (1984, 1987, 1988), Chamberlain and Zika (1992), Kozma (1990), McNeal et al. (1986), Mohr (1986), Mortimer and Lorence (1981), Mussen (1980, 1982), Harley and Lavery (1991), Ormel (1980), Palmore (1977), Stones et al. (1986, 1989, 1991) Tellegen et al. (1988) and Yardley and Rice (1991). Most of these authors stress the trait-character of subjective well-being, in particular Stones and Kozma who conclude that happiness can be raised only by psycho-therapy (1989: 534). Conclusions are typically based on rather fragmentary data, short follow-ups and dubious indicators of happiness.

I will now consider the matter in the light of all the data that is currently available. These data allow a test of three hypotheses involved in the theory that hapiness is a personal trait. These hypotheses are implied in the definition of trait above. The first hypothesis is that happiness is temporally stable (par. 2.1), the second that it is trans-situationally consistent (par. 2.2) and the third that it is internally caused (par. 2.3).

2.1. Temporal stability: Do the happy remain happy?

The notion of a personal 'trait' involves different assumptions, which tend to be confused in this discussion. One assumption is that some people are characteristically more happy than others. Even if living conditions were identical for everybody, there would be happy and unhappy people. When these people go through similar ups and downs in life, the difference remains; their happiness rises and drops in the same degree, but change starts at a different level. This view is pictured in figure 1a. Let's call this the *relative stability* of happiness.

The other assumption is that the appreciation of life is so much a dispositional matter that it hardly follows ups and downs at all. In this view happiness remains essentially at the same level, irrespective of the actual quality of life and changes for the better or worse. This more extreme view is depicted in figure 1b. I will refer to it as *absolute stability*.

This latter theory is at issue here. Theory 1b denies that improvement of living conditions adds to the subjective appreciation of life and thus predicts that a better society makes no happier citizens. Theory 1a does not. It only renounces the possibility that everybody can be made equally happy, social progress prolonging the difference between happy and unhappy at a higher average level.

Relative Stability

Relative temporal stability is mostly assessed by means of follow-up studies and expressed in overtime-correlations. An overtime-correlation of +0.90 means that the rankorder of happiness in a population has almost remained the same during the period studied. Several investigations have reported high overtime-correlations of happiness. These results are often cited.

In order to obtain a more complete view I gathered all studies that have ever assessed overtime-correlations of happiness. I found some hundred studies, of which 26 appeared to have used acceptable indicators of happiness. Together these studies yield 65 overtime-correlations: 30 on overall happiness, 25 on hedonic level and 6 on contentment. The time span of these studies varies from one month to forty years. The

(1a): Happiness varies with ups and downs in life, but interpersonal differences tend to remain.

(1b): Happiness remains essentially the same through time, both absolutely and relatively.

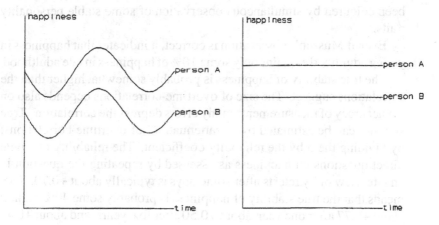

Fig. 1. Variants of the theory that happiness is a personal trait.

correlations are presented in exihibit 2 in a time diagram. The data are presented in more detail in appendix 1.

Stable on the Short Term, but not on the Long Run

Trait-theory is confirmed by the fact that overtime-correlations are almost all positive. However most of the correlations cannot be defined as 'high'. The range of the correlations is from −0.10 to +0.70, the average around +0.35.

It appears that the stability of happiness is a short-term matter. The highest correlations concern mainly time lags of several months; over-time correlations are around +0.60. Over the years the correlations drop considerably. After five years overtime-correlation is almost halved and varies around +0.30. Over periods of ten to fifteen years the correlation shrinks back to about +0.15. Extrapolation of this trend predicts complete disappearance of all overtime-correlation after twenty years. However, the only study that covered a longer period observed a slightly higher overtime-correlation. In Mussen's forty year follow-up the average correlation is +0.23. Possibly this is due to the measurement method used in that study. It assessed happiness by means of interviewer ratings rather than by means of self-reports. The interviewer ratings may have been coloured by simultaneous observation of some stable personality traits.

Even if Mussen's observation is correct, it indicates that happiness in young adulthood explains only some 10% of happiness in late adulthood.

The true stability of happiness is probably somewhat higher than the correlations suggest. The size of overtime-correlations depends also on the accuracy of measurement: many errors depress the correlation. True stability can be estimated by 'disattenuation' of overtime-correlations: by dividing them by the reliability coefficient. The reliability of single direct questions on happiness as assessed by repeating the question in an interview or by retests after some days is typically about +0.70. That means that the true stability of happiness is probably some 40% higher: about +0.77 after one year, about +0.50 after five years, and about +0.40 after ten years.

The decline of the overtime-correlations follows a curvilinear pattern. Stability drops sharply in the first few years, but stabilizes at a low level in the longer run. The asymptote is probably about +0.20. This suggests that there is some minor 'hard core'. However it is not at all sure that this hard core represents the hypothesized 'personality trait'. It could just as well be constancy in living conditions or constancy in traits other than happiness. We will deal further with this possibility in paragraph 2.3.

Overtime-correlations of measures of 'hedonic level' (largely Bradburn's Affect Balance Scale) are typically lower than those of the indicators of 'overall happiness' and 'contentment'. This is consistent with the view of happiness as an acquired attitude to which people tend to stick to cognitively, unless major changes lead to a reorientation. The relatively low stability of hedonic level of affect does not fit the theory that tendency to feel cheerful or not is largely inborn. This claim will be considered in more detail in 2.3 as well.

(2a): Predicted pattern: happiness remains stable over the years.

(2b): Observed pattern: happiness is not very stable in the long run.

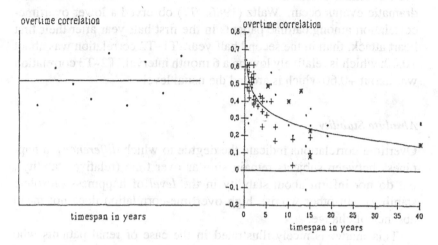

Fig. 2.   Overtime-correlations of happiness observed in 26 longitudinal studies. Data: Appendix 1: + = overall happiness · = affect level * = contentment.

Lower Stability through Serious Lifechange

If happiness is a trait, overtime-correlations must remain at the same level, even in periods of profound lifechange. If however happiness is essentially a judgement that is continually re-assessed, we can expect a drop in overtime-correlations in periods of transition. There are three reasons to expect this. First, transitions may involve a change in quality of life and hence invite a change in the evaluation of it. Secondly, new situations press towards a reorientation on life anyway. Thirdly, re-orientation typically involves some time of changing tentative judgements before the individual decides on a more definitive evaluation of this life. During this period the temporal stability of happiness is likely to be low as well.

Several studies have assessed overtime-correlations among subjects who went through some transition. Mostly the transitions considered are not very dramatic: leaving school, entering marriage, taking a new job, moving to an other house, etc. Overtime-correlations appear slightly lower among such transitions, but not much. (Data not shown). However, overtime-correlations do seem to be lower at times when really dramatic events occur. Waltz (1986: 77) observed a lower overtime-correlation among cardiac patients in the first half year after their first heart attack, than in the second half year. T1–T2 correlation was about +0.40; which is relatively low on a 6 month interval. T2–T3 correlation was about +0.60 which is around the usual level.

Absolute Stability

Overtime-correlations indicate the degree to which *differences* in happiness between subjects remain similar over time (relative stability), but do not inform about stability in the *level* of happiness (absolute stability). In other words: high overtime-correlation does not mean absence of change.

This matter is nicely illustrated in the case of renal patients who received a donor-kidney. The happiness of these patients increased dramatically after the transplant. When still on the waiting list only 31% saw themselves as happy, but one year after the transplant no less than 79% did so! This temporal upsurge of happiness is known as the 'Golden period'. Still the overtime-correlation in this period is quite sizable: r = +0.46 p < 0.001 (Simmons *et al.*, 1977: 61–62).

In a parallel study of kidney donors these investigators show in more detail how happiness changes after transplantion. Only 32% appear to have remained equally happy one year after the donation: 24% became less happy and 44% became more happy. Those initially least happy were most likely to have experienced a decrease in life-satisfaction, while those initially most happy had profited most (pp. 180–192). Thus the relative differences have been largely maintained, whereas the absolute levels of happiness have changed profoundly.

Happiness is Quite Variable

The easiest way to assess absolute stability of happiness is to ask people how happy they have been over the years. A common device for that purpose is the 'Life-Satisfaction Chart' (Kuhlen, 1948) on which respondents characterize their retrospective happiness by a line in a graph. If happiness is a trait, people must typically draw horizontal lines: if it is rather a state-like matter, deflections will be the rule. The latter pattern is by far the most common. Most people remember distinct differences in happiness. (Data not shown).

It is of course possible that reminiscences about happiness in earlier phases of life are inaccurate and that differences in earlier happiness tend to be over-estimated. Therefore we must also consider follow-up studies of present happiness. A good study of that kind was performed by Landua (1992). Landua analysed the yearly reponses on a 11 point life-satisfaction scale over a four-year period. He focused on 'substantial' changes; that is changes between four main categories (score 0–4, 5–6, 7–8 and 9–10). Only 10% of his respondents appeared to have stayed in the same satisfaction category for all four years; 90% had moved to another category. Landua observed quite radical changes: of the initially very unhappy movers (score 0–4) no less than 18% came to see themselves as very happy (score 9–10) in this four-year period. Similarly Heady and Wearing (1992: 126) found that about one third of their subjects in an 8 year panel study changed more then one standard deviation in both overall happiness and hedonic level.

Unhappiness less Constant than Happiness
If happiness is a fixed trait, dissatisfaction with life must be equally invariant as satisfaction. If however happiness is rather a judgement that is periodically reviewed, we can imagine that dissatisfaction is less of a lasting matter. We can expect so, because the discomfort of unhappiness involves a pressure to change; either to improve living-conditions or to revise ones judgement of life. On the other hand the happy are likely to maintain their judgement of life unless serious adversity urges a re-evaluation.

This implication can also be tested with the results of the 4-year follow up study mentioned above (Landua 1992); happiness must then be similar among 'stayers' and 'movers'. However, Landua observed that the unhappy make up a larger proportion of the movers than of the stayers (27% vs 12%).

Source of Stability can be Conditions for Happiness Rather than Happiness-as-such

Though less than expected, the constancy of happiness over time is still note-worthy. Does that mean that happiness is at least partly a personal trait? Not necessarily so. The statistical stability can also be the result of other things than an inner disposition to enjoy life.

Firstly, the correlations can be due to the stability of other personal characteristics other than happiness: f.e. to good health, a nice character and ability to deal with the problems of life. Such traits other than happiness can obviously add to the chance that things go well in life and hence that satisfaction with life tends to remain high. Happiness appears then as a stable trait, but is in fact an essentially variable state reproduced over and again.

Secondly, the overtime-correlation can be due to stability in living conditions. People who have a high income, a nice spouse and good connections mostly maintain these advantages over their lifetime. Sociologists have shown that there is much continuity in social inequalities.

Overtime-Correlation Disappears after Controls

In order to isolate these effects empirically, we must remove the influence of stable pre-conditions for happiness from the overtime-correlations. I know only of one study that involved such an analysis. Chiriboga (1984: 474) considered the stability of happiness over 11 years in a sample of people in transition. He controlled baseline personality and social status. He found hardly any overtime-correlation: ß = +0.02 among males and −0.18 among females. Not baseline-happiness appeared to predict happiness 11 years later, but baseline-personality; in particular earlier mental health and self-criticism predicted later happiness.

2.2. Situational Consistency: Are People Equally Happy in Fortune and Adversity?

If happiness is a trait-like disposition rather than a state-like evaluation of life, happiness must remain largely the same in different situations.

People living in good conditions can then be expected to be equally happy as people in bad conditions. Change for the better or worse will not render them any happier or unhappier. Some authors claim that this is exactly what empirical research has shown: a remarkable lack of correspondence between 'objective' living conditions and the 'subjective' appreciation of life. See Brickman *et al.* (1978: 925), Easterlin (1974) and Inglehart and Rabier (1985: 30).

Perceived Effects

A first test of this hypothesis is checking whether it fits common life-experience. This can be done by asking people whether major life-events in the past did affect their happiness at that time. De Frain and Ernst (1978: 988) asked parents about their adjustment to sudden death of their infant some years ago. These parents typically report a drastic drop in their personal happiness at the death of their infant, followed by a gradual recovery to the original level in 2 to 3 years. Likewise, studies with the above mentioned 'Life-Satisfaction Chart' show that people link up and downs in retrospective happiness with specific positive and negative times in their life (McKinley Runyan, 1979). Reminiscences may be inaccurate however, and biased by the evaluation of events. Therefore we must also consider situational correlates of present happiness.

Actual Effects

Comparisons of present happiness across situations show some striking non-differences. There is for instance little difference in happiness between rich and poor; at least in affluent welfare states. In present day Western nations happiness is neither related to age, sex nor education. Yet it is an exaggeration to say that happiness does not relate to any circumstances. Empirical research has identified several conditions where it does. Let's take a closer look at the available evidence:

Cross-Sections: Unfortunates Less Happy

First of all there is a wealth of cross-sectional studies that found less happiness among people in adverse conditions than in favourable ones.

For instance, people appear typically less happy in bad health than in good health and in isolation than in companionship. A problem in such comparisons is that living in either good or bad conditions may sometimes be a result of earlier happiness or unhappiness. Health and social integration depend to some extent on one's enjoyment of life (Veenhoven, 1988, 1989). Therefore it is better to focus on differences in living conditions that are clearly beyond the control of the individual.

Table 1 presents some data on the relation of happiness to uncontrollable hardship: 'widowhood', 'physical disability' and 'minority status'. In all cases adversity relates to a lower appreciation of life. The differences are greatest in the cases of recent personal disaster (miners' widows and recently paralyzed accident victims) and smallest in the case of long term disabled. This suggests that happiness drops drastically after serious adversity, but tends to revive in the long run. This is also more in line with the state-view on happiness than with the trait-view.

Follow-Ups: Change for the Worse Followed by Decline in Happiness
Methodologically it is of course preferable to assess the effects of fortune and adversity longitudually. Table 2 presents some relevant findings. Happiness appears consistently lower after life change for the worse. The effects remain visible over periods longer than a year.

It is worth noting that several of these studies control the effect of earlier personality (Eels, Chiriboga, Heady). This reduces the effect of life change on happiness, but does not wipe it out. Here again we see that happiness-as-such must be conceptually distinguished from happiness-related-personality.

Apparently happiness is not insensitive to fortune or adversity. People do adjust their evaluation of life if the actual quality of their life changes. That is not to say that happiness fluctuates with every move to the better or worse. Only serious shifts seem to bring about a re-orientation.

TABLE 1

Happiness of the unfortunate: some cross-sectional findings

Adversity	Indicator of happiness	Observed differences in happiness[1]		Population	Source
Bereaved					
Husband died in minefire 6 month ago	Question on happiness	widows: controls:	unhappy: 56% unhappy: 12%	Minerswives, USA, 1972 (N = 247)	Bahr & Harvey 1980: 24
	Cantril ladder	widows: controls:	modal happiness: 4 modal happiness: 7		
Wife died	Question on happiness	widower: married:	very happy: 20% very happy: 40%	60+ aged males USA, 1972/73/74 (N: 388)	Glenn, 1975: 596
Parent died	Cantril ladder	one parent died: both together:	mean happiness: 7.2 mean happiness: 7.4	Adolescents, Netherlands, 1985 (N = 2734)	Verkuyten & Veenhoven, 1988: 131
	Affect Balance Scale	one parent died: both together:	mean happiness: 6.1 mean happiness: 6.7		

Table 1 (continued)

Adversity	Indicator of happiness	Observed differences in happiness[1]		Population	Source
Problems in family					
Parents divorced	Affect Balance Scale	parents divorced: parents together:	mean happiness: 6.2 mean happiness: 6.7	Adolescents, Netherlands, 1985 (N = 2734)	Verkuyten & Veenhoven, 1988: 131
Handicapped child	Affect Balance Scale	handicapped child: matched controls:	mean happiness: 6.7; mean happiness: 8.4	Mothers, USA (N = 68)	Friedrich & Friedrich, 1981: 51
Husband unemployed	Affect Balance Scale	unemployed 1 employed 0	Gamma = −0.32 (p < 0.05)	Married wives, No chief wage earner, USA, 1960 (N = 1982, 62 of which had an unemployed husband)	Bradburn, 1969: 184

Table 1 (continued)

Adversity	Indicator of happiness	Observed differences in happiness[1]		Population	Source
Physically disabled					
Paralyzed accident victims, 1–12 month after injury	Question on happiness	disabled: controls:	mean happiness: 5.4 mean happiness: 7.0	Accident victims USA (N = 29) Controles picked from telephone directory. (N = 22)	Brickman et al. 1978: 921
Spinal cord injured, 20 yrs after injury	Affect Balance Scale	disabled: normals:	mean happiness: 5.0 mean happiness: 5.4	Injured: 40+ aged, Non instutionalized, USA (N = 100) Normals: 18+ aged population, USA (N = 6928)	Schulz & Decker 1985: 1167
Born handicapped	3 item index on satisfaction, mood and frustration	malformed: controls:	mean happiness: 7.4 mean happiness: 7.7	Handicapped: students and patients of a clinic. (N = 144) Controls: matched for age gender and situation (largely hospitalized as well) (N = 151)	Cameron et al., 1971: 641/2

Table 1 (continued)

Adversity	Indicator of happiness	Observed differences in happiness[1]		Population	Source
Minority status in society					
Black in the USA	Cantril ladder	Whites: Blacks:	mean happiness: 6.4 Mean happiness: 5.5	18+ aged USA 1973 (N = 1433)	Andrews & Withey, 1976: 323
Coloured in South Africa	5 item index of question on happiness and life-satisfaction	Whites: Indians: Coloureds: Africans:	mean happiness: 7.3 mean happiness: 6.9 mean happiness: 6.9 mean happiness: 5.4	Adults, South Africa, 1982/2 (N = 5587)	Moller, 1988: 73
Religious minority in neighbourhood, USA	6 item index of questions on happiness and mood	majority: minority:	unhappy: 16% unhappy: 23%	Adolescents, New York, USA, 1960 (N = 1618)	Rosenberg, 1962: 3
Immigrant worker in West-Germany	Question on satisfaction with life	German workers: Foreign workers:	mean happiness: 7.7 mean happiness: 6.9	Workers West Germany, 1980/82 (N = 1375)	Zapf & Brachtel, 1984: 294
	Question on happiness	German workers: Foreign workers:	unhappy: 4% unhappy: 18%		
Immigrant child in The Netherlands	Cantril ladder	Dutch children: Foreign children:	mean happiness: 7.7 mean happiness: 6.8	Secondary school pupils, Netherlands, 1986 (N = 261)	Verkuyten, 1986: 4
	Affect Balance Scale	Dutch children: Foreign children:	mean happiness: 6.6 mean happiness: 6.0		

[1] mean and modal happiness scores as transformed linearly to range 0–10

TABLE 2

Change in happiness following fortune and adversity: some longitudinal findings

Fortune/adversity	Time span	Indicator of happiness	Observed change in happiness	Population	Source
Unemployment					
Becoming unemployed	9 month: T1: 1963/1 T2: 1963/10	Affect Balance Scale	Happiness in average ridits on range 0–1: T1: employed: 0.49 T2: unemployed 0.36	Chief wage earners USA, 1963 (N = 931 of which 39 lost) their job between T1–T2	Bradburn, 1969: 189
	4 years: T1: 1977 T2: 1979 T3: 1981	Question on happiness	Significant drop in happiness among unemployed who became worse off financially. Not among other unemployed	Working adults, Nebraska, USA, 1977/8 (N = 444 of which 69 stopped working between T1 and T3)	Eels 1985: 156

Table 2 (continued)

Fortune/adversity	Time span	Indicator of happiness	Observed change in happiness	Population	Source
Unemployment					
Staying unemployed after job loss	6 months: T1: 1973/3 T2: 1973/4 T3: 1973/6 T4: 1973/9	Time sampling of mood (by diary)	Mean happiness of still unemployed on range 0–10 T1: 1 month after: 8.0 T2: 2 month after: 8.2 T3: 3 month after: 8.1 T4: 6 month after: 7.7	Unemployed, shortly after job loss Austria, 1974 ($N = 31$ of which 9 will still employed at T4)	Kirchler, 1985: 16
Staying unemployed after leaving school	2 years: T1: 1980 T2: 1981 T3: 1982	Depressive affect (score reversed) to indicate happiness	Mean happiness on range 0–10: T1: still in highschool: 6.4 T3: unemployed 3 years later: 5.8	School leavers, Australia, 1980–1982 ($N = 910$)	Feather & O'Brien, 1986: 132

Table 2 (continued)

Fortune/adversity	Time span	Indicator of happiness	Observed change in happiness	Population	Source
Bereavement					
Death of spouse	4 years: T1: 1977 T2: 1979 T3: 1980	Question on happiness	Those widowed became drastically less happy after bereavement, but partly recovered after 2 years	Adults, Nebraska, USA ($N = 1188$ of which 29 became widowed between T1 and T3)	Eels, 1985: 110
Divorce	4 years: T1: 1972 T2: 1976	Index of Depressive affect	Divorce is followed by an increase in depressive affect. T2 divorce status by T2 depression controlling T1 depression and prior conditions: $\beta = +0.10$	Marrieds, Chicago, USA ($N = 758$ of which 32 divorced between T1 and T2)	Menaghan 1986: 324
	4 years: T1: 1977 T2: 1979 T3: 1981	Question on happiness	Divorce is followed by change in happiness, but not always to the negative. Males and well educated get less happy, females and low educated get more happy.	Marrieds, Nebraska, USA ($N = 488$ of which 34 divorced T1 and T3)	Eells, 1985: 117

Table 2 (continued)

Summed life-events

Fortune/adversity	Time span	Indicator of happiness	Observed change in happiness	Population	Source
Negative event-score	11 years: T1: 1969 T2: 1971 T3: 1974 T4: 1976 T5: 1980	Question on happiness	Adverse events are followed by a drop in happiness; positive effects by a rise. The effects diminish through time T5 past years events by T5 happiness: $\beta = -0.42$ T4 past years events by T5 happiness: $\beta = -0.16$ T3 past years events by T5 happiness: $\beta = +0.00$	People in transition California, USA ($N = 163$)	Chiriboga 1982: 23
Positive event-score			T5 past years events by T5 happiness: $\beta = +0.30$ T4 past years events by T5 happiness: $\beta = +0.12$ T3 past years events by T5 happiness: $\beta = +0.09$ Beta's controled for T1 happiness as well as for personality and social status variables		
Net event-score (favourable minus adverse)	4 years: T1: 1983 T2: 1985 T3: 1987	Question on happiness asked in each interview	Earlier netscores (T1, T2) predict later happiness (T2, T3) even when the causal effect of happiness on life-events is removed. – Earlier eventscore $\longrightarrow$ Later happiness: $\beta L = +0.22$ – Earlier happiness $\longrightarrow$ Later eventscore: $\beta L = +0.18$ Standard maximum Likelihood Estimates (βL) obtained in LISREL analyses that also controled T1 personality and social status T2–T3 *Change* in net event-score explains *Change* in happiness: $R^2 = 0.51$	Adults Victoria, Australia ($N = 649$)	Heady & Veenhoven 1989: 119 Heady & Wearing 1988: 29

2.3. Inner Causation: Is Happiness Mere Psychology?

Trait theorists expect happiness to be temporally stable and situationally constant, because they believe that happiness is in some way 'built-in'. They presume the existence of an inner disposition to enjoy life or not. Such disposition has been conceived in several ways: as an innate affective 'temperament' and as more or less acquired cognitive inclination. There is more speculation on this matter than solid data. Let us take a look at a few relevant investigations.

Evidence for Existence of Innate Disposition

The theory of innate happiness presumes that a tendency to appreciate life is in some way wired in; possibly in the neuro-chemical structure of the pleasure centres in the brain. Two testable predictions can be derived from this theory: The first is that people who are alike genetically must also be alike in happiness, irrespective of upbringing and variation in living conditions. This prediction can be tested by comparing twins: preferably mono-zygotic and di-zygotic twins reared apart and reared together. The second prediction is that people who were happy as children must be happy in adulthood as well. This hypothesis can be tested by following people from the beginning of life; preferably from infancy on.

Comparison of Twins: Modest Correspondence in Happiness

Several studies have compared the well-being of twins, but only one of these used an indicator that meets my demands for the valid measurement of happiness. That is a study by Wierzibicki (1986) which measured hedonic level by means of a mood diary. Hedonic level appeared to be more alike among mono-zygotic twins ($r = +0.55$) than among di-zygotic twins ($r = +0.15$). This findings suggests some genetic influence, though only a modest one; there are still considerable mood differences among identical twins. However, it is not sure that happiness-as-such is the genetic factor. The correlation can also be due to effects on happiness of other innate characteristics.

Follow-Up from Birth on; No Constancy in Happiness
There is also only one long term study that has followed happiness from
infancy on. This is the famous Berkeley Guidance Study (Schaefer and
Bailey, 1963). In this developmental study hedonic level was assessed
in the first years of life. Hedonic level was rated several times on the
basis of expressive behaviour (laughing, crying etc.) These ratings were
made at regular visits of mother and child to an obstetric clinic. Twelve
ratings were made between birth and age 3. These ratings appeared
very stable over this period and could be regarded as a manifestation of
inborn cheerfulness.

Between age 12 and 18 these same subjects went through several
interviews and tests. Later on the protocols were used to derive indicators of adolescent happiness. A content analysis was performed by two
independant assessors who charcterized the subject in several dimensions. Two of these dimensions were 'gloomy' and 'not cheerful'. These
were combined in a sumscore that characterizes adolescent hedonic
level. This score appeared unrelated to average baby-cheerfulness:
$r = -0.11$ (ns). Another score representing adolescent contentment
(discontented, unhappy, dissatisfied, complaints) appeared not related
to baby-cheerfulness either: $r = -0.03$ (ns). Clearly this finding does
not fit the prediction that people born happy remain happy. Yet there
are methodological reasons to doubt the evidence: it is based on a very
small number of girls ($N = 11$).

These two tests do not support the theory of innate happiness. That
is in line with wider twin research, where cheerfulness does typically
not appear as a genetically transmitted propensity. In fact Buss and
Plomin (1984) identified only three temperaments for which an inherit-
ed contribution is likely to exist: emotionality, activity and sociability.
These characteristics may facilitate happiness, but do not constitute
happiness-as-such. Their effect on happiness is likely to be contingent
to situations.

Evidence for Dominance of Psychological Determinants

If innate dispositions to be happy are at best weak, it is still possible that we acquire a strong propensity of that kind. There is in fact a rich literature on how unhappy personalities develop. Traumatic experience and inappropiate learning are seen to produce distorted perception, unrealistic ambitions and inadequate coping. Chronic frustation and depressed affect is seen as the inevitable result. Even if external conditions are favourable, such inner handicaps would doom you to unhappiness. On the other hand good psychological health is depicted as a fairly sure ticket to happiness.

It is beyond doubt that inner characteristics influence happiness. Yet it is not so clear to what extent these dominate the appraisal of life, especially not among psychologically healthy people.

External Factors Play a Role

Several investigators have tried to grasp the relative impact of 'external' and 'internal' factors on happiness. *External factors* are usually split up in 'social resources' (income, education, status, social networks, etc.) and 'life-events' (illness, job loss, marriage, etc.). *Internal factors* are typically personality traits (extraversion, neuroticism, control orientation, etc.). The typical conclusion of such studies is that external factors explain less variance in happiness than one would expect and internal factors more.

The most sophisticated study of this kind is an Australian panel study by Heady and Wearing (1989, 1992), which also found that a sizeable part variance was explained by personality (35%). Yet that study also showed that social resources and life events make a difference over and above personality, and explain 7% additional variance.

These results are sometimes presented as evidence for the claim that happiness is mere psychology. The data do not justify that conclusion however.

Firstly, external factors still influence happiness independantly of personality. Secondly, the variance explained by external factors is probably greater than 7% the 7% which is left when personality factors are entered first.

Thirdly, these data probably underestimate the actual effects in the populations studied. Systematic measurement error tends to attenuate correlations with external factors, while boosting correlation with psychological variables (Moum, 1988).

Lastly, and most importantly, this pattern may say more about the societies in which these investigations took place than about the nature of happiness. The observations are made in affluent egalitarian and peaceful societies. Inner factors differentiate better between happy and unhappy in these societies, because external conditions are fairly good and equally distributed. Probably the relative impact of psychological factors is smaller in a social context of poverty, deprivation and upheavel.

'Inner Caused' Is not the Same as 'Immutable'

If there is some 'inner' happiness propensity, the next question is what that consists of precisely. Two kinds of psychological characteristics have been mentioned in that context: dispositions that more or less 'constitute' happiness and characteristics that typically 'facilitate' its achievement. Let's consider what qualities may be involved, and whether these are likely to fix happiness at a certain stable level.

Constituents of happiness. A possible inner constituent of happiness is the tendency to take a rosy look at everything, sometimes refered to as the 'Pollyanna tendency'. Such a personality trait obviously manifests in a more positive evaluation of life-as-a-whole. Pollyannaism is indeed correlated to happiness, but not very strongly (Matlin and Gawron, 1979). By itself it can therefore not be an inner anchor that fixes evaluations of life to the same level.

Another possible inner constituent of happiness is an 'attitude' towards one's life. As noted above, evaluations of life may crystallize in a stable set of beliefs. However, if such attitudes exist at all, they are unlikely to remain fixed forever. Elsewhere I have suggested that people stick to the same evaluation only if they feel no pressures for a re-evaluation (Veenhoven, 1991: 17). This view supports the notion that there is some inner happiness-set whilst remembering the evidence that happiness is not insentive to environmental change. As yet that presumed process of 'freezing' and 'unfreezing' of happiness attitudes has not been examined empirically.

Facilitators of happiness. Commonly mentioned inner facilitators of happiness are 'extraversion', 'inner-control' and 'hardiness'. These personality traits are believed to add to the chances to realize one's ambitions. In that context Heady and Wearing (1992: 95) showed for example that extraversion facilitates intimate relationships, which in turn makes life more enjoyable. 'Neuroticism' typically induces a constant stream of negative life-events. Again we must realize that these effects are context bound; inner control may facilitate happiness in an individualized society that allows choice, but may be detrimental to it in confined situations.

Such inner facilitators of happiness are not necessarily fixed traits themselves. People can become somewhat more extraverted and less neurotic during their life. Social improvements such as better mental health care may stimulate such changes. In the long term better social-isation and a safer society will also make the next generations better equiped psychologically to cope with the problems of modern life.

In summary: Even if there is a marked inner disposition to be happy or not, that does not mean a better society cannot make people any happier.

3. IS HAPPINESS A CULTURAL TRAIT?[4]

We now shift to the macro level and consider the claim that the appreciation of life is not really the result of an individual evaluation, but rather a reflection of collectively pre-conceived ideas. In this view happiness is a fixed social construction that has little to do with the variable realities of life. Therefore happiness would be largely insensitive to improvement of living conditions.

Differences in Happiness Between Nations
During the last decades, questions on happiness have figured in representative surveys in many countries. Comparison of the responses reveals striking differences. Table 3 presents the average scores on equivalent questions in 30 nations around 1980. Average happiness tends to be lower in developing countries than in rich industrialized nations. Average happiness is highest in the Netherlands (7.63 on a 10–0 scale) and lowest in India (5.16). Among the rich nations considerable differences exist as well. For instance Italians and the Japanese take less pleasure in life than Australians and the Swedes.

Similar differences in happiness have been observed in other cross-nation studies: in comparison between industrialized countries by Buchanan and Cantril (1953), Inkeles (1960, 1991) and Inglehart (1977/1992), and in global surveys by Cantril (1965) and Gallup (1976). These studies involved other indicators of happiness as well. The pattern of differences between countries appears almost the same when different measures of happiness are compared. See Veenhoven, 1993.

Explanations of Differences in Happiness Between Nations
There are three possible explanations for these differences: cultural bias in the measurements of happiness, differences in quality of living conditions and differences in view of life.

Measurement-bias. This explanation is that the seemingly identical questions on happiness work out differently accross countries. Possible sources of bias mentioned are: variation in social desirability distortion between countries, problems of precise translation and cultural variation in response tendencies. Elsewhere I have considered the empirical evidence for these claims. None of them was supported by the data (Ouweneel and Veenhoven, 1991; Veenhoven, 1993).

Societal quality. This explanation assumes that the differences in response to questions about happiness reflect true variation in appreciation of life. This variation is attributed to differences in 'quality' of the living conditions societies provide to their citizens, such as food and shelter, safety, adequate care for children, fit between socialized and

TABLE 3

Happiness in 30 nations around 1980

Taking all together, how happy would you say you are?				
	very	pretty fairly quite	neither/nor not too unhappy not at all	DK NA	standardized mean 10-0
India	6	31	62	1	5.16
Greece	10	40	48	2	5.60
White Russia	11	52	37	–	5.99
Portugal	11	70	21	–	6.18
Korea (South)	11	59	30	–	6.20
Mexico	26	34	37	3	6.31
Italy	10	65	23	2	6.47
Philippines	18	50	33	–	6.47
Hungary	11	66	22	2	6.60
Spain	20	58	22	2	6.84
Japan	15	62	16	8	6.94
Germany (West)	10	69	13	8	6.98
Switzerland	26	65	9	–	6.99
South Africa	27	54	18	2	7.07
Luxemburg	28	62	8	2	7.08
Singapore	32	58	9	–	7.15
Brazil	40	36	22	1	7.22
France	19	70	9	2	7.24
Finland	19	72	7	1	7.35
Norway	28	64	8	–	7.45
USA	31	60	9	1	7.55
Belgium	31	57	7	5	7.57
Sweden	29	66	4	2	7.62
Netherlands	44	50	6	–	7.63
Denmark	30	63	4	3	7.67
N. Ireland	39	55	5	1	7.74
Britain	38	57	4	1	7.74
Australia	34	61	4	1	7.75
Canada	35	61	4	–	7.76
Ireland	39	54	4	3	7.82
Iceland	43	53	4	1	7.96

Data: Veenhoven, 1993, table 1.1.1a+b+c

Standardized means computed on the basis of weights awarded to response categories by judges required behaviours and opportunities for self-actualization. Accounts of this kind have been proposed by Inglehart (1977) and Veenhoven (1984: ch.6). This explanation has also been used in accounts of differences in other aspects of well-being, such as cross-national differences in suicide, mental disorder and drug abuse (see e.g. Naroll, 1982). Basic postulates are that societies can be more or less effective in meeting human needs and that ineffective need gratification manifests itself in bad health, mental disturbance and dissatisfaction with life. In terms of trait theory this means that happiness is *not* consistent across situations.

National character. As we have seen the core of this explanation is that collective beliefs and values in a society mould individual evaluations of life. Some cultures are believed to predispose to a negative outlook on life, whereas others are said to foster a positive view. Various cultural differences have been mentioned in this context: Inglehart (1990: 30) suggests "that the culture component of these differences reflects the distinctive historical experience of the respective nationalities. Long periods of disappointed expectations give rise to cynical attitudes. These orientations may be transmitted from generation to generation through pre-adult socialisation". Religion has also been mentioned in this context. Calvinism is often said to breed unhappiness, because of its gloomy outlook on the future and its moral rejection of lust.

   Whatever the cultural mechanisms presumed, the underlying psychological assumption in all these reasonings is that happiness is largely a cognitive matter that is only loosely linked to real life-experience.

   If happiness is indeed a matter of national character, we can expect that it meets the three trait criteria at the collective level. This section examines whether that is the case or not. First I will inspect whether average happiness in countries remains the same over the years (temporal stability, section 3.1). Next I consider whether average happiness in nations is independant of the quality of living conditions in the country (situational consistency, section 3.2.). Finally I test some implications of the theory that happiness is a matter of collective outlook (inner causation: section 3.3.).

3.1. Temporal Stability: Do (Un)Happy Countries Remain (Un)Happy?

Time-series on average happiness are only available for some industrialized countries. In the USA happiness has been followed since 1945, in Japan since 1958 and in the EC countries since 1974. At the individual level that would be a significant time-lag, but at the societal level it is only a very short period. Next to these time-series (yearly surveys that use the same question) there are some more incidental data that allow a look at the temporal stability of public happiness. Data on happiness in nations were found in Veenhoven (1993).

Relatively Stability

The first comparative study on happiness in nations was performed in 1948 by Buchanan and Cantril (1953) among 9 countries. These same countries figure in the 1980 World Value Study. Though not identical, the measures of happiness (life-satisfaction) are quite alike. Table 4 presents the rank-orders. Four countries appear to have remained in the same position, five countries changed position by two or three steps. Norway and Mexico fell back, whereas Britain, France and Germany advanced in relative happiness. The rank-order correlation is +0.73.

Absolute Stability

In several countries happiness has remained at about the same level during the last decades. The USA is one of these: in 1948 36% of the Americans characterized themselves 'very happy' and 54% 'fairly happy'. Forty years later (1988) these percentages were 34% and 57% (Veenhoven, 1993: table 1.1.1a). In Japan happiness has remained at the same level as well in the years 1958–1988 (Veenhoven, 1993: table 1.2.1a).

However, there are also some countries where happiness has changed considerably. For instance, in 1954 26% of the Germans characterized themselves as unhappy, whereas in 1984 only 10% did so (Veenhoven, 1993: table 1.2.3). Likewise in Brazil ratings on the Cantril ladder rose from 4.6 in 1960 to 6.2 in 1975 (Veenhoven, 1993: table 1.3.1). Both

TABLE 4

Relative temporal stability of average happiness in nations

country	rank order of happiness	
	1948	1981
Australia	2	2/3
Britain (Great)	9	7
France	7/8	5
Germany (West)	4	1
Italy	7/8	8
Netherlands	5	6
Norway	1	2/3
Mexico	6	9
USA	3	4
rank order-correlation:	$r_s = +0.73$ ($p < 0.01$)	

Data: Veenhoven, 1993, table 1.2.1a and 1.2.2b.

Absolute values are not comparable, because questions
were not identical

these increases in happiness occurred in a period of marked economic development.

During the last decade happiness has increased slightly in most European countries. This increase is most pronounced in the originally least happy nations (France, Greece, Italy, Spain). This catching up of Mediterranean nations with North-West Europe is visible in several indicators of happiness (Veenhoven 1993: tables 1.1.1b, 1.1.2b and 2.2).

Again we must keep in mind that this data come, for the greater part, from affluent countries in an era of stability. The average happiness of citizens may be more variable in countries that provide less buffers and experience more turmoil.

3.2. Situational Consistency: Are People Equally Happy in Good and Bad Countries?

If happiness is a cultural stereotype rather than an individual evaluation, we can expect that it is largely unrelated to the quality of living conditions in the country. Consequently countries that provide good living conditions will not stand out by higher average happiness than countries of poor living conditions. Likewise changes to the good or the bad in countries will have little or no effect on the average happiness of citizens.

Cross-Sections: Higher Happiness in Countries that Provide Better Living Conditions

To check the first prediction I gathered data about the quality of living conditions for the 30 countries of which we have comparable happiness scores (the countries enumerated in table 3). I found comparable performance indicators on the *material comfort* these nations provide for their citizens, on the *freedom*, their political system allows, on the degree to which they save the pains of in*equality* and the degree to which they provide their citizens *access to knowledge*. Details about measurement can be found in appendix 2. These country characteristics were correlated with average happiness. The results are presented in table 5. All performance indicators appear to be related to average happiness. Economic affluence is the strongest predictor. Yet social equality and education relate to happiness independant of income per capita. Together they explain no less than 80% of the variance! An analysis of responses to another question (10 step life-satisfaction) in a slightly different nationset yields a similar result.

Follow-ups: Slight Effects of Economic Change in Rich Nations

A test of the prediction that happiness remains the same through prosperity and adversity requires time-series on happiness over periods in which marked changes occur such as wars, revolutions or economic crises. However the available time-series concern a period of peace and

TABLE 5

Average happiness and living conditions in 30 nations around 1980

Living conditions in countries	Correlation (r) with average happiness in countries		
	listwise ($N = 27$)		pairwise
	zero order	RGDP controlled	(N 23 to 27)
Material Comfort			
– Real income per capita	+0.71*	–	+0.70* ($N = 27$)
– Social security	+0.60*	+0.24	+0.53* ($N = 26$)
Social Equality			
– Women's emancipation	+0.77*	+0.67*	+0.62* ($N = 22$)
Freedom			
– Freedom of press	+0.55*	+0.28	+0.55* ($N = 27$)
– Political democracy	+0.57*	+0.02	+0.61* ($N = 23$)
Access to Wisdom			
– Education	+0.84*	+0.65*	+0.71* ($N = 27$)
– Media attendence	+0.54*	+0.07	+0.54* ($N = 27$)
Total variance explained:			
R^2	0.80*		

Data: Happiness: Table 3. Country characteristics: Appendix 2; * $p = < 0.01$

rather smooth economic growth. This seriously limits the possibilities to check the hypothesis.

Elsewhere I have considered the effects of postwar economic growth on average happiness in countries (Veenhoven, 1989). I observed that a doubling of the material standard of living was not parallelled by a doubling of average happiness in the already rich USA. Yet economic growth was followed by greater happiness in originally less affluent nations such as Brazil and also in West European nations. These latter cases falsify the theory that happiness is a national character trait. Together the findings suggest that people get happier when material living conditions improve, but that these increments are subject to the law of diminishing returns.

Together with Sasqia Chin Hon Foei I have also investigated the effects of the 1980–1982 economic recession in the EC countries. We found that this minor recession was followed by a minor drop in happiness at a 1 year interval. These effects were particularly clear in the countries that provide relatively little social security (e.g. Ireland), which means that they were least able to buffer the financial effects of economic fluctuation (Chin Hon Foei, 1989). A similar effect has been observed in Japan: the 1975 oil crisis was followed by a clear dip in average happiness. (Prime Ministers Office, 1987). Again it is clear that average happiness in the country is not a static matter.

3.3. Inner Causation: Individual Happiness Conditioned by Collective Outlook?

The theory that individual happiness is largely a matter of collective outlook can be checked in two ways: one way is to inspect whether happy and unhappy nations differ in relevant values and beliefs. Another way is to assess whether members of a same culture tend to be equally happy in spite of difference in living conditions.

Difference in Outlook Between Happy and Unhappy Nations

Above three hypotheses were mentioned in connection with national differences in outlook that may cause dissimilarity in happiness: 'moral appreciation of happiness', 'cynical attitudes' and 'calvinist religion'. Below I will test these hypotheses using data from the 1980 World Value Study.

Moral Appreciation of Happiness Unrelated to Level of Happiness
As suggested above, the differences in happiness between countries may be due to a difference in valuation of happiness: happiness acceptant cultures may allow more enjoyment of the same things, thereby fostering a more positive view on life. If so, happiness must be higher in countries that cherish happiness than in countries that deprecate it.

Testing this prediction requires that we measure moral appreciation of happiness in countries. I constructed an indicator of that matter on the basis of survey data. The European Value Study involved many questions about value preferences. In an earlier analysis of these data Halman (1987) distilled several value dimensions and computed average scores. Some of these dimensions are indicative of moral appreciation of pleasure and satisfaction. One such dimension is the tendency to approve of lust and pleasure as a guiding principle in matters of family, marriage, and sexuality. Halman refers to this dimension as 'Egoism'. A second dimension concerns enjoyment and comfort in the realm of work ethics. Halman refers to it as the 'Comfort/Materialistic' dimension. I added these two factor scores for each country and regarded the sum as a proxi of 'Moral Hedonism' in the country.

This indicator of moral hedonism is crossed with the level of happiness in the country. See figure 3. Average happiness appears not higher in the countries where hedonic values are most endorsed ($r = +0.03$). For instance, the three least happy nations are respectively low, medium, and high on hedonic value orientation. It is of course possible that other measures and other country-sets yield different results. Yet it must be noted that this explanation failed its first test.

No Consistent Attitudinal Cynism in Unhappy Nations

As noted above, Inglehart suggests that the relatively low happiness in the Mediterranian countries in Europe is the result of 'cynical attitudes' that may be rooted in earlier generations' disappointments. If that is true, unhappy countries must appear to be more cynical. The European Value Study involves two indicators that are relevant in this context: mistrust in fellow man and mistrust in society.

Mistrust in one's fellow men was measured by a single direct question: In general do you think that most people can be trusted? The responses were scored (1) can be trusted, (2) don't know and (3) better be careful. I crossed the average mistrust score per country with average happiness. In line with the hypothesis mistrust is highest in the least happy countries: $r = -0.59$.

Mistrust in society was measured by trust in social institutions. Respondents were asked to rate their trust in the following ten insti-

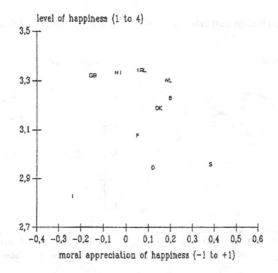

Fig. 3.   Happiness and moral appreciation of happiness 9 nations around 1980.
Data: European Value Survey (Halman *et al.*, 1987) r = +0.00.

tutions: the church, the army, the school, the law, the press, unions, the police, parliament, civil servants and big business. For each country an average trust score was computed. These scores were converted to mistrust and crossed with happiness. In this case a positive correlation appears. Mistrust is higher in the most happy nations: r = +0.35.

Inglehart's prediction is thus only partially confirmed: a cynical attitude towards fellow man is indeed related to unhappiness in the country, but a cynical attitude towards society is not. The absence of a correlation with mistrust in society is the more noteworthy in the context of Inglehart's suggestion that cynical attitudes result from earlier social disorganisation. If so, that must manifest itself in sceptism about society in the first place.

Calvinist Countries not Less Happy
The claim that the cultural heritage of Calvinism is predisposed to unhappiness can be easily checked. A look at table 3 shows that the countries where Protestantism dominates belong typically to the hap-

(4a): happiness and distrust in fellow man.   (4b): happiness and distrust in institution.

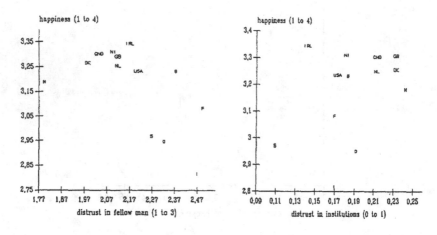

Fig. 4.   Happiness and attitudinal cynism 13 nations around 1980.
Data: European Value Survey: Halman, 1991.

piest group: Britain, Denmark, Iceland, Norway and Sweden. On the other hand happiness is typically low in Roman Catholic countries such as Belgium, France, Italy and Spain. Does that mean that the reverse is true, but that happiness is still conditioned by religious outlook? That does not seem to be the case either. The happiest country in table 3 is The Netherlands, which is religiously mixed.

Homogenity in Happiness within Cultures

If individual evaluations of life are heavily conditioned by collective outlook (rather than by individual reference), we can expect much homogenity in happiness within cultures. That homogenity must appear in similarity of happiness across social categories in countries. It must also manifest itself in similarity across borders between people reared in the same culture. For instance, the happiness of migrants must remain close to the level in their mother country and there must be little difference in average happiness between nations that share the same cultural heritage. Below I report some tests of these inferences.

Happiness of Students not Always Similar to Happiness of General Population

If individual happiness is largely a matter of collective values and beliefs, we can expect that all citizens in a country are effected by the prevailing outlook. Country differences observed in general population samples must then be reproduced in comparisons between specific social categories. For instance, if we focus on rich people only, we must find about the same difference in happiness between India and the Netherlands as reported in table 3, supposing that in both countries the rich look at their life through the same culturally coloured glasses as the non-rich.

This implication can best be tested by splitting up the data in table 3 by income, age and gender. However, this is easier said than done. Not all the data sets are available and categorizations are not identical. An easier way to do the same job is to compare average population means with mean happiness among university students. Data about happiness in university students in most of the countries in table 3 is available from a 39 nation study by Michalos (1991). University students are an attractive category for comparison in this context. Their social position is fairly similar in all countries.

The country differences in happiness among students appear not identical to the differences among general population samples. The differences are smaller and the rank order is not the same. In India and Mexico students are fairly happy, whereas the general population is not. In Thailand students are relatively least happy, whereas the general population average is modal. There are also consistent cases however: the Netherlands, USA, UK at the positive side and Japan, Korea and Greece at the negative side. These cases produce a correlation of +0.42 in this nation set. (Data not shown).

This finding means that shared views can at best determine average happiness in a country to a limited extent. Probably they do even less. The correspondence in happiness between students and the general population depends obviously on other things as well, in particular on societal characteristics, such as economic development, freedom and equality. Remember table 5.

Happiness of Migrants is Closer to Happiness in Homeland than to Happiness in Country-of-settlement

If Inglehart is right in that happiness is largely determined by "socialized attitudes" that are "transmitted through generations", we can expect that the happiness of migrants will be more similar to happiness in their country-of-origin than to average happiness in the country-of-settlement. Though living conditions may be different in the new country (mostly better), they are looked at from the same cultural perspective.

This prediction was tested in an analysis of studies in Australia and West Germany. Two Australian studies in the 1980's assessed the happiness of migrants from Britain, Greece, Germany, Italy, Netherlands and Yugoslavia. Data are summarized in table 6. Migrants appear about as happy as native Australians and differences among migrants are small. Yet table 6 also shows that there are marked differences in happiness between countries of origin. Happiness is clearly lower in Greece and Italy than in Australia. Only Britain, Ireland and The Netherlands are at the same level. Clearly migrants from unhappy countries are not saddled with a pessimistic outlook that prevents them from enjoying life as much as their new compatriots. A similar tendency can be observed in the results of two studies in West-Germany. Here again the happiness of migrants (from Greece, Italy, Spain, Turkey and Yugoslavia) is closer to the average in the host country than to the average in the mother land.

Cultural trait theory also predicts that the hierarchy of happiness in home countries must be reproduced among migrants. For that purpose rank order correlations were computed both in Australia and in West Germany, and the results are contradictary: in one study no correlation (r = +0.10 and +0.03), in the other a sizable (but still statistically insignificant) correlation: r = +0.58 and +0.50.

Happiness Is not the Same in East and West Germany

The theory that happiness is a cultural trait would also predict that East and West Germans are about equally happy. Germans share the same

TABLE 6
Life-satisfaction of migrants

Country of origin	Average life-satisfaction of migrants in country of settlement				average life-satisfaction of general population in country of origin
	Australia		Germany		
	1981[1] ($N = 246$)	1984[2] ($N = 656$)	1982[3] ($N = 770$)	1984[4] ($N = 1569$)	1981–1983
average life-satisfaction in country of settlement	7.6	7.9	7.7[5]	7.4	
Greece	7.6	7.4	7.2	7.1	5.9[6]
Germany	–	7.7	–	–	7.5[6]
Ireland	–	8.0	–	–	7.7[6]
Italy	7.9	7.7	6.9	7.6	6.7[6]
Netherlands	–	7.8	–	–	8.0[6]
Spain	–	–	7.1	8.2	6.2[7]
Turkey	–	–	6.2	6.9	< 5.0[8]
UK	8.0	8.0	–	–	7.6[6]
Yugoslavia	–	7.7	7.1	7.8	±5.0[9]
rank order-correlation: (r_s); migrant life-satisfaction by satisfaction in country of origin	+0.10 (ns)	+0.58 (ns)	+0.03 (ns)	+0.50 (ns)	

Data: Appendix 3 Lifesatisfaction scale 0–10

cultural heritage and speak the same language. The political separation
lasted only half a generation and did not cut off all cultural exchange.

The data clearly falsify that prediction. East Germans are less happy
than West Germans: in 1990 scores on a 11-step satisfaction scale were
respectively 6.0 and 7.3 in 1991 (Landua 1992: 33).

The current difference can be explained by poorer living conditions
in former East Germany. In the following decade successful resurrec-
tion will probably erase the dissimilarity in happiness.

Obviously one can think of more specifications of the theory that happiness is a matter of cultural outlook. In fact it is quite difficult to test
such a broad claim exhaustively. For the time being we must conclude
that these first tests provide little support.

4. DISCUSSION

The reason for this inquiry was the question whether improvement
of society can make citizens any happier. That question can now be
answered affirmatively. Happiness is not so invariable a matter that
it is insensitive to improvement or deterioration of living conditions.
Though people do not change their judgement of life every day at every
whim of fate, they do adjust the evaluation periodically and take major
life-changes into account. As such, happiness is a suitable endgoal for
social policy (though not necessarily the only one) and a useful indicator
of policy success.

This leads us to ask the question why is current opinion to the contrary? Four reasons seem to be involved, two technical distortions and
two ideological fallacies.

Firstly, the bulk of the available research findings seemed to indicate
that people tend to remain equally happy. As we have seen most follow-
up studies considered relative stability over short periods and found
surprisingly little change. The few long term studies seem to have been
snowed under. Absolute stability has not yet been considered.

Secondly, high relative stability rates have been found in studies that
use measures which tap broader aspects of psychological well-being

than just happiness. The much used Life-Satisfaction Index (Neugarten *et al.*, 1962) for instance also involves items about 'planning minded-ness', 'self-respect' and 'views on social progress'. These attitudes may be more fixed than happiness is.

Thirdly, the theory that happiness is a trait provides an easy expla-nation for the common observation that happiness is hardly linked to social positional variables such as income, education, sex and age: at least not in modern western nations. This finding was a surprise for most investigators who had hoped to demonstrate psychological con-sequences of social inequality. They were reluctant to conclude that present day western society is apparently so equal and affluent that traditional cleavages hardly matter any more. Therefore they rather attributed the non-difference to a presumed psychological insensitivity of the outcome-measure.

Lastly, there is scepticism about happiness that is rooted in long-standing discussions about value priorities. The Utilitarian position that happiness marks the ultimate value is not accepted by everybody and advocates of alternative value priorities tend to denounce happiness as 'fleeting' 'relative' and 'spoiling'. The idea that happiness is 'fixed' fits that negative view. Indications in that direction are therefore readily accepted.

5. CONCLUSION

Contrary to current opinion happiness is no trait; neither a personal trait nor a cultural trait. Happiness does *not* meet the classic three definitions of trait.

Firstly, *happiness is not temporally stable*. Individuals revise their evaluation of life periodically. Consequently their happiness rises and drops, both absolutely and relatively. Average happiness of nations appears not immutable either. Though stability prevails, there are cases of change.

Secondly, *happiness is not situationally consistent*. People are not equally happy in good or bad situations. Improvement or deterioration of life is typically followed by changes in the appreciation of it. This is also reflected at the collective level. Average happiness is highest in the countries that provide the best living conditions. Major changes in condition of the country affect average happiness of its citizens.

Lastly, *happiness is not entirerly an internal matter*. It is true that happiness roots to some extent in stable individual characteristics and collective orientations, but the impact of these inner factors is limited. They modify the outcome of environmental effects rather than dominating them.

These findings knock the bottom out of the argument that happiness is too static a matter to be influenced by social policy. There is thus still sense in pursuing greater happiness for a greater number.

The findings also refute the related claim that happiness is not a useful social indicator. Though happiness may be a slowly reacting instrument, it does reflect long-term change for better or worse.

APPENDIX 1
Overtime-correlation of happiness in 26 longitudinal studies

Subjects	Happiness measure	Happiness variant[1]	Time span in years	Overtime-correlation (in r)	Bibliografical source
60+ aged white unmarried females N = 42	10 item Affect Balance Scale	A	3	+0.38	Adams, 1988: 35
Highschool pupils, USA. Followed from age 12 to 15 N = 2213	6 item index of questions on happiness and mood	O	1 1,5 2,5 3,5	+0.61 +0.54 +0.45 +0.43	Bachman et al., 1970 (overtime-correlations provided by author)

Appendix 1 (continued)

Subjects	Happiness measure	Happiness variant[1]	Time span in years	Overtime-correlation (in r)	Bibliografical source
Highschool pupils, USA. Male and Female Followed from age 10 to 35 N = 160 Largely same subjects as studied by Tuddenham (below)	Rating of cheerfulness (vs gloomy) on the basis of interview protocols	A	6 6 15 15	+0.57 M +0.50 F +0.26 M +0.36 F	Block, 1971: 302–307
18+ aged, 2 communities, USA N = 547	Single question on happiness	O	0,6	+0.48	Bradburn & Caplovitz, 1965: 90[3]
People in transition, USA. High and low stressed N = 72	10 item Affect Balance Scale	A	2 5 7 11	+0.43 +0.40 +0.44 +0.20	Chiriboga, 1989: 65
People in transition, USA Males: N = 64 Females: N = 76	Single question on happiness	O	11 11	+0.03 M +0.18F	Chiriboga, 1982: 23
Males, Baltimore, USA N = 557	Single question on satisfaction with accomplishments	C	5,3 12,8	+0.49 +0.46	Costa et al., 1981: 81

Appendix 1 (continued)

Subjects	Happiness measure	Happiness variant[1]	Time span in years	Overtime-correlation (in r)	Bibliografical source
Mothers, USA. Followed 18 months after birth of first child $N = 105$	Single question on life-satisfaction	O	0,6 1,5	+0.61 +0.51	Crnic, 1984[2]
Elderly males, rural USA $N = 1319$	Single question on contentment (how things have worked out for your)	C	10	+0.40	Dobson, 1985: 124[3]
18+ aged, Nebraska, USA $N = 1188$	Single question on happiness	O	2 2 4	+0.41 +0.38 +0.34	Eels, 1985: 88
18–65 aged, Victoria, Austria $N = 649$	Single question on appreciation of life, asked twice each interview (7 step Delighted-Terrible about life)	O	2 4 6	+0.53 +0.42 +0.40	Heady, 1989[2]

Appendix 1 (continued)

Subjects	Happiness measure	Happiness variant[1]	Time span in years	Overtime-correlation (in r)	Bibliografical source
Volunteers, Canada N = 1000	Single question on appreciation of life (10 step Best-Worst Possible life)	O	7	+0.17	Harley & Laverly, 1991: 117
	Single question on life-satisfaction		7	+0.25	
65–95 aged, Canada. Living in old-age homes N = 55	10 item Affect Balance Scale	A	0,9	+0.27	Kozma & Stones, 1980: 911
	2 item index of questions on happiness 'at this moment of time' and over the past month'	O	0,9	+0.57	
18+ aged, Germany. Participants Socio-Economic Panel N = 7091	Single question on life-satisfaction (10 step satisfaction)	O	1 2 4 5	+0.46 +0.39 +0.34 +0.32	Landua, 1992[2]
Single males and couples, Baltimore, USA N = 459	10 item Affect Balance Scale	A	2	+0.51	McCrae & Costa, 1991: 229
	Single question on appre-ciation of life (7 step Delighted-Terrible Scale)	)	2	+0.51	

Appendix 1 (continued)

Subjects	Happiness measure	Happiness variant[1]	Time span in years	Overtime-correlation (in r)	Bibliografical source
University students, USA. Followed from entry	Single question on feeling happy	A	4 10 14	+0.33 +0.26	Mortimer & Lorence, 1981: 16[3]
			14	+0.14	
Mothers, Berkeley, USA. Followed from age ±30 to 70 (N = 53) (Guidance group); (N = 28) (Control group)	Rating of 'cheerfulness' by independent interviewers	A	±40 ±40	+0.28 G +0.27 C	Mussen *et al.*, 1980: 337
	Rating of 'satisfaction with lot' by independent interviewers	C	±40	+0.15 G	
15–60 aged, Netherlands N = 296	10 item Affect Balance Scale		1	+0.52	Ormel, 1980: 134
46–70 aged, Carolina, USA.	Single question on	O	2	+0.56	Palmore & Kivett, 1977: 314
Members of insurance association N = 502	Appreciation of life (10 step Best-Worst Possible life)		4	±0.40	

Appendix 1 (continued)

Subjects	Happiness measure	Happiness variant[1]	Time span in years	Overtime-correlation (in r)	Bibliografical source
Babies, Berkeley, USA. Followed from birth to age 3. Males (N = 27); Females (N = 27)	Time-sampling of cheerful utterances Ratings were made at regular visits at home and in clinic. Ratings were made at month: 10, 11, 12, 13, 14, 15, 18, 21, 24, 27, 30 and 36	A	0,4 0,8 1,7	+0.64 M +0.72 F +0.61 M +0.51 F +5.0 M +0.48 F	Schaefer & Baily, 1963: 29
Babies, Berkeley, USA. Followed from birth into adolescence (above sample, girls only) (N = 19)	Time-sampling of baby cheerfulness (above and extensive interviews on the basis of which a rating of adolescent 'cheerfulness' was made	A	±14	−0.11 F	Schaefer & Baily, 1963: 105
Basic school pupils, USA. Followed from grade 6 to 10 (N = 310)	4 item Rosenberg/Simmons Depression Scale	O	1 4	+0.42 +0.25	Simmons et al., 1987: 107

Appendix 1 (continued)

Subjects	Happiness measure	Happiness variant[1]	Time span in years	Overtime-correlation (in r)	Bibliografical source
Grandparents and grandchildren, USA (N = 1159)	10 item Affect Balance Scale	A	14	+0.32	Stacey & Gatz, 1991: 77
Highschoolseniors USA. Followed into adulthood. Males (N = 32); Females (N = 40). Largely same subjects as in Block (above)	Rating of cheerfulness (vs gloomy) on the basis of extensive interview protocols	A	19 19	+0.26 M +0.20 F	Tuddenham, 1959: 16
Highschool seniors, USA Followed into adulthood Males: N = 51 Females: N = 41	Single question of enjoyment and disapointments in life Single question on realisation of wants	O C	15 15 15 15	+0.10 M +0.19 F +0.23 M +0.08 F	Tuddenham, 1962: 666
30–50 aged, Netherlands. Employed and unemployed (N = 337)	10 item Affect Balance Scale	A	1	+0.48	Verkley & Stolk, 1989: 91
65+ aged, patients, USA. Geriatric and general medical clinic (N = 205)	10 item Affect Balance Scale	A	1,5	+0.32	Yeo et al., 1987: 256[3]

[1] O = Overall happiness, A = Affect, level C = Contentment

[2] Overtime correlations provided by author

[3] Overtime correlations computed from data in report

APPENDIX 2

Country-characteristics (used in figure 4)

Material comfort is measured by the real income per head. 'Real' income means that non-marked goods and services are taken into account as well, and that purchasing power differences are controlled for. Data was drawn from Summers and Heston (1988: 125). Next to income as such, I also considered income security. I expect this security to be higher in the so-called welfare states which guarantee their citizens a minimum material level of living. By lack of comparable measures for social security as such, in the countries at hand, I took proportions of government expenditures (minus defence) in the gross national product as a proxi. Data were drawn from IMF-statistics (IMF 1987) and Japanese government statistics (Min. of Finance Japan 1986).

Social equality was measured by inequality between the sexes. Emancipation of women was measured by Estes' (1984: 171; 184/5) Index of Women Status, which involves educational participation of women and womens' suffrage. Income equality was not used in this analysis by lack of comparable data.

Freedom was measured by freedom of press. Data on that matter from the early 1970's was found in Kurian (1979: 362). I also considered the political democracy in the country. For that purpose I took Estes' Index of Political Paticipation (Estes 1984: 175–187). This index involves independance of the country, presence and functioning of a parliamentary system and limitation of influence of the military.

Access to knowledge was measured by scope of education in the country and attendance to mass media. As an indicator of educational performance I took Estes' Education Index (Estes 1984: 169; 183/4). This index involves school enrolment, expenses on education and literacy. As an indicator of access to information from mass media we took the summed scores of daily newspaper circulation and the number of radio's as found in Kurian (1979: 347–359).

APPENDIX 3

Data about migrant happiness used in exhibit 10

1. Victoria Immigrant Survey, 1981, Secondary analysis, 1–9 Terrible-Delighted scale transformed lineary to 0–10.

2. Australian National Science Survey, 1984, Secondar analysis, 1–10 Dissatisfied-Satisfied scale transformed linearly to 0–10.

3. German Survey among foreign workers (Ausländerumfrage), 1982. Data reported in Zapf & Brachtl, 1984: 294, 0–10 Utmost dissatified-Utmost satisfied scale.

4.   German Socio-Economical Panel, first wave, 1984, Secondary analysis, 0–10 Utmost dissatisfied-Utmost satisfied scale.

5.   German Welfare Survey (Wohlfahrtssurvey) 1980. Data reported in Zapf & Brachtl 1984: 294.

6.   Eurobarometer 19, 1983. Data reported in Inglehart 1985: 12, 0–10 very dissatisfied-very satisfied scale.

7.   European Value Study 1981, Secondary analysis, 1–10 dissatisfied-satisfied scale transformed linearly to 0–10.

8.   Estimate on the basis of a cross-national study among university students in which Turkish students scored very low (4.2 on a 1–7 Terrible Delighted Scale) and lower than students in Greece, Spain and Yugoslavia (Michalos 1991: 83).

9.   Estimate on the basis of:

     a.   National sample in 1962 which observed a score 5.0 on a 0–10 Worst-Best Possible Life scale (Cantril, 1965: 258).

     b.   Cross-national study among 15–40 aged in 1967 in which Slovenia scored 5.06 on a 1–9 Worst-Best Possible Life scale (5.1 on 0–10 scale).

NOTES

[1] An earlier version of this paper was presented at the 12th World Conference of the International Sociological Association in Madrid, 1990.

[2] This study was supported by grant nr. 560–270–023 of the Nederlandse organisatie voor Wetenschappelijk Onderzoek (NWO).

[3] Part of the analyses were performed by Piet Ouweneel. I thank Joop Ehrhardt for his valuable comments.

[4] The analyses reported in this paragraph were made during my stay at the Wissenschaftzentrum für Sozialwissenschaften Berlin, November 1992.

REFERENCES

Adams, R. G.: 1988, 'Which comes first: poor psychological well-being or decreased friendship activity?' Activities, Adaptation and Aging 12, pp. 27–41.

Andrews, F. M. and Withey, S. B.: 1976, Social indicators of Well-Being (Plenum Press, New York).

Bahr, H. M. and Harvey, C. D.: 1980, 'Correlates of Morale among the newly widowed', Journal of Psychology 110, pp. 219–233.

Block, J.: 1971, Lives Through Time (Bancroft, Berkely, California), pp. 293–307.

Brachtel, W. and Zapf, W.: 1984, 'Stabilität und Wandel individueller Wohlfahrt: Panel Ergebnisse', in: Glatzer, W. and Zapf, W. (eds), Lebensqualität in der Bundesrepublik' Campus (Frankfurt/Main), pp. 323–342.

Bradburn, N. M.: 1969, The Structure of Psychological Well-Being (Aldine, Chicago).

Brickman, P. Coates, D. and Janoff Bullman, R.: 1978, 'Lottery winners and accident victims: Is happiness relative?', Journal of Personality and Social Psychology 36, pp. 917–927.

Brim, O. G. jr.: 1970, 'Personalty development as role-learning', in: Scott, W. R. (ed), Social Process and Social Structure (Holt, New York), pp. 158–169.

Buchanan, W. and Cantril, H.: 1953, How Nations See Each Other. A Study in Public Opinion (University of Illinois Press, Urbana, USA).

Buss, A. H. and Plomin, R.: 1975, A Temperament Theory of Personality Development (Wiley, New York).

Cameron, P. et al.: 1973, 'The life satisfaction of non-normal persons', Journal of Consulting and Clinical Psychology 41, pp. 207–214.

Cantril, H.: 1965, The Pattern of Human Concern (Rutgers University Press, New Brunswick, NJ).

Chamberlain, K. and Zika, S.: 1972, 'Stability and Change, in subjective well-being over short time periods', Social Indicator Research 26, pp. 101–117.

Chaplin, W. T. John O. P. and Goldberg L. R.: 1988, 'Conceptions of states and traits', Journal of Personality and Social Psychology 54, pp. 541–557.

Chin Hon Foei, S.: 1989, 'Life-satisfaction in the EC countries 1975–1984', in: Veenhoven, R. (ed), Did the Crisis Really Hurt? Effects of the 1980–1982 Economic Recession on Satisfaction, Mental Health and Mortality (Universitaire Pers Rotterdam, Den Haag).

Chiriboga, D. A.: 1982, 'Concistency in adult functioning: the influence of social stress', Aging and Society 2, pp. 7–29.

Chiriboga, D. A.: 1984, 'Social stressors as antecedents of change', Journal of Gerontology 39, pp. 468–477.

Chiriboga, D. A.: 1989, 'Stress and loss in middle age', in: Kalish, R. E. (ed), Midlife Loss: Coping Strategies (Sage, London).

Costa, P. T. et al.: 1987, 'Longitudinal analysis of psychological well-being in national sample: stability of mean levels', Journal of Gerontology 42, pp. 50–55.

Costa, P. T., McCrae, R. R. and Norris, A. H.: 1981, 'Personal Adjustment to aging: longitudinal prediction from neuroticism and extraversion', Journal of Gerontology 36, pp. 78–85.

Costa, P. T. and McCrae, R. R.: 1984, 'Concurrent validation after 20 years: the implications of personality stability for its assessment', in: Butcher, J. N. and Spielberger, C. D. (eds), Advances in Personality Assessment (Erlbaum, Hillsdale, New York), pp. 31–54.

Costa, P. T. and McCrae, R. R.: 1988, 'Personality in adulthood', Journal of Personality and Social Psychology 54, pp. 853–863.

Costa, P. T., McCrae, R. R. and Zonderman, A. B.: 1987, 'Environmental and dispositional influences on well-being longitudinal follow-up of an American national sample', British Journal of Psychology 78, pp. 299–306.

Dam van, M. Puyenbroek van, R. and Verschuren, P.: 1989, 'De centrum-periferie theorie, Intra – versus internationale determinanten van inkomensongelijkheid', Mens en Maatschappij 2, pp. 5–21.

Davis. J. A.: 1984, 'New money, an old man, lady and two's company: Subjective welfare in the NORC general Social Surveys 1972–1982', Social Indicators Reseach 15, pp. 319–356.

DeFrain, J. D. and Ernst, L.: 1978, 'The psychological effect of sudden infant death syndrome on surviving family members', Journal of Family Practice 6, pp. 985–989.

Diener, E., Larsen, R. J. and Emmons, R. A.: 1984, 'Bias in mood recall in happy and unhappy persons', Paper (American Psychological Association, Toronto).

Dobson, C.: 1985, 'Attitudes and Perceptions', in: Powers, E. A., Goudy, W. J. and Keith, P. M. (eds), Late Life Transitions (Kluwer Academic, Dordrecht), pp. 123–136.

Easterlin, R. A.: 1974, 'Does economic growth improve the human lot? Some empirical evidence', in: David P. A. and Melvin, W. R. (eds), Nations and Households in Economic Growth (Stanford University Press, Palo Alto, California, USA).

Eels, L. W.: 1985, The Effect of Role Change on Psysical Health, Mental Health and General Life-Satisfaction: A Panel Analysis [Dissertation] (University of Nebraska, Michigan).

Estes, R. J.: 1984, The Social Progress of Nations (Praeger, New York).

Feather, N. T. and O'Brien, G. E.: 1986, 'A longitudinal study of the effects of employment on schoolleavers', Journal of Occupational Psychology 59, pp. 121–144.

Friedrich, W. N. and Friedrich, W. L.: 1981, 'Psychological assets of parents of handicapped and non-handicapped children', American Journal of Mental Deficiency 85, pp. 551–553.

Gallup, G. H. and Kettering, C. F.: 1976, Human Needs and Satisfactions a Global Survey [Research Report] (C.F. Kettering Foundation and Gallup International Research Institutes).

George, V. and Lawson, R.: 1980, Poverty and Inequality in Common Market Countries (London: Routlegde and Kegan Paul, London).

Gergen, K. J.: 1972, 'Multiple identity: the happy healthy human being wears many masks', Psychology Today.

Glenn, N. D.: 1975, 'The contribution of marriage to the psychological well-being of males and females', Journal of Marriage and the Family 37, pp. 594–601.

Halman, L.: 1991, Waarden in de Westerse Wereld (Tilburg University Press, Tilburg).

Halman, L., Heunks, F., Moor, R. de and Zanders, H.: 1987, Traditie, Secularisatie en Individualisering (Tilburg University Press, Tilburg).

Harding, S.: 1985, 'Values and the nature of psychological well-being', in: Abrams, M. Gerard, D. and Timms, N. (eds), Values and Social Change in Britain (McMillan, London).

Harley, J. and Lavery, J. J.: 1991, 'The stability and sensitivity of subjective well-being measures'. Social Indicators Research 24, pp. 113–122.

Heady, B. and Veenhoven, R.: 1989, 'Does happiness induce a rosy outlook?', in: Veenhoven, R. (ed), How Harmful Is Happiness? (Universitaire Pers Rotterdam, The Netherlands).

Heady, B. and Wearing, A.: 1989, 'Personality: Life-events and subjective well-being: towards a dynamic equilibrium model', Journal of Personality and Social Psychology 57, pp. 731–734.

Heady B. and Wearing, A.: 1992, Understanding Happiness: A Theory of Subjective Well-Being (Longman Cheshire, Sydney, Australia).

Hornstra, R. K. and Klassen, D.: 1977, 'The course of depression', Comprehensive Psychiatry 18, pp. 119–125.

IMF: 1987, Government Finance Statistics Yearbook, vol. XI (Washington).

Inglehart, R.: 1977, The Silent Revolution (Princeton University Press, New Yersey, USA).

Inglehart, R.: 1990, Culture Shift in Advanced Industrial Society (Princeton University Press, New Yersey, USA).

Inkeles, A.: 1960, 'Industrial man: the relation of status of experience perception, and value', American Journal of Sociology 66, pp. 1–31.

Inkeles, A.: 1990/91, 'National character revisited', The Tocqueville Review 12, pp. 83–117.

Kirchler, E.: 1985, 'Jobloss and mood', Journal of Economic Psychology 6, pp. 9–25.

Kozma, A. et al. : 1990, 'Long- and short-term affective states in happiness', Social Indicators Research 22, pp. 119–138.

Kuhlen, R. G.: 1948, 'Age trends in adjustment during the adult years as reflected in happiness ratings', American Psychologist 3, p. 307.

Kurian, G. T.: 1979, The Book of World Rankings (McMillam Reference Books, London).

Landua, D.: 1992, 'Satisfaction changes', Social Indicators Research 26, pp. 221–241.

Lieberman, L. R.: 1970, 'Life satisfaction in the young and the old', Psychological Reports 27, pp. 75–79.

Matlin, M. W. and Gawron, V. J.: 1979, 'Individual differences in Polyannaisn', Journal of Personality Assesment 43, pp. 411–412.

McCrae, R. R.: 1984, 'Personality as a lifelong determinant of well-being', in: Malatesta, C. Z. and Izard, C. E. (eds), Emotioning Adult Development (Sage, Beverly Hills, California), pp. 143–153.

McCrae, R. R. and Costa, P. T.: 1990, 'Adding Liebe und Arbeit: the full five-factor model and well-being', Personality and Social Psychology Bulletin 17, pp. 227–232.

McKinley Runyan, W.: 1979, 'Perceived determinants of highs and lows in life-satisfaction', Developmental Psychology 15, pp. 331–333.

McNeil, J. K. Stones, M. J. and Kozma, A.: 1986, 'Subjective well-being in late life; issues concerning measurement and prediction', Social Indicators Research 18, pp. 35–70.

Meneghan, E. G. and Lieberman, M. A.: 1986, 'Changes in depression following divorces: a panel study', Journal of Marriage and the Family 48, pp. 319–328.

Michalos, A.: 1991, 'Global Report on Student Well-Being', Vol. I, 'Life satisfaction and Happiness' (Springer Verlag, New York).

Mohr, H. M.: 1986, Subjektives Wohlbefinden (Subjective well-being) [Paper] Presented at the Conference of the German Sociological Association, Hamburg.

Moller, V.: 1988, 'The relevance of personal domain satisfaction', South-Africa Tydskrif Sielkunde (S-Afr. Journal of Psychiatry), p. 74.

Mortimer, J. T. and Lorence, J.: 1981, 'Self-concept Stability and change from late adolescence to early adulthood', Research in Community and Mental Health 2, pp. 5–42.

Mussen, P., Honzik and Eichorn: 1982, 'Early adult antecedents of life satisfaction at age 70', Journal of Gerontology 37, pp. 316–322.

Mussen, P. Eichhorn, D. H. Honzik, M. P. Biebe, S. L. and Meredith, W.: 1980, 'Continuity and change in women's characteristics over four decades', International Journal of Behavioral Development 3, pp. 331–347.

Moum, T.: 1988, Yeah saying and mood-of-the-day effects in self reported quality of life, Social Indicators Research 20, pp. 117–139.

Naroll, R.: 1982, The Moral Order (London, Sage).

Neugarten, B. L. Hovinghurst, R. J. and Tobin, S. S.: 1961, 'The measurement of life-satisfaction', Journal of Gerontology 16, pp. 134–143.

Ormel, J.: 1980, Moeite met Leven of een Moeilijk Leven (Difficulty with Living or a Difficult Life) (Konstapel, Groningen, Holland).

Ostroot, N. and Snyder, W.: 1985, 'Measuring cultural bias in a cross-national study', Social Indicators Research 17, pp. 243–251.

Ouweneel, P. and Veenhoven, R.: 1991, 'Cross national differences in happiness: Cultural bias or societal quality', in: Bleichrodt, N. and Drenth, P. J. (eds), Contemporary Issues in Cross Cultural Psychology (Swets and Zeitlinger, Amsterdam/Lisse, The Netherlands), pp. 168–184.

Palmore, E. and Kivett, V.: 1977, 'Change in life-satisfaction: a longitudinal study of persons aged 46–70', Journal of Gerontology 32, pp. 311–316.

Prime Minister Office: 1987, Public Opinion Survey on the Life of the Nation (Foreign Press Center, Tokyo, Japan).

Rosenberg, M.: 1962, 'The dissonant religious context and emotional disturbance', American Journal of Sociology 68, pp. 1–10.

Schaefer, E. S. and Bayley, N.: 1963, 'Maternal behavior, child behavior, and their intercorrelations', Monographs of the Society for Research in Child Development 28(3).

Schulz, B. and Decker, S.: 1985, 'Long term adjustement to physical disability', Journal of Personality and Social Psychology 48, pp. 1162–72.

Simmons, R. G., Klein, S. D. and Simmons, R. C.: 1977, Gift of Life (Wiley, London).

Simmons, R. G. and Blyth, D. A.: 1987, Moving into Adolescence (Aldine de Gruyter, New York).

Stacey, A. and Gatz, M.: 1991, 'Cross-sectional agedifferences and longitudinal change on the Bradburn Affect Balance Scale', Journal of Gerontology 46, pp. 76–78.

Stones, M. J. and Kozma, A.: 1989, 'Happiness and activities in late life: a propensity formulation', Canadian Psychology 30, pp. 526, 537.

Stones, M. J., Kozma, A. Hannak, I. E. and Mc Kim, W. A.: 1991, 'The correlation coefficient and models of Subjective Well-Being', Social Indicators Research 24, pp. 317–327.

Summers, R. and Heston, A.: 1988, 'A new set of international comparisons of real product and price level estimates for 130 countries, 1950–1985', National Income and Wealth 34, pp. 1–25.

Tellegen, A. et al.: 1988, 'Personality similarity in twins reared apart and together', Journal of Personality and Social Psychology 54, pp. 1031–1037.

Tuddenham, R. D.: 1959, 'Constancy of personality ratings over two decades', Genetic Psychology Monographs 60, pp. 3–29.

Tuddenham, R. D.: 1962, 'Constancy of personal morale over a fifteen year interval': Child Devellopment 33, pp. 663–673.

United Nations: 1986, 1983/84 Statistical Yearbook (United Nations, New York).

Veenhoven, R.: 1984, Conditions of Happiness (Reidel, Dordrecht, Holland).

Veenhoven, R.: 1987, 'Cultural Bias in ratings of perceived life quality: a comment on Ostroot and Snyder', Social Indicators Research 19, pp. 329–334.

Veenhoven, R.: 1988, 'The utility of happiness', Social Indicators Research 20, pp. 33–354.

Veenhoven, R. (ed.): 1989, 'Did the crisis really hurt? Effects of the 1980–82 economic recession on satisfaction, mental health and mortality'. (Universitaire Pers Rotterdam, Rotterdam,)

Veenhoven, R. (ed.): 1989, How Harmfull is Happiness?: Consequences of Enjoying Life or Not (Universitaire Pers Rotterdam, Rotterdam).

Veenhoven, R.: 1991, 'Is happiness relative?', Social Indicators Research 24, pp. 1–34.

Veenhoven, R.: 1991, 'Questions on happiness, classical topics, modern answers, blind spots', in: Strack, F., Argyle, M. and Schwarz, N. (eds), Subjective Well-Being: In Interdisciplinary Perspective (London), pp. 7–26.

Veenhoven, R.: 1992, World Database of Happiness. Ongoing catalogue of research on subjective appreciation of life. Catalogue of correlates. Printout September 1992 (Erasmus University, Rotterdam, The Netherlands). Electronically published on ftp.eur.nl (pub\database.happiness\correlat).

Veenhoven, R.: 1993, Happiness in Nations (RISBO, Rotterdam). Electronically published on ftp.eur.nl (pub\database.happiness\nations).

Verkley, H. and Stolk, J.: 1989, 'Does happiness lead into idleness?', in: Veenhoven (ed), How Harmful is Happiness (Univ. Pers Rotterdam, Holland), pp. 79–93.

Verkuyten, M.: 1986, 'Opgroeien in den vreemde', Gezondheid en Samenleving 7, pp. 1–6.

Verkuyten, M. and Veenhoven, R.: 1988, 'Welbevinden van kinderen na echtscheding: een onderzoek onder adolescenten' ('Wellbeing of children after divorce: a study of adolescents'), Tijdschrift voor Sociale Gezondheidszorg 66, pp. 128–133.

Waltz, M.: 1986, 'A longitudinal study on environment and dispositional determinants of life quality: social support and coping with physical illness', Social Indicators Research 18, pp. 71–93.

Wierzbicki, M.: 1986, 'Similarity of monozygotic and dizigotic twins in level and lability of subclinically depresses mood', Journal of Clinical Psychology 42, 577–585.

Yardley, J. K. and Rice, R. W.: 1991, 'The relationship between mood and subjective well-being', Social Indicators Research 24, pp. 101–111.

Yeo, G. Ingram, L. Skunnic, J. and Crapo, L.: 1987, 'Effects of a geriatric clinic on functional health and well-being of elders', Journal of Gerontology 42, pp. 252–258.

Young, P. T.: 1937, 'Is cheerfullness-depression a general temperamental trait?: A study of moods in college students', Psychological Review 44, pp. 313–319.

Zapf, W. and Brachtel, W.: 1984, 'Gastarbeiter und Deutsche Bevölkerung', in: Glatzer, W. and Zapf, W. (eds), Lebensqualität in der Bundesrepublik (Campus, Frankfurt/Main), pp. 286–306.

Erasmus University of Rotterdam,
POB 1738
3000 DR Rotterdam,
The Netherlands

ROBERT A. CUMMINS

18. ON THE TRAIL OF THE GOLD STANDARD FOR SUBJECTIVE WELL-BEING

(Accepted 7 February 1995)

ABSTRACT. The absence of a 'gold standard' for subjective well-being has severely hampered the interpretation of data from empirical studies. This paper demonstrates a remarkable consistency among the results of 16 studies that have investigated 'life satisfaction' among large samples drawn from the general population. It is concluded that a population standard for 'life satisfaction' can be expressed as 75.0 ± 2.5 percent of the measurement scale maximum score.

INTRODUCTION

The most common statement in the quality of life literature is a lament at the lack of a 'gold standard', or some agreed statistic which could form the basis of comparison between empirical studies. In the absence of such a reference, studies are constrained by the need to rely either on internal comparisons or comparisons with others that have used an identical measurement procedure. Unfortunately, studies rarely use comparable measurement procedures and this lack of an empirical frame of reference has severely limited the interpretation of data relating to subjective well-being (SWB).

Despite these difficulties, some general characteristics of such data have been identified. Most notable is that they are not normally distributed but negatively skewed. This has been found almost irrespective of the measuring instrument, population sample, or nationality, as data presented later in this paper will detail.

In order to explain this phenomenon various hypotheses have been proposed. In 1954 Goldings found that college students rated themselves significantly above the scale mid-point on happiness. From these data he proposed a 'behavioral norm' for happiness which was hypothesised to lie within the band of 6.0 to 7.5 on a 9-point scale. The explanation offered for this distribution was that,

537

since happiness is positively valued in our culture, people select a happiness rating for themselves that is socially acceptable.

Subsequent research, however, has extended the form of this data distribution to include other personal attributes including perceived energy (Gill, 1984) and a wide variety of life satisfaction measures. Clearly, therefore, explanations for this phenomenon need to be broadly based.

Boucher and Osgood (1969) provided a different and more general perspective. They noted that people have a tendency to prefer the use of positive rather than negative concepts when evaluating words, and coined the 'Polyanna Hypothesis' to explain people's preference for the positive end of life satisfaction scales. Headey and Wearing (1988, 1992), on the other hand, have suggested the phenomenon is based on a need to maintain self-esteem through downward social comparisons and describe the negative skew in self-perceptions as providing a 'Sense of Relative Superiority'. So, does the positive distribution represent some actual tendency to 'look on the bright side of life' instead of a response to social expectations as suggested by Goldings?

Evidence in support of an internal, adjustable mechanism is presented by Muthny et al (1990) who compared life satisfaction between three different cancer groups and healthy controls. They found that, in terms of general life satisfaction, the group with the worst prognosis had the highest representation (33%) in the top category of 'very satisfied'; almost three times the percentage (13%) of healthy people who used this category. The authors comment, "This clearly points to the issue of comparison with internal standards and ideals; a patient who has faced death might more easily be satisfied with [objectively] bad conditions than a healthy man with high expectations towards quality of life" (p. 156).

This idea of adjustable internal standards is derivative from Helson's (1964) Adaptation Level Theory and has been used by a number of researchers, most notably Brickman et al. (1978), to explain the observation that sharp falls or rises in life satisfaction occasioned by a major life event are usually followed by a gradual return to original levels of subjective well-being. But what causes the adaptation level to be set within the positive side of the well-being continuum?

A variety of mechanisms have been suggested which could underpin and maintain a positive perception of self. Taylor *et al.* (1983) have proposed such devices as making social comparisons with less fortunate others, a selective focus on attributes that make the self appear advantaged, creating hypothetical worse-worlds, construing benefit from adverse events, and manufacturing unrealistic normative standards. To this list Headey and Wearing (1992) have added such processes as differential weightings of sub-roles in personal assessments of overall role performance and the use of restricted reference groups.

There is clearly no shortage of psychological devices to nominate for the role of negative-skew maintenance. Indeed, it seems likely that many act in concert to produce the end result. If this is true, then it is likely that the phenomenon represents a true reflection of self-perception, rather than a response to social acquiescence. The multiple nature of supporting devices may also reflect the psychological importance of maintaining positive self-regard.

The conclusions that may be drawn are threefold. Firstly that the existence of the negative skew in subjective quality of life data is ubiquitous. Secondly that a variety of psychological mechanisms have been identified as likely candidates to explain the production and maintenance of such high personal self-regard. Thirdly that the consistency of this phenomenon across widely differing studies would be evidence for the operation of a psychological set-point for feelings of personal well-being.

If these conclusions are valid, then one outcome might be a high level of consistency, from one population to another, in their absolute level of perceived life satisfaction. Should this prove to be the case, a single statistic could provide a reference point, or a 'gold-standard', for all empirical studies into life quality. Such an investigation is the purpose of this paper.

METHOD

In order to provide a large and relatively homogenous data base for this research, the 'normative' studies have been restricted to population samples from Western countries. Data from other countries are presented in comparison to these 'normative' statistics later in the paper.

Normative Studies

More than 1 000 articles and books pertaining to the broad literature on life quality were scanned for normative data that met the following criteria:

1. The scale used must measure perceived 'satisfaction' with either some statement of global life assessment, or with a number of life domains from which a mean score can be derived. Scales measuring happiness have been excluded.

2. Likert scales must be symmetric, ranging from strongly positive to strongly negative, around a neutral mean point.

3. The number of points on the scale must be known and the mean value stated.

4. Each sample must conform to the following specifications.

    (a) It must be drawn from countries with comparable cultures and socio-economic status. The actual samples were drawn from Australia, Canada, England, Norway, Sweden, and U.S.A.

    (b) It must not be selected on medical, psychiatric, or socio-economic criteria.

    (c) It must not be restricted to rural communities, but may be restricted to urban populations.

    (d) It must not include children or adolescents less than 17 years of age and must include adults less than 65 years of age.

    (e) The sample size must exceed 200.

Despite meeting these criteria, a few studies were excluded for the following reasons:

> Bortner and Hultsch (1970): The instructions to respondents combined the concepts of 'happiness' and 'satisfaction'.
>
> Hall (1973): Reports the same data as Abrams (1973) with slightly differing domain names and excluding the item 'being a housewife'.

Judge and Watanabe (1993): Combined responses to bipolar adjectives with a measure of global life satisfaction.

White (1992): Combined measures of domain satisfaction with a measure of general happiness.

Comparative Studies

The same collection of articles and books used to identify the normative studies, was also searched for data on population sub-samples. The criteria for their inclusion were the same as (1) and (2) of the normative studies. In addition, a minimum of three studies were required that presented data relevant to a common population subgroup.

RESULTS

Normative Studies

A total of 17 data sets were located that fulfilled all of the normative criteria. The samples and scale details are presented in Table I.

On the right-hand column of this table all scale scores have been converted to the common statistic "Percentage of Scale Maximum" (%SM), calculated through the formula (score -1) $\times$ 100/(number of scale points -1). There are two variations on the application of this formula. In situations where the scale starts from zero, instead of from one, the formula becomes % SM = score $\times$ 100/(number of scale points -1). If the scale starts from a number greater than one, due to the aggregation of scores from multiple items, then the aggregate score is initially divided by the number of items to restore a scale range that commences with one.

Observations on the Normative Studies

Non-probability samples

Three studies are included that restricted their samples to population sub-groups. In each case, the nature of the sample seems unlikely to have influenced the mean score significantly away from population norms.

TABLE I

Studies used for the normative comparisons

Study	Country	Sample	Scale (see below)	N	Mean score	% scale max
Abrams (1973)	England	Quota	A1	593	5.59[1]	76.5
Andrews & Withey (1976)	USA	Probability	A2	4,920	5.42	73.7
Andrews (1991)	USA	Probability				
		– 1972	A2	1,297	5.50	75.0
		– 1988	A2	616	5.80[2]	80.0
Atkinson (1982)	Canada	Probability	A3	2,129	8.69[3]	76.9
Brief et al. (1993)	USA	Probability	A4	443	7.19	79.9
Campbell et al. (1976)	USA	Probability	A5	2,134	5.5	75.0
Harris & Assoc. (1975)	USA	Probability	A6	1,457	13.35	74.2
Headey & Wearing (1994)	Australia	Probability	A7	619	6.97[2]	74.6
Hoyert & Seltzer (1992)	USA	Female	A8	5,900	4.0	75.0
Gove et al. (1983)	USA	Probability	A9	2,174	2.24	74.7
Mastekaasa (1992)	Norway	Never married[4]	A10	6,214	5.6	76.1
Mookherjee (1992)	USA	Probability	A11	2,529	17.97	78.4
Moum (1994)	Norway	Probability	A12	71,896	5.37	72.8
Oppong et al. (1988)	Canada	Probability	A13	421	3.87[5]	71.7
Palmore & Luikart (1972)	USA	Probability	A4	502	7.0	70.0
Roy Morgan Research (1993)	Australia	Probability	A14	1,217	6.67	70.9

[1] Average of two measures.

[2] Average of two responses to the question asked about 20 minutes apart.

[3] Average of 1977 and 1979 data.

[4] The sample was actually designated 'unmarried' but their youth (20–39y) would suggest that the vast majorty would never have been married.

[5] Average of 1984 and 1985 data

The scale descriptions are as follows:

A1 – (a) "All things considered, how satisified or dissatisfied are you overall with [domain]. Which number comes closest to how satisfied or dissatisfied you are?". The score was a composite from 12 life domains, each rated on a 7-point scale from 'completely satisfied' to 'completely dissatisfied'. (b) Towards the end of the interview, each respondent was asked to take into account all of the aspects of life that had been discussed and to use the scale to indicate satisfaction or dissatisfication with life as a whole.

A2 – "... we want to find out how you feel about various parts of your life, and life in this country as you see it. Please tell me the feelings you have now – taking into account what has happened in the last year and what you expect in the near future" (p. 19). "How do you feel about your life as a whole?", using a 7-point Delighted-Terrible scale.

A3 – "All things considered, how satisfied or dissatisfied are you with your life as a whole? Which number comes the closest to how you feel?, from 1 = 'completely dissatisfied' to 11 = 'completely satisfied'.

A4 – Global life satisfaction was measured using the Cantril Ladder (Cantril, 1965), a single-item, 10 point scale ranging from 0 ('worst possible life') to 9 ('best possible life').

A5 – "We have talked about various parts of your life, now I want to ask you about your life as a whole. How satisfied are you with your life as a whole these days?" (p. 33), using a 7-point Likert scale from 'completely dissatisfied' to 'completely satisfied'.

A6 – Life satisfaction Index (Neugarten *et al.*, 1961). The scale consists of 18 statements with which respondents agree or disagree. Scores can range from 0 to 18.

A7 – "How satisfied are you with your life as a whole ", scored on a 9-point Delighted-Terrible scale.

A8 – "On the whole, I am satisfied with myself" scored from "1-strongly disagree to 5-strongly agree" (p. 77).

A9 – "How satisfying do you find your life, very satisfying, pretty satisfying, not too satisfying, or not at all satisfying?" (p. 63).

A10 – "Thinking about how you feel about your life these days, are you generally satisfied, or are you generally dissatisfied?" The seven response categories were labelled from "extremely satisfied" to "extremely dissatisfied" (Mastekaasa, 1994).

11 – Composite seven item scale comprising: How happy the respondent was in general, and how satisfied he/she felt with their residence, non-work activities, family life, friendship, health and physical condition, and financial situation. Scored on a 3-point scale 'Not satisfied at all, somewhat satisfied, well satisfied'.

A12 – "When you think about the way your life is going at present, would you say that you are by and large satisfied with life or are you mostly dissatisfied" (p. 8), scored on a 7-point scale from 'extremely dissatified' to 'extremely satisfied'.

A13 – "How satisfied are you with your ____?" (p. 618), from 1-'very dissatisfied' to 5 (or 7) 'very satisfied'. The aggregate score was derived from seven domains as: house, family life, health and physical condition, amount of time for leisure and hobbies, friendships, standard of living, job satisfaction.

A14 – "How pleased are you with your life as a whole", using a 9-point Delighted-Terrible scale.

Hoyert and Seltzer (1992) selected an exclusively female sample. However, probability samples have tended to show a gender
difference in subjective well-being that is less than 2.5%, and which
favor either males (Mastekaasa, 1992) or females (Branholm and
Degerman, 1992; Shmotkin, 1990). One Australian study has
reported identical gender values for subjective well-being (Roy
Morgan Research, 1993). Table II will present data confirming the
absence of a gender difference in life satisfaction.

   Two other studies have included large samples that were selected
from people who have never married (Hughes and Gove, 1981;
Mastekaasa, 1992). These studies have been included on the basis
that the SWB scores of such persons tend to fall slightly below
people who are married and slightly above people who were once
married but now divorced or widowed (Hughes and Gove, 1981;
Ying, 1992). Thus it might reasonably be expected that the scores
from these studies would differ little from the adult population as a
whole.

Scales

Perhaps the most striking feature of the studies listed in Table I is the
diversity of their scales. Among the 16 studies, 14 different measures
of life satisfaction have been employed.

   Apart from Cantril's Ladder, used by two studies, and Neugarten's
Life Satisfaction Index, used by one, most others have employed
a variation on the Andrews and Withey (1976) global question
"How do you feel about your life as a whole?" scored on a 7-point
Delightful-Terrible scale. However, the extent of the variations on
this theme have been very considerable. Scales have ranged from a
minimum of three response points (Mookherjee, 1992) to a maximum of 11 (Atkinson, 1982). Some authors have reported a mean
response from two identical questions asked some 20 minutes or
so apart (Andrews, 1991; Headey and Wearing, 1994) while most
others ask the question only once.

   A number of authors reported using quite elaborate 'framing'
procedure for the question (e.g. Andrews and Withey, 1976; Moum,
1994). Framing procedures are used to define the context within
which the person is expected to respond, and again these differ
between studies to the point that the respondents' points of reference might be considered to have been very different. For example,

TABLE II

Sub-population comparisons

Sub-population and study	Country	Sample	Scale (see below)	N	Mean score	% Scale max.
Females						
Branholm &	Sweden	Married	B1	47	4.78	75.6[1]
Degerman (1992)			B2	47	5.05	81.0
Mastekaasa (1992)	Norway	Unmarried 20–39y	A10	2,089	5.50	75.0
Mookherjee (1992)	USA	Probability	A11	?[4]	17.97	78.4
Roy Morgan Research (1993)	Australia	Probability	A14	621	6.67	70.9
MEAN ± SD						75.7 ± 3.05
Aged >65y						
Adams (1969)	USA	Probability	A6	508	12.50	62.5
Andrews (1991)	USA	Probability	A2	25	5.8	80.0
Bowling (1990)	England	Low SES >85y	A6	662	13.30	66.5[1]
			B3	662	4.92	65.3
Bowling *et al.* (1991)	England	Low SES, 65–85y				
		Male	A6	186	12.86	64.3[3]
		Female	A6	279	12.38	61.9
		Low SES, >85y				
		Male	A6	166	11.68	58.4
		Female	A6	496	11.19	56.0
		Middle SES, 65–85y				
		Male	A6	95	13.80	69.0
		Female	A6	193	13.10	65.5
Harris & Assoc (1975)	USA	Probability	A6	2,797	12.20	67.8
Mookherjee (1992)	USA	Probability	A11	?[4]	18.01	78.6
MEAN ± SD						69.55 ± 7.15
Physical disability						
Krause (1992)	USA	Spinal injury >2y	B4	286	3.74	68.5
Schulz & Decker (1985)	USA	Spinal injury >20y	A6	100	11.76	59.8
Stensman (1985)	Sweden	Wheelchair users	B5	36	8.00	80.0
MEAN ± SD						69.4 ± 8.3
Chronic medical						
Baker & Intagliata (1982)	USA	Various disorders	B9	118	5.30	71.6
Ferrans & Powers (1992)	USA	Haemodialysis	B7	349	20.65	68.8

TABLE II Continued

Sub-population and study	Country	Sample	Scale (see below)	N	Mean score	% Scale max.
Huxley & Warner (1992)	USA	Low-income patients	B8	15	5.07	67.8
Kober et al. (1990)	USA	Liver disease	B6	12	4.00	50.0
	Germany	Liver disease	B6	9	4.50	58.3
MEAN ± SD						63.3 ± 8.01
Post-organ transplant						
Hicks et al. (1992)	USA	Liver >2yr	B7	17	21.60	72.0
Kober et al. (1990)	USA	Liver >2yr	B6	12	5.60	75.9
	Germany	Liver >2yr	B6	9	6.10	85.0
Koch & Muthny (1990)	Germany	Kidney	B10	761	3.71	67.8
Lough et al. (1985)	USA	Heart >6mo	B11	75	4.58	71.6
MEAN ± SD						74.5 ± 5.86
Intellectual disability						
Bramston (1994)	Australia	Mild/Moderate	B13	59	13.70	71.4
Cummins et al. (1994)	Australia	Mild/Moderate	B13	39	27.90	74.6
Schalock et al. (1989)	USA	Independent living	B12	25	2.54	76.8
MEAN ± SD						74.3 ± 2.19
Low income						
Andrews (1991)	USA	Probability	A2	67	5.40	73.3
Harris & Associates (1975)	USA	Probability	A6	?[5]	24.98	66.6
Mookherjee (1992)	USA	Probability	A11	?[4]	16.86	70.4
MEAN ± SD						70.1 ± 2.76
High income						
Andrews (1991)	USA	Probability	A2	71	6.00	83.3
Harris & Associates (1975)	USA	Probability	A6	?[5]	30.81	82.8
Mookherjee (1992)	USA	Probability	A11	?[4]	18.96	85.4
MEAN ± SD						83.8 ± 1.15
Whites (USA)						
Andrews (1991)	USA	Probability	A2	491	5.8	80.0
Harris & Associates (1975)	USA	Probability	A6	?[5]	29.80	80.0
Mookherjee (1992)	USA	Probability	A11	?[4]	18.10	79.3

TABLE II Continued

Sub-population and study	Country	Sample	Scale (see below)	N	Mean score	% Scale max.
MEAN ± SD						79.9 ± –
Blacks (USA)						
Andrews (1991)	USA	Probability	A2	53	5.6	76.7
Harris & Associates (1975)	USA	Probability	A6	?[5]	29.09	69.7
Mookherjee (1992)	USA	Probability	All	?[4]	17.14	72.4
MEAN ± SD						72.9 ± 2.91

[1] Where two different scales have been used on the same sample, a mean score for the scales in combination has been used in the calculation of the sub-population score.
[2] The sample contained 206 males and 241 females. The break-down for age-groupings is not stated.
[3] In calculating the sub-group mean for aged >65y, all six individual values from this study have been combined to yield a single score of 62.5% SM.
[4] The total probability sample for this study was 2,529 but the sub-population N was not stated.
[5] The total probability sample for this study was 1,457 but the sub-population N was not stated.

Scales A1 to A13 have been described below Table I. The other scale descriptions are as follows:
B1 – A 'Life Satisfaction Questionnaire' containing 8 items each scored on a 6-point scale from 'very dissatisfying' to 'very satisfying'.
B2 – Cantril Ladder based on 11 rungs.
B3 – Faces scale using 7 points on 5 items.
B4 – Life Situation Questionnaire containing eleven items scored on a 5-point satisifaction scale.
B5 – Single question on 'satisfaction with overall life quality' on an 11-point scale.
B6 – European Organization for Research and Treatment of Cancer Quality of Life Questionnaire; satisfaction with overall quality of life on a 7-point scale (Aaronson *et al.*, 1987).
B7 – Quality of Life Index, which used a formula of Importance × Satisfaction on an overall quality of life, 5-point scale, that ranged from 'very dissatisfied' to 'very satisfied'.
B8 – Quality of Life Profile (Oliver, 1988) containing 9 items on 7-point scales.
B9 Quality of Life Scale (Flanagan, 1978) containing 15 items on 7-point faces scales. "Which face comes closest to expressing how you feel about ...?"
B10 – An 8-item scale with each rated from 'very dissatisfied' to 'very satisfied' on 5-points.
B11 – "How satisfied are you with your current quality of life?" on a 6-point scale from 'Not at all satisfied' to 'very satisfied'.
B12 – Quality of Life Scale (Keith *et al.*, 1986) containing 28 items on a 3-point scale.
B13 – Comprehensive Quality of Life Scale – Intellectual Disability (Cummins, 1993) contains 7 domains scored using Importance × Satisfaction on a 5-point scale.

Andrews (1991) sets a complex frame which incorporates satisfaction with the person's own life, life for the national community, in the past, present and future (see A2, Table I). Others are more simple, concentrating on satisfaction with the person's life in the present (see A12, Table I) or even restricted to the person themselves (see A8, Table I). One (Roy Morgan Research, 1993) has used the context of how 'pleased' the person feels about their life. Still others are more general, stating frames such as 'all thing considered' (Atkinson, 1982).

Finally, there are differences in the dimension of 'satisfaction' to which the person responds. Most commonly people respond to a scale defined by 'completely dissatisfied' to 'completely satisfied'. However, the extended form of this scale has also been employed, using the 'Delighted-Terrible' anchors (e.g. Andrews and Withey, 1976), as has also the truncated form which ranges from 'very satisfying' to 'not at all satisfying' (Hughes and Gove, 1981). Others are as diverse as Cantril's Ladder which ranges from the 'worst possible life' to the 'best possible life', and the Life Satisfaction Index which contains statements to which the respondent agrees or disagrees.

All in all, there is remarkably little commonality in the methodology employed by these studies. Their single linking feature is that, in one way or another, they all enquire about the level of life satisfaction.

Calculation of a normative statistic

Table I presents the conversion of each data-set into the common statistic 'Percentage of Scale Maximum' (%SM). The data in this table have been generated through very diverse sample sizes, using widely differing techniques, as has been described in the previous section. Thus, there seems no compelling rationale to employ any weighting system to their combination. The arithmetic mean and standard deviation of the %SM values is 75.02 ± 2.74.

Comparative Sub-population Studies

Table II presents data organized under ten headings which represent population sub-groups.

As in the normative studies, there is little commonality among the measuring instruments other than the fact that they all measure life satisfaction by one means or another. Points to note in relation to each of the sub-groups are as follows:

Females:	The data indicate a mean and standard deviation which is very similar to the normative value.
Aged > 65 y:	The mean value of 69.55 lies within two standard deviations of the normative values but the degree of variation is considerable.
Physical disability:	The group data may be unduly elevated by the Stensman (1985) data indicating 80.0% satisfaction. The normal control group for this study scored 83%SM, but the precise nature of the question asked to generate these data is not stated. Nevertheless, even with the inclusion of this value, the mean score for the group lies around two standard deviations below the normative mean.
Chronic medical:	This very heterogeneous group display a high degree of variability and a mean that lies four standard deviations below the normative sample.
Post-organ transplant:	With one exception these values lie within, or in one case above, the normal range.
Intellectual disability:	All values lie within the normal range.
Low income:	All values lie towards the lower side of the normal range.
High income:	This is the only sub-group where all values lie above the normal range.
Whites (USA):	All values are firmly placed at the upper margin of the normal range.
Blacks (USA):	The values tend to lie below the normative mean.

TABLE III

Other countries

Study	Country	Sample	Scale	N	Mean score	% SM
Nathawat & Mathur	India	Housewives	A2	200	4.46	57.7
(1993)		Working women	A2	200	4.73	62.2
Shmotkin (1991)	Isreal	Males 21–59y	B2	?[1]	7.90	69.0
			A6		13.44	61.3
		Females 21-59y	B2		8.06	70.6
			A6		14.18	65.9
		Males 60–87y	B2		7.39	63.9
			A6		12.82	59.1
		Females 60–87y	B2		6.79	57.9
			A6		10.70	48.5
Makarczyk (1962)	Poland	Stratified quota	C1	2,387	3.60	65.0
Man (1991)	Hong Kong	Children 13y	A10	940	3.88	48.0
		Children 16y	A10	940	3.63	43.8
Moller (1988)	South Africa	Retired Zulu				
		<64y	C2	125	2.36	34.0
		>65y		127	2.73	43.3
Moller (1992)	South Africa	Black youth	C2	1,200	3.21	55.3

[1] The total sample for this study was 447 but the sub-sample N was not stated.

Scales A1 to A13 and B1 to B3 have been described below Tables I and II respectively. The other scale description is as follows:
C1 – "On the whole are you satisfied with life?" using a 5-point scale from 'definitely yes' to 'definitely no'.
C2 – "Taking all things together, how satisfied are you with your life as a whole these days?" using a 5-point scale from 'very dissatisfied' to 'very satisfied'.

Data from other Countries

Table III presents data from countries other than those included in either the normative or sub-population tables. As can be seen, the samples are extremely diverse and so no overall statistic has been calculated. It is notable, however, that the values generally lie well below the normative range.

The Satisfaction with Life Scale

A deliberate omission from previous tables has been data derived from the Satisfaction with Life Scale (Diener et al., 1985). The reason is that this scale appears to yield values that lie significantly below the other scales that have been reported.

Responses on Diener's scale are made to five items on a 7-point Likert format that is anchored by 'strongly disagree' and 'strongly agree'. Thus, scale scores may vary between 5 and 35. The statements that comprise this scale are as follows:

1. In most ways my life is close to ideal.

2. The conditions of my life are excellent.

3. I am satisfied with my life.

4. So far I have gotten the important things I want in life.

5. If I could live my life over, I would change almost nothing.

In 1993, Pavot and Diener published a compilation of data derived from the use of this scale. Including only those scores derived from the countries represented in Table I & II, the 22 values aggregate to a mean of 56.2%SM with a standard deviation of 13.3. The upper range extends to only 67%SM (college students and nuns) while the lower range extends to 24.3% (male prisoners) and 22.7%SM (medical inpatients). A total of six studies report on college students (mean = 63.6%SM), three on members of the adult work-force (mean = 64.2%SM), and three on medical patients/psychological clients (mean = 40.1%SM). It seems clear that this scale is yielding data which fall at least 10%SM points below those of comparable scales.

DISCUSSION

The main result to emerge from this paper is the finding that, despite the use of very different methodologies, the combination of data from 16 unrelated studies into life satisfaction has yielded a mean of 75.02%SM and a standard deviation of just 2.74.

One explanation for this result could be the existence of a psychological, homeostatic mechanism that maintains an average level of life-satisfaction at around 75%SM. This would be a highly adaptive device on a population basis ensuring that, under relatively stable but diverse living conditions, most people feel satisfied with their lives, thereby conferring a non-zero sum benefit on the population as a whole. Such a mechanism has been suggested previously (Headey and Wearing, 1988). However, it would clearly only apply on an averaged basis across populations. Many individuals or sub-population groups fall outside the normal range, defined by two standard deviations from the mean, as indicated by Table II.

The data presented in Table II, derived from non-probability samples, need to be interpreted cautiously. These studies do not generally have the advantage of large numbers of subjects, often were not intended to be representative even of their sub-population categorization as depicted in Table II, and have employed an even more diverse set of measuring instruments. Despite these caveats, some trends seem to be apparent.

Firstly it can be noted that some of these sub-groups do not differ from the normative range. This categorization applies to females, people who have survived an organ transplantation for a number of years, and people with a mild or moderate level of intellectual disability living in the community. In contrast, one group stands out as having a level of life satisfaction above the normative range. The three studies on people with higher-than-average income yielded a score of 83.8 ± 1.15, indicating a remarkable degree of consistency between the three sets of data.

On the downward side, people over the age of 65 years, people with a physical disability, or with a low income, are on the lower margins of the normal range. People with a chronic medical condition, on the other hand, have a mean value well below the two standard deviation range. In addition it would appear that blacks in the USA have a lower satisfaction than whites.

While there is a relatively high degree of variability within most of these sub-groups, the trends of these data do not seem surprising. This is encouraging for the idea that the %SM data are valid and that this measure of life satisfaction can be used to discriminate between people whose lives are objectively better or worse off than normal.

The two final sets of data are drawn from studies involving people from countries other than those used for the normative calculations, or from studies using the Satisfaction with Life Scale. Both yield values that lie well below the normative range. The reason for the former set is speculative at this stage. Whether people from these countries score lower due to cultural factors that influence their responding or whether their responses reflect a relatively lower standard of living remains to be determined. Similarly, the reason that Diener's scale produces such low values is unclear. It seems rather extraordinary that this scale should behave in a manner noticeably different from the multitude of others that have been cited, but the fact that it does is most interesting. Clearly there is some element in the format of this scale, such as reaction to the strong statements of positive life satisfaction that constitute the items, that causes people to respond differently from other scales.

One final statistic can be drawn from the data presented in Table II in support of an observation made by Headey and Wearing (1988). Since the human set-point for life satisfaction lies above the point of neutrality, ceiling effects should start to reduce sample variance as the sample means become higher. This has been tested through the calculation of a Spearman Rank Correlation Coefficient between the rank order of sub-population means in Table II against the rank order of their variance. This latter statistic was adjusted for absolute values by using the standard deviation divided by the mean. The resulting $r = 0.717$ ($N = 9$) is significant at $p < 0.05$. This result is further evidence of coherent variation among the sub-population %SM values listed in this table.

In terms of using the information presented in this paper to guide future studies, it is recommended that researchers standardize the form of their 'life satisfaction' question and the nature of their scale. In the absence of data indicating the superiority of one form of question over another, researchers who seek a global measure should consider using the original Andrews and Withey (1976) wording "How do you feel about your life as a whole?" It is further recommended that any variation on this wording, or the use of framing procedures for such a question, be constructed with a stated purpose. It is also recommended that, in the absence of alternative argument, researchers adhere to the original 7-point Delighted-Terrible scale.

The reason for this is that: (**a**) Adults, on average, could be expected to reliably locate their level of satisfaction on such a scale, (**b**) There are currently no data to indicate the reliability of scales that exceed 7-points. Moreover, Ramsay (1973) has argued, from a psychometric perspective, that using 7 categories on a Likert Scale provides very nearly as much precision of estimate as a corresponding continuous judgement task, and that increasing the number of categories beyond 7 is of little value in terms of increased precision of estimate. On the other hand, reducing the number of scale points below 7 is likely to reduce both validity (Andrews and McKennel, 1980) and discriminative power, (**c**) The words 'delighted-terrible' used as the scale reference-points, have been shown to produce greater discrimination than such other markers as 'very satisfied' and 'very unsatisfied' (Andrews and Withey, 1976).

It can also be observed that, if researchers are interested only in an overall life-satisfaction score, there seems little benefit in asking respondents multiple questions. It seems that a single question can yield reliable and valid data.

In considering the accuracy of the normative statistics that have been produced, it is clear that they must be viewed only as approximations. The use of multiple instruments, varying instructions to respondents, different populations and even nationalities, means that the data have been drawn from an extremely heterogeneous base. In addition, the simple arithmetic combination of mean values from studies with such differing sample sizes is clearly a crude method of averaging.

Because of these factors it is proposed that, as a working hypothesis, the life-satisfaction gold standard be considered as 75.0 ± 2.5%SM. This mean value closely approximates the calculated mean, and the range of two standard deviations includes all of the values in Table I. The utility of this proposition is that is exemplifies the approximate nature of the proposed standard in a way that is readily applied to future comparative studies.

To conclude that more research is needed seems rather obvious. At least now, however, the %SM statistic and the data presented in this paper may provide the rationale for comparative empirical studies based on population norms. One trail to the gold standard for life satisfaction is now open. The task of elaborating the hypothesised range of 75 ± 2.5%SM remains as a major challenge.

REFERENCES

Aaronson, N. K., W. Bakker, A. L. Stewart, F. S. A. M. Van Dam, Y. Van Zandwijk, Jr. and A. Kirkpatrick: 1987, 'Multidimensional approach to the measurement of quality of life in lung cancer clinical trials', in N. K. Aaronson and J. Beckmann (eds.), The Quality of Life of Cancer Patients (Raven Press, New York), pp. 63–82.

Adams, D. L.: 1969, 'Analysis of a life satisfaction index', Journal of Gerontology 24, 470–474.

Andrews, F. M.: 1991, 'Stability and change in levels and structure of subjective well-being: USA 1972 and 1988', Social Indicators Research 25, 1–30.

Andrews, F. M and A. C. McKennel: 1980, 'Measures of self-reported well being: Their affective, cognitive, and other components', Social Indicators Research 8, 127–155.

Andrews, F. M. and S. B. Withey: 1976, Social Indicators of Well-being: Americans' Perceptions of Life Quality (Plenum Press, New York).

Atkinson, T.: 1982, 'The stability and validity of quality of life measures', Social Indicators Research 10, 113–32.

Baker, F. and J. Intagliata: 1982, 'Quality of life in the evaluation of community support systems', Evaluation and Program Planning 5, 69–79.

Bortner, R. W. and D. F. Hultsch: 1970, 'A multivariate analysis of correlates of life satisfaction in adulthood', Journal of Gerontology 25, 41–47.

Boucher, J. and C. E. Osgood: 1969, 'The Pollyanna hypothesis', Journal of Verbal Learning and Verbal Behavior 8, 1–8.

Bowling, A.: 1990, 'Associations with life satisfaction among very elderly people living in a deprived part of inner London', Social Science and Medicine 31, 1003–1011.

Bowling, A., M. Farquhar and P. Browne: 1991, 'Life satisfaction and associations with social network and support variables in three samples of elderly people', International Journal of Geriatric Psychiatry 6, 549–566.

Bramston, P.: 1994, Personal communication.

Branholm, I. B. and E. A. Degerman: 1992, 'Life satisfaction and activity preferences in parents of Down's Syndrome children', Scandinavian Journal of Social Medicine 20, 37–44.

Brickman, P., D. Coates and R. Janoff-Bulman: 1978, 'Lottery winners and accident victims: Is happiness relative?', Journal of Personality and Social Psychology 36, 917–927.

Brief, A. P., A. H. Butcher, J. M. George and K. E. Link: 1993, 'Integrating bottom-up and top-down theories of subjective well-being: The case of health', Journal of Personality and Social Psychology 64, 646–654.

Campbell, A., P. E. Converse and W. L. Rodgers: 1976, The Quality of American Life (Russell Sage Foundation, New York).

Cantril, H.: 1965, The Pattern of Human Concerns (Rutgers University Press, New Jersey).

Cummins, R. A.: 1993, The Comprehensive Quality of Life Scale: Intellectual Disability. Fourth edition (School of Psychology, Deakin University, Melbourne).

Cummins, R. A., M. P. McCabe and Y. Romeo: 1994, 'The Comprehensive Quality of Life Scale – Intellectual Disability: Results from a Victoria Survey', Proceedings, 28th National Conference of the Australian Society for the Study of Intellectual Disability, pp. 93–98.

Diener, E., R. A. Emmons, R. J. Larson and S. Griffin: 1985, 'The satisfaction with life scale', Journal of Personality Assessment 49, 71–75.

Ferrans, C. E. and M. J. Powers: 1992, 'Psychometric assessment of the quality of life index', Research in Nursing and Health 15, 29–38.

Flanagan, J. C.: 1978, 'A research approach to improving our quality of life', American Psychologist 33, 138–147.

Gill, W. M.: 1984, 'Monitoring the subjective well-being of chronically ill patients over time', Community Health Studies 8, 288–296.

Goldings, H. J.: 1954, 'On the avowal and projection of happiness', Journal of Personality 23, 30–47.

Gover, W. R., M. Hughes and C. B. Style: 1983, 'Does marriage have positive effects on the psychological well-being of the individual?', Journal of Health and Social Behavior 24, 122–131.

Hall, J.: 1973, 'Measuring the quality of life using sample surveys', in J. Stober and D. Schumacher (eds.), Technology Assessment and Quality of Life (Elsevier, Amsterdam), pp. 93–102.

Harris, L. and Associates: 1975, The Myth and Reality of Aging in America. (National Council on Aging, Washington, DC).

Headey, B. and A. Wearing: 1988, 'The sense of relative superiority: Central to well-being', Social Indicators Research 20, 497–516.

Headey, B. and A. Wearing: 1992, Understanding Happiness: A Theory of Subjective Well-Being (Longman Cheshire, Melbourne).

Headey, B. and A. Wearing: 1994, Victorian Quality of Life Panel Study, personal communication.

Helson, H.: 1964, Adaption-Level Theory (Harper & Row, New York).

Hicks, F. D., J. L. Larson and C. E. Ferrans: 1992, 'Quality of life after liver transplant', Research in Nursing & Health 15, 111–119.

Hoyert, D. L. and M. M. Seltzer: 1992, 'Factors related to the well-being and life activities of family caregivers', Family Relations 41, 74–81.

Huxley, P. and R. Warner: 1992, 'Case management, quality of life and satisfaction with services of long-term psychiatric patients', Hospital and Community Psychiatry 43, 799–802.

Judge, T. A. and S. Watanabe: 1993, 'Another look at the job satisfaction-life satisfaction relationship', Journal of Applied Psychology 78, 939–948.

Keith, K. D., R. L. Shalock and K. Hoffman: 1986, Quality of life: Measurement and Programmatic Implications (Mental Retardation Services, Nebraska).

Kober, B., T. Kuchler, C. Broelsch, B. Kremer and D. Henne-Bruns: 1990, 'A psychological support concept and quality of life research in a liver transplantation program: An interdisciplinary multicenter study', Psychotherapy and Psychosomatics 54, 117–131.

Koch, U. and F. A. Muthny: 1990, 'Quality of life in patients with end-stage renal disease in relation to the method of treatment', Psychotherapy and Psychosomatics 54, 161–171.

Krause, J.S.: 1992, 'Life satisfaction after spinal cord injury: A descriptive study', Rehabilitation Psychology 37, 61–70.

Lough, M. E., A. M. Lindsey, J. A. Shinn and N. A. Stotts: 1985, 'Life satisfaction following heart transplantation', Journal of Heart Transplantation 4, 446–449.

Man, P.: 1991, 'The influence of peers and parents on youth life satisfaction in Hong Kong', Social Indicators Research 24, 347–365.

Makarczyk, W.: 1962, 'Factors affecting life satisfaction among people in Poland', Polish Sociological Bulletin 1, 105–116.

Mastekaasa, A.: 1992, 'Marriage and psychological well being: Some evidence on selection into marriage', Journal of Marriage and the Family 54, 901–911.

Mastekaasa, A.: 1994, Personal communication.

Moller, V.: 1988, 'Quality of life in retirement: A case study of Zulu return migrants', Social Indicators Research 20, 621–658.

Moller, V.: 1992, 'Spare time use and perceived well-being among black South African youth', Social Indicators research 26, 309–351.

Mookherjee, H. N.: 1992, 'Perceptions of well-being by metropolitan and non-metropolitan populations in the United States', Journal of Social Psychology 132, 513–524.

Moum, T.: 1994, 'Is subjective well-being a predictor of nonresponse in broad population surveys?', Social Indicators Research 32, 1–20.

Muthny, F. A., U. Koch and S. Stump: 1990, 'Quality of life in oncology patients', Psychotherapy and Psychosomatics 54, 145–160.

Nathawat, S. S. and A. Mathur: 1993, 'Marital adjustment and subjective well-being in Indian-educated housewives and working women', The Journal of Psychology 127, 353–358.

Neugarten, B. L., R. J. Havighurst and S. S. Tobin: 1961, 'The measurement of life satisfaction', Journal of Gerontology 16, 134–143.

Oliver, J.P.J.: 1988, 'The quality of life of the chronically mentally disabled', Research Progress Report, cited by P. Huxley and R. Warner: 1992, 'Case management, quality of life, and satisfaction with services of long-term psychiatric patients', Hospital and Community Psychiatry 43, 799–802.

Oppong, J. R., R. G. Ironside and L. W. Kennedy: 1988, 'Perceived quality of life in a centre-periphery framework', Social Indicators Research 20, 605–620.

Palmore, E. and C. Luikart: 1972, 'Health and social factors related to life satisfaction', Journal of Health and Social Behaviour 13, 68–80.

Pavot, W. and E. Diener: 1993, 'Review of the satisfaction with life scale', Psychological Assessment 5, 164–172.

Ramsay, J. O.: 1973, 'The effect of number of categories in rating scales on precision of estimation of scale values', Psychometrika 38, 513–532.

Roy Morgan Research: 1993, International Values Audit, 22/23 May (Roy Morgan Research Center, Melbourne).

Schalock, R. L., K. D. Keith, K. Hoffman and O. C. Karan: 1989, 'Quality of life: Its measurement and use', Mental Retardation 27, 25–31.

Schulz, R. and S. Decker: 1985, 'Long-term adjustment to physical disability: The role of social support, perceived control, and self-blame', Journal of Personality and Social Psychology 48, 1162–1172.

Schmotkin, D.: 1990, 'Subjective well-being as a function of age and gender: A multivariate look for differentiated trends', Social Indicators Research 23, 201–230.

Shmotkin, D.: 1991, 'The structure of the Life Satisfaction Index A in elderly Israeli adults', International Journal of Aging and Human Development 33 131–150.

Stensman, R.: 1985, 'Severely mobility-disabled people assess the quality of their lives', Scandinavian Journal of Rehabilitation Medicine 17, 87–99.

Taylor, S. E., J. V. Wood and R. R. Lichtman: 1983, 'It could be worse: Selective evaluation as a response to victimization', Journal of Social Issues 39, 19–40.

White, J. M.: 1992, Marital status and well-being in Canada – An analysis of age group variations', Journal of Family Issues 13, 390–399.

Ying, Y-W.: 1992, 'Life Satisfaction among San-Francisco Chinese-Americans', Social Indicators Research 26, 1–22.

School of Psychology,
Deakin University,
Victoria, 3125,
Australia

ROBERT A. CUMMINS

19. THE DOMAINS OF LIFE SATISFACTION: AN ATTEMPT TO ORDER CHAOS*

(Accepted 17 June 1996)

ABSTRACT. While life satisfaction is commonly measured as an aggregate of individual life domains, the characterisation of such domains is uncertain. This study attempts to group 173 different domains names derived from the literature under seven headings as used by the Comprehensive Quality of Life Scale (ComQol). It was found that 68% could be classified in this way. Moreover, due to the repeated use of some domain names, the ComQol classification included 83% of the total reported data. The ComQol domain data did not differ from single-item global measures of life satisfaction and the within-study variance was lower using the ComQol rather than the original domains. A hierarchy of domain satisfaction was found which was dominated by the domain of intimacy. The other ComQol domains were quite tightly clustered within a range of 1.08 standard deviations. No difference was found between normative data and data gathered from people with a chronic medical condition, but people selected on psychiatric criteria had a lower life quality, most particularly in the domain of intimacy. It is concluded that life satisfaction, and therefore subjective well-being, can be economically and validly measured through the seven ComQol domains.

INTRODUCTION

There are two basic approaches to the definition and measurement of subjective quality of life (QOL). One regards the construct as a single, unitary entity, while the other considers it to be composed of discrete domains.

An early example of the former approach has been incorporated into one of the most popular measurement instruments. Devised by Andrews and Withey (1976), it consists of the single question "How do you feel about your life as a whole?" with respondents using a Likert scale of life satisfaction/dissatisfaction. While this approach to subjective QOL measurement has proved very useful for

* I thank Natasha Cho, Poh Chua, Trudy Wallace and Lewi Yiolitis for their assistance in the production of this manuscript. The research was funded in part by grants from the Australian Research Council and the National Health and Medical Research Council.

Alex C. Michalos (ed.), Citation Classics from Social Indicators Research, 559–584.
© 2005 *Springer. Printed in the Netherlands.*

comparing population samples, it has limited utility for smaller group comparisons since it provides only a global measure of perceived well-being. The great majority of more recent definitions, models and instruments have attempted to break-down the QOL construct into constituent domains. There is little agreement, however, regarding either their number or scope.

The possible number of domains is large. If each term describing some aspect of the human condition is regarded as separate, then their number is very large indeed. But a more parsimonious view is that may terms share a great deal of their variance. Moreover, using the logic of the global measure, people should be able to synthesise a gestalt-view of how satisfied they are with the substantial divisions of their life. If we ask someone 'How satisfied are you with your health?', it seems reasonable to assume they can generate a response that bears a substantial relationship to an aggregate formed from their responses to individual components of the health construct.

Of course, the relationship between the gestalt and aggregate approach can never be perfect. Different people will use idiosyncratic groupings of life components to represent health and will weight these components in individual ways. Despite this the benefits of such a shorthand approach are substantial in reducing the number of questions concerning broad aspects of life to a manageable number. The extent to which any particular domain name is justifiable is an empirical issue. It should be possible to demonstrate that any named domain possess the normal requirements of reliability and validity required of all psychological measures. Moreover, any proposed set of domains should, in aggregate, encompass the entire construct of subjective life quality.

Cummins, McCabe, Romeo, and Gullone (1994) and Cummins (1996) have provided both empirical and theoretical argument for the use of seven domains, these being material well-being, health, productivity, intimacy, safety, community, and emotional well-being. In order to argue the case from the preceding literature, Cummins (1996) reviewed 27 definitions of life quality that attempted to iden-tify QOL domains. In summary, it was found that a clear majority supported five of the proposed domains. Eighty-five percent included emotional well-being (EMO) in some form (leisure, spiritual well-being, morale, etc.), 70% included health (HLTH), 70% social and family connections (intimacy- INT), 59% material wealth or well-being (MAT), and 56% work or other form of productive activity (productivity-PROD).

Further empirical support for the inclusion of these five domains is provided by data from surveys which asked respondents to indicate whether various domains of life are important to them. Four large population surveys provide relevant data. The earliest is by Abrams (1973) who found that the top four ranked domains are HLTH, INT, MAT and PROD. No domain directly relevant to EMO was included. In 1976, Campbell, Converse, and Rodgers asked people to rate domain importance on a five point scale. Expressed as a percentage of scale maximum for importance (the % scale maximum formula is provided in the Method section), items relevant to the domains scored HLTH- 91%, INT- 89%, MAT- 73%, PROD- 70%. Again, no domain directly relevant to EMO was included. Finally, Flanagan (1978) and Krupinski (1980) both asked respondents to rate domain importance. The percentage of people who ranked items relevant to each domain in the top two categories (very/extremely important; important/very important) were respectively: HLTH (97, −), INT (81, 80), EMO (86, 73), MAT (83, 70), and PROD (78, 55). From these data it can be safely concluded that the five domains are regarded as very important aspects of their lives by a large majority of people.

Cummins (1995) has proposed the two additional domains of safety and community. The domain of safety is intended to be inclusive of such constructs as security, personal control, privacy, independence, autonomy, competence, knowledge of rights, and residential stability. It is theoretically relevant to Antonovsky's (1987) Sense of Coherence, which refers to a disposition to look at life and its problems in a manner which makes coping easier by viewing the world as meaningful, comprehensible, and manageable.

Of the 27 definitions mentioned earlier, 22% identified a domain corresponding to safety. The terms used were: personal safety and justice (OECD, 1976), autonomy (Vitello, 1984), independence (Schalock, Keith, Hoffman, and Karan, 1989), stability (Borthwick-Duffy, 1990), a living environment that embraces security and autonomy (Stark and Goldsbury, 1990), and safety from harm and financial security (Halpern, 1993). It is interesting to note that, with the single exception of OECD, all of the other definitions pertained specifically to the life quality of people with an intellectual disability. This no doubt reflects the special concern that the safety domain has for the welfare of this particular group, but its influence is pervasive for the general population as well.

The seventh domain that is proposed is 'place in community'. This domain is intended to be inclusive of the constructs of social class, education, job status, community integration, community involvement, self-esteem, self- concept, and empowerment. This 'community' domain reflects the influence of large-scale social structures and pressures on QOL (Liem and Liem, 1978) and differs from the other 'social' domain in that intimacy is provided by family and friends, with no implied status hierarchy, while place in community reflects hierarchical position within community life that implies no intimacy.

Perhaps the strongest traditional linkage of this domain with QOL has been through its combination with material well-being to form the index Socio- Economic Status (SES). SES inevitably contributes significant variance to measures of life quality, and the relative importance of the social component has been nicely demonstrated in a review by Adler, Boyce, Chesney et al. (1994). They found the literature to support the SES-good health link more strongly within, rather than between, countries. This suggests that the active ingredient may be more associated with relative position on a social hierarchy than absolute wealth per se.

Of the 27 definitions mentioned earlier, 30% identified a domain corresponding to place in community. Most related to social relationships, activities or functioning (Felce and Perry, 1995; Hornquist, 1989; Schalock et al., 1989; Schumaker, Shea, Monfries, and Groth-Marnat, 1993; Stark and Goldsbury, 1990; Wenger, Mattson, Furberg, and Elinson, 1984), while Borthwick-Duffy (1990) referred to community involvement and Evans, Burns, Robinson, and Garrett (1985) to political activity and sporting activity.

In conclusion, there is a strong theoretical and empirical rationale for each of the seven domains that have been proposed. Whether they are too numerous or too few to represent life quality is an empirical question which can be approached in various ways. One is to determine whether the domains of life satisfaction that have been reported in the literature can be reasonably grouped under the seven proposed headings and, if they can, the empirical relationships of such domains to one another, and to other measures of life quality. This is the purpose of the investigation to be reported.

METHOD

The studies supplying the data for this research were located through the appraisal of over 1,500 articles that concerned the topic of life quality. From these, 152 articles were located that provided data on life satisfaction. In order for a study to be included in the following analysis it needed to supply the following:

1. Use of a scale containing a number of life domains.
2. The life domains, in aggregate, to represent a broad indication of life quality. Consequently, studies that restricted measurement to such areas as job satisfaction or institutional living were eliminated.
3. A minimum of three domains to be reported.
4. The response mode to be unequivocally that of life satisfaction. Responses to criteria of happiness were excluded.
5. A statement of the number of Likert scale points, the direction of scoring (e.g., 5 indicates high satisfaction), and a numerical average score to be provided for each domain.

A total of 32 studies were found that fulfilled all of the above criteria. Between them, those studies reported data on 173 different terms that had been used to describe domains of life satisfaction.

Each term was then classified according to whether or not it could be placed within one of the seven proposed domains: material well-being, health, productivity, intimacy, safety, community, and emotional well-being. Since these domains form the basis of the Comprehensive Quality of Life Scale (Cummins, 1993) they will be referred to as the ComQol domains. An initial classification of terms was made by myself. This was then checked by two colleagues familiar with ComQol and disagreement with individual item classifications were resolved through discussion.

The application of this classificatory scheme can be seen in Table I. Of the 173 available domain names, 68% were able to be categorized under one of the ComQol headings. In terms of the aggregate

351 domain names that had been utilized by the 32 studies, 83% were successfully classified. This process classified all of the domain names that had been used on more than two occasions, except for 'Police and Courts' which had been used three times.

Calculation of ComQol Domain Values

Between them, the 32 studies provided mean scores for each of the 351 domains presented in Table I. These domains, named by the original authors of each study, will be referred to as the original domains. The set of original domains from each study was standardised to the new ComQol domain values through the following process:

1. Each original domain mean was converted into a percentage of scale maximum score (%SM). This process expresses each original domain score as a percentage of the maximum score possible using the particular measurement scale. The formula is (mean score for the original domain − 1) × 100/ (number of scale points − 1). In using this formula the measurement scale must always commence at '1'. This is the most common form, where scales are typically scored on a 1–3, 1–5 or 1–7 point choice. However, two alternative methods forms are also used that require conversion before the formula can be applied.

   The first of these uses a scale that commences with zero. In this case '1' is added to both the mean score and each point on the scale before the formula is applied. For example, a mean value of 2.4 on a scale of 0–4 becomes a score of 3.4 on a scale of 1–5. The second alternative arises when a number of items have been combined to form the domain score. For example, five items, scored 1–5, have been combined such that an aggregate score is reported on a 5–25 scale. In this case the aggregate score and the number of scale points (25) are divided by the number of items before the formula is applied.
2. The original domains were grouped under the ComQol domain headings as indicated by Table I. These groupings were made by the process previously described.
3. If two or more original domains from a single study fell under a single ComQol domain, an average value was used.
4. The new ComQol domain values were used to calculated a mean and standard deviation for each study.

TABLE I

List of terms comprising each domain and their frequency (×) of occurrence.

Material well-being	Health	Productivity	Intimacy	Safety	Community	Emotional well-being
Car (1)	Health (22)	Achieve success (1)	Child interaction (1)	Amount of privacy (1)	Acq. and contacts (1)	Beautiful things (1)
Clothes (2)	Hlth./Funct. (2)	Activ. available (1)	Children (4)	Control (1)	Area you live in (2)	Comfort from religion (1)
Econ. situation (2)	Intellect. perfor. (1)	Employment (1)	Contact with family (1)	Control over life (1)	City (1)	Emot. adjustment (1)
Food (2)	Physical fitness (1)	House-work (1)	Family (7)	Contr. pers. circum. (1)	Clubs belong to (1)	Free-time activity (1)
Finances (11)	Phys. strength (1)	Job (11)	Family life (8)	Financial security (3)	Community (1)	Fun (4)
Finan. situation (1)	Personal health (2)	Paid employ. (2)	Family relations (3)	How handle probs. (1)	Country (1)	Hobbies (3)
Home (1)		School (2)	Friends (7)	Legal and safety (1)	District (2)	Leisure (13)
House (5)		Vocation (1)	Friendships (8)	Privacy (1)	Education (7)	Leisure activities (1)
House appearan. (1)		Vocat. situation (1)	Living partner (1)	Safety (5)	Education facilities (1)	Life opportunities (1)
Housing (4)		What accompl. (1)	Marriage (7)	Secure from crime (1)	Get on other peopl (2)	Non-work (1)
Income (2)		Work (10)	Number of friends (1)	Sec. of belongings (2)	Helping others (1)	Overall comfort (2)
Living situation (7)		Work and ed. (1)	Parenthood (2)		Location of home (1)	Psychol./Spiritual (2)
Mater. possss. (1)			Partner relationship(2)		Neighborhood (4)	Reading (2)
Pay (3)			Partnership (1)		People in comm. (1)	Recreation (4)
Place of resid. (1)			People live with (2)		People see socially (1)	Relax/Sitting around (1)
Quality of meals (1)			Relatives (3)		Rel. others in comm. (1)	Religion (8)
Savings (1)			Rel. with family (6)		Serv. and facilities (2)	Self (1)
Socio-economic (2)			Role in family (1)		Social life (3)	Self-acutalization (1)
Stand. of living (6)			Sex life (7)		Social relations (6)	Self-esteem (1)
			Spouse (3)		Social organisations (1)	Spare time (4)
			Time with friends (1)		Visiting (1)	Spiritual life (1)
			Wife/husband (1)			Sports or games (2)
						Take night out (1)
						Time to do things (1)
						Yourself (1)

Residual Terms: Ability to get around (1), Ability to manage self care (2), Amount you worry (1), Appearance (1), Basic child care (1), Being a housewife (1), Beliefs of the women's movement (1), Biculturality (1), Body (2), Bone marrow transplantation (1), Children's education (2), Consumption (1), Cultural life (1), Daily activities (1), Democratic standards (1), Eating (2), Follow politics/voting (1), Future (1), Government (2), Government handles economy (1), Grocery shopping (1), Halth care (2), House chores (1), Household maintenance (1), Housework (1), Immigration (1), Level of democracy (1), Life as a whole (1), Life in general (1), Life in the country (1), Life in USA (1), Living arrangements (1), Local council (1), Local government (2), Medical service (1), National Government (1), Number of others in home (1), Personal care (1), Place of living compared with hospital (2), Police and courts (3), Preparing/cooking food (1), Pressure at work (1), Psychiatric service (1), Relationship with sponsor (1), Resting (1), Shopping (1), Singlehood (1), Sleeping (1), Social work service (1), Space outside home (1), Television (1), Transportation (2), Travel (1), Trip to work (1). Welfare services (2), Your transplantation (1).

5. Each new ComQol domain value was expressed as a Z-score based on step 4.

As a consequence of the above process, each study could be described as a set of ComQol domains ranging in number from 3 to 7 (three was the minimum criterion for the inclusion of a study in the analysis and seven is the full set of ComQol domains). The domains in aggregate provided each study with a new mean and standard deviation, and each domain was described by both an absolute value (%SM) and a Z-score.

RESULTS

Table II indicates the studies that were incorporated into the analyses. Where studies reported data on multiple independent samples, these have been separately analysed. While it is realized that such samples cannot be independent of the study methodology, they can legitimately be used to provide comparative data on domains, and that is the primary purpose of this investigation. In situations where normative values needed to be derived (Table III), such samples were collapsed so that normative data was restricted to independent studies only.

From Table II it can be seen that the studies ranged from 1973 to 1994 and that while the great majority of the 68 samples were drawn from USA (43 or 64%), others were drawn from Britain (7), Canada (6), Sweden (4), Finland (4), Australia (1), Germany (1), Russia (1) and Thailand (1). The samples are essentially of four broad types: general population probability or quota samples, general population samples based on a variety of specific criteria, samples of people with chronic medical conditions, and samples comprising people with a chronic psychiatric impairment.

Standardization Effects on Normative Data

Cummins (1995) has reported that general population samples drawn from Western countries exhibit a standard range of scores that can be described as 75±2.5%SM. This prior analysis was based on large population samples and the data had usually been generated in response to a single global question along the lines of 'All things considered, how would you describe your life as a

TABLE II

Studies and sample characteristics.

Study	Country	Sample	No. subjects	No. original domains	No. ComQol domains	ComQol %SM Mean ± SD
Abrams (1973)	England	Quota	213	11	6	76.1 ± 6.10
		Quota	593	12	6	76.9 ± 7.68
Andrews (1991)	USA	1972 – whites	1165	24	7	72.9 ± 5.84
		1972 – blacks	115	24	7	70.2 ± 6.04
		1988 – low/low SES	67	24	7	70.2 ± 6.86
		– low/med. SES	103	24	7	73.8 ± 5.73
		– med./med. SES	122	24	7	76.2 ± 6.43
		– med./high SES	106	24	7	79.8 ± 4.12
		– high/high SES	71	24	7	79.3 ± 4.28
Andrews and Withey (1976)	USA	Probability – low/low SES	(3,802)	18	6	60.0 ± 11.49
		– low/med. SES	(3,802)	18	6	65.8 ± 9.92
		– med./med. SES	(3,802)	18	6	68.9 ± 10.11
		– med./high SES	(3,802)	18	6	72.5 ± 8.13
		– high/high SES	(3,802)	18	6	73.6 ± 7.68
Baker et al. (1992a)	USA	Chronic psychiatric	729	14	6	71.8 ± 2.44
Baker et al. (1992b)	USA	Bone marrow recipients	109	18	5	72.1 ± 3.94
Baker et al. (1994)	USA	Bone marrow recipients	120	18	5	73.3 ± 1.93
Baker and Intagliata (1982)	USA	Chronic medical	118	15	6	69.3 ± 4.43
Balatsky and Diener (1993)	Russia	College students	115	13	6	56.6 ± 9.37
Branholm and Degerman (1992)	Sweden	Male parent of disabled child	37	8	4	66.9 ± 8.89
		Female parent of disabled child	37	8	4	67.8 ± 10.26
		Male parent of non-dis. child	89	8	4	71.0 ± 6.94
		Female parent of non-dis. child	89	8	4	66.6 ± 9.30

TABLE II. Continued.

Study	Country	Sample	No. subjects	No. original domains	No. ComQol domains	ComQol %SM Mean ± SD
Campbell et al. (1976)	USA	Probability	2134	14	6	76.3 ± 5.36
Davis and Gerrard (1993)	USA	Psychiatric – group homes	234	14	5	60.1 ± 5.12
Fabien (1992)	USA	Psychiatric – employed	54	8	7	63.3 ± 3.91
		– unemployed	56	8	7	55.5 ± 11.20
Ferrans and Powers (1992)	USA	Hemodialysis – lower income	(341)	4	4	70.9 ± 8.64
		– higher income	(341)	4	4	(74.3 ± 8.27)
Haavio-Mannila (1971)	Finland	City – males	(948)	3	3	66.3 ± 8.46
		– females	(948)	3	3	66.8 ± 4.65
		Rural – males	(948)	3	3	50.8 ± 10.25
		– females	(948)	3	3	57.2 ± 9.25
Hall (1973)	England	Quota	213	11	6	73.7 ± 6.80
		Quota	593	11	6	76.2 ± 9.23
Headey and Wearing (1992)	Australia	Probability	502	23	6	69.6 ± 4.51
Hicks et al. (1992)	USA	Liver transplant – < 24 mo	18	4	4	76.9 ± 5.81
		–> 24 mo	17	4	4	73.4 ± 7.68
Holahan and Gilbert (1979)	USA	Career women	15	4	3	64.6 ± 8.99
		Other employed women	26	4	3	84.5 ± 4.04
Huxley and Warner (1992)	USA	Chronic psychiatric	68	9	7	64.2 ± 4.84
		Low inc., non-psychiat. patients	15	9	7	71.4 ± 13.13
Koch and Muthny (1990)	Germany	Renal transplant	761	8	4	63.6 ± 6.39
Krause (1992)	USA	Spinal cord injury >2y	286	11	7	66.7 ± 5.37
Leelakulthanit and Day (1993)	USA	Probability	331	13	6	72.9 ± 4.46
Lehman et al. (1982)	USA	Psychiatric – residential	278	11	7	66.6 ± 9.67

TABLE II. Continued.

Study	Country	Sample	No. subjects	No. original domains	No. ComQol domains	ComQol %SM Mean ± SD
Lehman et al. (1992)	USA	Psychiatric – males	(469)	7	6	60.1 ± 3.55
		– females	(469)	7	6	62.0 ± 3.55
Michalos (1980)	Canada	Non-academic university staff	357	12	7	69.3 ± 4.34
Michalos (1985)	USA	Undergraduate students	682	12	7	63.0 ± 10.00
Oppong et al. (1988)	Canada	Probability – City 1984	421	7	5	71.7 ± 6.38
		– City 1985	(166)	7	5	71.7 ± 6.38
		Large country town	(166)	7	5	74.6 ± 8.59
		Small country town	(166)	7	5	72.5 ± 4.59
		Remote area	(166)	7	5	65.0 ± 11.32
Robinson (1977)	USA	Probability – males	43	22	4	88.1 ± 6.25
		– females	97	22	4	81.1 ± 2.49
		Employed – males	520	18	5	68.4 ± 8.56
		– females	697	18	5	68.8 ± 9.94
Simpson et al. (1989)	England	Psychiatric – hospital	11	10	7	44.5 ± 6.07
		– hostel	10	10	7	55.9 ± 4.66
		– group home	13	10	7	67.7 ± 12.29
Sullivan et al. (1992)	USA	Psychiatric – outpatient	101	4	3	67.2 ± 6.32
Warner and Huxley (1993)	USA	Psychiatric – residential	13	10	7	55.7 ± 12.80
		– outpatient exp.	16	10	7	64.9 ± 9.42
		– outpatient cont.	40	10	7	65.9 ± 4.76
Ying (1992)	USA	Chinese-Americans	142	8	3	69.9 ± 3.34

Note: Where the 'No. of subjects' appears in brackets it indicates that the sub-group Ns were not available.

whole?'. It is therefore of interest to determine whether general population surveys that use domains instead of single items yield a similar distribution of scores. It is also important to determine whether such data are significantly altered through the conversion from original to ComQol domains.

In order to measure these relative influences Table III has been prepared. The criteria of a sample N>200 and a restriction to data from Western countries has been maintained in accordance with Cummins (1995). The data listed in the ComQol column are the same as those provided in Table II with the following exceptions. For Andrews and Withey (1976) the data from their single summary table (p. 241) were used. In addition, the two entries for Andrews (1991) are the aggregate white/black data from 1972 and the aggregate socioeconomic data from 1988. The %SM scores in the 'single item' column of Table III are restricted to studies that provided data on both life domains and a single global question of life satisfaction.

The first comparison is restricted to just the five studies that are represented in the single item column with a mean of 76.3 ± 2.55. The comparable mean values are 72.5 ± 2.86 for the five original means and 74.5 ± 2.99 for the ComQol means. A comparison between these three sets of data indicates that the ComQol data do not differ from either the original [$t(8) = 0.973$] or single item data [$t(8) = 1.142$]. However, the single item data are significantly higher than the original domains [$t(8) = 1.983, p < 0.05$]. If the full data set of 11 independent studies is used to compare the original and ComQol data, then again there is no significant difference [$t(20) = 1.634$]. The coefficient of variation comparisons indicate higher variance within the original domain data [$t(20) = 4.450, p < 0.001$].

General Population Domain Values

The studies listed in Table II were separated into three groups: those selected on medical criteria, on psychiatric criteria, and the remainder. This latter group contained samples defined as probability and quota general population samples (see Table III), as well as samples selected on criteria of being parents, Chinese-American, geographic location, university staff or students, being employed, black or white American, and socio-economic status. It is assumed that this diverse

TABLE III

The comparative influence of domain grouping on normative data.

Study	Original[a] %SM Mean ± SD	CV	ComQol[b] %SM Mean ± SD	CV	Single item %SM
Abrams (1973a)	74.0 ± 8.50	11.5	76.1 ± 5.57	7.3	–
Abrams (1973b)	75.1 ± 8.84	11.8	76.9 ± 7.01	9.1	77.8
Andrews (1991) (1972)	70.2 ± 10.96	15.6	72.8 ± 5.93	7.6	75.0
Andrews (1991) (1988)	72.8 ± 10.91	15.0	76.4 ± 4.97	6.5	80.0
Andrews and Withey (1976)[c]	69.0 ± 3.95	5.7	70.0 ± 4.60	6.6	73.7
Campbell et al. (1976)	75.4 ± 8.01	10.6	76.3 ± 4.90	6.4	75.0
Hall (1973a)	71.3 ± 9.44	13.2	73.7 ± 6.21	8.4	–
Hall (1973b)	73.9 ± 11.34	15.3	76.2 ± 8.43	11.1	–
Headey and Wearing (1992)	65.1 ± 9.03	13.9	69.6 ± 4.11	5.9	–
Leelakulthanit and Day (1993)	67.3 ± 10.78	16.0	72.9 ± 4.05	5.6	–
Oppong (1988) (City 1984)	70.7 ± 7.17	10.1	69.0 ± 7.46	10.8	–
	71.3 ± 3.29	12.6 ± 3.08	73.6 ± 3.00	7.8 ± 1.89	76.3 ± 2.55

Coefficient of Variation (CV) = $^{SD}/_{mean}$ × 100.

Note: [a] Calculated using all of the original domains.
[b] Calculated using the new ComQol domains.
[c] Taken from the authors' summary table.

collection of samples, in aggregate, is fairly representative of the adult population at large.

The ComQol domains calculated from these collective general population studies were examined to test two hypotheses. The first was that a hierarchy of domain satisfaction could be established. The second was that the hierarchy would change between groups reporting high or low levels of life satisfaction.

The data to test these hypotheses are presented in Table IV. Mean values for each domain are presented at four levels of overall life satisfaction as determined by each study's ComQol mean (see Table II). The choice of these levels was determined on the basis of 70%SM being the lowest point of the normal distribution as defined by two standard deviations from the mean (75 $\pm$ 2.5%SM)(Cummins, 1995). It was predicted that any shift in domain ranking due to overall level of life satisfaction would be likely to occur around this point. For this analysis, the general population studies from Table II were placed into one of four groups depending on whether their means lay in the range of $\geq$74, 73–70, 69–67, or $\leq$66%SM. The ComQol domain values for each study were then distributed within each group as shown in Table IV.

Table IV depicts the distribution of ComQol domains between four levels of overall life satisfaction. It can be seen that while most cells in this table contain five or more values, the two domains of safety and community contain some cell sizes of only 3 or 4. In the Multivariate Analyses of Variance (MANOVAs) to follow, these two domains have been excluded from the analysis.

A groups MANOVA yielded a Pillais criterion which was significant [F(15, 72) = 3.040, p < 0.001]. Univariate ANOVAs within each domain were all significant and, as can be seen from the mean values in Table IV, each domain showed a fairly uniform pattern of decline from group $\geq$74 to group $\leq$66. There is no real evidence of a change in this pattern around the 70%SM. The only possible exception is material well-being that actually increased from the 73–70 group to the 69–67 group but the difference between these two was not significant [t(18) = 1.490]. The most marked difference within each group was caused by the intimacy domain which was significantly higher than all of the others (minimum p < 0.01).

TABLE IV

ComQol domain values from general population samples.

	Group							
	≥74		73–70		69–67		≤66	
Domain	N	Mean ± SD	N	Mean ± SD	N	Mean ± SD	N	Mean ± SD
MAT	8	72.39 ± 5.01	13	65.24 ± 6.19	7	68.99 ± 3.16	7	59.64 ± 6.75
HLTH	8	79.33 ± 2.66	12	74.59 ± 2.72	5	70.96 ± 4.42	5	64.58 ± 5.26
PROD	11	78.73 ± 2.98	13	69.80 ± 3.94	8	66.01 ± 3.58	12	57.18 ± 8.38
INT	11	86.75 ± 3.84	13	81.48 ± 5.14	8	79.63 ± 5.11	12	73.26 ± 7.14
SAF	3	76.13 ± 0.98	7	71.44 ± 2.64	3	63.60 ± 3.70	3	52.77 ± 2.54
COMM	9	76.58 ± 6.02	8	71.76 ± 5.06	4	63.10 ± 5.13	3	57.33 ± 10.33
EMO	11	75.55 ± 8.76	13	69.83 ± 4.40	7	63.49 ± 4.39	12	60.93 ± 9.18

MAT = Material, HLTH = Health, PROD = Productivity, INT = Intimacy, SAF = Safety, COMM = Community, EMO = Emotional well-being.

A groups MANOVA computed on the Z-scores failed to reach significance [$F(15, 72) = 1.207$] indicating that the magnitude of the domains relative to their own study mean did not change between the four groups. This pattern can be clearly seen in Figure 1 which also shows the consistently high relative levels of intimacy which range from +1.54 to +1.29. The other domain to produce consistently positive Z-scores was health, with values ranging from +0.51 to +0.23. The other five domains produced consistently negative Z-scores except for one minor positive deviation for material well-being.

A further observation on the data in Table IV can be made with respect to the degree of variance. When the standard deviations for each domain are expressed as coefficients of variation, the mean group data are as follows: (≥74) = 5.61 ± 3.44, (73–70) = 6.01 ± 2.04, (69–67) = 6.02 ± 1.12, (≤66) = 11.67 ± 4.56. This latter group has a significantly higher coefficient of variation than all of the other three groups, the minimum difference being with the 69–67 group, yielding $t(12) = 2.601$, $p < 0.05$.

Table V indicates domain comparisons between the normative data and samples chosen on either medical or psychiatric criteria (see Table II). The normative data have been drawn only from the 11 studies providing N>200 probability or quota samples drawn from the general adult population listed in Table III. One datum for each

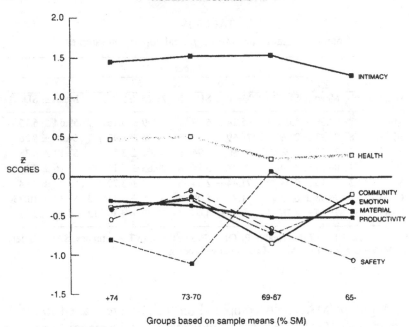

Figure 1. General population samples compared on Z-scores.

domain has been derived from each study. A groups MANOVA was confined to material, health, productivity, intimacy and emotion due to insufficient data in the other two domains. The Pillais criterion indicated a significant effect [$F(10, 42) = 3.837, p < 0.001$]. Univariate ANOVAs revealed that the psychiatric scores were less than those of normal adults and, in the case of intimacy, were also less than the chronic medical. In terms of the normal adult vs. chronic medical differences, only the health domain was significantly different.

An interaction of groups with the intimacy domain was also apparent. While intimacy was significantly higher than all other domains within both the normal adult group [minimum difference was with health, $t(19) = 3.379, p < 0.01$] and the chronic medical group [minimum difference was with emotional well-being, $t(14) = 2.594, p < 0.05$], it did not differ from other domains in the psychiatric group.

A groups MANOVA based on the Z-scores was significant [$F(10, 78) = 3.709, p < 0.001$]. Subsequent ANOVAs within each domain revealed that only intimacy changed across the three groups [$F(2,42)$

TABLE V

Domain satisfaction for comparative groups.

Domain	Normal adult		Chronic medical		Psychiatric	
	N	Mean ± SD	N	Mean ± SD	N	Mean ± SD
MAT	11	69.11 ± 2.71	5	66.88 ± 5.93	16	58.03 ± 8.60
HLTH	10	75.51 ± 5.21	8	68.54 ± 5.70	15	63.80 ± 7.20
PROD	11	74.61 ± 5.54	4	66.48 ± 7.75	13	59.55 ± 13.98
INT	11	82.78 ± 4.47	8	78.49 ± 6.97	15	61.55 ± 9.51
SAF	3	69.90 ± 5.15	3	70.70 ± 1.85	13	64.18 ± 9.73
COMM	10	71.86 ± 2.97	1	72.50 ±	15	61.01 ± 9.17
EMO	11	69.44 ± 6.38	8	71.20 ± 3.82	14	63.46 ± 6.78
MEAN[a]	7	73.32 ± 4.87	7	70.68 ± 4.11	7	61.65 ± 2.32

[a] Calculated from the domain mean values.

$= 21.457$, $p < 0.001$]. Scheffe tests revealed no difference in intimacy between the normal adult and chronic medical groups, but a markedly lower value for the psychiatric group. This indicates a shift in the relative domain ordering within the psychiatric group such that intimacy was no longer pre-eminent (Figure 2).

Other Putative Domains

Below Table I is a list of the 56 domain names not included in the ComQol categories. While many of these terms seem to be highly individualistic, some may be grouped to form domains different from ComQol.

The first of these might be called 'Government'. It includes the terms 'Democratic Standards', 'Government', 'Government Handles Economy', 'Level of Democracy', 'Local Council', 'Local Government', 'National Government', and 'Police and Courts'. Five studies (Abrams, 1973; Andrews, 1991; Hall, 1973; Headey and Wearing, 1992; Lelakulthanit and Day, 1993) contributed eight independent population samples which, between them, contained 16 scores attributed to the above domain names. The mean life satisfaction score for these eight studies, calculated from their ComQol domain scores, was $74.21 \pm 2.35\%SM$. The mean score derived from the 16 Government domains was 55.55 ± 6.52. The equiva-

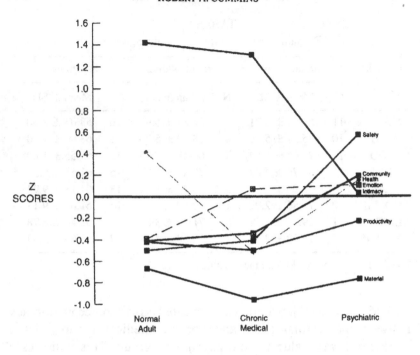

Figure 2. Population groups compared on Z-scores.

lent Z-score, calculated against the ComQol study mean scores, was −3.63 ± 1.46.

Two other possible domains were considered. The first was 'Community Services' comprising the domain names 'Medical Service', 'Psychiatric Service', 'Social Work Service', and 'Welfare Services'. Unfortunately these domain were almost all contained within psychiatric group studies and so population values could not be calculated. The final domain to be considered was 'Life Maintenance' comprising the domains 'Grocery Shopping', 'House Chores', 'Household Maintenance', 'Housework', 'Personal Care', 'Preparation/Cooking Food', and 'Shopping'. Unfortunately all except one of these domains had been used only once in a single study (Robinson, 1977) so that comparative data could not be generated.

DISCUSSION

The main result to emerge from this analysis is that the domains of life satisfaction are not equally perceived. The domain of intimacy clearly receives a higher rating of satisfaction than all of the other domains, almost irrespective of the sample characteristics of the respondents; the exception being people with a psychiatric impairment. This finding, of a hierarchy in domain satisfaction within the general population, has a number of interesting implications for quality of life measurement. Before discussing these issues, however, it is necessary to consider whether the methodology employed for this study has been likely to impose biases on the reported analyses.

The first issue concerns the selection of articles for this study. This is of interest because the available literature is far larger than that captured for the current analysis. The method of selection was biased only in so far as the articles and books located formed the basis of a collection that has been compiled through the combined activities of Deakin University researchers and graduate students over a number of years. As such it is biased to articles with a high citation index and the particular research interests of the contributors. Otherwise the selection criteria seem unremarkable.

The second methodological issue concerns the sorting of reported domains into the seven ComQol categories. Can the initial decision to use the seven ComQol domains be justified and has the sorting of reported domain names been valid?

The justification for the establishment of seven ComQol domains has been argued both here and elsewhere. In brief, Cummins et al. (1994) presented a description of the process whereby college students successfully sorted domain names under the putative ComQol headings and the subsequent verification analysis. Cummins (1996) has also presented a detailed review, which appears in abbreviated form in the introduction to this paper, from which it is concluded that each of the seven domains can be justified from the literature. Finally, data are presented in the ComQol manual (Cummins, 1993) and elsewhere (Cummins, McCabe, Romeo et al., 1996) that support the psychometric utility of the seven domains. Despite this, the question as to the appropriate number of domains must remain open. While, in my view, the most useful number is unlikely to drop below seven based on the data currently to hand, the number could be extended.

The current analysis explored one such possibility drawn from the residual terms not included under any ComQol heading. This domain was termed 'Government' and yielded a mean value of 55.55 ± 6.52%SM, some eight standard deviations below the population mean of 75.0 ± 2.5%SM (Cummins, 1995). It is not recommended that this domain or its constituent terms be used in QOL measurement, at least within the Western cultures to which these data refer. Not only would the inclusion of such a domain exert a strong negative bias on life satisfaction measurement, but also people generally report these aspects of life to be unimportant to them personally (e.g., Andrews and Withey, 1976; Flanagan, 1978; Howieson and Carroll, 1991).

The other issue regarding the generation of the ComQol domain data reported in this study is whether the original domain names have been validly sorted. It is a matter of interpretation as to what terms can be subsumed within each of the ComQol domains. The categorization presented in Table I is consistent with my view of what each ComQol domain embraces based on the original data analysis that gave rise to those domains in the first place (Cummins et al., 1994). This view could be open to challenge from two directions. The first would be based on an alternative sorting of the original domain names presented to Table I. I will be pleased to provide the original domain data calculated for this paper to anyone who wishes to attempt this task. The second challenge to the conclusion of seven domains could come from a more refined analysis of the terms comprising each domain. This could determine whether intra-domain groupings can be formed which would indicate the presence of alternative domain or sub-domain structures.

And so to the analysis of the data presented in this paper. The first mater examined (Table III) was whether the overall life satisfaction data calculated from aggregating the new ComQol domains was different from that using either single item, global life satisfaction data, or that derived from the aggregated original domains. The answer was in the negative; the ComQol domain data were not significantly different from either of the other two data sets. However, there was a fairly consistent tendency for the ComQol means to lie above the original domain data and below that of single-items. Thus, an expanded data set may reveal a significant difference, particularly with the single-item data where only five studies were available for comparison. Notwithstanding this, use of the original domains did produce a significantly lower value than the single-items (72.5 vs. 76.3). Thus, the process of standardising to ComQol domains has avoided a situation where the single-item and domain-measures of life satisfaction differ significantly from one another. This is probably an advantage from a psychometric viewpoint since it implies a more homogeneous set of measures. The reason the original domains produced a lower mean value is due to the inclusion of domains with which people are relatively less satisfied. Most of the domains listed as 'residuals' in Table I had values that lay below the mean of their study, as evidenced by the data for 'Government' discussed earlier.

It is also notable that the amount of within-study variance, as measured through coefficients of variation, was significantly lower using the ComQol rather than the original domains. This would seem advantageous in situations where such scales are being used to detect between-group differences or treatment effects. In summary, these data indicate a possible psychometric advantage to the use of ComQol domains over those that were originally employed.

In comparing the ComQol domains across groups differing in levels of life satisfaction, the data in Table IV indicate a high level of inter-domain consistency. There was also no evidence of change in the relative ordering of the domains as they moved through the 'lower-normal' value of 70.0%SM (Cummins, 1995) with the possible exception of material well-being, but the degree of change in this domain was non-significant around the 70% point. This is an important finding since it implies that the ComQol domains exhibit a robust relationship to one another when applied to population groups that differ markedly in their levels of life satisfaction. It is also evident from the Z-scores depicted in Figure 1, that the two domains of intimacy and health lay consistently above the study mean, while the other five domains lay consistently below. Most remarkable in this respect was intimacy which lay from 1.29 to 1.53 standard deviations above the mean for each of the four levels of overall life satisfaction.

This result has obvious implications for the construction of life satisfaction scales. The larger the proportion of scale items that relate to satisfaction with family and friends, the higher will be the overall life satisfaction score. Conversely, as has been previously noted, the inclusion of items relating to 'Government' or many of the other items residual to Table I will produce a lower life satisfaction score. This leads to a consideration of whether the other ComQol domains are introducing strong sources of bias. With the exception of intimacy, the domain Z-scores depicted in Figure 1 lie within 1.02 standard deviations of one another. It is concluded that none of these six domains induce a strong source of bias to the overall life satisfaction score. Moreover, since intimacy must, presumably, be included as a key domain to the measurement of overall life satisfaction it would seem that the seven ComQol domains represent a suitable group for the construction of a life satisfaction scale.

A final observation with regard to the data in Table IV is that the domains in the studies depicting low overall life satisfaction (group ≤65) had a higher level of within-domain variance. The simplest explanation of this would be a greater spread of study-mean values below than above the range of 67–73%SM. However this appears not to be the case. The study means in group (≥74) ranged up to a maximum of 88.1%SM while those in group (≤66) ranged down to a minimum of 50.8%SM. This indicates a comparative range of 14.1%SM and 15.2%SM respectively. An alternative explanations is an actual increase in the variability of domain values within studies where the overall level of life satisfaction lies at or below 67%SM. It is notable that this value is approximately three standard deviations from the general population standard of 75 ± 2.5%SM and may indicate the emergence of abnormal domain inter-relations at such low levels. This may imply that caution is required in applying the principles of scale construction and domain behaviour outlined in this paper to samples of very low life satisfaction.

The data from Table V compare the normal population samples with people who have a chronic medical condition or a psychiatric impairment. The lack of any overall difference in life satisfaction between the normative and medical-group data may seem surprising. Indeed a glance at Table II shows that of the nine samples selected on medical criteria only three had means lying below 70%SM. These data should be noted well by authors who use such devices as Quality Adjusted Life Years (QALYs) as a measure of life quality. As has been argued elsewhere (e.g., Cummins, 1996), objective medical criteria of functional status, however measured, have little relationship to subjective well-being.

The psychiatric group had significantly lower overall life quality scores than either of the other two groups. Moreover, as can most clearly be seen from the Z-scores depicted in Figure 2, the domain of intimacy no longer retained its pre-eminence. These data are consistent with the loss of intimacy as a buffer against diminished life circumstances.

In sum, this investigation has provided substantial support for the idea that the satisfaction, and therefore subjective well-being, can be efficiently and comprehensively measured through the seven domains of ComQol. A previous paper (Cummins, 1995) claimed a population standard for life satisfaction of $75 \pm 2.5\%SM$. The current data from Table III indicate that single-item measures of global life satisfaction lie slightly above this figure, while an average based on ComQol domains are slightly lower. The mean of these two methods yields an average of 74.95 while each method yields a standard deviation of 2.55 and 3.00 respectively. The suggested value of $75 \pm 2.5\%SM$, as an approximate standard for life satisfaction, appears to have been confirmed provided that measurement is made using either a single-global item or the seven domains of ComQol.

REFERENCES

Abrams, M.: 1973, 'Subjective social indicators', Social Trends 4, pp. 35–50.
Adler, N. E., T., Boyce, M. A. Chesney, S. Cohen, S. Folkman, R. L. Kahn, and S. L. Syme: 1994, 'Socioeconomic status and health: The challenge of the gradient', American Psychologist 49, pp. 15–24.
Andrews, F. M.: 1991, 'Stability and change in levels and structure of subjective well-being: USA 1972 and 1988', Social Indicators Research 25, pp. 1–30.
Andrews, F. M. and S. B. Withey: 1976, Social Indicators of Well-being: Americans' Perceptions of Life Quality (Plenum Press, New York).
Antonovsky, A.: 1987, Unraveling the Mystery of Health (Jossey-Bass, San Francisco).
Baker, F. and J. Intagliata: 1982, 'Quality of life in the evaluation of community support systems', Evaluation and Program Planning 5, pp. 69–79.
Baker, F., D. Jodrey and J. Intagliata: 1992a, 'Social support and quality of life of community support clients', Community Mental Health Journal 28, pp. 397–411.

Baker, F., B. Curbow, and J. R. Wingard: 1992b, 'Development of the satisfaction with life domains scale for cancer', Journal of Psychosocial-Oncology 10, pp. 75–90.

Baker, F., J. R. Wingard, B. Curbow, J. Zabora, D. Jodrey, L. Fogarty and M. Legro: 1994, 'Quality of life of bone marrow transplant long-term survivors', Bone Marrow Transplantation 13, pp. 589–596.

Balatsky, G. and E. Diener: 1993, 'Subjective well-being among Russian students', Social Indicators Research 28, pp. 225–243.

Borthwick-Duffy, S. A.: 1990, 'Quality of life of persons with severe or profound mental retardation' in R. L. Schalock (ed.), Quality of Life: Perspectives and Issues (American Association on Mental Retardation, Washington), pp. 177–189.

Branholm, I., and E. Degerman: 1992, 'Life satisfaction and activity preferences in parents of Down's syndrome children', Scandinavian Journal of Social Medicine 20, pp. 37–44.

Campbell, A., P. E. Converse, W. L. Rodgers: 1976, The Quality of American Life: Perceptions, Evaluations, and Satisfactions (Russel Sage Foundation, New York).

Cummins, R. A.: 1993, The Comprehensive Quality of Life Scale: Adult. 4th Edition (ComQol-A4) (School of Psychology, Deakin University, Melbourne).

Cummins, R. A.: 1995, 'On the trail of the gold standard for life satisfaction', Social Indicators Research 35, pp. 179–200.

Cummins, R. A.: 1996, 'Assessing quality of life', in R. I. Brown (ed.), Quality of Life for Handicapped People (Chapman & Hall, London), in press.

Cummins, R. A., M. P. McCabe, Y. Romeo, and E. Gullone: 1994, 'The comprehensive quality of life scale: Instrument development and psychometric evaluation on tertiary staff and students', Educational and Psychological Measurement 54, pp. 372–382.

Cummins, R. A., M. P. McCabe, Y. Romeo, S. Reid, and L. Waters: 1996, 'An initial evaluation of the Comprehensive Quality of Life Scale: Intellectual disability', International Journal of Disability, Development and Education (in press).

Davis, A. H. and C. Gerrard: 1993, 'Resident satisfaction with community residential care placement', Research on Social Work Practice 3, pp. 91–102.

Evans, D. R., J. E. Burns, W. E. Robinson and O. J. Garrett: 1985, 'The Quality of Life questionnaire: A multidimensional measure', American Journal of Community Psychology 13, pp. 305–322.

Fabian, E. S.: 1992, 'Longitudinal outcomes in supported employment: A survival analysis', Rehabilitation Psychology 37, pp. 23–35.

Felce, D. and J. Perry: 1995, 'Quality of life: Its definition and measurement', Research in Development Disabilities 16, pp. 51–74.

Ferrans, C. E., and M. J. Powers: 1992, 'Psychometric assessment of the Quality of Life Index', Research in Nursing and Health 15, pp. 29–38.

Flanagan, J. C.: 1978, 'A research approach to improving our quality of life', American Psychologist 33, pp. 138–147.

Haavio-Mannila, E.: 1971, 'Satisfaction with family, work, leisure and life among men and women', Human Relations 24, pp. 585–601.

Hall, J.: 1973, 'Measuring the quality of life using sample surveys', in G. J. Stober, and D. Schumacher (eds.), Technology Assessment and Quality of Life (Elsevier, Amsterdam), pp. 93–102.

Halpern, A. S.: 1993, 'Quality of life as a conceptual framework for evaluating transition outcomes', Exceptional Children 59, pp. 486–499.

Headey, B., and A. Wearing: 1992, Understanding Happiness: A Theory of Subjective Well-being (Longman Cheshire, Melbourne).

Hicks, F. D., J. L. Larson, and C. E. Ferrans: 1992, 'Quality of life after liver transplant', Research in Nursing & Health 15, pp. 111–119.

Holahan, C. K. and L. A. Gilbert: 1979, 'Interrole conflict for working women: Careers versus jobs', Journal of Applied Psychology 64, pp. 86–90.

Hornquist, J. O.: 1989, 'Quality of life: Concept and assessment', Scandinavian Journal of Social Medicine 18, pp. 69–79.

Howieson, N. and J. Carroll: 1991, 'Satisfaction with life and satisfaction with community', Paper presented at the September 1991 Australian Psychological Society Conference, Adelaide.

Huxley, P., and R. Warner: 1992, 'Case management, quality of life and satisfaction with services of long-term psychiatric patients', Hospital and Community Psychiatry 43, pp. 799–802.

Koch, U., and F. A. Muthny: 1990, 'Quality of life in patients with end-stage renal disease in relation to the method of treatment', Psychotherapy and Psychosomatics 54, pp. 161–171.

Krause, J. S.: 1992, 'Life satisfaction after spinal cord injury: A descriptive study', Rehabilitation Psychology 37, pp. 61–70.

Krupinski, J.: 1980, 'Health and quality of life', Social Science and Medicine 14A, pp. 203–211.

Leelakulthanit, O. and R. Day: 1993, 'Cross-cultural comparisons of quality of life of Thais and Americans', Social Indicators Research 30, pp. 49–70.

Lehman, A. F., N. C. Ward, and L. S. Linn: 1982, 'Chronic mental patients: The quality of life issue', American Journal of Psychiatry 139, pp. 1271–1276.

Lehman, A. F., J. G. Slaughter, and C. P. Myers: 1992, 'Quality of life experiences of the chronically mentally ill: Gender and stages of life effects', Evaluation and Program Planning 15, pp. 7–12.

Liem, R., and J. Liem: 1978, 'Social class and mental illness reconsidered: The role of economic stress and social support', Journal of Health and Social Behavior 19, pp. 139–156.

Michalos, A. C.: 1980, 'Satisfaction and happiness', Social Indicators Research 8, pp. 385–422.

Michalos, A. C.: 1985, 'Multiple Discrepancies Theory (MDT)', Social Indicators Research 16, pp. 347–413.

Oppong, J. R., R. G. Ironside, and L. W. Kennedy: 1988, 'Perceived quality of life in a centre-periphery framework', Social Indicators Research 20, pp. 605–620.

Organization for Economic Cooperation and Development: 1976, Measuring Social Well-being (Author, Paris).

Robinson, J. P.: 1977, How Americans Use Time: A Social-psychological Analysis of Everyday Behavior (Praeger, New York).

Schalock, R. L., K. D. Keith, K. Hoffman, and O. C. Karan: 1989, 'Quality of life: Its measurement and use', Mental Retardation 27, pp. 25–31.

Schumaker, J. F., J. D. Shea, M. M. Monfries, and G. Groth-Marnat: 1993, 'Lone-
liness and life satisfaction in Japan and Australia', The Journal of Psychology
127, pp. 65–71.

Simpson, C. J., C. E. Hyde, and E. B. Faragher: 1989, 'The chronically mentally ill
in community facilities: A study of quality of life', British Journal of Psychiatry
154, pp. 77–82.

Stark, J. A. and T. Goldsbury: 1990, 'Quality of life from childhood to adulthood',
in R. L. Schalock (ed.), Quality of Life: Perspectives and Issues (American
Association on Mental Retardation, Washington), pp. 71–83.

Sullivan, G., K. B. Wells, and B. Leake: 1992, 'Clinical factors associated with
better quality of life in a seriously mentally ill population', Hospital and Community Psychiatry 43, pp. 794–798.

Vitello, S. J.: 1984, 'Deinstitutionalization of mentally retarded persons in the
United States: Status and trends', in J. M. Berg (ed.), Perspectives and Progress
in Mental Retardation, Volume 1 (International Association for the Scientific
Study of Mental Deficiency, New York), pp. 345–349.

Warner, R., and P. Huxley: 1993, 'Psychopathology and quality of life among
mentally ill patients in the community: British and U.S. samples compared',
British Journal of Psychiatry 163, pp. 505–509.

Wenger, N. K., M. E. Mattson, C. D. Furberg, and J. Elinson: 1984, 'Assessment
of quality of life in clinical trials of cardiovascular therapies', American Journal
of Cardiology 54, pp. 908–913.

Ying, Y.: 1992, 'Life satisfaction among San Francisco Chinese-Americans',
Social Indicators Research 26, pp. 1–22.

School of Psychology
Deakin University
Victoria 3125
Australia

3. Developing measures of perceived life quality: Results from several national surveys (1974)
Frank M. Andrews and Stephen B. Withey

Social Indicators Research **1** (1974) 1–26. *All Rights Reserved*
Copyright © 1974 by D. Reidel Publishing Company, Dordrecht-Holland

4. The quality of life in large American cities: Objective and subjective social Indicators (1975)
Mark Schneider

Social Indicators Research **1** (1975) 495–509. *All Rights Reserved*
Copyright © 1975 by D. Reidel Publishing Company, Dordrecht-Holland

5. Quality of life (1975)
Storrs McCall

Social Indicators Research **2** (1975) 229–248. *All Rights Reserved*
Copyright © 1975 by D. Reidel Publishing Company, Dordrecht-Holland

6. Does money buy satisfaction? (1975)
Otis Dudley Duncan

Social Indicators Research **2** (1975) 267–274. *All Rights Reserved*
Copyright © 1975 by D. Reidel Publishing Company, Dordrecht-Holland

7. On the multivariate structure of wellbeing (1975)
Shlomit Levy and Louis Guttman

Social Indicators Research **2** (1975) 361–388. *All Rights Reserved*
Copyright © 1975 by D. Reidel Publishing Company, Dordrecht-Holland

8. The structure of subjective well-being in nine western societies (1979)
Frank M. Andrews and Ronald F. Inglehart

Social Indicators Research **6** (1979) 73–90.   0303-8300/79/0061-0073$01.80
Copyright © 1979 by D. Reidel Publishing Co., Dordrecht, Holland, and Boston, U.S.A.

9. Measures of self-reported well-being: Their affective, cognitive and other components (1980)
Frank M. Andrews and Aubrey C. McKennell

Social Indicators Research 8 (1980) 127–155. 0303-8300/80/0082-0127$02.90
Copyright © 1980 by D. Reidel Publishing Co., Dordrecht, Holland, and Boston, U.S.A.

10. Satisfaction and happiness (1980)
Alex C. Michalos

Social Indicators Research 8 (1980) 385–422. 0303–8300/80/0084-0385$03.80
Copyright © 1980 by D. Reidel Publishing Co., Dordrecht, Holland, and Boston, U.S.A.

11. The stability and validity of quality of life measures (1982)
Tom Atkinson

Social Indicators Research 10 (1982) 113–132. 0303-8300/82/0102-0113$02.00
Copyright © 1982 by D. Reidel Publishing Co., Dordrecht, Holland, and Boston, U.S.A.

12. The analysis and measurement of happiness as a sense of well-being (1984)
Richard Kammann, Marcelle Farry and Peter Herbison

Social Indicators Research 15 (1984) 91–115. 0303–8300/84/0152–0091$02.50.
© 1984 by D. Reidel Publishing Company.

13. Multiple discrepancies theory (MDT) (1985)
Alex C. Michalos

Social Indicators Research 16 (1985) 347–413. 0303–8300/85.10
© 1985 by D. Reidel Publishing Company.

14. A review of research on the happiness measures: A sixty second index of Happiness and mental health (1988)
Michael W. Fordyce

Social Indicators Research 20 (1988) 355—381.
© 1988 by Kluwer Academic Publishers.

15. Top-down versus bottom-up theories of subjective well-being (1991)
Bruce Headey, Ruut Veenhoven and Alex Wearing

Social Indicators Research **24**: 81—100, 1991.
© 1991 *Kluwer Academic Publishers. Printed in the Netherlands.*

16. Assessing subjective well-being: progress and opportunities (1994)
Ed Diener

Social Indicators Research **31**: 103—157, 1994.
© 1994 *Kluwer Academic Publishers. Printed in the Netherlands.*

17. Is happiness a trait? (1994)
Ruut Veenhoven

Social Indicators Research **32**: 101–160, 1994.
© 1994 *Kluwer Academic Publishers. Printed in the Netherlands.*

18. On the trail of the gold standard for subjective well-being (1995)
Robert A. Cummins

Social Indicators Research **35**: 179–200, 1995.
© 1995 *Kluwer Academic Publishers. Printed in the Netherlands.*

19. The domains of life satisfaction: An attempt to order chaos (1996)
Robert A. Cummins

Social Indicators Research **38**: 303–328, 1996.
© 1996 *Kluwer Academic Publishers. Printed in the Netherlands.*

Author Index

Subject Index

10-step elation-depression, 283
11-point Fordyce scale, 382
11-point happy/unhappy scale, 19
11-point response scale, 263
11-point satisfaction scales, 177, 186
3-point happiness measure, 208
3-point happiness scale, 20
3-point satisfaction measure, 207
3-step happiness, 287
7-point delighted-terrible response
     scale, 202
7-point delighted-terrible scale (DT
     scale), 11, 177, 186, 283
7-point satisfaction scale, 17
7-step happiness rating scale, 282, 287,
     290
9-point delighted-terrible scale, 404,
     543
AAAS science, 62
absence of health concerns, 388
absolute stability, 509, 520
abstracting services, 5
acceptability of scientific theories, 1
acceptance and rejection, 69
access to knowledge, 529
accurate perceptions, 26
achievements and life satisfactions,
     257
achievers, 249, 250, 251, 253
acting, 194
acting happy, 453
action readiness, 27, 437, 456
activation of the autonomic system,
     437
active, 19
actual changes in the QOL measures,
     275
adaptation, 21, 125
adaptation-level theory, 226, 256, 538
additive combination of affective
     responses, 105
adjustment, 434
adjustment to physical disability, 534
adult antecedents of life satisfaction,
     534

adversity relates to a lower
     appreciation of life, 492
advertising, 257
affect, 191
affect and memory, 466
affect balance scale, 281, 287, 288, 374
affect is an effect of cognitive, 349
affect neg, 198
affect pos, 197
affect-cognition ratios, 17, 207, 209,
     211
affection, 27
affective, v, 16, 194, 195
affective and cognitive indicators, 270
affective component, 287
affective reactions, 76, 200
affective response, 77, 79
affective space is bipolar, 303
Affectometer 1, 2, 18, 282, 287, 288,
     290, 293, 298, 302
Affectometer 2, 18, 374
age, 26
aggregate objective social indicators,
     113
air quality, 119
allocate credit, 6
ambiguities of citation practices, 4
American structure, 185
American values, 100
amount of fun, 10
anger, 19, 27
anglophone and francophone
     differences, 218
anxiety, 19, 280
anxiety-adjustment, 281
avowed happiness, 32
applied research, 462
appraisals of publications, 7
approximate standard for life
     satisfaction, 581
area lived in, 319
area of concern, 70
article citation counts, vii
arts and humanities citation index, 2
arts and humanities journals, 2
aspiration, 25, 114, 224, 249, 255

Social Indicators Research Series

23. A. Dannerbeck, F. Casas, M. Sadurni and G. Coenders (eds.): *Quality-of-Life Research on Children and Adolescents*. 2004   ISBN 1-4020-2311-1
24. W. Glatzer, S. von Below and M. Stoffregen (eds.): *Challenges for Quality of Life in the Contemporary World*. 2004   ISBN 1-4020-2890-3
25. D.T.L. Shek, Y. Chan and P.S.N. Lee (eds.): *Quality of Life Research in Chinese, Western and Global Contexts*. 2005   ISBN 1-4020-3601-9
26. A.C. Michalos (ed.): *Citation Classics from Social Indicators Research*. The Most Cited Articles Edited and Introduced by Alex C. Michalos. 2005
     ISBN 1-4020-3722-8